Acute Pain Medicine

Acute Pain Medicine

Edited by

Chester C. Buckenmaier III, MD
Professor of Anesthesiology, Director, Defense and Veterans Center for Integrative Pain Management, Uniformed Services University of the Health Sciences

Michael Kent, MD
Assistant Professor of Anesthesiology, Duke University Medical Center

Jason C. Brookman, MD
Attending Staff Anesthesiologist, North American Partners in Anesthesia, Director of Regional Anesthesia and Acute Pain Medicine, Department of Anesthesia, Sinai Hospital of Baltimore

Patrick J. Tighe, MD
Associate Professor of Anesthesiology, University of Florida College of Medicine

Edward R. Mariano, MD
Professor of Anesthesiology, Perioperative and Pain Medicine, Palo Alto Veterans Affairs Health Care System, Stanford University School of Medicine

David A. Edwards, MD, PhD
Assistant Professor of Anesthesiology, Pain Medicine, Neurological Surgery, Chief, Division of Pain Medicine, Vanderbilt University Medical Center

AAPM
American Academy of Pain Medicine

OXFORD
UNIVERSITY PRESS

OXFORD
UNIVERSITY PRESS

Oxford University Press is a department of the University of Oxford. It furthers the University's objective of excellence in research, scholarship, and education by publishing worldwide. Oxford is a registered trade mark of Oxford University Press in the UK and certain other countries.

Published in the United States of America by Oxford University Press
198 Madison Avenue, New York, NY 10016, United States of America.

CIP data is on file at the Library of Congress
ISBN 978–0–19–085664–9

Contents

Foreword

Case-based medical education enjoys the unique distinction not only of enjoying increasing popularity in the past decade but also of being the original method employed 5000 years ago in Egypt for medical education (mostly about acute trauma management). This brief foreword will note the millennia-long importance of case-based learning in medicine and also point out why this method is as popular as ever despite the advent of quantitative "evidence-based" medicine, including randomized controlled trials (RCTs), meta-analyses, and big data.

The past two decades have witnessed great strides in medical education. A sea change has taken place from emphasizing rote memorization of curricular content to a practical focus on achieving real-world competencies in clinical decision-making amid complex, changing, incomplete, or imprecise information. Supporting this revolution have been advances in case-based learning and educational neuroscience, the latter providing brain imaging and neuroendocrine characterization of the learner. Case-based learning benefits from the instinctive empathy and identification with those around us that are hardwired within all of us in our neuromatrix and mirror neuron systems, that secure our emotional identification with real or simulated patients.

This innovative volume edited by Drs. Chester Buckenmaier III, Michael Kent, Jason C. Brookman, Patrick J. Tighe, Edward R. Mariano, and David Edwards applies case-based learning to the practice of the subspecialty of acute pain medicine. It does so in a consistent and compelling fashion by presenting key diagnostic and therapeutic features for a variety of the postoperative and posttraumatic situations facing those practicing acute pain medicine. Mirroring the ancient Egyptian papyrus purchased by and named after Edwin Smith, a 19th-century collector, many cases in this book benefit from recent advances in military medicine. Examples include ultrasound imaging applied in the field to facilitate regional anesthesia, and multimodal analgesia so as to decrease reliance on morphine.

The concept of case-based learning is ancient. The earliest known writings about any medical practices were copied onto papyrus by an Egyptian scribe around 1500 BCE. Textual and grammatical analyses indicate much of the material copied by that scribe originated between 3000 and 2500 BCE. The 48 cases in the Edwin Smith papyrus were composite cases mostly involving surgical treatment of traumatic injury, although breast cancer and lumbar vertebral strain were mentioned. Cases were presented in anatomic sequence beginning at the crown of the skull and proceeding caudally. The papyrus ends abruptly in midsentence during an account of a man with acute low back strain, in whom the diagnosis is confirmed by worsening of pain upon straight leg raising. Although the types of trauma presented are those commonly seen in battle, these cases may also have been intended to instruct doctors treating workers injured in building the pyramids. As with the structured presentations in the present volume, each case in the Edwin Smith papyrus was presented in a standard format: location, examination, diagnosis, whether treatment should be attempted, and if so, the nature of that treatment.

A myriad of injuries (including surgical excisions) and other causes of acute pain such as sciatica or headache have been described—often vividly—throughout much of the world's literature and biography, including autobiography. Indeed, a cuneiform pharmacopeia produced in Sumeria on a clay tablet about the same epoch as the Edwin Smith papyrus described ingredients of prescriptions but with minimal clinical correlation. But if we wish to focus on the concept that individual cases can and should be used as evidence to inform medical training and decision-making, we need only look to the system of medicine as practiced in ancient Greece around 400 BCE, recounted by Socrates in Plato's Dialogues as assembled by Osler. The practice of medicine in ancient Greece was two-tiered. Slaves received formulaic symptom-based remedies dispensed hurriedly in crowded dispensaries. Freemen (citizens) were examined and interviewed at length, often in the presence of their families to encourage a thoughtful and holistic view of their problems. State physicians treating slaves and freemen were respected and paid well. They had, however, to undergo an annual review convened by the community they served, at which time patients (or their survivors) described individual cases, indicating the physician's competence or lack thereof. Of this process, Socrates asked, "If you and I were physicians, and were advising one another that we were competent to practice, should I not ask you, and would you not ask me, Well, what about Socrates himself, has he not good health? And was anyone else ever been known to be cured by him, whether slave or freeman?"

Fast-forward to the 21st century. How is it possible—given our instant access to more information than all medical libraries, journals, and registries together offered until very recently—that case-based learning is still an integral part of medical education? Why hasn't it become obsolete, rendered superfluous by the rise of evidence-based medicine? The answer is that evidence-based medicine emerged in the late 20th century to help policymakers wisely allocate resources to meet the public health needs of national populations. Yet as Katherine M. Keyes and Sandro Galea have observed, "Population health manifests as a continuum [and] we can predict health in populations with much more certainty than we can predict health in individuals." Louis Lasagna, writing just before the modern inflection point of increasing numbers of RCTs and meta-analyses, pointed out that RCTs were typically implemented in selected homogeneous populations without significant comorbidities, with few if any concurrent medications, who were recruited and followed attentively—all very different from the real world of everyday practice. Howard S. Frazier and Frederick Mosteller have emphasized that "the physician serves as advocate for the personal goals and subjective preferences of individual patients, not for classes of patients or for society as a whole." In 2017, writing in the prestigious *New England Journal of Medicine*, Thomas Frieden, a former director of the US Centers for Disease Control and Prevention, called for the use of multiple sources of evidence beyond RCTs to aid in the evaluation of health effects, patient preferences, and costs of treatments. In other words, the dominant position of the RCT, and aggregation of RCTs through meta-analyses, to inform educators and policy makers is being eroded. Increasingly, thought leaders are voicing concerns that such approaches fail to offer clinicians clear direction amid the everyday uncertainty and incompleteness of information characteristic of individualized or personalized care. Anesthesiology Board examiners recognize this shortfall, too, and still require real-time, in-person oral examination of candidates confronted with cases designed to convey complex, often deteriorating patients who must be managed with incomplete information, or who respond atypically to standard interventions.

As medical education enters the 21st century, it is heartening to see that case-based medicine is alive and well, allowing educators to assess the diverse levels of preparation of trainees and offer them living scenarios to best prepare them to practice acute pain medicine swiftly and skillfully. Drs. Buckenmaier, Kent, Brookman, Tighe, Mariano, and Edwards and their contributors are to be commended for advancing a powerful didactic tradition as old as recorded history.

Daniel Carr

Preface

Welcome to *Acute Pain Medicine*. The textbook aims to serve as a clinical guide in acute pain medicine, spanning both perioperative and nonperioperative inpatient pain conditions. At the beginning of this effort, the editors compiled an essential list of topics in acute pain medicine that spanned interventional, pharmacologic, and diagnostic considerations. This expansive list was then matched against some of the most common acute pain conditions (surgical and nonsurgical) to provide context for such concepts. For each acute pain condition, a case is presented, followed by questions and answers that focus on the patient factors, interventional considerations, and postoperative/immediate analgesic strategies. In order to capture the diverse set of strategies and opinions, authors were selected from a diverse set of institutions.

In addition to this case-based approach, this text includes an updated version of the *Military Advanced Regional Anesthesia and Analgesia Handbook* (MARAA II) originally spearheaded in 2008 by Colonel (Retired) Chester Buckenmaier III, MD. Dr Buckenmaier returns as the section editor for this update of a cornerstone bedside tool for learners and practitioners alike.

The *Military Advanced Regional Anesthesia and Analgesia Handbook* (MARAA) was originally developed as a supplement to *Emergency War Surgery—Third United States Revision*. In *Emergency War Surgery*, regional anesthesia is described as "a 'field friendly' anesthetic requiring minimal logistical support while providing quality anesthesia and analgesia on the battlefield." Although the MARAA text was conceived and executed in support of military healthcare providers caring for combat wounded, the lessons and techniques herein are no less effective or important for civilian trauma. New chapters have been added, and original anatomic renderings have been provided to supplement new techniques that have arisen since the original text was published, providing a useful resource for managing the pain of battlefield and civilian trauma.

We hope you enjoy this reference.

Chester C. Buckenmaier III
Michael Kent
Jason C. Brookman
Patrick J. Tighe
Edward R. Mariano
David Edwards

Contributors to Sections I and II

Chidi Ani, MD
Assistant Professor
Department of Anesthesiology and Perioperative Medicine
Oregon Health and Science University
Portland, OR

Vikram Bansal, MD
Assistant Professor of Clinical Anesthesiology
Department of Anesthesiology
Vanderbilt University Medical Center
Nashville, TN

Jack M. Berger, MS, MD, PhD
Department of Anesthesiology
Keck School of Medicine of USC
LAC+USC Medical Center
Los Angeles, CA

Jill Berlin, MD
CA-2 Anesthesiology Resident
Yale University School of Medicine
Department of Anesthesiology
Yale-New Haven Hospital
New Haven, CT

Karen Boretsky, MD
Lecturer in Anesthesia
Harvard Medical School
Director, Perioperative Regional Anesthesia Program
Boston Children's Hospital
Boston, MA

W. Michael Bullock, MD, PhD
Assistant Professor of Anesthesiology
Duke University Medical Center
Durham, NC

David Byrne, MD
Department of Anesthesiology
Vanderbilt University Medical Center
Nashville, TN

Rishi Chokshi, MD
Fellow
Division of Regional Anesthesia and Acute Pain Management
Department of Anesthesiology and Critical Care Medicine
Johns Hopkins University
Baltimore, MD

Danielle Cobb, MD
Fellow; Acute & Perioperative Pain Medicine
Department of Anesthesiology
The University of Florida College of Medicine
Gainesville, FL

Lori Ann Dangler, MD, MBA
Associate Professor
Anesthesiology and Perioperative Medicine
University of Texas–MD Anderson Cancer Center
Houston, TX

Melanie Julia Donnelly, MD
Associate Professor
Department of Anesthesiology
University of Colorado
Aurora, CO

David A. Edwards, MD, PhD
Assistant Professor of Anesthesiology and Neurological Surgery Chief
Division of Pain Medicine
Department of Anesthesiology
Vanderbilt University Medical Center
Nashville, TN

Nabil Elkassabany, MD, MSCE
Associate Professor
Director; Sections of Regional and Orthopedic Anesthesiology
Department of Anesthesiology and Critical Care
University of Pennsylvania
Philadelphia, PA

Clint Elliott, MD
Director
Regional Anesthesiology and Acute Pain Medicine Fellowship
Ochsner Medical Center
New Orleans, LA

James Flaherty, MD
Assistant Professor
Department of Anesthesiology
University of Minnesota
Minneapolis, MN

Ian M. Fowler, MD
Pain Medicine Center
Department of Anesthesiology
Naval Medical Center
San Diego, CA

Andrew D. Franklin, MD
Department of Anesthesiology
Vanderbilt University Medical Center
Nashville, TN

Jeffrey Gonzales, MD, MA
Staff Anesthesiologist
Guardian Anesthesia Services
Parker, CO

Julio A. Gonzalez-Sotomayor, MD
Associate Professor
Department of Anesthesiology and Perioperative Medicine
Oregon Health and Science University
Portland, OR

Roxana Grasu, MD
Associate Professor of Anesthesiology
Department of Anesthesiology, Perioperative Medicine and Critical Care
The University of Texas MD Anderson Cancer Center
Houston, TX

Roy Greengrass, MD
Department of Anesthesiology and Perioperative Medicine
Mayo Clinic
Jacksonville, FL

Padma Gulur, MD
Professor of Anesthesiology
Duke University Medical Center
Durham, NC

Thomas Halaszynski, DMD, MD, MBA
Professor of Anesthesiology
Senior Director of Regional Anesthesia and Orthopedic Surgery
Yale University School of Medicine
Department of Anesthesiology
Yale-New Haven Hospital
New Haven, CT

Steven R. Hanling, MD
Department of Anesthesiology and Perioperative Medicine
Medical College of Georgia
Augusta University
Augusta, GA

Brian E. Harrington, MD
Staff Anesthesiologist
Billings Clinic Hospital
Billings, MT

Sharon Jiang, MD
Keck School of Medicine
University of Southern California
Los Angeles, CA

Francis Wickham Kraemer III, MD
Associate Professor
Department of Anesthesiology and Critical Care
Perelman School of Medicine
University of Pennsylvania
Philadelphia, PA

J. Matthew Kynes, MD
Department of Anesthesiology
Vanderbilt University Medical Center
Nashville, TN

James Kyunghoon Kim, MD
Assistant Professor
Department of Anesthesiology
University of Virginia School of Medicine
Charlottesville, VA

Alicia Lopez Warlick, MD
Department of Anesthesiology
USAP Colorado
Greenwood Village, CO

Edward R. Mariano, MD, MAS
Professor of Anesthesiology, Perioperative and Pain Medicine
Stanford University School of Medicine
Veterans Affairs Palo Alto Health Care System
Palo Alto, CA

M. Stephen Melton, MD
Assistant Professor
Department of Anesthesiology
Duke University Medical Center
Durham, NC

Carrie Menser, MD
Assistant Professor
Department of Anesthesiology
Division of Pediatric Anesthesia
Vanderbilt University Medical Center
Nashville, TN

Linh T. Nguyen, MD
Associate Professor
Department of Anesthesiology and Perioperative Medicine
The University of Texas MD Anderson Cancer Center
Houston, TX

Luke Nicholson, MD
Department of Orthopedic Surgery
LAC+USC Medical Center
Los Angeles, CA

Karen C. Nielsen, MD
Associate Professor
Department of Anesthesiology
Duke University Medical Center
Durham, NC

Aaron Persinger, MD
Staff Anesthesiologist
US Anesthesia Partners Colorado
Englewood, CO

C. Ryan Phillips, MD
Pain Medicine Center
Department of Anesthesiology
Naval Medical Center
San Diego, CA

Sally Raty, MD, MHA
Professor of Anesthesiology
Department of Anesthesiology, Perioperative Medicine and Critical Care
The University of Texas MD Anderson Cancer Center
Houston, TX

Albert Robinson III, MD
Associate Professor
Department of Anesthesiology
The University of Florida College of Medicine
Gainesville, FL

Sydney E. Rose, MD
Assistant Professor
Department of Anesthesiology and Perioperative Medicine
Oregon Health and Science University
Portland, OR

Deva Sharma, MD
Fellow of Hematology and Oncology
Department of Medicine
Division of Hematology/Oncology
Vanderbilt University Medical Center
Nashville, TN

Uma Shastri, MD
Assistant Professor of Clinical Anesthesiology
Department of Anesthesiology
Vanderbilt University Medical Center
Nashville, TN

Christopher Sobey, MD
Assistant Professor
Department of Anesthesiology
Division of Pain Medicine
Vanderbilt University Medical Center
Nashville, TN

Jenna Sobey, MD
Assistant Professor
Department of Anesthesiology
Division of Pediatric Anesthesia
Vanderbilt University Medical Center
Nashville, TN

Michale Sofer, MD
Associate Professor
Department of Anesthesiology and Critical Care
Perelman School of Medicine
University of Pennsylvania
Philadelphia, PA

Jose M. Soliz, MD
Associate Professor
Department of Anesthesiology and Perioperative Medicine
The University of Texas MD Anderson Cancer Center
Houston, TX

Richa Wardhan, MD
Clinical Assistant Professor
University of Florida School of Medicine
Department of Anesthesiology
Gainesville, FL

Elizabeth H. Wilson, MD
Assistant Professor
Department of Anesthesiology
University of Wisconsin Hospital Clinics
Madison, WI

Contributors to Section III (MARAA)

The Military Advanced Regional Anesthesia and Analgesia Handbook represents a highly cooperative effort among many authors working together to write and edit chapters. The editors wish to acknowledge the authors who updated and revised the original MARAA Handbook for this publication as well as the contributors to the first edition, published in 2008.

Authors of the Military Advanced Regional Anesthesia and Analgesia Handbook, 2nd edition

Michael R. Anderson, MD
Assistant Professor
Department of Anesthesiology, Perioperative and Pain Medicine
Icahn School of Medicine at Mount Sinai

Hisani Brandon-Edwards, MHA, RN-BC
Acute Pain Nurse Research Manager
Henry M. Jackson Foundation for the Advancement of Military Medicine

Robert Henry Burch III, MD
Captain, Medical Corps, US Army
Walter Reed National Military Medical Center
Regional Anesthesia & Acute Pain Medicine Fellow

Kenneth D. Candido, MD
Professor of Clinical Anesthesiology
Clinical Professor of Surgery
University of Illinois, Chicago
Chairman, Department of Anesthesiology
Advocate Illinois Masonic Medical Center

Michael Carreras, MD
Ocala Regional Medical Center

Lauren Devine, PharmD
Clinical Pharmacist
Cardiology/Cardiac ICU
Massachusetts General Hospital
Boston, MA

Sandeep T. Dhanjal, MD
Section Chief, Regional Anesthesiology and Acute Pain Medicine
Department of Anesthesiology
Brooke Army Medical Center

Ryan Derby, MD
Clinical Assistant Professor
Stanford University

Hesham Elsharkawy, MD, MBA, MSc
Staff, Department of General Anesthesiology and Outcomes Research
Anesthesiology Institute
Associate Professor of Anesthesiology
CCLCM of Case Western Reserve University

Ralf E. Gebhard, MD
Professor of Anesthesiology
Professor of Orthopedics and Rehabilitation
Department of Anesthesiology, Perioperative Medicine and Pain Management
University of Miami-Miller School of Medicine

Harold J. Gelfand, MD
Commander, U.S. Navy
Assistant Professor of Anesthesiology
Uniformed Services University of Health Sciences
Director Acute Pain Medicine and Regional Anesthesia
Walter Reed National Military Medical Center

Ki Jinn Chin, MBBS
Associate Professor, Anesthesia
University of Toronto
Fellowship Coordinator, Toronto Western Hospital
Regional Anesthesia Fellowship Program Director, Toronto Western Hospital

James H. Kim, MD
Assistant Professor
Department of Anesthesiology
University of Virginia School of Medicine

Teresa Kusper, DO
Department of Anesthesiology
Advocate Illinois Masonic Medical Center

Jonathan D. Lin, MD
Program Director, Regional Anesthesia and Acute Pain Medicine Fellowship
Assistant Professor of Anesthesiology and Critical Care Medicine
The Johns Hopkins Hospital

Richard Marks, MD
Attending Anesthesiologist
Department of Anesthesiology, Perioperative Care and Pain Medicine
NYU Langone Health
NYU School of Medicine

M. Steve Melton, MD
Assistant Professor
Department of Anesthesiology
Duke University Medical Center

Andres Missair, MD, EDRA
Chief, Acute Pain Service
Asst. Chief of Service, Anesthesiology & Pain
Bruce Carter Miami VA Healthcare System
Associate Professor
Department of Anesthesiology
University of Miami

Daniel Moy, MD
CA-2 Resident
Stanford University

Karen C. Nielsen, MD
Associate Professor
Department of Anesthesiology
Duke University Medical Center

Aurora Naa-Afoley Quaye, MD
Assistant in Anesthesia
Department of Anesthesia, Critical Care and Pain Medicine
Massachusetts General Hospital
North Shore Medical Center Salem Hospital
Boston, MA

Rosemary C. Polomano, PhD, RN, FAAN
Associate Dean for Practice and Professor of Pain Practice
University of Pennsylvania School of Nursing
Professor of Anesthesiology and Critical Care (Secondary)
University of Pennsylvania Perelman School of Medicine
Adjunct Professor, Uniformed Services University
Graduate School of Nursing

G. Ryan Pomicter, MD
Assistant Professor of Anesthesiology
Uniformed Services University of the Health Sciences

Russel J. Roberts, PharmD, BCCCP, FCCM
Clinical Pharmacy Manger
Cardiology, Critical Care and Infectious Diseases
Massachusetts General Hospital
Boston, MA

Deborah A. Romeo, MD
Assistant Professor
Anesthesia and Perioperative Medicine
Division of Pediatric Anesthesia
Medical University of South Carolina

Gregory D. Schnepper, MD
Assistant Professor
Anesthesia and Perioperative Medicine
Medical University of South Carolina

Cynthia H. Shields MD
Colonel (Retired), Medical Corps US Army
Associate Professor Anesthesiology
Uniformed Services University of the Health Sciences

Eellan Sivanesan, MD
Assistant Professor, Division of Pain Medicine
Department of Anesthesiology and Critical Care Medicine
Johns Hopkins School of Medicine

Susan M. Steele, MD
Staff Anesthesiologist
Mission Community Anesthesia Specialists
Mission Hospital

Alex Toyoda, PharmD
Attending Clinical Pharmacist
Cardiology/Cardiac ICU
Massachusetts General Hospital
Boston, MA

Uchenna O. Umeh, MD
Assistant Professor
Assistant Regional Anesthesia Fellowship Director
Department of Anesthesiology, Perioperative Care and Pain Medicine
NYU Langone Health
NYU School of Medicine

Sylvia H. Wilson, MD
Associate Professor
Department of Anesthesia and Perioperative Medicine
Medical University of South Carolina

Models

Pierre-Etienne Cagniart, MD
Lieutenant Commander, Medical Corps, US Navy

Kathryn M. Eliasen, MD
Captain, Medical Corps, US Army

Illustrations

Michael K. Sracic, MD, MS, FACOEM
Lieutenant Commander, Medical Corps (UMO/DMO), United States Navy
Command Surgeon
Naval Special Warfare Group FOUR

Authors of the Military Advanced Regional Anesthesia and Analgesia Handbook, 1st edition

Gregory Applegate, DO
Major, Medical Corps, US Army

Todd Carter, MD
Lieutenant Colonel, Medical Corps, US Air Force

John Chiles, MD
Colonel (Retired), Medical Corps, US Army

James E. Cox, MD
Colonel (Retired), Medical Corps, US Air Force

Scott Croll, MD
Lieutenant Colonel, Medical Corps, US Army

Steve Cohen, MD
Colonel, Medical Corps, US Army

John Dunford, MD
Assistant Professor of Anesthesiology, Uniformed Services University of the Health Sciences

Eric Elster, MD, FACS
CAPT, MC, United States Navy
Professor and Chairman
Department of Surgery
Uniformed Services University of the Health Sciences
Walter Reed National Military Medical Center

Carlo Franco, MD
Associate Professor of Anesthesiology and Anatomy
Rush University Medical Center

Bill Fritz, MD
Conemaugh Health System

Kurt Grathwohl, MD
Lieutenant Colonel, Medical Corps, US Army

Scott Griffith, MD
Major, Medical Corps, US Army

Stephen M. Klein, MD
Associate Professor of Anesthesiology
Duke University Medical Center

Robert S. Lennon, DO
Brigadier General (Retired), Medical Corps, US Army
Associate Professor, Mayo Clinic Medical School

Courtney Lennon
Ensign, Medical Corps, US Navy

Robert Lennon, JD
Ensign, Medical Corps, US Navy

Randall Malchow, MD
Colonel, Medical Corps, US Army

Greg Malone, MD
Captain, Medical Corps, US Air Force

Geselle McKnight, CRNA, MSN
Walter Reed Army Medical Center

Brian McMillan, MD
Major, Medical Corps, US Army

Jonathon Rogers, MD
Captain, Medical Corps, US Air Force

Christine Rupprecht, RN, MSN
Walter Reed Army Medical Center

Cynthia Shields, MD
Colonel, Medical Corps, US Army

Sean Shockey, MD
Major, Medical Corps, US Army

Kenneth Son, MD
Lieutenant Commander, Medical Corps, US Navy

Alexander Stojadinovic, MD, MBA, FACS
Medical Director, Healthcare Management Service
Amerigroup, Anthem, Inc.
Professor of Surgery (Hon)
Colonel, United States Army, Medical Corps (Ret)

Amy Vertrees, MD
Captain, Medical Corps, US Army

Ann Virtis, MD
Colonel (Retired), Medical Corps, US Air Force

Ronald White, MD
Major, Medical Corps, US Army

Alon P. Winnie, MD
Professor of Anesthesiology
Northwestern University Medical Center

Production Assistant

Christian Calilung, MS
Project Coordinator
Henry M. Jackson Foundation for the Advancement of Military Medicine
Defense and Veterans Center for Integrative Pain Management

Models

Michael Adams, MD

Brian McLean, MD

Aidan Shields

Michael Shigemasa

Necia Williams, MD

Section I

The Practice of Acute Pain Medicine

Acute Pain Medicine Services: Structure and Procedures

Alicia Lopez Warlick, W. Michael Bullock, and Padma Gulur

1

1. Staffing Models and Suggested Facilities

The implementation of an acute pain service (APS) requires appropriate medical professionals and facilities to allow for optimal patient care. These resources include adequate medical staff, equipment, patient care areas, and a modality for necessary documentation.[1]

A successful acute pain practice is often run in conjunction with a strong regional anesthesia service to provide patients with a multimodal approach to perioperative analgesia.

Multimodal analgesia, in addition to oral and intravenous medications, may incorporate neuraxial and peripheral nerve catheters. These catheters have been essential in decreasing opiate consumption, improving pain scores, and improving functional outcomes.

Regional anesthesia procedures are associated with potential complications, including local anesthetic systemic toxicity (LAST), high spinal anesthesia, pneumothorax, and arterial puncture. Routine monitors, including pulse oximetry, noninvasive blood pressure, and electrocardiography, are essential and should be used in all cases to identify problems and prevent injury. If sedation is used, regular monitoring of oxygenation and ventilation is necessary to detect hypoventilation or airway obstruction. If available, capnography is useful to ensure ongoing ventilation. Supplemental oxygen should be routinely administered in the setting of sedation because hypoxia will worsen the negative chronotropic and inotropic effects in LAST.[2]

Regional anesthesiology procedures may have potential complications and can be performed in a specialized area, termed the *block area*, a preoperative space where supplies, drugs, block equipment, and monitors are organized. This area allows the block team to place blocks and catheters in a timely manner to minimize the use of costly operating room time. The block team consists of the regional anesthesiologist, providers such as residents and nurse anesthetists, and specialized block nurses.[9]

A typical block area also contains specialized equipment necessary for the performance of the block, including echogenic needles, nerve block catheter kits, nerve stimulators, and ultrasound machines. Nerve stimulators have been a useful method for nerve localization over the past 3 decades and, despite low sensitivity, remain a clinically useful tool with high specificity in detecting intraneural placement of a needle tip.[3] Recently, ultrasound has replaced nerve stimulation, and the use of ultrasound-guided regional anesthesia has gained great popularity. Ultrasound-guided regional anesthesia has been shown to decrease the amount of local anesthetic needed to achieve a successful block.[4] Furthermore, ultrasound has been helpful in minimizing the risk of inadvertent vascular puncture.[5]

In addition to specialized equipment, the block area will have access to commonly used local anesthetics and additives. Epinephrine, a reliable and sensitive marker to determine intravascular injection, is one such additive. It is routinely added to local anesthetic solutions for peripheral nerve block placement as the detection of intravascular injection of local anesthetic alone drops significantly in patients who are sedated.[6,7]

It is imperative that any block area where regional anesthesia procedures are performed is adequately equipped with emergency airway equipment (e.g., self-inflating bag-valve mask, suction, airways and endotracheal tubes, and laryngoscopes) and resuscitation drugs, including lipid emulsion for rescue from LAST. Given the infrequent incidence of LAST, a checklist that outlines the tenets of treatment may be helpful. In a simulated environment, trainees using the American Society of Regional Anesthesia and Pain Medicine (ASRA) checklist completed more critical steps in the management of LAST than did trainees who did not use the checklist.[8]

2. Acute Pain Service

The APS extends to inpatient floors where patients with indwelling peripheral nerve or neuraxial catheters, or with complicated pain management plans, may require continued support from acute pain specialists. A designated workspace for the APS is helpful to facilitate patient care, including activities such as rounding and handoffs between care team members. Moreover, patients who have indwelling peripheral nerve and epidural catheters require special nursing care by practitioners who are knowledgeable about the care of these devices as well as the specialized monitoring required by these patients. Nurses on these units should be able to readily recognize the signs of local anesthetic toxicity or oversedation.

Patients may benefit from prolonged analgesia via continued use of peripheral nerve catheters attached to disposable infusion pumps upon discharge to the outpatient setting. Once discharged, patients must be able to contact providers at any time in case of urgent complications, such as LAST, catheter dislodgement, or equipment malfunction while these nerve catheters are in place. All outpatients with nerve catheters should be contacted daily to ensure completion of therapy, including removal of catheters and resolution of motor and sensory block.

Finally, a system must exist that allows for patient care documentation, including procedure notes, daily progress notes, and outpatient follow-up. Electronic medical records are widely used and can be helpful in facilitating handoffs between patient care teams.

3. Daily Procedures

Multiple components make up the daily procedures of an acute pain medicine service. These daily procedures can be categorized into 3 time intervals: preoperative, intraoperative, and postoperative. *Preoperative considerations* include the timing of the block, help from ancillary staff, patient monitoring, and location of the block placement. Because a timely start is important in the operating room, the patient must arrive early enough to be checked into the block area. The surgeon should examine the patient and mark the surgical site before the performance of the block. Check-in, examination, and site marking will help minimize the occurrence of wrong-sided blocks. Ideally, check-in and marking should be finished at least 30 minutes before the start of the surgical procedure. This will allow the anesthesiologist enough time to assess the patient and perform the block. Once the patient is ready for the regional procedure, confirmation of site and laterality by the anesthesiologist and another licensed provider is performed to further minimize occurrence of wrong-sided blocks. In addition, the provider should assist the anesthesiologist in performing the block by helping to position the patient, adjusting the ultrasound, administering the local anesthetic, and monitoring the patient. This provider should be a block nurse, as supported by studies which have shown that having a block team with devoted regional anesthesia nurses improves the efficiency and safety of the procedure.[9]

Regardless of the location of the block, premedication is used to maximize patient comfort, such as anxiolytics and opioids. Monitoring is necessary to manage any hemodynamic changes from the premedications or from procedural complications. *Intraoperative considerations* often dictate the anesthetic technique. The regional anesthetic can be used as the primary anesthetic technique, or the block can be performed for postoperative pain management as part of the comprehensive anesthetic plan. Factors to consider include the use of a tourniquet, patient positioning, and patient comorbidities. Tourniquet pain may influence anesthetic technique. Sedated patients begin to exhibit pathophysiologic changes from the tourniquet at approximately 45 minutes after tourniquet inflation.[10] Patients will exhibit tourniquet pain and accompanying physiologic responses despite regional anesthesia, which can only be mitigated by deep sedation, general anesthesia, or spinal anesthesia. The inability to prevent tourniquet pain with local anesthesia is thought to be due to the relative resistance of the smaller, unmyelinated C-fibers to local anesthesia.[11] Therefore, a general or spinal anesthetic should be given for any surgery with an anticipated tourniquet inflation time longer than 45 minutes. Surgical factors, including patient positioning (prone, beach-chair, supine, etc.), anticipated blood loss, and length of operative procedure, also influence anesthetic technique. In addition, patient comorbidities greatly influence the anesthetic technique. A comprehensive and thoughtful plan requires careful evaluation of all intraoperative considerations.

Postoperative considerations include patient safety, education, and follow-up. Patients with functioning nerve blocks generally recover quickly in the postanesthesia care unit (PACU). PACU stay is frequently short as patients have minimal pain and a lower incidence of postoperative nausea and vomiting. Ambulatory patients may be discharged with a continuous nerve catheter, but this is dependent on caregiver support and follow-up care. Hospitalized patients should be formally handed over to the APS, an invaluable resource that has been shown to improve pain outcomes.[12,13] Regardless of postoperative destination, patients must be educated consistently and clearly about block safety, catheter management, and proper use and cessation of narcotic and nonnarcotic pain medications.

4. Suggestions on Integrating and Reporting to Wider Medical Systems

An APS provides a unique dimension to patient care, but unfortunately, few studies support improved outcomes as most research has focused on narrow perspectives such as patient-controlled analgesia or direct cost-effectiveness. Traditionally, APSs have focused on alleviating pain measured by subjective pain scores; however, achieving appropriate analgesia to facilitate functional recovery is critical.

Many services are limited to managing neuraxial and regional catheters placed on the day of surgery, while others may also focus on multimodal analgesic protocols started on the day of surgery or immediately after surgery. For pain services focused on functional recovery, the scope should broaden to encompass preoperative patient optimization, pain management throughout the inpatient period, and restoration of functionality in the home environment.

5. Importance of Measuring Outcomes

Measuring and reporting outcomes is important in the evolving healthcare landscape as reliance on pain scores alone is unlikely to show value. Patient-reported outcomes measured by Hospital Consumer Assessment of Healthcare Providers and Systems (HCAHPS) also have limitations. HCAHPS pain-related questions are vague or misleading, including "During this hospital stay, did you need medicine for pain?" "During this hospital stay, how often was your pain well controlled?" and "During this hospital stay, how often did the hospital staff do everything they could to help you with your pain?" These survey questions raise significant concerns about unduly influencing prescribing practices. Current prescribing practices may be contributing to the prescription opioid epidemic, for which the Centers for Disease Control and Prevention (CDC) recently released safe prescribing guidelines that emphasize the need for caution.[14] As such, healthcare providers are faced with the conundrum of appropriate opioid prescribing despite fiscal pressure to improve patient-reported outcomes on pain treatment satisfaction.

The Centers for Medicare and Medicaid Services (CMS) initially stated that opioids should not be considered the basis of pain management, and hence the preceding questions do not adversely impact pain practice.[15] Subsequently, however, CMS removed the questions based on findings from the Hospital Outpatient Prospective Payment System and Ambulatory Surgical Center Payment System final rule for calendar year 2017. Omitting these questions will remove the financial link in the Hospital Value-Based Purchasing program.[16] They are developing new, replacement questions about pain management; therefore, providers who practice acute pain medicine must help define outcomes and consistent measures for reporting.

6. Measure and Report Key Outcomes

Key measures include pain intensity and analgesic utilization. These measures are important especially given concerns with the prescription opioid epidemic. Patient-reported outcomes are primarily guiding treatment. Current patient measures are often unidimensional.

Unidimensional pain intensity scales such as the Numerical Rating Scale or Visual Analog Scale, primarily used in inpatient assessments, are inherently subjective. The subjectivity of these assessments and wide variability in interpretation of these scales by both patients and providers lead to significant gaps in understanding and treatment. Multidimensional pain scales such as the Brief Pain Inventory or the McGill Pain Questionnaire that address pain with movement and rest, pain interference, functionality, sleep, and psychological interplay are more valid and accurate representations of the impact of pain.[17]

Analgesic utilization should be expressed in standard terms for optimal patient care, especially when opioids are administered. Equianalgesic tables that convert patient-administered opioids into oral morphine equivalents should be incorporated into the electronic medical record and electronic order systems to ensure standard comparison. Additionally, measures of functional status, such as the Banner Mobility Assessment Tool mobility level or the A-test, should be integrated.[18,19] Furthermore, use of measures such as diffuse noxious inhibitory control or conditioned pain modulation can aid providers in assessing the risk of progression of acute pain to chronic pain.[19]

7. Demonstrate Value

An APS should focus on patient-centered healthcare and demonstrate value-based care efforts to remain relevant in the changing healthcare landscape. Ensuring that major outcome metrics are measured, collected, and reported is instrumental in demonstrating value. Key performance indicators should include cost-effectiveness measures, both direct and indirect, such as impact on length of stay, emergency room visits, and readmissions. This information should be made available to all personnel at the departmental level and to all collaborating/referring services via a pain management dashboard for analysis and improvement (Figure 1.1). In addition, hospital administrators should receive a quarterly report on patient outcomes through direct and indirect efforts of the APS for further analysis.

8. Align to Organizational Goals

Outcome metrics reported by an APS should align with the organization's clinical and financial goals. Currently, length of stay, 30-day readmission rates, 30-day emergency department visits, and HCAHPS scores are among the most common outcomes important to health systems. These metrics are evolving as a result of the CMS's Quality Payment Program (MACRA). These quality measures will support MACRA's 2 tracks—the Merit-Based Incentive Payment System (MIPS) and the Advanced Alternative Payment Models (APMs). By choosing to participate in APMs, a group will earn an incentive payment for using an innovative payment model. A group that chooses to participate in MIPS will earn a performance-based payment adjustment. These tracks will be chosen based on practice size, specialty, location, or patient population.[20]

An APS may generate APMs though collaboration with surgeons in Enhanced Recovery After Surgery (ERAS) pathways and partnership with palliative care and other stakeholders to generate chronic disease management. Furthermore, collaboration with medicine services to optimize care of patients admitted for nonsurgical management of low back pain would be high yield. Low back pain has a significant economic impact in the United States, with total costs related to this condition exceeding $100 billion per year.[21]

DukeHealth

Discharge Annual Summary

Year of Discharge Dtm	Encounters Per Day	Encounter Days	Total Encounters	% Opioid Tolerant	LOS	% ED visits	% 30 Day Readmit Thru ED	% 30 Day Readmit	% 30 day Mortality	% Staff Do Everything "Always" Help w/Pain	% Pain "Always" Controlled
2013	2.3	229	523	29.4%	8.15	31.0%	10.3%	15.9%	0.0%	78.0%	58.0%
2014	2.5	306	763	38.8%	7.55	28.0%	7.9%	16.1%	0.0%	76.0%	54.0%
2015	3.7	82	300	36.0%	6.81	24.0%	8.7%	11.3%	0.0%	71.0%	51.0%

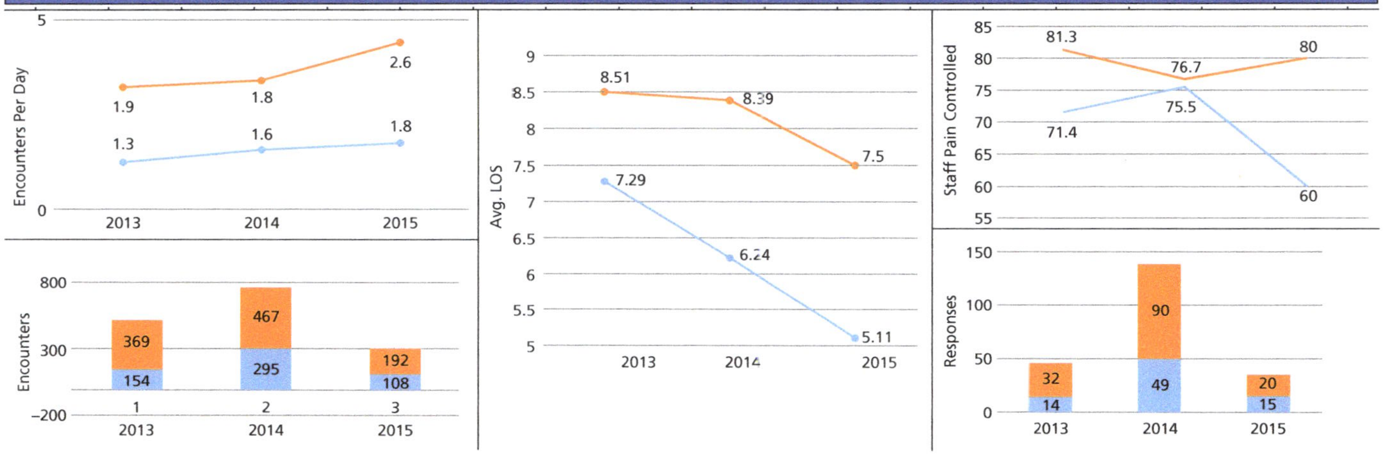

Figure 1.1 Sample pain management dashboard used at Duke Health by the Inpatient Acute Pain Service.

9. Conclusions

Implementation of an APS can beneficially impact patient outcomes and hospital systems. Designing an infrastructure that allows the service to thrive is essential. This includes personnel, space, equipment, and a collaborative culture. The service must be able to function in all 3 perioperative periods with the goal of functional restoration. Goals and outcomes measured by the APS should align with those of the hospital. Outcomes should be continually measured and practice refined to deliver better patient care and show value to both patients and the hospital.

References

1. Schuler M, Becker A, Lindena G, Mattenklodt P. [Treatment of elderly with chronic pain in geriatric care and pain therapy facilities in Germany. Survey results]. *Schmerz*. 2015;29(4):422–430.
2. Heavner JE, Dryden CF Jr, Sanghani V, Huemer G, Bessire A, Badgwell JM. Severe hypoxia enhances central nervous system and cardiovascular toxicity of bupivacaine in lightly anesthetized pigs. *Anesthesiology*. 1992;77(1):142–147.
3. Tsai TP, Vuckovic I, Dilberovic F, Obhodzas M, Kapur E, Divanovic KA, et al. Intensity of the stimulating current may not be a reliable indicator of intraneural needle placement. *Reg Anesth Pain Med*. 2008;33(3):207–210.
4. Casati A, Baciarello M, Di Cianni S, Danelli G, De Marco G, Leone S, et al. Effects of ultrasound guidance on the minimum effective anaesthetic volume required to block the femoral nerve. *Br J Anaesth*. 2007;98(6):823–827.
5. Barrington MJ, Watts SA, Gledhill SR, Thomas RD, Said SA, Snyder GL, et al. Preliminary results of the Australasian Regional Anaesthesia Collaboration: a prospective audit of more than 7000 peripheral nerve and plexus blocks for neurologic and other complications. *Reg Anesth Pain Med*. 2009;34(6):534–541.
6. Moore JM, Liu SS, Neal JM. Premedication with fentanyl and midazolam decreases the reliability of intravenous lidocaine test dose. *Anesth Analg*. 1998;86(5):1015–1017.
7. Guinard JP, Mulroy MF, Carpenter RL, Knopes KD. Test doses: optimal epinephrine content with and without acute beta-adrenergic blockade. *Anesthesiology*. 1990;73(3):386–392.
8. Neal JM, Hsiung RL, Mulroy MF, Halpern BB, Dragnich AD, Slee AE. ASRA checklist improves trainee performance during a simulated episode of local anesthetic systemic toxicity. *Reg Anesth Pain Med*. 2012;37(1):8–15.
9. Russell RA, Burke K, Gattis K. Implementing a regional anesthesia block nurse team in the perianesthesia care unit increases patient safety and perioperative efficiency. *J Perianesth Nurs*. 2013;28(1):3–10.
10. Kam PC, Kavanagh R, Yoong FF. The arterial tourniquet: pathophysiological consequences and anaesthetic implications. *Anaesthesia*. 2001;56(6):534–545.
11. Gissen AJ, Covino BG, Gregus J. Differential sensitivities of mammalian nerve fibers to local anesthetic agents. *Anesthesiology*. 1980;53(6):467–474.
12. Lee A, Chan SK, Chen PP, Gin T, Lau AS, Chiu CH. The costs and benefits of extending the role of the acute pain service on clinical outcomes after major elective surgery. *Anesth Analg*. 2010;111(4):1042–1050.
13. Tighe P, Buckenmaier CC III, Boezaart AP, et al. Acute pain medicine in the United States: a status report. *Pain Med*. 2015;16(9):1806–1826.
14. www.cdc.gov/drugoverdose/pdf/guidelines.
15. Tefera L, Lehrman WG, Conway P. Measurement of the patient experience: clarifying facts, myths, and approaches. *JAMA*. 2016;315(20):2167–2168. doi:10.1001/jama.2016.1652
16. https://www.federalregister.gov/documents/2016/11/14/2016-26515/medicare-program-hospital-outpatient-prospective-payment-and-ambulatory-surgical-center-payment.
17. Boynton T, et al. Banner Mobility Assessment Tool for Nurses: instrument validation. *Am J SPHM*. 4(3):86–92. 2014.
18. Vojnosanit Pregl. The A-test: assessment of functional recovery during early rehabilitation of patients in an orthopedic ward—content, criterion and construct validity. 2014;71(8):715–722. PMID: 25181829

19. Yarnitsky D, et al. Conditioned pain modulation (the diffuse noxious inhibitory control-like effect): its relevance for acute and chronic pain states. *Curr Opin Anaesthesiol.* 2010 Oct;23(5):611–615. doi:0.1097/ACO.0b013e32833c348b
20. https://www.cms.gov/Medicare/Quality-Initiatives-Patient-Assessment-Instruments/Value-Based-Programs/MACRA-MIPS-and-APMs/MACRA-MIPS-and-APMs.html.
21. Katz JN. Lumbar disc disorders and low-back pain: socioeconomic factors and consequences [review]. *J Bone Joint Surg Am.* 2006;88(suppl 2):21–24.

2

Economics of Acute Pain Medicine

Brian E. Harrington and Edward R. Mariano

1. Introduction

Acute pain is a common and anticipated consequence of surgical interventions. It is usually directly associated with tissue damage, is expected to fade with tissue healing, and resolves within days to weeks. Despite being generally self-limited, however, acute pain can profoundly impact the perioperative period and alter patient well-being. In recent decades, numerous insights have been made into the significance of acute pain and its management. During this same period, the economics of healthcare have assumed increasing importance as an ever-growing proportion of US gross domestic product (GDP) is spent on healthcare (essentially doubling since 1980 to approximately 17.8% in 2015).[1] The topic of healthcare economics is particularly prominent in the United States, which already spends about 50% more on healthcare than comparable developed countries and is projected to spend 20% of GDP on healthcare by the year 2025.[1]

Surprisingly, despite compelling interest and importance, our insights into healthcare economics of acute pain medicine remain relatively primitive. Publications specifically concerning the economics of acute pain medicine are particularly scarce. In a comprehensive review of acute pain management, the Australian and New Zealand College of Anaesthetists and Faculty of Pain Medicine collected the available scientific evidence through August 2014.[2] Although the entire analysis by Schug and colleagues yielded more than 750 evidence-based "key messages," there were only 4 regarding economic considerations (Box 2.1). It is noteworthy that each of these was based on "new" evidence that had become available since publication of these researchers' previous edition in 2010.

Box 2.1 Summary of Key Messages: Economic Considerations in Acute Pain Management

1. Patients highly value well-controlled pain.
2. Long-term economic consequences from the progression of acute to chronic pain can be significant.
3. Costs from patient-controlled analgesia errors can be considerable; the most common high-cost errors arise from staff communication error and operator error.
4. There are different measures of economic assessment and analysis used in healthcare; no one method is most appropriate.[2]

This chapter will attempt to expand on and update previously published summaries and will consider the economics of acute pain medicine primarily in terms of costs and benefits. Rather than concentrate on any specific measures of economic assessment and analysis, the chapter will focus on general concepts that apply to virtually all clinical settings. Details regarding healthcare finances will only be considered indirectly, as they are tremendously situational, rapidly changing, and simply beyond the scope of this discussion.

2. The Modern Focus on Acute Pain

As alluded to in the introduction, the past several decades have witnessed significant improvements in the prevention and treatment of acute postoperative pain. Developments such as patient-controlled analgesia, continuous epidural analgesia, and minimally invasive surgical techniques have led to dramatic breakthroughs in patient care. Through such successes, it has become the standard of care that severe acute postoperative pain can and should be effectively managed.

Around the recent turn of the century, a number of initiatives were introduced that were intended to help close the gap between potential and actual patient care regarding acute pain. Some notable efforts include the following:

1999—Adopting the concept from the American Pain Society, the Veterans Health Administration called for pain to be treated as the "fifth vital sign" and required the use of the Numeric Rating Scale for all clinical encounters.[3] This resulted in an organized effort to detect and quantify pain, and included a mandate to treat specific levels of pain (e.g., pain scores of 4 or greater out of 10).

2000—The US Congress designated the 10 years beginning January 1, 2001, as the "Decade of Pain Control and Research." Although this push was primarily directed toward inadequacies in chronic, irreversible, and palliative pain management, it signaled a new level of federal engagement in pain medicine.[4]

2001—The Joint Commission on Accreditation of Healthcare Organizations (JCAHO, now known simply as the Joint Commission) introduced new pain management standards that required facilities to better assess and treat pain. Notably, an article in the *Journal of the American Medical Association* that introduced these new standards described poor pain control as "unethical, clinically unsound, and *economically wasteful*" (italics added).[5]

2002—Building on the increased focus on pain management, work began on the development of the Hospital Consumer Assessment of Healthcare Providers and Systems (HCAHPS) survey. This survey includes several pointed questions that assess a patient's experience with pain management. The HCAHPS survey has since become an important metric in patient care and is variously tied to reimbursement.

Along with many others, these milestones were instrumental in substantially raising the profile of acute (and chronic) pain management. Today, the treatment of pain has widely come to be considered a fundamental human right.[6] Currently, it can be said that there is a strong mandate for the optimal management of pain.

Despite heightened awareness and clinical advancements, however, contemporary patient surveys suggest that acute pain continues to be inadequately controlled. A recent survey of American patients indicated that there has been little improvement in acute pain control over the past 20 years.[7] In this survey of 300 random American adults who had undergone surgery within the past 5 years, 86% reported pain after surgery, with fully 75% of these experiencing moderate to extreme levels of pain (levels that were commonly still present after discharge). These disappointing findings likely indicate deficiencies in compliance with accepted approaches. This concern is supported by indirect evidence indicating that multimodal analgesia (MMA) is not being provided when indicated. Ladha and colleagues looked at the perioperative use of MMA in a large database of appropriate surgical patients and found that only 54.2% had received 2 or more nonopioid analgesics.[8] The adoption of "value-based" payment models (e.g., bundled payments) is intended to accelerate the adoption of best practice initiatives such as MMA.

3. Core Concepts in Acute Pain Medicine

Efforts directed toward discerning the optimal management of acute pain have progressed on many fronts. The American Society of Anesthesiologists (ASA) Committee on Standards and Practice Parameters (representing the medical specialists most intimately involved in acute pain management) published practice guidelines on acute pain management in the perioperative setting in 2004 and again in 2012.[9] Expanding on the ASA guidelines, the American Pain Society (with input from the ASA and American Society of Regional Anesthesia and Pain Medicine) recently published even more current guidelines in 2016.[10] In these and other publications, several concepts are emphasized that represent the core of modern acute pain management.

3.1. Multimodal analgesia

Perhaps the most fundamental advance in the management of acute pain in recent years has been the concept of MMA.[11] In this paradigm, combinations of analgesic agents are administered to take advantage of additive and possibly synergistic effects while decreasing dose-related side effects. Options may also include physical (e.g., transcutaneous electrical nerve stimulation) and cognitive-behavioral modalities. The multitude of available agents (acetaminophen, nonsteroidal anti-inflammatory drugs, local anesthetics, ketamine, etc.) presents numerous possible combinations of analgesics. Through the use of alternative nonopioid analgesic agents, an opioid-sparing effect is a common goal of the MMA approach.

At this point, the role of opioids for pain control deserves special comment. Opioids have long been appreciated as effective analgesics, particularly for acute pain. It is not surprising, therefore, that an increased reliance on them was the initial response to recent mandates to improve pain control. This approach to acute pain management has proven to be unsatisfactory on several levels. Unfortunately, these drugs are associated with a high incidence of opioid-related adverse drug effects (ORADEs). The increased use of opioids is thereby naturally expected to increase the rate of nausea (and vomiting), increase the frequency of pruritis, and decrease bowel motility. On further analysis, such "minor" ORADEs have been shown to exert significant negative effects on acute perioperative recovery, length of stay, and overall costs of care.[12] Furthermore, despite efforts at proper titration, the increased use of opioids has also been associated with increased rates of such major adverse effects as opioid-associated sedation and respiratory depression.[13] Last, the recent "opioid epidemic" has raised further concerns regarding opioid prescribing for acute pain management. Recent data indicate that the transition from acute to chronic opioid use is more common in the perioperative period than formerly appreciated.[14] These as well as other issues with opiates (e.g., diversion) strongly further support the concept of opioid-sparing MMA.

However, it must be appreciated that in the evolving realm of MMA there are not yet any "gold standards."[15] Nevertheless, current ASA guidelines recommend the use of multimodal pain management therapy "whenever possible."[9]

3.2. Pain protocols

Unsurprisingly, the severity and nature of postoperative pain are ultimately dependent on the specific surgical procedure performed. A growing body of evidence also indicates that the effectiveness of analgesics is dependent on the nature of the surgical procedure. These observations form the basis for designing evidence-based, procedure-specific pain management protocols (which can be further refined through the inclusion of patient-specific features such as pediatrics).

The PROSPECT (PROcedure-SPECific Postoperative Pain ManagemenT) initiative is an international effort to develop procedure-specific management recommendations.[16] The PROSPECT Working Group consists of an international panel of anesthesiologists and surgeons and has published evidence-based guidelines for a number of procedures (www.postoppain.org).

In a closely related development, the desire to optimize and accelerate recovery for common surgical procedures has resulted in several enhanced recovery after surgery (ERAS) protocols. Although these are not exclusively concerned with pain management, acute pain control is recognized as one of 5 key components of ERAS protocols and is considered a prerequisite for other clinical advantages of ERAS such as early mobility and minimization of hospital-acquired adverse events. Accelerated clinical care, including effective pain management, has been encouraged as a further means to address the opioid epidemic (mentioned in the "Multimodal Analgesia" section of this chapter).[17]

3.3. Pain management as a service

In the 1980s, the concept of the acute pain service (APS) was developed in response to both humanitarian and pragmatic concerns regarding deficiencies in pain management.[18] Although there is still no consensus regarding the optimal structure or function of an APS, its primary purpose remains all-day, everyday accountability for acute pain management within an institution. Essential functions of an APS include (1) the promotion of evidence-based care of pain, (2) the development of pain management protocols and guidelines, and (3) the management of advanced analgesic techniques (e.g., continuous regional anesthesia). The ASA Task Force on Acute Pain Management specifically recommends that "anesthesiologists providing perioperative analgesia services should do so within the framework of an Acute Pain Service."[9]

In 2009, a nationwide survey indicated that 74% of hospitals in the United States (and fully 96% of American university/teaching hospitals) had an organized APS.[19] With anesthesiology personnel involved in 95% of these services, virtually all American anesthesiology residents will have significant exposure to the organized APS model during residency training.

Each of the 3 key concepts mentioned in this section has been considered from an economic perspective. It should be noted, however, that such studies have often been inconclusive, open to valid criticism, and can certainly be said to illustrate the difficulties inherent in studying in isolation a single element of complex systems.

From its inception, MMA has long been thought of in terms of value.[20] Although evidence is limited and studies have a great deal of heterogeneity, it is widely thought that optimal MMA has the potential to decrease healthcare costs (primarily through opioid sparing and a decreased incidence of dose-related adverse drug effects).[11]

Economic analyses of procedure-specific pain protocols have been nearly uniformly favorable. A recent analysis of a clinical pathway for total knee arthroplasty, for example, noted several patient benefits as well as a reduction in direct costs.[21] Similarly, a meta-analysis of enhanced recovery for colorectal surgery concluded that implementation of ERAS pathways optimized utilization of healthcare resources.[22] These and other studies robustly support the ERAS concept of accelerating the return of baseline function.[23]

Studies of the economic impact of the APS have been mixed.[24] Systematic reviews of studies published through the first decade of the 2000s are acknowledged as being hampered by poor-quality evidence.[25,26] However, a more recent analysis of studies published between 2005 and 2012 concluded that using an APS resulted in 17.4% cost savings (primarily through shorter hospital stays and lower readmission rates).[27]

4. Fundamentals of Healthcare Economics: The Value Equation

> Price is what you pay, value is what you get.
>
> Warren Buffett, American investor

The fee-for-service payment model so commonly encountered in healthcare clearly rewards volume of care, often with little regard for outcomes, complications, or expenditures. In recent years, there have been concerted efforts to promote alternative incentives in healthcare. The result has been termed the *value agenda* or the *transition from volume to value*.[28] "Value-based" models intend to promote efficient, high-quality care at a lower cost. Ideally, metrics can be developed that will also allow for individualized patient-centered care.

While the concept of value is ultimately in the eye of the beholder (i.e., the consumer—which can include patients, physicians, healthcare systems, payers, and even society as a whole), it is often expressed mathematically as simply:

Value = Benefits/Costs

Box 2.2 Definitions of Health Economic Assessment Measures (from Schug et al.).

- **Cost-effectiveness analysis:** Consequences are measured in natural units such as life years gained, disability days avoided, or cases detected.
- **Cost-utility analysis:** Consequences are measured in terms of preference-based measures of health such as quality-adjusted life years or disability-adjusted life years.
- **Cost-benefit analysis:** Consequences are valued in monetary units.
- **Cost-minimization analysis:** Consequences of compared interventions are equivalent (in terms of clinical efficacy and tolerability) and only relative costs are compared.
- **Cost-outcome description:** Costs are measured in monetary value and health effects are measured in natural units (e.g., ICU days saved, patient satisfaction).

This definition of value warrants a few comments. First, it should be noted that value is a concept that lacks specific units and is not always monetary. Second, costs can be extremely complex and must be considered from the various perspectives of healthcare stakeholders (patients, for example, often consider the value of lower pain levels [benefit] relative to adverse drug effects such as nausea [cost]).[29] Third, while value is certainly increased by providing the same benefit at lower cost or increased benefit at the same cost, *relative* values remain extremely difficult to compare (e.g., the costs of acute pain management compared with those for cancer treatment or childhood immunizations—in other words, given the reality of limited healthcare resources, is acute pain medicine "worth it"?). Finally, the value of acute pain medicine has proven to be particularly challenging to determine since upfront costs are frequently associated with significant "downstream" benefits (many of which are reflected in an absence of adverse events).

The assessment of value in healthcare can be expressed in many ways (Box 2.2). Although consensus has been reached on definitions, economic terms are frequently used inexactly in the literature. A detailed consideration of these terms can be found in other sources.[30] Practitioners should be aware that no single economic assessment measure is considered superior to another.

5. Benefits and Costs of Acute Pain Management

5.1. Benefits of acute pain management

Effective treatment of acute pain has been shown to result in numerous benefits. These can be broadly categorized as follows.

5.1.1. Improved patient experience of care

Improving the individual patient experience of care constitutes one-third of the "triple aim" of modern healthcare, with the other aims being reduction in the costs of care and improved public health.[31] Acute postoperative pain has long been known to be a major concern for surgical patients. Although surveys have repeatedly demonstrated substantial patient "willingness to pay" for antiemetic interventions, a comparative survey has shown the prevention of postoperative pain to be valued by patients twice as highly as the prevention of postoperative nausea and vomiting.[32]

Adequate pain control is clearly associated with patient satisfaction.[33] Analysis of HCAHPS surveys demonstrates a high correlation between global satisfaction with care and "always" receiving good pain control ($r > .84$)[34]

5.1.2. Systematic efficiency

Despite efforts at cost control, medicine remains an extremely labor- and resource-intensive industry. Any factors that adversely impact the smooth and efficient delivery of surgical care can be anticipated to have a negative economic effect.

A major impact of acute postoperative pain control is in the facilitation of throughput within a facility. Effective pain control, particularly through the use of regional anesthesia, has been shown to facilitate postanesthesia care unit (PACU) bypass, decrease the duration of PACU stay, and promote timely discharge. This may benefit a facility in terms of reducing usage of staff overtime. Although the overall economic impact of these effects is often debatable, they certainly offer the potential to decrease utilization of healthcare personnel (particularly in the ambulatory surgery setting). Perhaps a more tangible example of improved throughput is the opioid-sparing pain management seen in ERAS protocols for colorectal surgery, which improve bowel motility and significantly reduce hospital length of stay.[35]

In the ambulatory surgery setting, effective pain control can also reduce unanticipated admissions and readmissions. Pain has been shown to be the most common cause for these major inefficiencies, which incur significant costs.[36]

5.1.3. Fewer acute complications

Minor complications associated with pain and its management are common in the acute postoperative setting. Opioids, effective and having low acquisition costs, are frequently utilized as first-line agents but are associated with a high incidence of economically significant minor adverse effects (e.g., nausea and vomiting) that can accumulate and have a substantial impact on postoperative recovery.[37] Optimal pain management, as through MMA, can be expected to reduce the incidence of these minor complications.

Although it may seem intuitive that effective postoperative analgesia should result in a lower incidence of major postoperative complications, efforts to analyze this issue have been constrained by the available evidence (which has often been of low quality) and limitations of existing data and methods.[38] The relatively low incidence of major adverse events renders most studies underpowered to detect statistically significant effects. The strongest evidence for a beneficial effect of pain management appears to be a reduction in major pulmonary complications, particularly in elderly patients.[39]

5.1.4. Less chronic morbidity

Reducing the incidence of the pain-related inability to participate in timely postoperative rehabilitation programs certainly has the potential to result in faster and more complete recovery with less work loss and less reduction in productivity. However, the greatest potential benefit associated with optimal acute pain management may be in difficult-to-measure longer-term benefits.

Perhaps most promising is the potential for optimal acute pain management to prevent persistent postsurgical pain (PPSP). Not surprisingly, chronic pain has been shown to be associated with tremendous economic costs.[40] PPSP appears to be much more common than generally appreciated (Table 2.1), and its prevention has been referred to as the "Holy Grail of anesthesiology."[41] While association should not be confused with causation, intense acute postoperative pain has

Table 2.1:
Incidence of PPSP After Various Interventions

Limb amputation	60%–80%
Total hip arthroplasty	30%
Hysterectomy	5%–30%
Caesarean section	10%
Breast surgery	20%–50%
Groin hernia surgery	10%
Sternotomy	20%
Thoracotomy	25%–60%

Source: Perkins F, Kehlet H. Chronic pain as an outcome from surgery: a review of predictive factors. *Anesthesiology*. 2000;93:1123–1233.

been shown to be one of the most predictive factors in the development of PPSP.[42,43] There is great hope that optimal acute pain management may be the key to prevention of PPSP.

Finally, one of the most intriguing topics in recent years has been the possible role of postoperative pain control in reducing the incidence of cancer recurrence.[44] Although studies to date in this regard have been mixed, they have been encouraging enough to warrant further investigation.

5.2. Costs of acute pain medicine

Most analyses of healthcare costs attempt to measure the financial costs associated with medical resource utilization. Such direct costs include materials, labor, and facility expenditures. Examples of commonly tracked direct costs include the following.

5.2.1. Material costs, including drugs, supplies, and equipment

While drug costs for acute pain medicine have usually been shown to be nominal,[33] recent developments such as liposomal bupivacaine have challenged this assumption (and prompted cost-benefit analyses of this and other relatively expensive agents). Competition among vendors has turned the acquisition of supplies (like block trays and infusion tubing) into prime opportunities for cost savings. Progress in acute pain medicine has been accompanied by requirements for more advanced equipment such as continuous infusion devices and ultrasound imaging systems.

5.2.2. Labor costs consist of the time and effort expended by the individuals involved in the management of pain

This includes the time required to initiate (e.g., to perform a regional block) and manage pain over time (e.g., pain rounds and telephone care). The savings in labor costs have been a major driver in the development of the familiar physician-led APS team model.

5.2.3. Facility costs range from obvious expenditures such as physical space (e.g., a block room or APS office) to provision of dictation services and electronic medical records

However, as challenging as it may be to determine direct costs, it is certainly even more difficult to measure indirect costs. Indirect costs are those related to the consequences of acute pain management and can include any number of concerns. Adverse drug effects (ADEs), for example, are a type of indirect cost that may be tied to MMA, yet Hoffer and colleagues recently found marked deficiencies in reporting of ADEs in studies of gabapentin and pregabalin for postoperative pain.[45] A recent study estimated that the indirect costs from adverse effects associated with intravenous patient-controlled analgesia can be twice the direct costs of this relatively straightforward technique.[46] Complications and medicolegal liability associated with peripheral nerve blocks can be considered another form of indirect cost. Uncontrolled pain may generate indirect costs on an inpatient basis (e.g., additional resources, longer hospital stay, need for posthospital institutionalized care) or outpatient basis (e.g., family member taking time off work, prolonged disability). Given the financial constraints in modern healthcare, it is prudent to consider all potential cost "centers" along with strategies to decrease the cost of care when planning to present a proposal to establish a new APS to hospital administrators.

Finally, while healthcare costs are most commonly measured in monetary terms, it is important to appreciate that there are many other types of costs (such as the emotional cost incurred by patients in the form of discomfort or anxiety related to pain or procedures). Given the multiple types of costs involved in healthcare, it is easy to appreciate why healthcare costs are extremely complex and notoriously difficult to accurately measure. Once again, this discussion is not intended be a comprehensive consideration of such costs, but rather a broad overview of the concepts involved.

6. Future Directions in Acute Pain Medicine

Predicting the future course of acute pain medicine is extremely challenging. In the rapidly shifting landscape of modern healthcare, economics (to say nothing of economic uncertainty) are playing a growing role. As has been seen in the past, acute pain medicine is particularly susceptible to disruptive innovation such as novel analgesic approaches and minimally invasive surgical techniques.

At present, it appears most likely that acute pain medicine will continue to build on recent successes. Momentum currently exists across several directions.

6.1. Evolution of the acute pain service

Although the APS has achieved widespread adoption—especially in academic settings—it has often proven difficult to link this allocation of resources with economic benefit. This appears to be leading to a transition of APS resources into efforts with more tangible economic metrics.

One example is the merging of anesthesiology resources into accelerated recovery programs. Pain control is an essential component of enhanced recovery programs, which can often readily demonstrate economic benefits (e.g., decreased length of stay). Surveys of Danish anesthesiology departments between 2000 and 2009 indicate that there was a decline in the number of formal APSs during that interval. This was accompanied by a steady increase in anesthesiology resources directed into accelerated multimodal rehabilitation (ERAS) programs (especially for orthopedic and abdominal surgeries). Although there are several possible reasons for these observed changes, the most likely cause of this transition from APS to ERAS services appears to be a more efficient and justifiable use of limited resources.[47]

Another, more recent, development has been the transitional pain service (TPS). The goal of the TPS is to identify and optimally treat patients at risk for PPSP, with the ultimate objective of preventing the *transition* of acute to chronic pain.[48] Anesthesiologists have taken the lead in the multidisciplinary TPS at Toronto General Hospital, which has already yielded preliminary data for some anticipated outcomes (including substantial cost savings).

6.2. Integration of acute pain medicine into value-based care models

Economic pressures (e.g., bundled payment models) promise to increasingly force value-based practice (i.e., better outcomes at lower cost). To remain competitive, physicians will need to identify opportunities to improve care (the near-universal adoption of the electronic medical record and healthcare informatics should facilitate this process). The continuous analysis of costs and benefits associated with value-driven outcomes can effectively direct efforts to improve care. In this paradigm, acute pain management cannot be separated from the entire process of care and will need to be closely integrated into the team-based care network.

A recent publication by Lee and colleagues nicely illustrates a value-driven program.[49] In this study, 2 of the most important baseline processes were to (1) identify the greatest opportunities for cost reduction and outcome optimization, and (2) use value-driven outcomes to improve care. Only one of the 3 selected clinical improvement projects involved acute pain management (total joint replacement). In this instance, although pain management was but a single aspect of multidisciplinary care, it comprised several critical components along the entire clinical pathway (spinal anesthesia, a multimodal pain protocol, and the daily assessment of pain). Over the 1-year study period, a composite quality index for total joint replacement increased from 54% to 80% (a 50% improvement) while direct costs fell by 7%.

6.3. High-quality research

Many unanswered questions remain regarding the optimal management of acute pain. Of 32 recommendations recently published by the American Pain Society regarding the management of postoperative pain, only 4 were supported by high-quality evidence (in contrast, 11 were made on the basis of low-quality evidence).[10] Appropriately, urgent calls have

Box 2.3 Current Research Gaps for Acute Postoperative Pain Management in Adults

- Sensitivity of behavioral assessment scales for nonverbal adults and preverbal children to detect changes resulting from pain treatment
- Assessment criteria to identify when and how to transition from acute surgical pain care to primary care and when referral to a pain specialist should be considered for persistent postsurgical pain management
- Differential outcome effects of neuraxial analgesia by surgery site
- Comparative benefits and harms of treatments by gender, race, ethnicity, age, history of substance abuse, history of chronic pain, and other specific characteristics or comorbidities
- Optimal pharmacologic and biobehavioral approaches in all phases of care for patients with opioid tolerance
- Evidence of treatments by type of pain [e.g., tissue-specific (muscle, visceral, joint), nociceptive, neuropathic, and central sensitization)
- Head-to-head studies of analgesics from the same drug class and from differing drug classes (e.g., tapentadol to other opioids, pregabalin or gabapentin to opioid analgesics)
- Clinical harm of nonsteroidal anti-inflammatory drugs, intra-articular opioids, and local anesthetics on bone or soft tissue healing in randomized controlled studies
- Optimal multimodal combinations (e.g., epidurals with opioids and local anesthetics, systemic opioids and other agents such as dexmedetomidine, intravenous vs. perineural dexamethasone)
- Duration of opioid treatment following inpatient discharge and optimal tapering strategies
- Approaches and outcomes of preemptive analgesia on long-term outcomes (defined as techniques that reduce central sensitization preventing development of subacute and chronic pain)

been made for improvements in acute pain trial designs and reporting.[50] Following publication of its recommendations, the American Pain Society went on to form an interdisciplinary panel to review the available evidence. The panel found much of the evidence regarding acute pain management to be weak and identified key unanswered questions (Box 2.3).[51]

Areas of intense research currently include the expansion of procedure-specific protocols as well as the optimal anticipation and prevention of pain (particularly PPSP). It is widely anticipated that current research can help provide a stronger evidence base for these pressing clinical issues. Growing economic pressures will likely mean that efforts to control pain will also be accompanied by robust economic analysis, ensuring that pain can be controlled in an efficient and cost-effective manner.

7. Conclusions

Recent decades have seen vast improvements in the management of acute pain, which have been shown to result in multiple patient benefits. This progress has been accompanied by the simultaneous growth of economic forces in healthcare, which promise to play an increasingly prominent role in patient care.

Despite the ability to control acute perioperative pain, clinical care continues to fall short of its perceived potential. The optimal management of acute postoperative pain is a topic of intense clinical investigation and remains a major challenge for our times.

8. Summary

- The management of acute pain has become an important metric in the analysis of modern patient care.
- The economics of healthcare are being increasingly defined in terms of value, which will demand better outcomes at lower cost.

- Effective acute pain management has been clearly shown to result in numerous patient benefits that have the potential to add value to the continuum of care.
- The optimal management of acute pain will involve the further development and the adoption of evidence-based patient- and procedure-specific protocols.
- Acute pain management is inseparable from other aspects of perioperative medicine and seems likely to be increasingly integrated into the entire process of care.
- The economic analysis of acute pain medicine has only begun and warrants further study.

References

1. Keehan S, Stone D, Poisal J, et al. National health expenditure projections, 2016–25: price increases, aging push sector to 20% of economy. *Health Aff (Millwood)*. 2017;36:553–563.
2. Schug S, Palmer G, Scott D, et al. *APM:SE Working Group of the Australian and New Zealand College of Anaesthetists and Faculty of Pain Medicine (2015), Acute Pain Management: Scientific Evidence*. 4th ed. Melbourne: ANZCA and FPM. 2015.
3. Morone N, Weiner D. Pain as the 5th vital sign: exposing the vital need for pain education. *Clin Ther*. 2013;35:1728–1732.
4. Brennan F. The US congressional "Decade on Pain Control and Research" 2001–2011: a review. *J Pain Palliat Care Pharmacother*. 2015;29:212–227.
5. Phillips D. JCAHO pain management standards are unveiled. *JAMA*. 2000;284:428–429.
6. Brennan F, Carr D, Cousins M. Access to pain management—still very much a human right. *Pain Med*. 2016;17:1785–1789.
7. Gan T, Habib A, Miller T, et al. Incidence, patient satisfaction, and perceptions of post-surgical pain: results from a US national survey. *Curr Med Res Opin*. 2014;30:149–160.
8. Ladha K, Patorno E, Huybrechts K, et al. Variations in the use of perioperative multimodal analgesic therapy. *Anesthesiology*. 2016;124:837–845.
9. American Society of Anesthesiologists Task Force on Acute Pain Management. Practice guidelines for acute pain management in the perioperative setting: an updated report by the American Society of Anesthesiologists Task Force on Acute Pain Management. *Anesthesiology*. 2012;116:248–273.
10. Chou R, Gordon D, de Leon-Casasola O, et al. Guidelines on the management of postoperative pain. Management of postoperative pain: a clinical practice guideline from the American Pain Society, the American Society of Regional Anesthesia and Pain Medicine, and the American Society of Anesthesiologists' Committee on Regional Anesthesia, Executive Committee, and Administrative Council. *J Pain*. 2016;17:131–157.
11. Buvanendran A, Kroin J. Multimodal analgesia for controlling acute postoperative pain. *Curr Opin Anaesthesiol*. 2009;22:588–593.
12. Kane-Gill S, Rubin E, Smithburger P, et al. The cost of opioid-related adverse drug events. *J Pain Palliat Care Pharm*. 2014;28:282–293.
13. Vila H, Smith R, Augustyniak M, et al. The efficacy and safety of pain management before and after implementation of hospital-wide pain management standards: is patient safety compromised by treatment based solely on numerical pain ratings? *Anesth Analg*. 2005;101:474–480.
14. Shah A, Hayes C, Martin B. Characteristics of initial prescription episodes and likelihood of long-term opioid use—United States, 2006–2015. *Morb Mortal Wkly Rep*. 2017;66:265–269.
15. Dahl J, Nielsen R, Wetterslev J, et al. Post-operative analgesic effects of paracetamol, NSAIDs, glucocorticoids, gabapentinoids and their combinations: a topical review. *Acta Anaesthesiol Scand*. 2014;58:1165–1181.
16. Joshi G, Schug S, Kehlet H. Procedure-specific pain management and outcome strategies. *Best Pract Res Clin Anaesth*. 2014;28:191–201.
17. Stone A, Wick E, Wu C, Grant M. The US opioid crisis: a role for enhanced recovery after surgery. *Anesth Analg*. 2017;125:1803–1805.
18. Tawfic Q, Faris A. Acute pain service: past, present and future. *Pain Manag*. 2015;5:47–58.
19. Nasir D, Howard J, Joshi G, Hill G. A survey of acute pain service structure and function in United States hospitals. *Pain Res Treat*. 2011;2011:934932.

20. Kehlet H, Dahl J. The value of "multimodal" or "balanced analgesia" in postoperative pain treatment. *Anesth Analg.* 1993;77:1048–1056.
21. Duncan C, Moeschler S, Horlocker T, et al. A self-paired comparison of perioperative outcomes before and after implementation of a clinical pathway in patients undergoing total knee arthroplasty. *Reg Anesth Pain Med.* 2013;38:533–538.
22. Adamina M, Kehlet H, Tomlinson G, et al. Enhanced recovery pathways optimize health outcomes and resource utilization: a meta-analysis of randomized controlled trials in colorectal surgery. *Surgery.* 2011;149:830–840.
23. Carli F. Physiologic considerations of enhanced recovery after surgery (ERAS) programs: implications of the stress response. *Can J Anesth.* 2015;62:110–119.
24. Sun E, Dexter F, Macario A. Can an acute pain service be cost-effective? *Anesth Analg.* 2010;111:841–844.
25. Werner M, Soholm L, Rotboll-Nielsen P, Kehlet H. Does an acute pain service improve postoperative outcome? *Anesth Analg.* 2002;95:1361–1372.
26. Lee A, Chan S, Chen P, et al. Economic evaluations of acute pain service programs: A systematic review. *Clin J Pain.* 2007;23:726–733.
27. Korczak D, Kuczera C, Rust M. Acute pain treatment on postoperative and medical non-surgical wards. *GMS Health Technol Asses.* 2013;9:Doc05.
28. Porter M, Lee T. The strategy that will fix health care. *Harv Bus Rev.* 2013;91:50–70.
29. Kissin I. Patient-controlled-analgesia analgesimetry and its problems. *Anesth Analg.* 2009; 108:1945–1949.
30. Husereau H, Drummond M, Petrou S, et al. Consolidated Health Economic Evaluation Reporting Standards (CHEERS) statement. *Pharmacoeconomics.* 2013;31:361–367.
31. Berwick D, Nolan T, Whittington J. The triple aim: care, health, and cost. *Health Aff.* 2008;27:759–769.
32. van den Bosch J, Bonsel G, Moons K, Kalkman C. Effect of postoperative experiences on willingness to pay to avoid postoperative pain, nausea, and vomiting. *Anesthesiology.* 2006;104:1033–1039.
33. Koo P. Addressing stakeholders' needs: economics and patient satisfaction. *Am J Health-Syst Pharm.* 2007;64(suppl 4):S11–S15.
34. Gupta A, Daigle S, Mojica J, Hurley R. Patient perception of pain care in hospitals in the United States. *J Pain Res.* 2009;2:157–164.
35. Adamina M, Kehlet H, Tomlinson G, et al. Enhanced recovery pathways optimize health outcomes and resource utilization: a meta-analysis of randomized controlled trials in colorectal surgery. *Surgery.* 2011;149:830–840.
36. Coley K, Williams B, DaPos S, et al. Retrospective evaluation of unanticipated admissions and readmissions after same day surgery and associated costs. *J Clin Anesth.* 2002;14:349–353.
37. Philip B, Reese P, Burch S. The economic impact of opioids on postoperative pain management. *J Clin Anesth.* 2002;14:354–364.
38. Liu S, Wu C. Effect of postoperative analgesia on major postoperative complications: a systematic update of the evidence. *Anesth Analg.* 2007;104:689–702.
39. Shea R, Brooks J, Dayhoff N, Keck J. Pain intensity and postoperative pulmonary complications among the elderly after abdominal surgery. *Heart Lung.* 2002;31:440–449.
40. Gaskin D, Richard P. The economic costs of pain in the United States. *J Pain.* 2012;13:715–724.
41. Cohen S, Raja S. Prevention of chronic postsurgical pain: the ongoing search for the Holy Grail of anesthesiology. *Anesthesiology.* 2013;118: 241–243.
42. Grosu I, de Kock M. New concepts in acute pain management: strategies to prevent chronic postsurgical pain, opioid-induced hyperalgesia, and outcome measures. *Anesthesiology Clin.* 2011;29:311–327.
43. Clarke H, Poon M, Weinrib A, et al. Preventive analgesia and novel strategies for the prevention of chronic post-surgical pain. *Drugs.* 2015;75:339–351.
44. Byrne K, Levins K, Buggy D. Can anesthetic-analgesic technique during primary cancer surgery affect recurrence or metastasis? *Can J Anaesth.* 2016;63:184–192.
45. Hoffer D, Smith S, Parlow J, et al. Adverse event assessment and reporting in trials of newer treatments for post-operative pain. *Acta Anaesthesiol Scand.* 2016;60:842–851.
46. Palmer P, Ji X, Stephens J. Cost of opioid intravenous patient-controlled analgesia: results from a hospital database analysis and literature assessment. *Clinicoecon Outcomes Res.* 2014;6:311–318.

47. Nielsen P, Christensen P, Meyhoff C, Werner M. Post-operative pain treatment in Denmark from 2000 to 2009: a nationwide sequential survey on organizational aspects. *Acta Anaesthesiol Scand*. 2012;56:686–694.
48. Katz J, Weinrib A, Fashler S, et al. The Toronto General Hospital Transitional Pain Service: development and implementation of a multidisciplinary program to prevent chronic postsurgical pain. *J Pain Res*. 2015;8:695–702.
49. Lee V, Kawamoto K, Hess R, et al. Implementation of a value-driven outcomes program to identify high variability in clinical costs and outcomes and association with reduced cost and improved quality. *JAMA*. 2016;316:1061–1072.
50. Fabritius M, Wetterslev J, Dahl J, Mathiesen O. An urgent call for improved quality of trial design and reporting in postoperative pain research. *Acta Anaesthesiol Scand*. 2017;61:8–10.
51. Gordon D, deLeon-Casasola O, Wu C, et al. Research gaps in practice guidelines for acute postoperative pain management in adults: findings from a review of the evidence for an American Pain Society clinical practice guideline. *J Pain*. 2016;17:158–166.

Section II

Case-Based Acute Pain Medicine

3

Total Shoulder Arthroplasty

Christopher Sobey and David Byrne

Case Scenario

A 65-year-old man presents for a left total shoulder arthroplasty. His medical history includes hypertension, hyperlipidemia, obstructive sleep apnea, and obesity. His BMI is 37, and his creatinine is 1.0.

1. Patient Factors

1.1. Obstructive sleep apnea

1.1.1. What are the diagnostic criteria for obstructive sleep apnea?

According to the American Academy of Sleep Medicine, obstructive sleep apnea (OSA) is characterized by recurrent partial or complete obstruction (hypopnea/apnea) of the upper airway during sleep. Hypopnea and apnea are defined in 3 ways: (1) a decrease in amplitude of >50% on a valid measurement of breathing, (2) associated with an oxygen desaturation, or (3) associated with an electroencephalogram (EEG) arousal. The events last for 10 seconds or more.

To fulfill the criteria for OSA, excessive daytime sleepiness and/or unrefreshing sleep with impaired daytime function is present in patients demonstrating 5 or more obstructive events per hour on overnight monitoring. Severity of disease is based on the number of sleep-related obstructive breathing events per hour and is termed the *apnea hypopnea index* (AHI): 5 to 15 = mild, 15 to 30 = moderate, >30 = severe.

Screening for OSA can be performed by nocturnal pulse oximetry by measuring transient desaturations (>4% from baseline) that occur after hypopnea and apnea. The reference standard for sleep apnea recording is overnight polysomnography, which includes measurement of airflow and respiratory effort, pulse oximetry, and often body position.

One simple validated tool to assess for presence of OSA without undergoing formalized testing involves the STOP-Bang criteria. This tool includes the following questions:

1. Do you **S**NORE loudly (louder than talking or loud enough to be heard through closed doors)? Do you often feel **T**IRED, fatigued, or sleepy during daytime? Has anyone **O**BSERVED you stop breathing during your sleep?
2. Do you have or are you being treated for high blood **P**RESSURE?
3. **B**MI more than 35 kg/m^2?
4. **A**GE over 50 years old?
5. **N**ECK circumference >16 inches (40 cm)?
6. **G**ENDER: Male?

The STOP-Bang score was validated in obese and morbidly obese surgical patients, with a score of 4 having a sensitivity of 88% while a score of 6 is more specific.

Further Reading

American Academy of Sleep Medicine Task Force. Sleep-related breathing disorders in adults: recommendations for syndrome definition and measurement techniques in clinical research. *Sleep*. 1999;22:667–689.

Chung F, Yang Y, Liao P. Predictive performance of the STOP-Bang score for identifying obstructive sleep apnea in obese patients. *Obes Surg*. 2013 Dec;23(12):2050–2057.

McNicholas WT. Diagnosis of obstructive sleep apnea in adults. *Proc Am Thorac Soc*. 2008;5(2):154–160.

1.1.2. Describe the risk of adverse events regarding perioperative analgesia in patients with obstructive sleep apnea

OSA is associated with a number of comorbidities, including cardiovascular disease, arrhythmia, stroke, obesity, metabolic syndrome, insulin resistance, and depression. When untreated, OSA can lead to uncontrolled hypertension, heart failure (cor pulmonale), and premature death. In the perioperative setting, OSA presents unique challenges with respect to mask ventilation, tracheal intubation, increased airway collapsibility, sensitivity to central nervous system depressants, and difficulty with postextubation ventilation.

In regard to perioperative management of patients with OSA, one should focus on optimization of associated comorbidities, preparing for a potential difficult airway, guarding against aspiration, and avoidance of factors that contribute to respiratory depression. In 2012, the Society for Ambulatory Anesthesia issued a consensus statement addressing appropriate patient selection for adult patients scheduled for ambulatory surgical procedures. Authors advised that OSA patients with controlled comorbidities can be reasonable candidates for ambulatory procedures if their pain can be appropriately managed with minimal or no postoperative opioids.

Epidemiologic evidence suggests that OSA in combination with other serious comorbidities, such as renal or cardiovascular disease, is among conditions that predispose patients for opioid-induced ventilatory impairment (OIVI) in the postoperative period. Use of opioid analgesics worsens postoperative sleep-disordered breathing in OSA patients. Important components of OSA, like sleep fragmentation and intermittent hypoxia, may enhance pain behavior and also increase sensitivity to opioid analgesia. Patients suffering from sleep-disordered breathing may present with increased sensitivity to both central (i.e., sedation, diminished central respiratory drive) and peripheral (i.e., increased airway collapsibility) effects of opioids. Incidence of perioperative OIVI ranges between 0.1% and 37% depending on diagnostic criteria.

Further Reading

Joshi GP, Ankiechetty SP, Gan TJ, Chung F. Society for Ambulatory Anesthesia consensus statement on preoperative selection of adult patients with obstructive sleep apnea scheduled for ambulatory surgery. *Anesth Analg.* 2012;115(5):1060–1068.

Lam KK, Kunder S, Wong J, Doufas AG, Chung F. Obstructive sleep apnea, pain, and opioids: is the riddle solved? *Curr Opin Anaesthesiol.* 2016 Feb;29(1):134–140.

Liao P, Yegneswaran D, Vairavanathan S, Zilberman P, Chung F. Postoperative complications in patients with obstructive sleep apnea: a retrospective matched cohort study. *Can J Anesth.* 2009;56:819–828.

Stierer TL. Obstructive sleep apnea, sleep disorders, and perioperative considerations. *Anesthesiol Clin.* 2015 Jun;33(2):305–314.

1.1.3. What analgesic strategies/considerations may minimize the risk of adverse events in patients with obstructive sleep apnea?

The perioperative management of patients with OSA should emphasize the use of regional anesthesia and anesthetic medications (anesthetics/sedatives/analgesics) that minimize respiratory depression, such as dexmedetomidine or ketamine. Similarly, opioid-sparing adjuvants such as nonsteroidal anti-inflammatory drugs (NSAIDs), acetaminophen, or anticonvulsants can be helpful in providing adequate analgesia postoperatively. It is prudent to avoid or use minimal benzodiazepine for premedication due to increased risk of postoperative airway obstruction and respiratory depression. Postoperatively, continuous positive airway pressure (CPAP) or nasal/oral airways should be available, and the patient should be in an upright, lateral, or slightly reclined position.

Use of short-acting analgesics such as remifentanil has demonstrated rapid recovery, better oxygenation saturation profile, and shorter postoperative length of stay. However, due to its short half-life, patients often will demonstrate inadequate pain control without additional analgesics or regional anesthesia.

The Society for Ambulatory Anesthesia has developed the following consensus recommendations for patients with OSA in the outpatient setting:

1. Use STOP-Bang as screening due to its high sensitivity.
2. If you suspect OSA, treat the patient as if he or she has the diagnosis.
3. If painful outpatient surgeries cannot be done with opioid-sparing techniques, recommend deferring to an inpatient setting.

Further Reading

Chung SA, Yuan H, Chung F. A systematic review of obstructive sleep apnea and its implications for anesthesiologists. *Anesth Analg.* 2008;107:153–163.

Joshi GP, Ankiechetty SP, Gan TJ, Chung F. Society for Ambulatory Anesthesia consensus statement on preoperative selection of adult patients with obstructive sleep apnea scheduled for ambulatory surgery. *Anesth Analg.* 2012;115(5):1060–1068.

2. Surgical and Regional Anesthesia Considerations

2.1. Describe the innervation of the shoulder, including soft tissues and joint structures

Refer also to Figure 3.1.

- *Anterior glenohumeral joint*:
  - Subscapular nerve (C5-C6): The subscapular nerve arises from the proximal posterior cord of the brachial plexus and provides innervation to the subcorticoid bursa, subscapularis muscle, and teres major
  - Anterior branch of axillary nerve (C5-C6): The axillary nerve is the terminal branch of the posterior cord originating at the level of the axilla and separates into an anterior and an posterior branch. The anterior branch winds around the surgical neck of the humerus whereas the posterior branch pierces the deep fascia and proceeds posteriorly. The anterior branch further divides into a medial and a lateral branch to supply the anterior shoulder joint. The medial portion of the anterior branch supplies the inferior anterior capsule of the glenohumeral joint and parts of the axillary recess. The lateral branch runs along the inferior edge of the subscapular muscle to innervate the humeral aspect of the anterior capsule.
  - Lateral pectoral nerve (C5-C6): The lateral pectoral nerve arises from the lateral cord and runs laterally toward the coracoid process innervating the subacromial bursa and anterior acromioclavicular joint.
- *Posterior glenohumeral joint*:
  - Suprascapular nerve (C5-C6): The suprascapular nerve arises from the upper trunk with one branch innervating the coracohumeral ligament and its adjacent capsular region, and the other branch innervating the subacromial bursa and posterior aspect of the acromioclavicular joint capsule. It also supplies the main muscular branch to the supraspinatus muscle and the infraspinatus muscle.
  - Posterior branch of the axillary nerve: Small branches of the posterior branch of the axillary nerve contribute to innervation of the posterior shoulder joint.

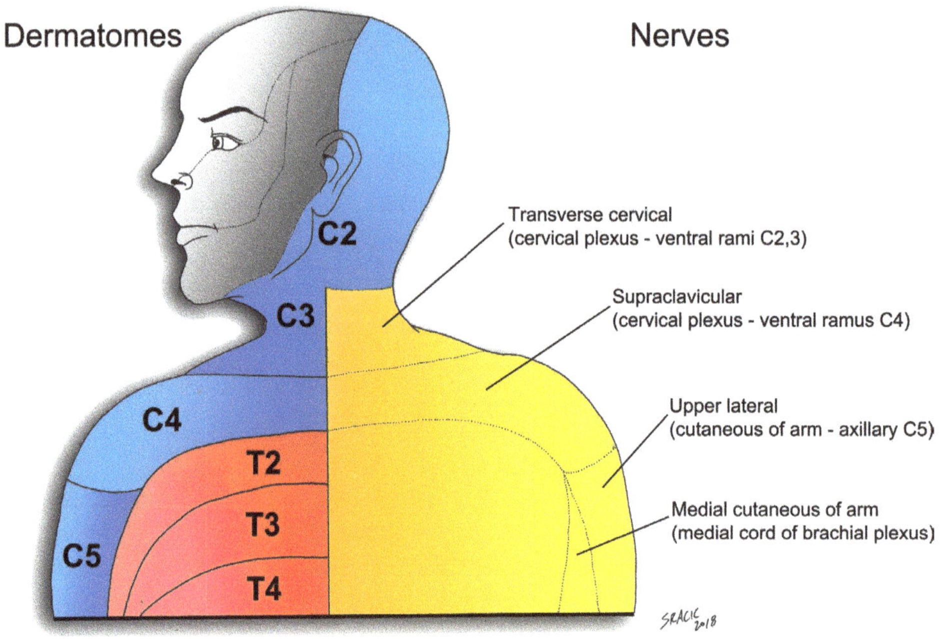

Figure 3.1 Innervation of the shoulder.

This article was published in *Continuing Education in Anaesthesia Critical Care & Pain*, 8, Christian L. Beecroft and David M. Coventry, Anaesthesia for Shoulder Surgery, 193–198, Copyright Elsevier (2008).

- *Muscular innervation*:
  - Axillary nerve (C5-C6) supplies the deltoid and teres minor.
  - Long thoracic nerve (C5-C7) supplies the serratus anterior.
  - Suprascapular nerve (C5-C6) supplies the supraspinatus and infraspinatus muscle.
  - Subscapular nerves arise from the posterior cord and supply the subscapularis muscle and the teres major.
  - Musculocutaneous nerve (C5-C7) supplies the biceps muscle.
  - Dorsal scapular nerve (C5) supplies the rhomboid major and minor.

Further Reading

Aszmann OC, Dellon AL, Birely BT, McFarland EG. Innervation of the human shoulder joint and its implications for surgery. *Clin Orthop Relat Res*. 1996 Sep;330:202–207.

2.2. Describe the surgical steps when performing a total shoulder arthroplasty

Following induction of general anesthesia and intubation, the patient is placed in the beach-chair position, elevating the scapula on the operative side, with the affected arm completely free off the edge of the table. After sterile prep and drape, a longitudinal anterior incision is made from the coracoid process superiorly to the lateral edge of the biceps. There is then dissection down between the deltoid and pectoralis major muscle, and the cephalic vein is identified and mobilized laterally. The conjoint tendon is exposed, and incision of the deltopectoral fascia is performed to expose the subscapularis tendon. The biceps tendon is tagged with a suture and tenotomized. Partial release of the deltoid muscle at its insertion on the humerus is performed on the superior aspect if needed for exposure. Dissection continues and the joint capsule is opened, protecting the axillary nerve as it travels around the neck inferior to the capsule. The humeral head is externally rotated, and the canal finder of the humerus is inserted at the superior aspect. The humeral head is cut with a jog, protecting the rotator cuff tendons, followed by reaming of the humeral canal. The last reamer is left in the humerus to protect it from fracture. Subsequently, retractors are placed to expose the glenoid fully. The glenoid is prepared using reamers and sized with the appropriate glenoid trial component. Reduction of the joint with trial components is performed to test fit. The trial components are then removed and the definitive inserted components are fixed. A hemovac is inserted, thorough irrigation of wounds performed, and layered closure of incisions performed. Sterile dressings are applied at the conclusion of the procedure.

Further Reading

Al-Taki M. Total shoulder replacement. In: Saghieh S, Weinstein SL, Hoballah JJ, eds. *Operative Dictations in Orthopedic Surgery*. New York, NY: Springer Science+Business Media; 2013:277–279.

2.3. What is the utility of regional anesthesia in the perioperative management in total shoulder arthroplasty?

While minor procedures of the shoulder such as arthroscopy can be performed under regional anesthesia alone, for larger surgical interventions such as total shoulder arthroplasty or surgeries of longer duration, a combination of general and regional anesthesia may be more appropriate. Most commonly, an interscalene approach to the brachial plexus is performed to provide anesthesia of the necessary dermatomes and underlying structures (Figure 3.2). Blocks can be performed as single injections or continuous infusions with the placement of indwelling catheters.

Postoperatively, severe pain following total shoulder arthroplasty is common, and multiple studies have found that the addition of regional techniques as part of the anesthetic plan demonstrates significant benefits. The addition of regional anesthesia not only has the ability to provide significant analgesia, both at rest and with movement, but also allows for earlier mobilization and improvement in range of motion. Use of continuous interscalene nerve blocks has also

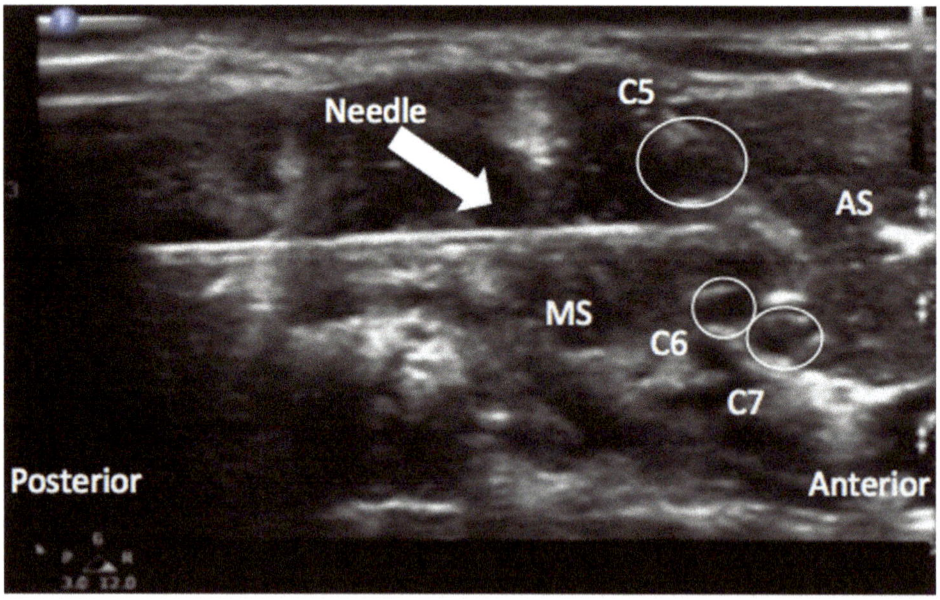

AS – Anterior Scalene; MS – Middle Scalene

Figure 3.2 Interscalene block ultrasound.

Reproduced with permission from Brian Allen, MD, Vanderbilt University Medical Center, Department of Anesthesia.

demonstrated reduction in postoperative opioid requirement, reduction in opioid-related side effects, and decreased time to discharge. More recently, with the utilization and refinement of upper extremity perineural local anesthetic infusions, surgeons have begun to perform total shoulder arthroplasties in the outpatient setting as well.

In preparing for regional anesthesia for shoulder surgery, surgical and patient factors should be considered. One concern, in particular, relates to the impact of hemidiaphragmatic paralysis in perineural blocks performed above the clavicle due to the proximity of the phrenic nerve. While phrenic nerve palsy following interscalene blockade is often transient, care must be taken in patients with significant pulmonary comorbiditities, obesity, or obstructive sleep apnea. Prospective and retrospective studies often find no significant incidence of dyspnea in patients receiving interscalene blocks, but such studies often exclude patients with these comorbidities.

The most common presentation is subjective dyspnea; however, numerous studies have shown that only a portion of dyspneic patients following interscalene blockade have phrenic nerve involvement. Thus, providers performing interscalene blockade must also remain vigilant of other causes of dyspnea.

A variety of strategies have been used to minimize the incidence of phrenic nerve palsy in patients receiving interscalene blockade. Studies examining decreased volume, decreased concentration, and differing sites of injection (e.g., periplexus) have shown a decreased but not zero incidence of phrenic nerve palsy. Of note, the use of ultrasound has been instrumental in applying such techniques, allowing for direct visualization and precise application of local anesthetic. In order to avoid phrenic nerve palsy, alternative perineural blocks may be considered. A combined suprascapular and axillary nerve block (either single injection or continuous infusion) has been documented as a reasonable analgesic alternative in patients undergoing total shoulder arthroplasty who cannot tolerate phrenic nerve palsy.

Further Reading

Auyong DB, Yuan SC, Choi DS, Pahang JA, Slee AE, Hanson NA. A double-blind randomized comparison of continuous interscalene, supraclavicular, and suprascapular blocks for total shoulder arthroplasty. *Reg Anesth Pain Med.* 2017 May/Jun;42(3):302–309.

Beecroft CL, Coventry DM. Anaesthesia for shoulder surgery. *Contin Educ Anaesth Crit Care Pain.* 2008;8:193–198.

Bishop JY, Sprague M, Gelber J, et al. Interscalene regional anesthesia for shoulder surgery. *J Shoulder Elbow Surg.* 2006 Sept–Oct;15(5):567–570.

Brandl F, Taeger K. The combination of general anesthesia and interscalene block in shoulder surgery [in German]. *Anaesthesist.* 1991;40:537–542.

El-Boghdadly K, Chin KJ, Chan VWS. Phrenic nerve palsy and regional anesthesia for shoulder surgery: anatomical, physiologic, and clinical considerations. *Anesthesiology.* 2017 Jul;127(1):173–191.

Ilfeld BM, Vandenborne K, Duncan PW, et al. Ambulatory continuous interscalene nerve blocks decrease the time to discharge readiness after total shoulder arthroplasty: a randomized, triple-masked, placebo-controlled study. *Anesthesiology.* 2006;105:999–1007.

Ilfeld BM, Wright TW, Enneking FK, Morey TE. Joint range of motion after total shoulder arthroplasty with and without a continuous interscalene nerve block: a retrospective, case-control study. *Reg Anesth Pain Med.* 2005;30:429–433.

Ilfeld BM, Wright TW, Enneking FK, et al. Total shoulder arthroplasty as an outpatient procedure using ambulatory perineural local anesthetic infusion: a pilot feasibility study. *Anesth Analg.* 2005;101:1319–1322.

Rohrbaugh M, Kentor ML, Orebaugh SL, Williams B. Outcomes of shoulder surgery in the sitting position with interscalene nerve block: a single-center series. *Reg Anesth Pain Med.* 2013;38:28–33.

Shah A, Nielsen KC, Braga L, Pietrobon R, Klein SM, Steele SM. Interscalene brachial plexus block for outpatient shoulder arthroplasty: postoperative analgesia, patient satisfaction and complications. *Indian J Orthop.* 2007;41:230–236.

Stunder O, Rasul R, Chiu YL, et al. Peripheral nerve blocks in shoulder arthroplasty: how do they influence complications and length of stay? *Clin Orthop Relat Res.* 2014 May; 472:1482–1488.

Sviggum HP, Jacob AK, Mantilla CB, Schroeder DR, Sperling JW, Hebl JR. Perioperative nerve injury after total shoulder arthroplasty: assessment of risk after regional anesthesia. *Reg Anesth Pain Med.* 2012;37:490–494.

Tetzlaff JE, Yoon HJ, Brems J. Interscalene brachial plexus block for shoulder surgery. *Reg Anesth.* 1994;19:339–343.

Urmey WF, Talts KH, Sharrock NE. One hundred percent incidence of hemidiaphragmatic paresis associated with interscalene brachial plexus anesthesia as diagnosed by ultrasonography. *Anesth Analg.* 1991;72:498–503.

Verelst P, Van Zundert A. Respiratory impact of analgesic strategies for shoulder surgery. *Reg Anesth Pain Med.* 2013;38:50–53.

2.4. What are general considerations in providing optimal perioperative analgesia in obese patients?

In planning for postoperative analgesia in an obese patient for operations such as total shoulder arthroplasty, it is generally recommended to utilize analgesic options that will maximize analgesia and minimize sedation and respiratory compromise. Reducing reliance on medications that diminish respiratory drive, such as opioids, is suggested. Continuous regional blockade using perineural catheters confers significant analgesia for multiple days postoperatively and is opioid-sparing. Patients can ambulate postoperatively with the perineural catheter in place receiving a continuous infusion from an infusion pump. Commonly used infusion devices include elastomeric balloon pumps, which are simple to use and disposable, or reusable electronic pumps. Combining regional anesthesia with multimodal analgesic regimens, including NSAIDs, antineuropathic agents, acetaminophen, and others, allows adequate pain relief during the most acute phase of recovery, without resulting in depressed sensorium.

2.5. What are the benefits of regional anesthesia in obese patients?

The overall number of obese and overweight individuals worldwide has grown rapidly in the last 3 decades, and management of this condition has become an increasingly regular consideration in anesthetic techniques. In obese patients undergoing total shoulder arthroplasty, optimization of analgesia utilizing regional anesthesia is of paramount importance due to the increased risks of postoperative respiratory complications in the obese population especially in opioid-based analgesic regimens. Utilizing regional anesthesia in the obese population offers several advantages, including minimizing airway intervention, less cardiopulmonary depression, improved postoperative analgesia, decreased opioid consumption, and decreased postoperative nausea and vomiting. All these factors combine to result in decreases in postanesthesia care unit and hospital length of stay. Regional blocks have been associated with improved postoperative analgesia, particularly when long-acting local anesthetics or continuous peripheral nerve blocks are used.

2.6. What are the technical challenges and their impact in regard to utilizing regional anesthesia in obese patients?

Performing regional anesthesia in the obese population can be technically challenging. These challenges are related to difficulties in patient positioning, identifying the usual bony and muscular landmarks, and the depth of needle penetration. Consequently, an increased incidence of failed blocks has been shown in obese patients compared with similar, normal-weight patients. Nielsen et al. demonstrated that obesity is associated with higher block failure and complication rates in surgical regional anesthesia in ambulatory setting. In more than 9000 patients reviewed, 31.3% had a BMI of 30 or higher. Obese patients were 1.62 times more likely to have a failed block, and the unadjusted rate of acute complications was higher in obese patients. However, when compared with patients with normal BMI, overweight and obese patients were found to have similar postoperative pain at rest, unanticipated admissions, and overall satisfaction.

Further Reading

Adams JP, Murphy PG. Obesity in anaesthesia and intensive care. *Br J Anaesth*. 2000;85:91–108.

Coveney E, Weltz CR, Greengrass R, Iglehart JD, Leight GS, Steele SM, Lyerly HK. Use of paravertebral block anesthesia in the surgical management of breast cancer: experience in 156 cases. *Ann Surg*. 1998;227:496–501.

D'Alessio JG, Rosenblum M, Shea KP, Freitas DG. A retrospective comparison of interscalene block and general anesthesia for ambulatory surgery shoulder arthroscopy. *Reg Anesth*. 1995;20:62–68.

Ingrande J, Brodsky JB, Lemmens HJM. Regional anesthesia and obesity. *Curr Opinion Anaesthesiol*. 2009;22:683–686.

Lynch EP, Welch KJ, Carabuena JM, Eberlein TJ. Thoracic epidural anesthesia improves outcome after breast surgery. *Ann Surg*. 1995;222:663–669.

Nielsen JC, Guller U, Steele SM, et al. Influence of obesity on surgical regional anesthesia in the ambulatory setting: an analysis of 9,038 blocks. *Anesthesiology*. 2005 Jan;102(1):181–187.

Pusch F, Freitag H, Weinstabl C, Obwegeser R, Huber E, Wildling E. Single-injection paravertebral block compared to general anaesthesia in breast surgery. *Acta Anaesthesiol Scand*. 1999;43:770–774.

Urmey WF, McDonald M. Hemidiaphragmatic paresis during interscalene brachial plexus block: effects on pulmonary function and chest wall mechanics. *Anesth Analg*. 1992; 74:352–357.

Clinical Scenario

The patient receives a continuous interscalene catheter preoperatively and undergoes an uneventful general anesthetic with endotracheal intubation. Postoperatively, the patient is placed on an analgesic regimen of acetaminophen, celecoxib, and oxycodone to supplement his perineural infusion

3. Postoperative Pain Management

3.1. What is the salient physiology of prostaglandin synthesis as it relates to nociceptive signaling?

Prostaglandins are made from arachadonic acid, which, following tissue damage, is cleaved from phospholipids in the cell membrane by phospholipase A2 (PLA2). Cyclooxygenase (COX) enzymes then catalyze the formation of prostanoid

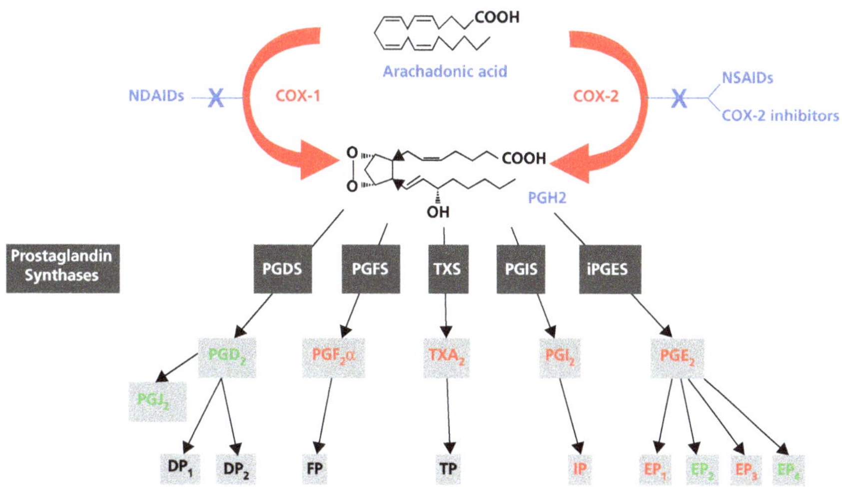

Figure 3.3 Prostanoid cascade.

Bingham S, Beswick, PJ, Blum, DE, Gray NM, Chessell IP. The role of cylooxygenase pathway in nociception and pain. *Semin Cell Dev Biol.* 2006 Oct; 17(5):544–554.

precursors, PGG_2 and PGH_2, from arachadonic acid. These precursors are then converted to biologically active prostaglandins called prostanoids: PGD_2, PGE_2, PGF_2, PGI_2 (prostacyclin), and thromboxane A2 (TXA_2). There are multiple tissue-specific prostaglandin synthases that convert precursors to biologically active prostaglandins. Such a diversity in synthases results in difficult targets for therapeutic intervention. The COX pathway, however, is more standardized between tissues, where differential tissue expression and induction patterns of these enzymes and receptors play a major role in determining the cellular effects of prostanoids.

Prostanoids can act both peripherally and centrally. In the periphery, they increase sensitivity of peripheral terminals of high-threshold pain fibers by producing a protein kinase A–mediated phosphorylation of sodium channels. This increases excitability, reduces the pain threshold, and potentiates the action of pain-producing stimuli from heat or irritant molecules. Centrally, prostanoids can exaggerate responses to both painful and innocuous stimuli, reduce glycine-mediated inhibitory pathways in the spinal cord, and alter neurotransmitter release. Inhibiting prostanoid production is the primary analgesic mechanism of NSAIDs (Figure 3.3).

Further Reading

Bingham S, Beswick, PJ, Blum, DE, Gray NM, Chessell IP. The role of cylooxygenase pathway in nociception and pain. *Semin Cell Dev Biol.* 2006 Oct;17(5):544–554.

Samad TA, Sapirstein A, Woolf CJ. Prostanoids and pain: unraveling mechanisms and revealing therapeutic targets. *Trends Mol Med.* 2002 Aug;8(8):390–396.

Zeilhofer H. Prostanoids in nociception and pain. *Biochem Pharmacol.* 2007 Jan;73(2):165–174.

3.2. Describe the primary physiologic differences between nonselective and selective NSAIDs

COX-1 and COX-2 have 60% amino acid sequence homogeny; however, they vary in their gene expression profiles, kinetic properties, and synthase interactions. COX-1 is constitutively expressed and produces prostanoids that are involved with continuous regulation (gastrointestinal [GI] mucosal protection, control of renal blood flow, platelet aggregation), while COX-2 expression is inducible through cytokine influences including interleukin-1beta (IL-1beta), interleukin

15, TNF-alpha, as well as lipopolysaccharides. Whereas nonselective NSAIDs decrease prostaglandin and thromboxane levels associated with the GI, platelet, renal, and inflammatory systems, COX-2 selective inhibition is more isolated to the inflammatory cascade and kidneys.

Further Reading

Bombardier C, Laine L, Reicin A, Shapiro D, Burgos-Vargas R, Davis B, et al. Comparison of upper gastrointestinal toxicity of rofecoxib and naproxen in patients with rheumatoid arthritis;VIGOR study group. *N Engl J Med.* 2000;343:1520–1528.

Bresalier RS, Sandler RS, Quan H, Bolognese JA, Oxenius B, Horgan K, et al. Cardiovascular events associated with rofecoxib in a colorectal adenoma chemoprevention trial. *N Engl J Med.* 2005;352:1092–1102.

Nutt DJ. Discontinuation ofVioxx. *Lancet.* 2005;365(9453):28.

Schnitzer TJ, Burmester GR, Mysler E, Hochberg MC, Doherty M, Ehrsam E, et al. Comparison of lumiracoxib with naproxen and ibuprofen in the Therapeutic Arthritis Research and Gastrointestinal Event Trial (TAR-GET), reduction in ulcer complications: randomised controlled trial. *Lancet.* 2004;364:665–674.

Solomon SD, McMurray JJV, Pfeffer MA, Wittes J, Fowler R, Finn P, et al. Cardiovascular risk associated with celecoxib in a clinical trial for colorectal adenoma prevention. *N Engl J Med.* 2005;352:1071–1080.

Szczeklik E. Nizankowska G. Bochenek, et al. Safety of a specific COX-2 inhibitor in aspirin-induced asthma. *Clin Exp Allergy.* 2001;31:219–225.

Warner TD, Mitchell JA. Cyclooxygenases: new forms, new inhibitors, and lessons from the clinic. *FASEB J.* 2004;18:790–804.

3.3. What are commonly used perioperative NSAIDs, including common dosing?

- *Acetaminophen*: Mechanism of action is not completely understood. It has been demonstrated to centrally inhibit nociception via the COX pathway, reinforce descending serotonin inhibitory pathways, trigger indirect activation of cannabinoid receptors, and inhibit nitric oxide pathways via NMDA or substance P. It is available in IV, rectal, or oral formulations. Peaks 45 to 60 minutes after oral administration. Dosing for adults weighing at least 50 kg: 650 mg to 1 g q4-6 hours to a maximum of 4 g/d. If patient weighs less than 50 kg, use 10 to 15 mg/kg.
- *Ketorolac* (Toradol): 15 mg IM/IV q6h, maximum daily dose of 60 mg/d. PO dosing 10 mg q4-5h. Duration of dosing not to exceed 5 days. Higher doses associated with GI and surgical site bleeding.
- *Celecoxib* (Celebrex): 200 mg qday or BID; 400 mg × 1 can be used for acute pain.
- *Diclofenac*: Nonselective, oral: 50 mg PO q8-12h or 75 mg q12h. Extended-release form available at 100 mg qday. Intravenous: 37.5 mg q6h (maximum 150 mg/d).
- *Ibuprofen*: Nonselective NSAID, racemic mixture, only (+)S isomer is active, (–R) isomer is inactive but can be converted to (–)S isomer. Dosing 400 to 800 mg q6-8h. Maximum: 3200 mg/d.
- *Naproxen*: 250 to 500 mg PO q12h. Maximum 1500 mg/d. May have the least cardiovascular risk of all NSAIDs.
- *Meloxicam* (Mobic): 7.5 to 15 mg PO qday. No need for dose adjustments in patients with mild to moderate renal impairment.

Further Reading

Boulton-Jones JM, Geddes CG, Heinzel G, Türch D, Nehmiz G, Bevis PJ. Meloxicam pharmacokinetics in renal impairment. *Br J Clin Pharmacol.* 1997 Jan;43(1):35–40.

Howard, S. Perioperative intravenous acetaminophen and NSAIDs. *Pain Med.* 2011;12:961–981.

Trelle S, Reichenbach S, Wandel S, et al. Cardiovascular safety of non-steroidal anti-inflammatory drugs: network meta-analysis. *BMJ.* 2011;342:c7086.

3.4. Describe the unique risks of NSAIDs as related to antiplatelet function, bone healing, cardiovascular risk, and gastrointestinal risk

Antiplatelet Function: Aspirin and nonaspirin NSAIDs inhibit platelet COX, blocking the formation of TXA_2, which acts as a potent vasoconstrictor and platelet aggregator. These medications increase systemic bleeding propensity by impairing thromboxane-dependent platelet aggregation, resulting in a prolonged bleeding time. Aspirin use can increase risk of spontaneous bleeds (both GI and intracranial) as well as increase surgical bleeding complications. There are conflicting data regarding nonaspirin NSAIDs and perioperative bleeding risk, but risk appears to be dependent on specific NSAID use.

It has been shown that selective COX-2 inhibitors do not significantly increase the risk of intraoperative bleeding, postoperative bleeding, or blood loss, as they exert no significant effect on platelet function. Therefore, perioperative, single-dose, or short course of COX-2 inhibitors can be safely used in individuals who are undergoing surgery.

Bone Healing: The initial local inflammation generated at the site of injury is considered a key factor in bone healing cascade. Cytokines play an essential role in the induction of downstream responses after injury, signaling chemotaxis of inflammatory cells, enhancing extracellular matrix synthesis, stimulating angiogenesis, and recruiting endogenous fibrogenic cells to the injury site. Excessive inflammation may also be detrimental to bone healing. Prolonged administration of NSAIDs has been shown to interfere with a successful bone healing response, but current evidence supports the view that NSAID administration is safe in the setting of anticipated primary bone healing (absolute stability) as well as during the first week during secondary bone healing (callous formation).

Prostaglandins and COX-2 in the early inflammatory phase of fracture repair regulate critical subsequent events during endochondral bone formation, including early chondrogenesis and hypertrophy. NSAIDs, including selective COX inhibitors, can be utilized following fracture in short duration. These drugs should be reconsidered and possibly avoided in patients with other risk factors for delayed fracture healing or if the fracture shows signs of delayed union or nonunion.

Cardiovascular Risk: All NSAIDs have been determined to increase cardiovascular risks; however, traditional nonselective COX inhibitors demonstrate less risk than selective COX-2. Rofecoxib (Vioxx) was withdrawn in 2004 due to an increased risk of cardiovascular events. There is still no consensus regarding the cause, although many mechanisms have been proposed. The imbalance of vasoconstrictive and pro-aggregatory TXA_2 and vasodilating and antiaggregatory PGI_2 is one consideration. Selective COX-2s reduce endothelium-derived and COX-2-derived protective PGI_2, but, in contrast to classical NSAIDs, would leave COX 1 derived thromboxane unchanged. The majority of available evidence suggests that sparing PGI_2 synthesis should reduce the risk of unwanted cardiovascular effects. Another proposed mechanism for the increase in cardiovascular risk is the reduced oxygen free radical antioxidant capacity, which can lead to accumulation of oxidized LDL. Nonetheless, NSAIDs have been associated with increased risk of cardiovascular events (especially cardiovascular thrombotic events, atrial tachyarrhythmias, and ventricular tachyarrhythmias) during the perioperative period.

Renal Risk: Nonsteroidal anti-inflammatory drugs can lead to acute kidney injury in the perioperative setting, resulting in considerable morbidity to the patient, increased length of stay, and additional utilization of healthcare resources. Prostaglandins, especially PGE_2 and prostacyclin (PGI_2), play an important role in controlling renal blood flow and glomerular filtration rate due primarily to their vasodilator properties at the afferent arterioles. While healthy individuals can take normal doses of NSAIDs without adverse effects, those with some degree of baseline renal impairment and those put in other situations that reduce renal blood flow and glomerular filtration rate are at risk for further reduction and acute kidney injury. Under conditions of decreased renal perfusion, the production of renal prostaglandins serves as an important compensatory mechanism. For example, major surgery decreases renal function secondary to stimulation of the adrenosympathetic system and the renin-angiotensin system. Other factors in the perioperative period that increase risk for acute kidney injury include general anesthesia, hypovolemia, and nephrotoxic drugs like aminoglycosides. Additionally,

NSAIDs interact unfavorably with some commonly prescribed medications, including loop diuretics, angiotensin-converting enzyme inhibitors, and angiotensin receptor blockers, leading to reduced effectiveness, along with increased risk of renal impairment.

For those with chronic kidney disease, a further reduction in renal blood flow resulting from decreased prostaglandin synthesis can lead to acute kidney injury, sodium retention, edema, hypertension, and hyperkalemia. While no epidemiologic studies support definitive accelerated progression of chronic kidney disease with regular-dosed NSAID use, empirical perioperative practice dictates caution in this setting, especially given that chronic kidney disease is a risk factor for acute kidney injury.

Gastrointestinal Protection: COX-2 selective NSAIDs have been demonstrated to be less irritating to GI mucosa, producing fewer incidents of abdominal discomfort, gastritis, and ulcerations. The TARGET study showed that lumiracoxib was associated with a three- to fourfold reduction in serious GI complications compared with its traditional NSAID comparators. The VIGOR study showed a 50% relative risk reduction for GI complications for rofecoxib compared with naproxen.

Other Effects: COX-2 selective NSAIDs demonstrate less bronchoconstriction risk in the patient population with aspirin-induced asthma and less depression of platelet function (aggregation and hemostasis).

Further Reading

Bresalier RS, Sandler RS, Quan H, Bolognese JA, Oxenius B, Horgan K, et al. Cardiovascular events associated with rofecoxib in a colorectal adenoma chemoprevention trial. *N Engl J Med.* 2005;352:1092–1102.

Gerstein NS, Gerstein WH, Carey, MC, et al. The thrombotic and arrhythmogenic risks of perioperative NSAIDs. *J Cardiothorac Vasc Anesth.* 2014;28(2):369–378.

Geusens P, Emans PJ, de Jong JJ, van den Bergh J. NSAIDs and fracture healing. *Curr Opin Rheumatol.* 2013;25(4):524–531.

Giannoudis PV, Hak D, Sanders D, Donohoe E, Tosounidis T, Bahney C. Inflammation, bone healing, and anti-inflammatory drugs: an update. *J Orthop Trauma.* 2015;29(suppl 12):S6–S9.

Jaquenod M, Rönnhedh C, Cousins MJ, Eckstein RP, Jordan V, Mather LE, Power I. Factors influencing ketorolac-associated perioperative renal dysfunction. *Anesth Analg.* 1998 May;86(5):1090–1097.

Nderitu P, Doos L, Jones PW, Davies SJ, Kadam UT. Non-steroidal anti-inflammatory drugs and chronic kidney disease progression: a systematic review. *Fam Pract.* 2013 Jun;30(3):247–255. doi:10.1093/fampra/cms086. Epub 2013 Jan 8. Review.

Plantinga L, Grubbs V, Sarkar U, Hsu CY, Hedgeman E, Robinson B, Saran R, Geiss L, Burrows NR, Eberhardt M, Powe N; CDC CKD Surveillance Team. Nonsteroidal anti-inflammatory drug use among persons with chronic kidney disease in the United States. *Ann Fam Med.* 2011 Sep–Oct;9(5):423–430.

Schafer AI. Effects of nonsteroidal antiinflammatory drugs on platelet function and systemic hemostasis. *J Clin Pharmacol.* 1995;35:209–219.

Solomon SD, McMurray JJV, Pfeffer MA, Wittes J, Fowler R, Finn P, et al. Cardiovascular risk associated with celecoxib in a clinical trial for colorectal adenoma prevention. *N Engl J Med.* 2005;352:1071–1080.

Teerawattananon C, Tantayakom P, Suwanawiboon B, Katchamart W. Risk of perioperative bleeding related to highly selective cyclooxygenase-2 inhibitors: a systematic review and meta-analysis. *Semin Arthritis Rheum.* 2016 Jul 20. pii: S0049-0172(16)30123-8

Vioxx: an unequal partnership between safety and efficacy. *Lancet.* 2004;364:1287–1288.

Walter MF, Jacob RF, Day CA, Dahlborg R, Weng Y, Mason RP. Sulfone COX-2 inhibitors increase susceptibility of human LDL and plasma to oxidative modification: comparison to sulfonamide COX-2 inhibitors and NSAIDs. *Atherosclerosis.* 2004;177:235–243.

3.5. Describe the effectiveness of adding NSAIDs to postoperative analgesic regimens in regard to postoperative opioid use and pain burden

Use of NSAIDs has been shown to be effective both as a primary analgesic option and in combination with other analgesics, reducing the opioid requirement in most of the clinical trials with a 30% to 50% sparing effect on morphine consumption. Beneficial effects have also been shown outside of analgesia. NSAIDs have been shown to significantly decrease postoperative nausea and vomiting by 30%, nausea alone by 12%, vomiting alone by 32%, and sedation by 29%. However, in various studies there has been questionable significant improvement in the incidence of pruritus, urinary retention, and respiratory depression with the addition of NSAIDs.

Many different surgical procedures have demonstrated benefits with the perioperative addition of NSAIDs. In patients undergoing extracorporeal lithotripsy, patients administered diclofenac sodium received a greater number of shock waves, required less fentanyl, and showed a marginal improvement in hemodynamic stability and oxygenation during ambulatory nonimmersion extracorporeal shock wave lithotripsy. Women undergoing cesarean delivery demonstrated significantly lower pain scores, less opioid consumption, and less drowsiness/sedation when receiving perioperative NSAIDs. There has been concern based on experimental studies that NSAIDs have a detrimental effect on soft-tissue-to-bone healing; however, a retrospective review performed by Blomquist et al., demonstrates that short-term postoperative treatment with nonsteroidal agents did not influence functional outcome after arthroscopic Bankart procedures.

Opioids may be considered more potent analgesics than NSAIDs, although historical data for these 2 drug classes yield similar numbers needed to treat. The addition of NSAIDs to an opioid-based perioperative regimen has demonstrated to consistently reduce morphine requirements and opioid-related side effects. As an example, administration of parecoxib sodium with patient controlled analgesia (PCA) with morphine resulted in significantly improved postoperative analgesic management as defined by reduction in opioid requirements, lower pain scores, reduced time on PCA morphine, and higher global evaluation ratings. In multiple studies, use of COX-2 selective agents has demonstrated analgesic efficacy in spine surgery, otolaryngologic surgery, orthopedic surgery, breast surgery, robotic prostatectomy, and gynecologic surgery.

Further Reading

Blomquist J, Solheim E, Liavaag S, Baste V, Havelin LI. Do nonsteroidal anti-inflammatory drugs affect the outcome of arthroscopic Bankart repair? *Scand J Med Sci Sports*. 2014;24(6):e510–e514.

Buvanendran A, Tuman KJ, McCoy DD, Matustic B, Chelly JE. Anesthetic techniques for minimally invasive total knee arthroplasty. *J Knee Surg*. 2006;19(2):133–136.

Cepeda MS, Carr DB, Miranda N, Diaz A, Silva C, Morales O. Comparison of morphine, ketorolac and their combination for postoperative pain: results from a large, randomized, double blind trial. *Anesthesiology*. 2005;103(6):1225–1232.

Elia N, Lysakowski C, Tramér MR. Does multimodal analgesia with acetaminophen, nonsteroidal antiinflammatory drugs, or selective cyclooxygenase-2 inhibitors and patient-controlled analgesia morphine offer advantages over morphine alone? Meta-analyses of randomized trials. *Anesthesiology*. 2005;103(6):1296–1304.

Fredman B, Jedeikin R, Olsfanger D, Aronheim M. The opioid sparing effect of diclofenac sodium in outpatient extracorporeal lithotripsy (ESWL). *J Clin Anesth*. 1993;5(2):141–144.

Gärtner R, Kroman N, Callesen T, Kehlet H. Multimodal prevention of pain, nausea and vomiting after breast cancer surgery. *Minerva Anestesiol*. 2010;76(10):805–813.

Jensen K, Kehlet H, Lund CM. Postoperative recovery profile after elective abdominal hysterectomy: a prospective, observational study of a multimodal anaesthetic regime. *Eur J Anaesthesiol*. 2009 May;26(5):382-8.

Kehlet H, Dahl JB: The value of "multimodal" or "balanced analgesia" in postoperative pain treatment. *Anesth Analg*. 1993;77(5):1048–1056.

Long J, Lewis S, Kuklo T, Zhu Y, Riew KD. The effect of cyclooxygenase-2 inhibitors on spinal fusion. *J Bone Joint Surg Am*. 2002;84–A:1763–1768.

Malan TP Jr, Marsh G, Hakki SI, Grossman E, Traylor L, Hubbard RC. Parecoxib sodium, a parenteral cyclooxygenase-2 selective inhibitor improves morphine analgesia and is opioid sparing following total hip arthroplasty. *Anesthesiology*. 2003;98(4):950–956.

Marret E, Kurdi O, Zufferey P, Bonnet F. Effects of nonsteroidal antiinflammatory drugs on patient-controlled analgesia morphine side effects: meta-analysis of randomized controlled trials. *Anesthesiology*. 2005;102(6):1249–1260.

Trabulsi EJ, Patel J, Viscusi ER, Gomella LG, Lallas CD. Preemptive multimodal pain regimen reduces opioid analgesia for patients undergoing robotic-assisted laparoscopic radical prostatectomy. *Urology*. 2010;76(5):1122–1124.

Turan A, Emet S, Karamanlioglu B, Memis D, Turan N, Pamukcu Z. Analgesic effects of rofecoxib in ear-nose-throat surgery. *Anesth Analg*. 2002; 95(5):1308–1311.

Zeng AM, Nami NF, Wu CL, Murphy JD. The analgesic efficacy of nonsteroidal anti-inflammatory agents (NSAIDs) in patients undergoing cesarean deliveries: a meta analysis. *Reg Anesth Pain Med*. 2016;41(6):763–772.

4

Distal Radius Fracture

Sharon Jiang, Jack M. Berger, and Luke Nicholson

Case Scenario

A healthy, 55-year-old white woman falls on an outstretched right upper extremity while walking on a slippery surface and goes to the emergency room complaining of isolated right wrist pain. Radiographs are obtained, and she is diagnosed with a right distal radius fracture. She is otherwise healthy without any pertinent surgical or medical history. She undergoes uncomplicated open reduction and internal fixation of the right distal radius the following day through a volar approach to the radius using a locking plate and screws. A splint is placed postoperatively and is maintained until she is seen in clinic 2 weeks later, when her sutures are removed and she is converted to a removable wrist splint for 4 weeks. Occupational therapy is begun after 2 weeks to aid in postoperative recovery.

1. Distal Radius Fractures

1.1. What is the epidemiology of distal radius fractures?

Fractures of the distal end of the radius are among the most commonly encountered fractures in the emergency department, with an annual incidence of more than 600,000. These fractures occur in a bimodal age distribution as the result of high-energy injuries in young patients and low-energy falls in elderly patients. Frequently the result of decreased bone mineral density in the elderly population, distal radius fractures account for 18% of all fractures in the over-65 age group and affect women over 65 years of age 4.88 times more frequently than men. Recent literature suggests that the incidence of distal radial fractures has been increasing, likely as a result of the increased activity of elderly patients.

Further Reading

Baron JA, Karagas M, Barrett J, Kniffin W, Malenka D, Mayor M, Keller RB. Basic epidemiology of fractures of the upper and lower limb among Americans over 65 years of age. *Epidemiology*. 1996 Nov;7(6):612–618.

Koval K, Haidukewych GJ, Service B, Zirgibel BJ. Controversies in the management of distal radius fractures. *J Am Acad Orthop Surg*. 2014 Sep;22(9):566–575.

Nellans KW, Kowalski E, Chung KC. The epidemiology of distal radius fractures. *Hand Clin*. 2012;28(2):113–125.

1.2. What must be evaluated for distal radius fractures?

A thorough physical examination of patients with a distal radius fracture must identify open fractures, degree of soft tissue swelling, and associated injuries, as each of these may dictate the need for and urgency of surgical management. A "dinner fork" deformity typically accompanies the most common type of distal radius fracture, the dorsally angulated fracture referred to as a Colles fracture. Commonly associated injuries include scaphoid fracture (indicated by snuffbox tenderness), scapholunate dissociation (found on ulnarly deviated wrist radiographs), distal radioulnar instability (in more proximal fractures), and radial head fractures (indicated by point tenderness at the elbow). Radiographic examination should include an evaluation for intra-articular involvement, displacement, angulation, shortening, comminution, and involvement of the ulnar styloid.

1.3. How are distal radius fractures classified?

A variety of descriptions and classification systems exist to categorize distal radius fractures in an effort to guide management options. Common eponyms used to refer to distal radius fractures include the following:

1. Colles fracture: Dorsally angulated fracture resulting from a fall onto an outstretched palm. Represents more than 90% of all distal radius fractures.
2. Smith fracture: A volarly angulated ("reverse Colles") fracture resulting from a fall onto a flexed wrist. Though uncommon, this fracture pattern is inherently unstable and requires open reduction and internal fixation to restore stability.
3. Barton fracture: A fracture associated with radiocarpal subluxation or dislocation. An uncommon but inherently unstable fracture pattern that generally requires open reduction and internal fixation.
4. Chauffeur's fracture: A radial styloid avulsion fracture resulting from rapid ulnar deviation at the wrist. Treatment depends on degree of instability and an evaluation for scapholunate dissociation, which may accompany a radial styloid fracture.

Classification systems, commonly used in the research setting to describe distal radius fractures, include the following:

1. Frykman classification: Based on articular involvement of the radiocarpal and distal radioulnar joints, as well as the presence of a distal ulna fracture.
2. Fernandez classification: Represents a description of the mechanism of injury, including bending, shearing, compression, and avulsion fractures.
3. OTA classification: Evaluates the extent of articular involvement of the radiocarpal joint with an emphasis on number of fracture fragments.

1.4. Describe the management of distal radius fractures

Management options for distal radius fractures vary widely and are influenced by multiple patient- and fracture-specific variables. Important patient factors include age and activity level, with older, more sedentary patients often benefiting from nonoperative management. Fracture variables that increase the likelihood of instability and thereby increase the need for surgery include significant angulation, intra-articular extension, fracture comminution, and concomitant ulnar styloid fractures.

1. Nonoperative: Nonoperative treatment of distal radius fractures is commonly indicated for nondisplaced fractures and fractures occurring in elderly, sedentary patients or in those with medical problems precluding operation. Nonoperative treatment typically consists of closed reduction under local or regional anesthetic, followed by application of an above-elbow splint that is replaced with a molded cast after resolution of soft-tissue swelling—typically about 1 week. See section 2.1.
2. Open reduction internal fixation: Since the advent of locking plate technology, open reduction and internal fixation has become widely used and is the most common means to surgically stabilize a distal radius fracture. Approaches to the distal radius typically include the volar Henry approach between the flexor carpi radialis and brachioradialis tendons, and the dorsal approach between the third and fourth extensor compartments of the wrist. Open reduction and internal fixation is typically performed under regional or general anesthesia with use of an above-elbow tourniquet. Postoperatively, patients are typically immobilized with a splint until seen in clinic, when they are transitioned to a brace or cast after swelling resolution. A specific type of internal fixation that has gained popularity in recent years

is dorsal bridge plating, during which a plate is applied to the dorsum of the wrist to span the joint and prevent any wrist motion. The plate remains in place for 3 months until the fracture is healed, and then removed under a separate anesthetic to allow for wrist motion.

3. External fixation: Typically reserved for complex intra-articular fractures not amenable to anatomic reduction using locking plate technology or fractures accompanied by severe soft tissue injury, external fixation involves placement of pins outside of the zone of injury that are connected by external rods to stabilize across the fracture site. While still commonly utilized for fractures with severe soft tissue injury, external fixation is increasingly being replaced by dorsal bridge plating.
4. Percutaneous fixation: Percutaneous fixation of distal radius fractures is performed using stainless steel Kirschner wires that are placed across the fracture site percutaneously after closed reduction is performed. The Kirschner wires are left in place for 4 to 6 weeks and typically removed in clinic; however, they may be removed in the operating room if they are left under the skin for aesthetic reasons. Postoperative immobilization with Kirschner wires in place typically consists of a splint or cast.

Further Reading

Alluri RK, Hill JR, Ghiassi A. Distal radius fractures: approaches, indications, and techniques. *J Hand Surg Am.* 2016 Aug;41(8):845–854.

1.5. What is the typical postoperative management?

Patients who undergo closed reduction are typically followed with weekly radiographs for 1 month to monitor for displacement that may necessitate operative intervention. Splints and casts used for patients undergoing both nonoperative and operative treatment are typically discontinued after 6 weeks. Occupational therapy is an important component of recovery as both wrist stiffness and digital stiffness are common after prolonged periods of immobilization. In addition, the occupational therapist plays an important role in desensitization for patients with complex regional pain syndrome. Weight bearing is typically resumed after 6 weeks, with a full return to activity at around 3 months. Medical comorbidities such as diabetes may necessitate prolonged immobilization or non-weight-bearing restrictions to confirm complete healing.

1.6. What are the prevalence and causes of compartment syndrome in the upper extremity?

While uncommon, compartment syndrome of the upper extremity may lead to significant morbidity. The overall incidence of compartment syndrome in both upper and lower extremities is quoted as 3.1 per 100,000 population per year, with younger age being the most important risk factor. The true incidence of upper extremity compartment syndrome is unclear; however, the majority of cases are due to either distal radius fractures or diaphyseal forearm fractures. Within the upper extremity, the forearm is more commonly affected. Causes of upper extremity compartment syndrome include fracture, crush injury, reperfusion injury in the setting of arterial disruption, and burns.

Compartment syndrome is managed with emergent fasciotomy to decompress the afflicted compartments. If the diagnosis of compartment syndrome is delayed or missed, irreversible muscle and nerve injury will result in permanent severe dysfunction. *Volkmann contracture* refers to the sequela of a missed volar forearm compartment syndrome.

Further Reading

Botte MJ, Gelberman RH. Acute compartment syndrome of the forearm. *Hand Clin.* 1998;14(3):391.

Duckworth AD, McQueen MM. The diagnosis of acute compartment syndrome: a critical analysis review. *JBJS Rev.* 2017 Dec;5(12):e1.

Kalyani BS, Fisher BE, Roberts CS, Giannoudis PV. Compartment syndrome of the forearm: a systematic review. *J Hand Surg Am.* 2011;36:535–543.

1.7. What is the pathophysiology of compartment syndrome in the upper extremity?

The upper arm contains 15 anatomical compartments (upper arm, 2; forearm, 3; hand, 10) that are encased within fascial linings. The pathophysiology of compartment syndrome is a complex interplay between both compartmental and system blood pressures. However, the final common pathway is cellular anoxia and death.

Following a corresponding insult, intracompartmental pressure increases lead to vein compression and increased interstitial edema. Continued progression leads to a threshold whereby the arteriovenous gradient is insufficient and ischemia occurs. Numerous ischemic mediators (i.e., hydrogen ions, bradykinin, serotonin, etc.) lead to nociceptor activation and contribute to reported pain symptoms.

Further Reading

Elliott KG, Johnstone AJ. Diagnosing acute compartment syndrome. *J Bone Joint Surg Br.* 2003;85(5):625.

Prasarn ML, Ouellette EA. Acute compartment syndrome of the upper extremity. *J Am Acad Orthop Surg.* 2011 Jan;19(1):49–58.

1.8. What are important diagnostic considerations when there are concerns for compartment syndrome?

Early diagnosis is critical in the setting of acute compartment syndrome. Diagnosis is largely based on clinical variables such as the presence of pain out of proportion to clinical examination, pallor, paresthesia, paralysis, and pulselessness. However, the majority of these symptoms lack sensitivity and specificity and, if present, occur during the late stages of ischemia. The most sensitive and commonly utilized clinical sign is pain with passive stretch of a muscle in the involved compartment.

In scenarios where the diagnosis is still in question, particularly in the management of obtunded patients unable to cooperate with examination, intracompartmental pressure may be measured. Current guidelines suggest that the diagnosis of compartment syndrome is suggested by a compartment 30 mmHg within diastolic pressure or an absolute pressure of 30 mmHg.

Further Reading

Kistler JM, Ilyas AM, Thoder JJ. Forearm compartment syndrome: evaluation and management. *Hand Clin.* 2018 Feb;34(1):53–60.

2. Regional Anesthesia Considerations

2.1. What kind of perineural interventions can be considered for the initial closed or operative management of distal radius fracture?

Distal radial fractures often lead to significant pain following the initial trauma, reduction, and fixation. The use of brachial plexus peripheral nerve blocks can provide excellent anesthesia and analgesia for these fractures. Most commonly, supraclavicular, infraclavicular, and axillary brachial plexus blocks can provide excellent nonopioid analgesia during this period. The interscalene approach, while effective, is less commonly performed for distal radius fracture. Both the supraclavicular and infraclavicular approaches are amenable to continuous catheter placement. However, while axillary blockade can provide anesthesia for distal radius fractures, it is not suitable for continuous catheterization.

2.2. At what locations should such peripheral nerve techniques be employed?

While performance of perineural interventions can occur in the field or prehospital setting, this practice is rare and more applicable to austere environments. However, following admission to the emergency room, these blocks can be performed to provide analgesia for fracture reduction. If the patient is not going to be taken to the operating room, single-shot injections will suffice for the closed reductions. If, instead, the patient is expected to undergo operative fixation within 24 hours, then a continuous peripheral nerve block catheter can be inserted to allow for continuous local anesthetic infusion or bolus reactivation at the time of surgery.

2.3. What considerations occur when choosing between supraclavicular and infraclavicular brachial plexus blocks in patients with distal radius fractures?

Perineural blockade maintains an established role in managing acute pain following the operative fixation of distal radius fractures. In a study by Galos et al., 40 patients with distal radius fractures were randomized to receive general anesthesia or a brachial plexus block. Patients who received a brachial plexus block utilized fewer opioids and had shorter postanesthesia care unit stays and lower immediate pain scores. In regard to placement of continuous perineural catheters for distal radius fractures, current data are unclear in regard to benefit. In a study by Ganta et al., 50 patients were randomized to receive either a single injection or continuous infraclavicular block. Of note, while all pain scores were lower in the continuous catheter group, statistical significance was not achieved. Additionally, no difference in opioid use was observed. Significant limits of this study included no functional measures of pain (pain with movement, sleep quality, etc.), and patients with preexisting pain and opioid use were excluded. Such a study highlights the need for individualized analgesic planning depending on patient and surgical factors.

At present, no consistent evidence establishes superiority or lack thereof when comparing infraclavicular (IC) to supraclavicular (SC) blockade. In a systematic review performed by Park et al., sensory loss in 4 distributions was analyzed as the primary outcome between IC and SC blockade. While IC blockade resulted in less incomplete ulnar sensory loss, no other significant differences were noted in block quality, onset, and time to perform. Significant differences were isolated to expected above-the-clavicle (i.e., SC block) effects such as phrenic nerve palsy, Horner's syndrome, and paresthesia during needle placement.

Further Reading

Egol KA, Soojian MG, Walsh M, Katz J, Rosenberg AD, Paksima N. Regional anesthesia improves outcome after distal radius fracture fixation over general anesthesia. *J Orthop Trauma.* 2012 Sep;26(9):545–549.

Galos DK, Taormina DP, Crespo A, Ding DY, Sapienza A, Jain S, Tejwani NC. Does brachial plexus blockade result in improved pain scores after distal radius fracture fixation? A randomized trial. *Clin Orthop Relat Res.* 2016 May;474(5):1247–1254.

Ganta A, Ding D, Fisher N, Lavery J, Jain S, Tejwani NC. Continuous infraclavicular brachial block versus single-shot nerve block for distal radius surgery: a prospective randomized control trial. *J Orthop Trauma.* 2018 Jan;32(1):22–26.

Park SK, Lee SY, Kim WH, Park HS, Lim YJ, Bahk JH. Comparison of supraclavicular and infraclavicular brachial plexus block: a systematic review of randomized controlled trials. *Anesth Analg.* 2017 Feb;124(2):636–644.

2.4. What are the strategies to reduce the occurrence of secondary perineural catheter failure in distal upper extremity surgery?

Surgeries involving the distal forearm or hand often include numerous neurotomes, osteotomes, and dermatomes. For example, numerous surgeries involving the wrist require blockade of the median, radial, and ulnar nerves, including the cutaneous nerves of the forearm (radial, musculocutaneous, and medial antebrachial nerves). When a primary block is placed, a larger volume of high-concentration local anesthetic is placed around a plexus or grouping of nerves to provide complete blockade. However, a continuous infusion provides a lower volume and lower concentration of local anesthetic such that when the primary block subsides, not all nerve distributions may be anesthetized. This scenarios is termed *secondary failure.*

While the true incidence is unclear, both the infraclavicular and supraclavicular approaches to the brachial plexus are susceptible to secondary failure with perineural catheter placement as neither approach consistently provides complete blockade of all nerve distribution in the distal upper extremity. One recently described approach, the costoclavicular approach to the brachial plexus, may mitigate the risk of secondary failure. Performance of this technique is done with the patient in the supine position with the arm slightly abducted. An ultrasound probe is placed parallel to the clavicle and the axillary artery is visualized. Unlike the paracoracoid infraclavicular approach, all 3 cords of the brachial plexus are positioned lateral to the axillary artery and encased within a single connective tissue compartment. Placement of local anesthetic and/or perineural catheter allows contact with all three cords of the brachial plexus in a single space, theoretically decreasing the chance for secondary failure.

Further Reading

Boezaart AP, Dell PC2. Secondary block failure for upper extremity surgery: less is not more. *J Hand Surg Am*. 2014 Sep;39(9):1887–1888.

Li JW, Songthamwat B, Samy W, Sala-Blanch X, Karmakar MK. Ultrasound-guided costoclavicular brachial plexus block: sonoanatomy, technique, and block dynamics. *Reg Anesth Pain Med*. 2017 Mar/Apr;42(2):233–240.

3. Complications of Distal Radius Fractures

3.1. What are some long-term complications of distal radius fractures?

Distal radius fractures may be associated with a range of complications, including but not limited to carpal tunnel syndrome, malunion, persistent wrist pain, and complex regional pain syndrome (CRPS I). Carpal tunnel syndrome may occur acutely at the time of injury and is more common with high-energy injuries. Urgent carpal tunnel release is indicated in the setting of acute carpal tunnel syndrome. Malunion is most common following nonoperative management of displaced distal radius fractures and may result in chronic distal radioulnar joint instability and pain. Persistent wrist pain, particularly ulnar-sided wrist pain, is common in both operatively and nonoperatively managed distal radius fractures, and is commonly attributed to occult damage to the triangular fibrocartilage complex. Finally, CRPS I is a disabling condition that may follow both operatively and nonoperatively managed distal radius fractures; it is discussed in further detail later in this chapter.

Further Reading

Davis DI, Baratz M. Soft tissue complications of distal radius fractures. *Hand Clin*. 2010;26(2):229–235.

3.2. What is the role of psychosocial variables in general outcomes following distal radius fractures?

Among a variety of psychosocial variables, depression has emerged as a significant mediator following distal radius fracture. In a study of 228 patients older than 55 years, Yeoh et al. demonstrated that the presence of depression had a significant role in portending a poor outcome. A significant portion of patients older than 55 years with low-energy distal radius fracture experienced depression. A positive screen for depression indicated by a Center for Epidemiologic Studies Depression Scale score ≥16 was associated with higher rates of complications at 3 months. When compared with other covariates, depression was the most important predictor of functional outcomes and disability 1 year after DRF. These findings may illustrate and explain challenges for patients with depression during recovery from DRF. Data support that outcomes after DRF can be related to biopsychosocial factors, specifically depression. It is important for healthcare providers, patients, and caretakers to be aware of the potential impact of depression on patient recovery and outcomes because both patients and healthcare providers may alter their treatment and expectations accordingly.

Further Reading

Yeoh JC, Pike JM, Slobogean GP, O'Brien PJ, Broekhuyse HM, Lefaivre KA. Role of depression in outcomes of low-energy distal radius fractures in patients older than 55 years. *J Orthop Trauma*. 2016;30(5):228–233.

3.3. What is acute neuropathic pain?

The International Association for the Study of Pain (IASP) defines neuropathic pain as pain caused by a lesion or dysfunction of the nervous system. A variety of other pain subtypes exist, including nociceptive and inflammatory pain, which arise from tissue damage such as that produced by trauma, surgery, childbirth, or invasion of tissue by a tumor. However, neuropathic pain results from damage to a nerve or from changes in the nervous system itself. While neuropathic pain is often considered a chronic condition, a variety of medical (e.g., cancer, disc herniation, herpes zoster) and surgical conditions (e.g., amputation) causing neuropathic pain occur in the acute setting. Following surgery, the incidence of acute neuropathic pain ranges from 1% to 10% depending on surgical type and the screening tool utilized.

Further Reading

Gray P. Acute neuropathic pain: diagnosis and treatment. *Curr Opin Anaesthesiol.* 2008 Oct;21(5):590–595.

3.4. How is acute neuropathic pain diagnosed?

Although no definitive symptomology or test can establish the diagnosis of acute neuropathic pain, a variety of clinical variables and neuropathic pain questionnaires can alert physicians. These may include the following:

- Pain that is sharp, episodic, or burning in quality
- Reported pain in an anatomic region that is without sensation
- Pain out of proportion (length or intensity) to initial insult
- Pain that is difficult to control with standard therapies
- Allodynia, or loss of sensation on physical examination

Numerous neuropathic pain scales have been developed, but none has undergone validation in the acute setting (Table 4.1). At present, it is unclear whether such screening tools are useful in the acute or subacute setting following surgery given the presence of confounding surgical nociceptive pain. However, in a study of 100 patients undergoing video-assisted thoracic surgery (video-assisted thoracoscopic surgery or thoracotomy, patients who screened positively via the Leeds Assessment of Neuropathic Symptoms and Signs in the immediate

Table 4.1:
Neuropathic pain screening tools

Scale	Number of Items	Measurement of Symptoms	Measurement of Signs
Leeds Assessment of Neuropathic Symptoms and Signs (LANSS)	7	Yes	Yes
painDETECT	9	Yes	No
Douleur Neuropathique en 4 (DN4)	7	Yes	Yes
ID Pain	6	Yes	No
Neuropathic Pain Questionnaire	12	Yes	No
PROMIS Neuropathic Pain Quality	5	Yes	No

postoperative period were noted to have a higher probability of displaying neuropathic pain symptoms 3 months postoperatively.

Further Reading

Mulvey MR, Bennett MI, Liwowsky I, Freynhagen R. The role of screening tools in diagnosing neuropathic pain. *Pain Manag.* 2014 May;4(3):233–243.

4. Complex Regional Pain Syndrome Type I

4.1. What are the criteria for diagnosing CRPS I?

CRPS I may follow a variety of inciting events; however, 55% to 60% of the time, it is preceded by a traumatic event, with distal radius fractures being the most common. The incidence of CRPS I varies widely in the current literature, ranging from 1% to 37% due to different criteria used by the authors.

Consistent with its subtype of neuropathic pain, CRPS occurs when trauma of the extremity leads to sympathetic denervation distal to the site of injury. Sympathetic denervation leads to vasodilation and release of inflammatory mediators followed by hypersensitivity of the distal vasculature and sensory nerves to adrenergic stimulation, resulting in peripheral autonomic dysfunction.

In 1994, the IASP first characterized CRPS and listed the diagnostic criteria as follows:

1. The presence of an initiating noxious event, or a cause of immobilization (not required for diagnosis as 5% to 10% of patients will not have this)
2. Continuing pain, allodynia (perception of pain from a nonpainful stimulus), or hyperalgesia (an exaggerated sense of pain) in which the pain is disproportionate to the inciting event
3. Evidence at some time of edema, changes in skin blood flow, or abnormal sudomotor activity in the region of pain
4. The diagnosis is excluded by the existence of any condition that would otherwise account for the degree of pain and dysfunction.

However in 2007, Bruehl and Harden et al. proposed a more specific set of criteria based on 4 major clusters of signs and symptoms: sensory, vasomotor, edema/sudomotor, and motor/trophic (Table 4.2).

These criteria later evolved into the Budapest consensus criteria for the clinical diagnosis of CRPS I (Box 4.1).

The severity of pain in CRPS I exceeds the expected clinical course of the inciting event in both magnitude and duration. CRPS I is a common problem with a population-based rate of 5.5 per 100,000 person-years in a North American study and 26.2 per 100,000 person-years in a 2014 European study.

Table 4.2:
Four categories of CRPS signs and symptoms

Sensory	Hyperesthesia/hyperalgesia (to pinprick) and/or allodynia (to light touch and/or temperature sensation and/or deep somatic pressure and/or joint movement)
Vasomotor	Temperature asymmetry (>1°C) and/or skin color changes and/or skin color asymmetry
Sudomotor/edema	Edema and/or sweating changes and/or sweating asymmetry
Motor/trophic	Decreased range of motion and/or motor dysfunction (weakness, tremor, dystonia) and/or trophic changes (hair, nail, skin)

Box 4.1 Budapest Consensus Criteria for CRPS

All of the following statements must be met:

1. The patient experiences continuing pain that which is disproportionate to any inciting event.
2. For the clinical diagnosis of CRPS, the patient must report at least 1 symptom in 3 of the 4 categories (the more stringent research criteria require at least 1 symptom in all 4 categories).
3. For the clinical diagnosis of CRPS, the patient must display at least 1 sign at the time of evaluation in 2 of the 4 categories (the more stringent research criteria require at least 1 sign in 3 of the 4 categories).
4. There is no other diagnosis that better explains the signs and symptoms.

Further Reading

Harden RN, Bruehl S, Perez RS, et al. Validation of proposed diagnostic criteria (the "Budapest criteria") for complex regional pain syndrome. *Pain*. 2010;150(2):268–274.

Harden RN, Bruehl S, Stanton-Hicks M, Wilson PR. Proposed new diagnostic criteria for complex regional pain syndrome. *Pain Med*. 2007;8(4):326–331.

Merskey H, Bogduk N. *Classification of Chronic Pain: Descriptions of Chronic Pain Syndromes and Definitions of Pain Terms*. Seattle, WA: IASP Press; 1994.

4.2. What is the incidence of CRPS I following nonoperative of DRF?

In a 2014 study, Jellad et al. looked at the incidence of CRPS I after nonoperative treatment of DRF. Patients suffering from extra-articular DRF underwent conservative treatment with close reduction and cast immobilization for 6 weeks, with rehabilitation sessions beginning 7 days prior to cast removal. Ninety (90) patients met inclusion criteria, with 34 men and 56 women with a mean age of 51.6 ± 17.3 years. Using criteria according to Veldman et al., CRPS I was diagnosed in 32.2%, or 29 patients, including 6 men and 23 women. The average time until CRPS I onset was 21.7 ± 23.7 days after cast removal. All patients completed the follow-up period of 9 months. Of note, CRPS I occurred frequently at the third and fourth week after cast removal. The primary predictors for the development of CRPS I included female sex, social stressors, trauma of low and medium energy, and impairment of physical quality of life and wrist function.

The severity of early pain has also been linked to the development of CRPS I. In a 2014 prospective cohort study, a sample of 1549 patients with wrist fracture and managed nonsurgically was assessed within 1 week of DRF incidence and followed up 4 months later. One in 26 patients, or 3.8%, developed CRPS within 4 months of nonsurgically managed wrist fracture. A simple assessment of pain intensity (0–10 numerical rating scale) provided the level of discrimination.

Further Reading

Jellad A, Salah S, Ben Salah Frih Z. Complex regional pain syndrome type I: incidence and risk factors in patients with fracture of the distal radius. *Arch Phys Med Rehabil*. 2014;95(3):487–492.

Moseley GL, Herbert RD, Parsons T, Lucas S, Van Hilten JJ, Marinus J. Intense pain soon after wrist fracture strongly predicts who will develop complex regional pain syndrome: prospective cohort study. *J Pain*. 2014;15(1):16–23.

Veldman P, Reynen H, Arntz I, et al. Signs and symptoms of reflex sympathetic dystrophy: prospective study of 829 patients. *Lancet*. 1993;342:1012–1016.

4.3. What is the incidence of CRPS I following surgical treatment of distal radius fractures?

Although wrist fracture is considered an initiating trauma for CRPS I, few studies have comprehensively evaluated factors associated with the occurrence of CRPS I after the surgical treatment of a DRF. In 2014 prospective observational study, Roh et al. evaluated the factors that influence the occurrence of CRPS I after the surgical treatment of a DRF. Six months after surgery, patients were evaluated using the Budapest diagnostic criteria. Among the 477 patients with a surgically treated DRF, 42 (8.8%) satisfied the Budapest criteria for CRPS I.

The criteria for operative treatment in this study were radial shortening of >5 mm, dorsal angulation of >10° or volar angulation of 20° in wrist lateral radiographs, radial inclination of <10° in wrist postero-anterior view, or an articular step-off of >2 mm. Patients undergoing volar plating were treated with a short-arm splint for 2 weeks followed by a removable short-arm brace for around 2 weeks as required by the patients. Patients who underwent closed reduction and external fixation were treated with a short-arm splint for 2 weeks, and the external fixator was removed after 5 weeks from surgery, followed by a removable brace as required.

Postoperative care consists of wrist range-of-motion exercises initiated immediately after the removal of the splint in the case of internal fixation or immediately after the removal of the frame in the case of external fixation. Patients were instructed to perform daily activities after splint removal and to use the wrist brace as required only for physical labor using the hand. All patients had formal physiotherapy and were given a standardized home exercise program.

Risk factors for the development of CRPS I included high-energy injuries, comminuted fractures, older age, and female sex.

Further Reading

Roh YH, Lee BK, Noh JH, et al. Factors associated with complex regional pain syndrome type I in patients with surgically treated distal radius fracture. *Arch Orthop Trauma Surg*. 2014;134(12):1775–1781.

4.4. What is the pathophysiology of CRPS I?

4.4.1. Pathophysiology of CRPS: glial cell and cytokines

Numerous etiologic pathophysiologic events have been incriminated in development of CRPS, including inflammation, autoimmune responses, abnormal cytokine production, sympathetic-sensory disorders, altered blood flow, and central cortical reorganization (Figure 4.1).

Within the past decade, there has been increasing recognition that microglia and astrocytes are far more than simply "housekeepers" for neurons. Activation of glia can create and maintain enhanced pain states such as neuropathic pain, and compromise the efficacy of morphine and other opioids for pain control. Interestingly, glia will become increasingly activated in response to repeated administration of opioids. While glial cells have little to no role in pain under basal conditions, activated glia induce the release of pro-inflammatory cytokines, neuronal chemokines, and neurotransmitters from damaged, dying, and dead neurons.

Understanding CRPS pathophysiology is crucial to developing effective treatments. A number of studies have specifically examined the associations between CRPS and pro-inflammatory and anti-inflammatory cytokines. A 2010 review of current literature found that compared with pain-free controls and non-CRPS pain patients, CRPS patients have significant increases in pro-inflammatory cytokines (TNF-α, interleukin-1β, interleukin-2, and interleukin-6) in local blister fluid, circulating plasma, and cerebrospinal fluid. TNF-α is a key cytokine because it not only has direct pro-nociceptive actions but also induces production of other cytokines involved in inflammation, including interleukin-1β and interleukin-6. The administration of infliximab, a monoclonal antibody against TNF-α, may produce notable reductions in CRPS symptoms in some patients. CRPS patients also seem to have reduced systemic levels of anti-inflammatory cytokines such as interleukin-10 compared with controls, which may also contribute to

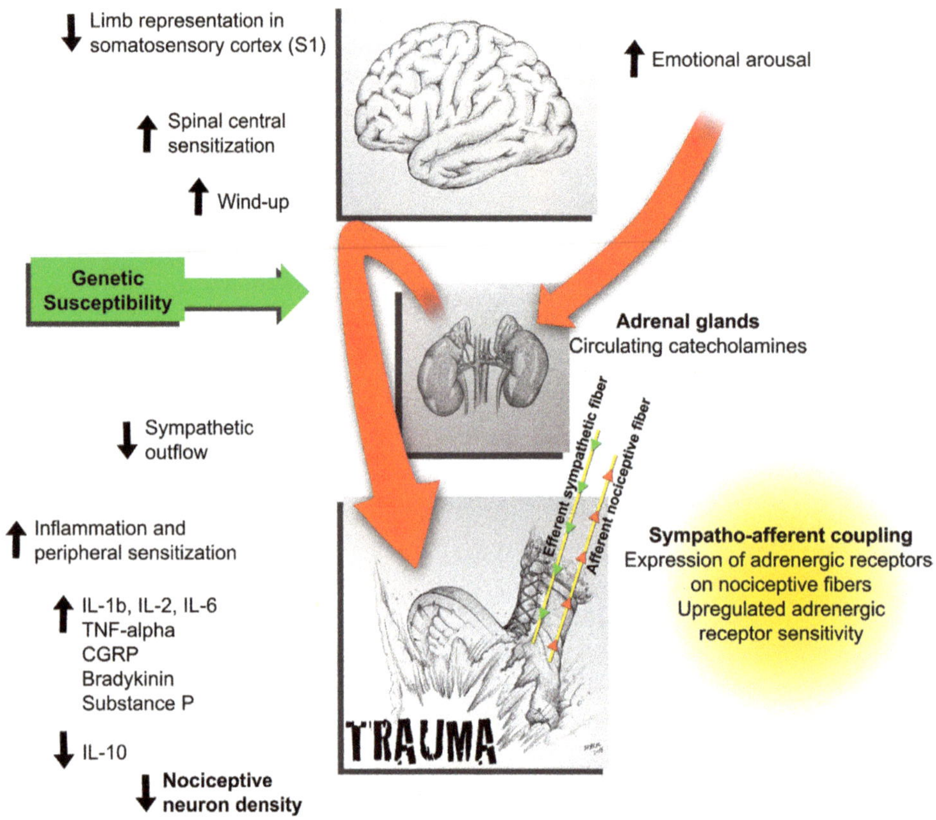

Figure 4.1 A speculative model of interacting mechanisms involved in CRPS and summary of all the multifactorial pathophysiologic mechanisms that may contribute to the disorder. These may include peripheral and central sensitization, inflammation, altered sympathetic and catecholaminergic function, reduced representation of the affected limb in the somatosensory cortex, genetic factors, and psychophysiologic interactions. The degree to which individual mechanisms contribute to CRPS may differ from one patient to another and even within one patient over time. Modified from Bruehl S. An update on the pathophysiology of complex regional pain syndrome. *Anesthesiology*. 2010;113(3):713–25.

increased inflammation in the condition. CRPS-I patients with hyperalgesia had significantly higher plasma levels of soluble TNF-α receptor type I than did CRPS patients without hyperalgesia. Neuropathic pain patients with allodynia display a higher plasma TNF-α level than do similar patients without allodynia.

4.4.2. Animal models for elucidating the pathophysiology of CRPS

A mouse model of tibia fracture/cast immobilization showed the principal stigmata of CRPS observed in humans. Mice were randomly allocated to the control or the fracture/cast group. Mice were then anesthetized with 1.5% isoflurane and underwent a closed distal tibia fracture using a hemostat. Then the hind limb was wrapped in casting tape so the hip, knee, and ankle were all fixed. The cast extended from the metatarsals of the hind paw up to a spica formed around the abdomen. A window was left open over the dorsal paw and ankle to prevent constriction when postfracture edema developed. After the procedure, the mice were given subcutaneous buprenorphine (0.05 mg/kg) and enrofloxacin (5 mg/kg) for the next 2 days, as well as normal saline (1.5 ml once) for postoperative analgesia, prevention of infection, and dehydration. Mice were inspected daily to ensure the cast was positioned properly through the 3-week period of cast immobilization.

Based on behavioral observations, this study focused on 3 potential neurobiological substrates: the amygdala, for its role in processing threatening stimuli, mood, fear, emotional memory, anxiety, and the emotional-affective dimension of pain; and the perirhinal cortex and hippocampus, for their roles in memory. Collectively, data from this study provide unique evidence for structural and biochemical changes in the brain that accompany selective measures of anxiety, working memory, and social memory impairment in a mouse model of tibia fracture/cast immobilization.

These findings have clear clinical implications for the CRPS patient, since, in addition to elucidating some of the supraspinal correlates of the syndrome, they support the potential use of therapeutic interventions that not only directly target sensory input and other peripheral mechanisms but also attempt to ameliorate the pain experience by modifying its associated cognitive and emotional comorbidities. Findings show that the histologic changes indicative of increased dendritic complexity occur in the amygdala and perirhinal cortex in the absence of increased synaptophysin, an indirect measure of synaptic numbers. Furthermore, synaptophysin levels are decreased in the hippocampus isolated from CRPS mice and trended toward lower levels in homogenates of tissue from the perirhinal cortex and amygdala.

Further Reading

Borchers AT, Gershwin ME. Complex regional pain syndrome: a comprehensive and critical review. *Autoimmun Rev*. 2014;13(3):242–265.

Bruehl S. An update on the pathophysiology of complex regional pain syndrome. *Anesthesiology*. 2010;113(3):713–725.

Tajerian M, Leu D, Zou Y, et al. Brain neuroplastic changes accompany anxiety and memory deficits in a model of complex regional pain syndrome. *Anesthesiology*. 2014;121(4):852–865.

4.5. Describe the initial management of CRPS I

Current pharmacotherapeutic approaches to attenuate spinal pain amplification mechanisms include the use of clonidine and antidepressants, local anesthetics, ketamine, intravenous (IV) lidocaine, NSAIDs, gabapentin, and/or pregabalin. Recommendations for CRPS include the regimen should be individualized for the patient; initial treatment modalities should be the simplest and least invasive; management of mild to moderate pain should include an NSAID (COXIB) and/or acetaminophen if possible (COX-3 inhibitor); when pain persists despite adequate adjunct treatment or increases, an opioid may be considered.

A 2010 comprehensive literature review by Perez evaluated the efficacy of all therapies for CRPS I and developed evidence-based guidelines for treatment and prevention. The recommendations include adequate perioperative analgesia, limitation of operating time, and limited use of a tourniquet. Additionally, to reduce pain in CRPS I patients, there are a few indications: administration of a subanesthesic dose of ketamine, 600 to 1800 mg gabapentin daily for the first 8 weeks, and 10–20 mg of IV ketanserine. There may also be a role for corticosteroids, bisphosphanates, calcium channel blockers, and free radical scavengers (DMSO and N-acetylcysteine).

To prevent the occurrence of CRPS I after wrist fractures, vitamin C is recommended but not proven. A prospective randomized, controlled multicenter dose-response study by Zollinger et al. showed decreased rates of CRPS I in DRF patients who were treated with vitamin C for 50 days after injury. However, a 2015 meta-analysis of randomized controlled trials indicated a low overall quality of the evidence for vitamin C preventing the development of CRPS I in patients with DRF. Secondary prevention of CRPS I via use of regional anesthetic techniques such as brachial plexus blockade, epidural anesthesia, stellate ganglion blocks, and IV regional anesthesia with clonidine has yet to be shown.

Further Reading

Evaniew N, Mccarthy C, Kleinlugtenbelt YV, Ghert M, Bhandari M. Vitamin C to prevent complex regional pain syndrome in patients with distal radius fractures: a meta-analysis of randomized controlled trials. *J Orthop Trauma*. 2015;29(8):e235–241.

Perez RS, Zollinger PE, Dijkstra PU, Thomassen-Hilgersom IL, Zuurmond WW, Rosenbrand KC, Geertzen JH. Evidence based guidelines for complex regional pain syndrome type 1. *BMC Neurol*. 2010 Mar 31;10:20.

Zollinger PE, Tuinebreijer WE, Breederveld RS, Kreis RW. Can vitamin C prevent complex regional pain syndrome in patients with wrist fractures? A randomized, controlled, multicenter dose-response study. *J Bone Joint Surg Am*. 2007;89(7):1424–1431.

5

Arthroscopic Shoulder Surgery

M. Stephen Melton, James Kyunghoon Kim, and Karen C. Nielsen

Case Scenario

A 62-year-old, obese man presents for outpatient arthroscopic rotator cuff repair (RCR) and biceps tenodesis. He has a medical history significant for smoking, nonobstructive coronary artery disease, and controlled hypertension on lisinopril.

1. Introduction

Shoulder arthroscopy is a common elective ambulatory surgery procedure performed for a multitude of surgical indications, including rotator cuff tears, instability, and stiffness. Patients may present for surgery after acute or chronic injury. The spectrum of patient comorbidities reflects a diverse patient population from teenagers to elderly adults, and from the athletic to the inactive. Significant postoperative pain associated with these procedures necessitates an adequate multimodal analgesic plan to optimize patient satisfaction, recovery, and rehabilitation. Peripheral nerve blockade (PNB) is commonly performed for intraoperative anesthesia and/or postoperative analgesia. This chapter will review pertinent patient- and surgery-specific considerations for outpatient shoulder arthroscopy anesthesia and postoperative analgesia.

Further Reading

Jain NB, Higgins LD, Losina E, Collins J, Blazar PE, Katz JN. Epidemiology of musculoskeletal upper extremity ambulatory surgery in the United States. *BMC Musculoskelet Disord.* 2014;15(1):4.

Robinson JC, Brown TT, Whaley C, Bozic KJ. Consumer choice between hospital-based and freestanding facilities for arthroscopy: impact on prices, spending, and surgical complications. *J Bone Joint Surg Am.* 2015;97(18):1473–1481.

Warrender WJ, Syed UAM, Hammoud S, et al. Pain management after outpatient shoulder arthroscopy. *Am J Sports Med.* 2016;20(1):036354651666790.

2. Preoperative Evaluation: Patient-Related Considerations for Multimodal Perineural Analgesia

2.1. What are considerations for patients with cardiac history undergoing shoulder arthroscopy?

Patients with a history of cardiac disease should be evaluated and managed preoperatively in accordance with the American College of Cardiology/American Heart Association guidelines for noncardiac surgery. Decisions pertaining to anticoagulation and PNB should be managed according to these guidelines in addition to the American Society of Regional Anesthesia and Pain Medicine (ASRA) Evidence-Based Guidelines. Aspirin and nonsteroidal anti-inflammatory drugs (NSAIDs) do not have to be held prior to performing PNB. In some cardiac patients, aspirin should be continued perioperatively, if surgical bleeding risk allows. Consultation with the patient's cardiologist and surgeon is appropriate to make this determination. Herbal medications, which may influence bleeding, such as ginseng and ginkgo biloba, should be held.

Angiotensin converting enzyme inhibitors and angiotensin receptor blockers may be associated with a more profound degree of anesthesia-induced hypotension. Consideration should be given to holding these medications the morning of surgery. For shoulder surgery, the beach-chair position (BCP) with decreased venous return to the heart may exacerbate this hypotension. The physiology of the BCP presents a certain level of risk for cerebral hypotension. Avoidance of volatile anesthetics by utilizing ISB with propofol sedation and spontaneous respiration via a natural airway may reduce the risk of ischemic neurologic injury.

Further Reading

Horlocker TT, Wedel DJ, Rowlingson JC, et al. Regional anesthesia in the patient receiving antithrombotic or thrombolytic therapy: American Society of Regional Anesthesia and Pain Medicine Evidence-Based Guidelines (Third Edition). *Reg Anesth Pain Med.* 2010;35(1):64–101.

Koh JL, Levin SD, Chehab EL, Murphy GS. Neer Award 2012: cerebral oxygenation in the beach chair position: a prospective study on the effect of general anesthesia compared with regional anesthesia and sedation. *J Shoulder Elbow Surg.* 2013;22(10):1325–1331.

Fleisher LA, Fleischmann KE, Auerbach AD, et al. 2014 ACC/AHA Guideline on Perioperative Cardiovascular Evaluation and Management of Patients Undergoing Noncardiac Surgery. *J Am Coll Cardiol.* 2014;64(22):1–107.

Rohrbaugh M, Kentor ML, Orebaugh SL, Williams B. Outcomes of shoulder surgery in the sitting position with interscalene nerve block: a single-center series. *Reg Anesth Pain Med.* 2013;38(1):28–33.

2.2. What are pulmonary-specific concerns associated with shoulder arthroscopy?

If ISB is a part of the anesthesia plan, patients should be able to tolerate an approximate 25% decrease in pulmonary function secondary to phrenic nerve block and resultant hemidiaphragmatic paresis. In patients with moderate to severe pulmonary dysfunction, this risk may outweigh the benefit of ISB and continuous interscalene brachial plexus block (CISB).

Further Reading

Urmey WF, McDonald M. Hemidiaphragmatic paresis during interscalene brachial plexus block: effects on pulmonary function and chest wall mechanics. *Anesth Analg.* 1992;74(3):352–357.

2.3. What is the mechanism for hemidiaphragmatic paresis after ISB?

A potential disadvantage of ISB and CISB is a transient ipsilateral hemidiaphragmatic paresis from spread of LA to the phrenic nerve. Ipsilateral hemidiaphragmatic paresis inhibits normal lung expansion, as a result of the paralyzed hemidiaphragm moving in a paradoxical cephalad direction during inspiration. Previous studies have confirmed that concomitant paralysis of the ipsilateral hemidiaphragm is an unavoidable consequence of ISB when typical volumes of LA (10–45 mL) are used. Even ultra-low volumes of LA (5 mL) placed under ultrasound guidance are associated with a 45% incidence of hemidiaphragmatic paresis. Lower anesthetic concentrations may reduce the incidence of hemidiaphragmatic paresis. Five minutes after ISB and resultant hemidiaphragmatic paresis, Urmey and McDonald found that nonobese participants had a 27% decrease in forced vital capacity (FVC) and a 26% decrease in forced expiratory volume in 1 second (FEV1). Subsequent investigation in nonobese participants demonstrated that the magnitude of this reduction reached a plateau at 15 minutes with no significant change in FVC and FEV1 between 15 and 30 minutes. Further, ISB local anesthetic (LA) injection volume (20 mL versus 45 mL) produced no significant difference in onset or degree of pulmonary dysfunction over time. Extrafascial injection, as opposed to intrafascial injection between the fifth and sixth cervical roots, may be associated with reduced incidence of hemidiaphragmatic paresis and preservation of pulmonary function. Extrafascial CISB catheter tip location was associated with decreased incidence of hemidiaphragmatic paresis, but there was no difference in functional respiratory outcomes. Hemidiaphragmatic paresis is typically limited to LA duration of action. Fortunately, persistent phrenic nerve paresis is rare, with a reported incidence of 0.048% in one investigation. While symptomatic cervical spine disease was found to be a risk factor for the development of persistent phrenic nerve paresis, the etiology is multifactorial. Persistent phrenic nerve paresis remains a perplexing complication of ISB, and many questions remain unanswered.

Further Reading

Albrecht E, Bathory I, Fournier N, Jacot-Guillarmod A, Farron A, Brull R. Reduced hemidiaphragmatic paresis with extrafascial compared with conventional intrafascial tip placement for continuous interscalene brachial plexus block: a randomized, controlled, double-blind trial. *Br J Anaesth*. 2017;118(4):586–592.

al-Kaisy AA, Chan VW, Perlas A. Respiratory effects of low-dose bupivacaine interscalene block. *Br J Anaesth*. 1999;82(2):217–220.

Borgeat A, Perschak H, Bird P, Hodler J, Gerber C. Patient-controlled interscalene analgesia with ropivacaine 0.2% versus patient-controlled intravenous analgesia after major shoulder surgery: effects on diaphragmatic and respiratory function. *Anesthesiology*. 2000;92(1):102–108.

Cuvillon P, Le Sache F, Demattei C, et al. Continuous interscalene brachial plexus nerve block prolongs unilateral diaphragmatic dysfunction. *Anaesth Crit Care Pain Med*. June 2016.

Jules-Elysee K, Reid SC, Kahn RL, Edmonds CR, Urban MK. Prolonged diaphragm dysfunction after interscalene brachial plexus block and shoulder surgery: a prospective observational pilot study. *Br J Anaesth*. 2014;112(5):950–951.

Pakala SR, Beckman JD, Lyman S, Zayas VM. Cervical spine disease is a risk factor for persistent phrenic nerve paresis following interscalene nerve block. *Reg Anesth Pain Med*. 2013;38(3):239–242.

Palhais N, Brull R, Kern C, et al. Extrafascial injection for interscalene brachial plexus block reduces respiratory complications compared with a conventional intrafascial injection: a randomized, controlled, double-blind trial. Colvin L, ed. *Br J Anaesth*. 2016;116(4):531–537.

Pere P, Pitkänen M, Rosenberg PH, Bjorkenheim JM, Linden H, Salorinne Y, Tuominen M: Effect of continuous interscalene brachial plexus block on diaphragm motion and on ventilatory function. *Acta Anaesthesiol Scand*. 1992;36:53–57.

Riazi S, Carmichael N, Awad I, Holtby RM, McCartney CJL. Effect of local anaesthetic volume (20 vs 5 ml) on the efficacy and respiratory consequences of ultrasound-guided interscalene brachial plexus block. *Br J Anaesth*. 2008;101(4):549–556.

Sala-Blanch X, Lázaro JR, Correa J, Gómez-Fernandez M. Phrenic nerve block caused by interscalene brachial plexus block: effects of digital pressure and a low volume of local anesthetic. *Reg Anesth Pain Med*. 1999;24(3):231–235.

Sinha SK, Abrams JH, Barnett JT, et al. Decreasing the local anesthetic volume from 20 to 10 mL for ultrasound-guided interscalene block at the cricoid level does not reduce the incidence of hemidiaphragmatic paresis. *Reg Anesth Pain Med*. 2011;36(1):17–20.

Urmey WF, Gloeggler PJ. Pulmonary function changes during interscalene brachial plexus block: effects of decreasing local anesthetic injection volume. *Reg Anesth*. 1993;18(4):244–249.

Urmey WF, McDonald M. Hemidiaphragmatic paresis during interscalene brachial plexus block: effects on pulmonary function and chest wall mechanics. *Anesth Analg*. 1992;74(3):352–357.

Urmey WF, Talts KH, Sharrock NE. One hundred percent incidence of hemidiaphragmatic paresis associated with interscalene brachial plexus anesthesia as diagnosed by ultrasonography. *Anesth Analg*. 1991;72(4):498–503.

Wong AK, Keeney LG, Chen L, Williams R, Liu J, Elkassabany NM. Effect of local anesthetic concentration (0.2% vs 0.1% ropivacaine) on pulmonary function, and analgesia after ultrasound-guided interscalene brachial plexus block: a randomized controlled study. *Pain Med*. 2016;17(12):2397–2403.

2.4. Will pulmonary dysfunction be more pronounced in obese subjects after ISB?

In obese patients, due to restrictive pulmonary mechanics, the perception of reduced breathing associated with hemidiaphragmatic paresis may be more profound. This may be exacerbated in obese patients undergoing general anesthesia with a volatile anesthetic in conjunction with ISB. Specific benefits of ISB, including avoidance of volatile anesthetics, potential avoidance of airway manipulation, and reduced opioid consumption, must be weighed against the risks of ISB in obese patients.

When compared with a nonobese group, obese subjects undergoing ISB and sedation for arthroscopic shoulder surgery demonstrated greater reductions in pulmonary function. Lung parameters decreased 28% to 40% in obese participants compared with 21% to 31% in the normal-weight participants. Neither time (30 minutes vs. postanesthesia care unit [PACU]) nor position (sitting vs. supine) affected this relationship. Changes in pulmonary function were not associated with increased breathlessness, and despite their persistence in the PACU, there were no delays in readiness for discharge or respiratory-related issues identified during overnight stays or follow-up phone calls.

Further Reading

Melton MS, Monroe HE, Qi W, Lewis SL, Nielsen KC, Klein SM: Effect of interscalene brachial plexus block on the pulmonary function of obese patients: a prospective, observational cohort study. *Anesth Analg*. 2017; 125:313–319.

2.5. How will obstructive sleep apnea syndrome affect preoperative planning?

In patients with moderate to severe obstructive sleep apnea (OSA), the appropriateness of shoulder arthroscopy and rotator cuff repair (RCR) in the outpatient setting may be questioned due to the potential increased risk of postoperative respiratory adverse events. While the effects of ISB/CISB and resultant hemidiaphragmatic paresis on OSA are unknown, the possible avoidance of general anesthesia (airway manipulation, volatile anesthetics, etc.) and reduced opioid consumption achieved with regional anesthesia as part of a multimodal postoperative analgesic regimen are beneficial in patients with OSA.

Further Reading

Borgeat A, Perschak H, Bird P, Hodler J, Gerber C. Patient-controlled interscalene analgesia with ropivacaine 0.2% versus patient-controlled intravenous analgesia after major shoulder surgery: effects on diaphragmatic and respiratory function. *Anesthesiology*. 2000;92(1):102–108.

Joshi GP, Ankichetty SP, Gan TJ, Chung F. Society for Ambulatory Anesthesia consensus statement on preoperative selection of adult patients with obstructive sleep apnea scheduled for ambulatory surgery. *Anesth Analg*. 2012;115:1060–1068.

2.6. What if a patient has preexisting numbness or tingling in the hand and/or cervical spine disease?

A history and physical exam that document baseline neurologic assessment of the extremity are important. Cervical spine imaging, if available, should be reviewed. For some patients, the preoperative workup may include an electromyogram, while for others this will not be available or will not be necessary. The etiology of neurologic symptoms should be evaluated and discussed with the patient and surgeon. Decisions to incorporate or exclude PNB as part of the anesthesia plan should be made with the patient and surgeon, after the etiology or potential etiology is understood. Preexisting neuropathy may not be worsened by PNB, but outcomes tend to be worse when neurologic dysfunction occurs in the presence of preexisting neuropathy. It is important to review with the patient the possibility of postoperative neurologic symptoms (PONS) such as numbness, tingling, and/or weakness in the surgical extremity, which may occur after surgery, with or without ISB. The incidence of PONS after regional anesthesia in the literature is multifactorial, and reported numbers vary based on block type, procedure type, patient reported versus elicitation of symptoms, absence or presence of physical exam, follow-up, means of diagnosis, and so forth. In a study analyzing 1505 consecutive patients receiving continuous interscalene analgesia, 106 (7.3%, 95% CI 6.0%–8.7%) patients reported numbness or tingling in the arm or side of the neck, weakness in the hand, or pain in the forearm/hand persisting beyond 1 month. Forty-seven (3.2%, 95% CI 2.4%–4.3%) patients' symptoms persisted beyond 3 months, 26 (1.8%, 95% CI 1.2%–2.6%) patients' symptoms persisted beyond 6 months, and 11 (0.7%, 95% CI 0.4%–1.4%) patients' symptoms persisted beyond 12 months. Of these 11 patients, 6 had a clear cause unrelated to the nerve block, and in the remaining 5 the etiology was undetermined. In a study by Borgeat et al., minor neurologic complications (paresthesias, dysesthesias, pain not related to surgery) after ISB for shoulder surgery were observed in 14.0%, 7.9%, 3.9%, 0.9%, and 0.2% of patients at 10 days, 1, 3, 6, and 9 months, respectively. Two patients (0.2%) had sensory-motor deficit, which necessitated 19 and 28 weeks to recover, with electromyography suggestive of partial axonotmesis. Persistent paresthesias, dysesthesia, or pain not related to surgery after ISB need to be evaluated as specific treatment may be required.

Further Reading

Borgeat A, Ekatodramis G, Kalberer F, Benz C. Acute and nonacute complications associated with interscalene block and shoulder surgery: a prospective study. Anesthesiology. 2001;95:875–880.

Fredrickson MJ, Leightley P, Wong A, Chaddock M, Abeysekera A, Frampton C. An analysis of 1505 consecutive patients receiving continuous interscalene analgesia at home: a multicentre prospective safety study. *Anaesthesia*. 2016;71(4):373–379.

Neal JM, Barrington MJ, Brull R, et al. The Second ASRA Practice Advisory on Neurologic Complications Associated With Regional Anesthesia and Pain Medicine: Executive Summary 2015. Reg Anesth Pain Med. 2015 Sep-Oct;40(5):401-30.

2.7. What should be considered when evaluating patients for continuous perineural infusions?

Preoperative decisions for perineural interscalene catheter placement include surgical, medical, and social considerations. Postoperative analgesia should anticipate postoperative pain demand and complement surgical- and patient-specific issues. After minor arthroscopic shoulder surgery, the addition of a continuous interscalene ropivacaine infusion to a single-injection ISB demonstrated a reduction in pain scores during the first 24 hours and opioid consumption during the first 2 days. In patients undergoing RCR, CISB has demonstrated improved analgesia, fewer sleep disturbances, increased patient satisfaction, and reduced opioid requirements and opioid related side effects as compared with single-injection ISB up to 7 days. After shoulder adhesive capsulitis manipulation, a pilot study found that CISB was associated with lower average/dynamic pain scores, decreased opioid requirements, fewer awakenings from pain, and improved shoulder range of motion during and up to 12 weeks.

While surgery-specific factors might make CISB attractive, medical circumstances, including but not limited to anticoagulation, pulmonary function, obesity, and OSA, must be suitable and stable for continuous perineural analgesia in the home environment. Social elements, however, may not allow for the safety of LA infusion at home: patients with cognitive dysfunction, which may make assessment of pain and complications difficult; unreliability of patients (patients with drug dependency or psychiatric disorders may not follow instructions); patients without a home support system (patients living alone or without a continual caretaker, in a dorm, or patients caring for a dependent spouse); and patients in whom the continuous infusion may make ambulation difficult. Finally, does a current or heightened risk of postoperative neurologic symptoms exclude a potentially more invasive continuous catheter technique and render continuous sensory block unfavorable? Risks and benefits of continuous interscalene analgesia must be carefully evaluated, after discussion with the patient and surgical team.

Further Reading

Borgeat A, Schappi B, Biasca N, Gerber C. Patient-controlled analgesia after major shoulder surgery: patient-controlled interscalene analgesia versus patient-controlled analgesia. *Anesthesiology*. 1997;87(6):1343–1347.

Fredrickson MJ, Ball CM, Dalgleish AJ. Analgesic effectiveness of a continuous versus single-injection interscalene block for minor arthroscopic shoulder surgery. *Reg Anesth Pain Med*. 2010;35(1):28–33.

Greengrass RA, Nielsen KC: Management of peripheral nerve block catheters at home. *Int Anesthesiol Clin*. 2005;43:79–87.

Ilfeld BM, Morey TE, Wright TW, Chidgey LK. Continuous interscalene brachial plexus block for postoperative pain control at home: a randomized, double-blinded, placebo-controlled study. *Anesth Analg. 2003 Apr;96(4):1089-95.*

Malhotra N, Madison SJ, Ward SR, Mariano ER, Loland VJ, Ilfeld BM. Continuous interscalene nerve block following adhesive capsulitis manipulation. *Reg Anesth Pain Med.* 2013;38(2):171–172.

Neal JM, Barrington MJ, Brull R, et al. The Second ASRA Practice Advisory on Neurologic Complications Associated With Regional Anesthesia and Pain Medicine: Executive Summary 2015. Reg Anesth Pain Med. 2015 Sep-Oct;40(5):401-30.

Salviz EA, Xu D, Frulla A, et al. Continuous interscalene block in patients having outpatient rotator cuff repair surgery: a prospective randomized trial. *Anesth Analg.* 2013; 117(6):1485–1492.

3. Intraoperative Management: Surgical/Regional Anesthetic Considerations for Multimodal Perineural Analgesia

3.1. What are anesthetic options for patients undergoing shoulder arthroscopy and RCR?

Comorbidities, airway, aspiration risk, anticoagulation status, preexisting neuropathies, patient position, and case duration are critical factors in evaluating anesthetic management for shoulder surgery. Most commonly, surgery for RCR is performed under a general anesthetic or sedation in combination with an ISB. ISB is typically performed at the C5-C6 root/superior trunk level of the brachial plexus. It provides both brachial (C5-C7) and cervical (C3-C4) plexus blockade. Incomplete blockade of the inferior trunk (C8, T1) is not uncommon. ISB is performed as a single injection or as a continuous catheter technique under ultrasound or nerve stimulation guidance, or a combination of the two. Benefits include potential avoidance of volatile anesthetics, reduced opioid consumption and opioid-related side effects, and improved postoperative analgesia and rehabilitation. Alternative PNB techniques available for postoperative analgesia are discussed later in the chapter.

Further Reading

Franco CD, Williams JM. Ultrasound-guided interscalene block: reevaluation of the "stoplight" sign and clinical implications. *Reg Anesth Pain Med.* 2016;41(4):452–459.

Hadzic A, Williams BA, Karaca PE, et al. For outpatient rotator cuff surgery, nerve block anesthesia provides superior same-day recovery over general anesthesia. *Anesthesiology.* 2005;102(5):1001–1007.

Malhotra N, Madison SJ, Ward SR, Mariano ER, Loland VJ, Ilfeld BM. Continuous interscalene nerve block following adhesive capsulitis manipulation. *Reg Anesth Pain Med.* 2013;38(2):171–172.

3.2. What side effects and complications are associated with ISB?

Common side effects associated with ISB/CISB result from LA spread to adjacent nerves, including (1) the phrenic nerve, resulting in diaphragmatic paresis; (2) the recurrent laryngeal nerve, resulting in hoarseness/difficulty swallowing; and (3) the superficial cervical plexus, resulting in Horner's syndrome with nasal congestion, ipsilateral partial ptosis, miosis, and conjunctival hyperemia. These side effects, while most prevalent with the initial bolus for surgical anesthesia, may persist with continuous perineural infusions and should be discussed with patients preoperatively. Motor-sensory block of the hand has been described as unsatisfactory by patients with an ISB/CISB. Potential complications include transient/permanent nerve injury, persistent phrenic nerve paresis, pneumothorax, bleeding, infection, epidural/spinal/subdural injection, intravascular injection, and LA toxicity. Contralateral spread has also been described with CISB.

Further Reading

Dooley J, Fingerman M, Melton S, Klein SM. Contralateral local anesthetic spread from an outpatient interscalene catheter. *Can J Anesth/J Can Anesth.* 2010;57(10):936–939.

Fredrickson MJ, Abeysekera A, Price DJ, Wong AC. Patient-initiated mandatory boluses for ambulatory continuous interscalene analgesia: an effective strategy for optimizing analgesia and minimizing side-effects. *Br J Anaesth.* 2011;106(2):239–245.

Fredrickson MJ, Price DJ. Analgesic effectiveness of ropivacaine 0.2% vs 0.4% via an ultrasound-guided C5–6 root/superior trunk perineural ambulatory catheter. *Br J Anaesth. 2009 Sep;103(3):434-9.*

Shin H-J, Na H-S, Oh A-Y, et al. A prospective, randomized and controlled study of interscalene brachial plexus block for arthroscopic shoulder surgery: a comparison of C5 and conventional approach, a CONSORT-compliant article. *Medicine (Baltimore).* 2016;95(37):e4921.

3.3. What alternatives are there to classical ISB?

In an effort to potentially reduce these side effects, alternative PNB techniques or approaches to the brachial plexus may be performed. The C5 approach for ISB provides effective postoperative pain after arthroscopic shoulder surgery for rotator cuff tears and minimizes lower brachial plexus (C7, C8, and T1) blockade, avoiding prolonged numbness and weakness of the arm/hand. Low-dose interscalene approaches at C7 or supraclavicular approaches may reduce the possibility of hemidiaphragmatic paresis, but they do not exclude this possibility. Low interscalene, supraclavicular approaches may sacrifice the analgesia in an effort to reduce potential phrenic nerve paresis. Alternatively, suprascapular nerve blocks, combined supraclavicular and suprascapular nerve blocks, or combined suprascapular and axillary nerve blocks (shoulder block) of varying approaches may be performed. In patients undergoing general anesthesia for arthroscopic shoulder surgery, combined ultrasound-guided supraclavicular and suprascapular (suprascapular groove) nerve blocks demonstrated equivalent postoperative pain scores at 6, 12, and 24 hours; similar time to first request for morphine; and similar total morphine consumption during the first 24 hours compared with ISB. Combined ultrasound-guided suprascapular and axillary nerve blocks provided nonequivalent analgesia compared with ISB with increased mean opioids intraoperatively and in the PACU, higher pain scores in the PACU and at the 6-hour time point, but lower pain scores at the next data collection time point at 24 hours. Mean opioid consumption was not reported at 6- and 24-hour time points. There were no differences at 7 days.

Ultrasound-guided suprascapular nerve block alone, using an anterior approach, in patients undergoing arthroscopic shoulder surgery demonstrated noninferior pain control, superior unimpaired grip strength, and an absence of ISB-related side effects including hoarseness, Horner's syndrome, and dyspnea, compared with ISB, and subjects reported greater satisfaction and were more likely to recommend this anesthetic technique. When compared with ISB placed with neurostimulation, suprascapular nerve block performed intraoperatively by the surgical team utilizing a landmark-based technique was associated with greater pain and opioid consumption in the PACU, but there was no difference in mean pain scores or opioid consumption at other time points (6 hours, postoperative days [] 1, 2, and 7 after surgery). Of note, successful continuous suprascapular nerve catheters, as an analgesic supplement to single-injection supraclavicular nerve blocks, were described in case reports of 2 patients after shoulder arthroscopy. An additional stated advantage of suprascapular and axillary nerve blocks is the demonstrated hand sparing, a source of patient dissatisfaction. However, if patients are given preoperative counseling regarding the presence of this side effect, a notable decrease in patient satisfaction does not occur. Furthermore, a continuous interscalene ropivacaine infusion has a low incidence of significant distal motor block, as patients can usually use the operative hand on POD 1. When questioned about dissatisfaction of an ambulatory CISB with ropivacaine 0.2%, only 2 of 100 patients reported arm weakness.

Combined infraclavicular-suprascapular blocks have also been proposed as a potential diaphragm-sparing technique. The infraclavicular approach targets the posterior and lateral cords, which would anesthetize the axillary nerve (anterior/posterior shoulder joint innervation), as well as the subscapular and lateral pectoral nerves (anterior shoulder joint innervation), whereas the suprascapular nerve block anesthetizes the posterior shoulder. Future randomized trials are required to validate the efficacy of this combined approach for shoulder surgery analgesia. Finally, selective targeting of shoulder innervation using intermuscular plane injections such as the subscapularis and sub-omohyoid planes has been proposed. Dispersion of LA along the ventral surface of subscapularis muscle blocks both axillary and subscapular nerves; below the sub-omohyoid, the suprascapular nerve; and the addition of the pectoral nerve (PECS-1) block to anesthetize the lateral pectoral nerve, if the acromio-clavicular joint is being operated upon. Combined subscapularis plane and sub-omohyoid plane injections were proposed to serve as an alternative to peripheral nerve blocks for shoulder analgesia, with minimal impact on phrenic nerve function. However, further comparative trials will be needed to evaluate this method in relation to other analgesic modalities.

Further Reading

Desroches A, Klouche S, Schlur C, Bauer T, Waitzenegger T, Hardy P. Suprascapular nerve block versus interscalene block as analgesia after arthroscopic rotator cuff repair: a randomized controlled noninferiority trial. *Arthroscopy*. 2016;32(11):2203–2209.

Elsharkawy HA, Abd-Elsayed AA, Cummings KC, Soliman LM. Analgesic efficacy and technique of ultrasound-guided suprascapular nerve catheters after shoulder arthroscopy. *Ochsner J*. 2014;14(2):259–263.

Fredrickson M, Borgeat A. Continuous interscalene block is preferable to the "shoulder block" for postoperative analgesia following shoulder surgery. *Anaesth Intensive Care*. 2008;36(1):119–120; author reply 120–121.

Koh WU, Kim HJ, Park HS, Choi WJ, Yang HS, Ro YJ. A randomised controlled trial comparing continuous supraclavicular and interscalene brachial plexus blockade for open rotator cuff surgery. *Anaesthesia*. 2016;71(6):692–699.

Marty P, Rontes O, Delbos A. A comparison of combined suprascapular and axillary nerve blocks to interscalene block: interpret with caution. *Reg Anesth Pain Med*. 2017;42(2):273–274. doi:10.1097/AAP.0000000000000551

Matsumoto D, Suenaga N, Oizumi N, Hisada Y, Minami A. A new nerve block procedure for the suprascapular nerve based on a cadaveric study. *J Shoulder Elbow Surg*. 2009;18(4):607–611. doi:10.1016/j.jse.2009.01.005

Pitombo PF, Barros RM, Matos MA, Módolo NSP. Selective suprascapular and axillary nerve block provides adequate analgesia and minimal motor block: comparison with interscalene block. *Braz J Anesthesiol*. 2013;63(1):45–51.

Price D. It's not just about the diaphragm. *Reg Anesth Pain Med*. 2017;42(3):416–417. doi:10.1097/AAP.0000000000000597

Price D. Optimizing the combined suprascapular and axillary nerve (SSAX) block. *Reg Anesth Pain Med*. 2017;42(1):122. doi:10.1097/AAP.0000000000000518

Renes SH, van Geffen GJ, Rettig HC, Gielen MJ, Scheffer GJ. Minimum effective volume of local anesthetic for shoulder analgesia by ultrasound-guided block at root C7 with assessment of pulmonary function. *Reg Anesth Pain Med*. 2010;35(6):529–534.

Reply to Dr Price. *Reg Anesth Pain Med*. 2017;42(1):123. doi:10.1097/AAP.0000000000000530

Reply to Marty et al. *Reg Anesth Pain Med*. 2017;42(2):274–275. doi:10.1097/AAP.0000000000000557

Ryu T, Kil BT, Kim JH. Comparison between ultrasound-guided supraclavicular and interscalene brachial plexus blocks in patients undergoing arthroscopic shoulder surgery: a prospective, randomized, parallel study. *Medicine (Baltimore)*. 2015;94(40):e1726.

Shin H-J, Na H-S, Oh A-Y, et al. A prospective, randomized and controlled study of interscalene brachial plexus block for arthroscopic shoulder surgery: a comparison of C5 and conventional approach, a CONSORT-compliant article. *Medicine (Baltimore)*. 2016;95(37):e4921.

Siegenthaler A, Moriggl B, Mlekusch S, et al. Ultrasound-guided suprascapular nerve block, description of a novel supraclavicular approach. *Reg Anesth Pain Med*. 2012;37(3):325–328. doi:10.1097/AAP.0b013e3182409168

Sondekoppam RV, Lopera-Velasquez L-M, Naik L, Ganapathy S. Subscapularis and sub-omohyoid plane blocks: an alternative to peripheral nerve blocks for shoulder analgesia. *Br J Anaesth*. 2016;117(6):831–832. doi:10.1093/bja/aew370

Trabelsi W, Ben Gabsia A, Lebbi A, Sammoud W, Labbène I, Ferjani M. Suprascapular block associated with supraclavicular block: an alternative to isolated interscalene block for analgesia in shoulder instability surgery? *Orthop Traumatol Surg Res*. 2017;103(1):77–83.

Tran DQ, Aliste J, Elgueta MF, Finlayson RJ. Reply to Dr Price. *Reg Anesth Pain Med*. 2017;42(3):417–418. doi:10.1097/AAP.0000000000000582

Tran DQH, Elgueta MF, Aliste J, Finlayson RJ. Diaphragm-sparing nerve blocks for shoulder surgery.—PubMed—NCBI. *Reg Anesth Pain Med*. 2017;42(1):32–38.

Verelst P, van Zundert A. Respiratory impact of analgesic strategies for shoulder surgery. *Reg Anesth Pain Med*. 2013;38(1):50–53.

Wiegel M, Moriggl B, Schwarzkopf P, Petroff D, Reske AW. Anterior suprascapular nerve block versus interscalene brachial plexus block for shoulder surgery in the outpatient setting: a randomized controlled patient- and assessor-blinded trial. *Reg Anesth Pain Med*. 2017;42(3):310–318.

3.4. What are the disadvantages of alternative techniques?

As compared with an ISB, selective blockade of the suprascapular and axillary nerves will leave several nerves unblocked: upper subscapular (teres major), lower subscapular, thoracodorsal (latissimus dorsi), and lateral and medial pectoral nerves, which are involved in most shoulder surgeries. As a result, selective blockade of the suprascapular and axillary nerves does not provide dense motor blockade of the upper arm and shoulder girdle necessary for surgical anesthesia and, potentially, adequate postoperative analgesia and protection of the surgical repair. However, in patients undergoing total shoulder arthroplasty, mean pain scores and 24-hour opioid consumption for continuous interscalene, supraclavicular, and suprascapular blocks, respectively, were not significantly different. Fewer adverse effects (Horner's syndrome, dyspnea, and hoarseness) were noted in the suprascapular group when compared with the interscalene group.

Further Reading

Auyong DB, Yuan SC, Choi DS, Pahang JA, Slee AE, Hanson NA. A double-blind randomized comparison of continuous interscalene, supraclavicular, and suprascapular blocks for total shoulder arthroplasty. *Reg Anesth Pain Med*. 2017;42(3):302–309.

Desroches A, Klouche S, Schlur C, Bauer T, Waitzenegger T, Hardy P. Suprascapular nerve block versus interscalene block as analgesia after arthroscopic rotator cuff repair: a randomized controlled noninferiority trial. *Arthroscopy*. 2016;32(11):2203–2209.

Elsharkawy HA, Abd-Elsayed AA, Cummings KC, Soliman LM. Analgesic efficacy and technique of ultrasound-guided suprascapular nerve catheters after shoulder arthroscopy. *Ochsner J*. 2014;14(2):259–263.

Fredrickson M, Borgeat A. Continuous interscalene block is preferable to the "shoulder block" for postoperative analgesia following shoulder surgery. *Anaesth Intensive Care*. 2008;36(1):119–120; author reply 120–121.

Wiegel M, Moriggl B, Schwarzkopf P, Petroff D, Reske AW. Anterior suprascapular nerve block versus interscalene brachial plexus block for shoulder surgery in the outpatient setting: a randomized controlled patient- and assessor-blinded trial. *Reg Anesth Pain Med*. 2017;42(3):310–318.

3.5. What volume and concentration should be utilized to maximize postoperative analgesia associated with single-injection and continuous catheter ISB techniques?

Single-injection block duration is influenced by both LA volume and concentration, a finding in opposition to the current trend to use lower volumes for ultrasound-guided regional anesthesia. Increasing the volume of ropivacaine 0.375% from 10 to 40 mL was estimated to increase median (quartiles) block duration from 10.0 (9.5–11.5) to 15.0 (10.75–21) hours. Similarly, increasing the concentration of 20 mL ropivacaine from 0.375% to 0.75% was estimated to increase median (quartiles) block duration from 10.75 (9.75–14.0) to 13.75 (10.5–21.0) hours. Nonetheless, 5 mL of 0.5% ropivacaine did not reduce block quality as assessed by pain scores, sleep quality, and total morphine consumption up to 24 hours after surgery in comparison with 20 mL of 0.5% ropivacaine. However, ISB was not utilized as a surgical block.

Successful surgical anesthesia with ultrasound-guided ISB for shoulder arthroscopy can be accomplished with 5 mL of 0.75% ropivacaine (100%, 95% CI 74.1%–100%) without clinically apparent deterioration in block onset or duration. However, because the lower limit of the CI may be associated with a 25% failure rate, no meaningful statement regarding any difference in block duration between 5 mL or >5 mL of LA can be made from this study. Additionally, a low volume of LA may not yield adequate motor relaxation in all patients whereas a higher volume of LA may result in a more expeditious onset and more consistent duration of blockade.

When used for surgical anesthesia for shoulder arthroscopies in the ambulatory setting, a 20-mL volume in an ultrasound-guided ISB preserved greater handgrip strength on the ipsilateral side in the PACU compared with 40 mL without significant decrease in block success, duration of analgesia, and patient satisfaction. While readiness for surgical anesthesia was achieved sooner with 20 mL 1% ropivacaine, postoperative analgesia mean duration (SD) was similar with 20 mL of 3 ropivacaine concentrations (11.5 [5] h, 10.7 [2] h, and 10 [2.4] h with 0.5%, 0.75%, and 1% concentrations, respectively). Similar efficacy for surgical anesthesia and postoperative analgesia has been demonstrated between 30-mL equal concentrations of ropivacaine and bupivacaine, and increasing the concentration of ropivacaine from 0.5% to 0.75% failed to improve the onset or duration (mean >12 hours) of ISB.

In an effort to determine the volume and concentration of ropivacaine that would prevent recovery room pain after shoulder surgery under general anesthesia and CISB, the ED(vol)50/ED(vol)95 of ropivacaine 0.5%, was determined to be 2.7/20.5 mL, and the ED(conc)50/ED(conc)95 of ropivacaine 20 mL was 0.15/0.34%. As such, 20 mL of 0.375% ropivacaine (ED[vol]95 and ED[conc]95) prevented recovery room pain in approximately 95% of patients. If sonographic images and/or needle-to-nerve or catheter-to-nerve proximity are less than ideal, such that LA deposition is less accurate, a larger volume of LA may be required. With the administration of a larger volume of LA, placement accuracy may be less critical.

Further Reading

Casati A, Fanelli G, Aldegheri G, et al. Interscalene brachial plexus anaesthesia with 0.5%, 0.75% or 1% ropivacaine: a double-blind comparison with 2% mepivacaine. *Br J Anaesth.* 1999;83(6):872–875. doi:10.1093/bja/83.6.872

Fredrickson MJ, Abeysekera A, White R. Randomized study of the effect of local anesthetic volume and concentration on the duration of peripheral nerve blockade. *Reg Anesth Pain Med.* 2012;37(5):495–501. doi:10.1097/AAP.0b013e3182580fd0

Fredrickson MJ, Smith KR, Wong AC. Importance of volume and concentration for ropivacaine interscalene block in preventing recovery room pain and minimizing motor block after shoulder surgery. *Anesthesiology.* 2010;112(6):1374–1381. doi:10.1097/ALN.0b013e3181d6929d

Gautier P, Vandepitte C, Ramquet C, DeCoopman M, Xu D, Hadzic A. The minimum effective anesthetic volume of 0.75% ropivacaine in ultrasound-guided interscalene brachial plexus block. *Anesth Analg.* 2011;113(4):951–955. doi:10.1213/ANE.0b013e31822b876f

Klein SM, Greengrass RA, Steele SM, D'Ercole FJ, Speer KP, Gleason DH, DeLong ER, Warner DS: A comparison of 0.5% bupivacaine, 0.5% ropivacaine, and 0.75% ropivacaine for interscalene brachial plexus block. *Anesthe Analg.* 1998;87:1316–1319.

Maalouf DB, Dorman SM, Sebeo J, et al. Prospective, randomized double-blind study: does decreasing interscalene nerve block volume for surgical anesthesia in ambulatory shoulder surgery offer same-day patient recovery advantages? *Reg Anesth Pain Med.* 2016;41(4):438–444. doi:10.1097/AAP.0000000000000418

Riazi S, Carmichael N, Awad I, Holtby RM, McCartney CJL. Effect of local anaesthetic volume (20 vs 5 ml) on the efficacy and respiratory consequences of ultrasound-guided interscalene brachial plexus block. *Br J Anaesth.* 2008;101(4):549–556. doi:10.1093/bja/aen229

3.6. Are there perineural LA additives that can be utilized to prolong postoperative analgesia associated with PNB?

In order to provide evidence for a perineural mechanism of action, studies involving perineural LA additives to prolong postoperative analgesia should ideally comprise perineural treatment groups, intravenous systemic control groups, and saline control groups. Further, such additives should be preservative-free. Many trials to date investigating perineural additives are conflicting in terms of these additives' efficacy to prolong postoperative analgesia and their systemic or perineural mechanism of action. Certainly, the idea of achieving extended analgesia with a single-injection technique is attractive as compared with the disadvantages of continuous catheter techniques, including time for placement, management, follow-up, leakage, catheter disconnection, pump malfunction, and cost. Research is ongoing into the combined administration of midazolam-clonidine-buprenorphine-dexamethasone to ropivacaine for ISB in shoulder surgery. In terms of perineural dexamethasone administered in combination with LA, conflicting results on its site of action, potential neurotoxicity, and off-label use support the intravenous administration of dexamethasone as a suitable alternative to improve postoperative analgesia following arthroscopic shoulder surgery. Interestingly, a common preoperative antiemetic 4-mg intravenous dose of dexamethasone was shown to be comparable to a 10-mg dose in its systemic analgesic effect in patients undergoing shoulder arthroscopy with ISB.

Further Reading

Chalifoux F, Colin F, St-Pierre P, Godin N, Brulotte V. Low dose intravenous dexamethasone (4 mg and 10 mg) significantly prolongs the analgesic duration of single-shot interscalene block after arthroscopic shoulder surgery: a prospective randomized placebo-controlled study. *Can J Anesth/J Can Anesth*. 2017;64(3):280–289. doi:10.1007/s12630-016-0796-6

Desmet M, Vanneste B, Reynvoet M, et al. A randomised controlled trial of intravenous dexamethasone combined with interscalene brachial plexus blockade for shoulder surgery. *Anaesthesia*. 2015;70(10):1180–1185. doi:10.1111/anae.13156

Ilfeld BM. Continuous peripheral nerve blocks: an update of the published evidence and comparison with novel, alternative analgesic modalities. *Anesth Analg*. 2017;124(1):308–335. doi:10.1213/ANE.0000000000001581

Neal JM, Rathmell JP, Rowlingson JC. Publishing studies that involve "off-label" use of drugs: formalizing Regional Anesthesia and Pain Medicine's policy. *Reg Anesth Pain Med*. 2009;34(5):391–392.

Williams BA, Ibinson JW, Mangione MP, Scanlan RL, Cohen PZ. Clinical benchmarks regarding multimodal peripheral nerve blocks for postoperative analgesia: observations regarding combined perineural midazolam-clonidine-buprenorphine-dexamethasone. *Pain Med*. 2015;16(1):1–6. doi:10.1111/pme.12599

YaDeau JT, Gordon MA, Goytizolo EA, et al. Buprenorphine, clonidine, dexamethasone, and ropivacaine for interscalene nerve blockade: a prospective, randomized, blinded, ropivacaine dose-response study. *Pain Med*. 2016;17(5):940–960. doi:10.1093/pm/pnv010

3.7. How do surgical position and anesthetic choice affect intraoperative blood pressure management?

Requests for blood pressure reduction in an effort to reduce bleeding and obscuring arthroscopic visualization are not uncommon. In the BCP, blood pressure readings at the arm may not reflect postural cerebral perfusion. The brachial mean arterial pressure and the estimated temporal mean arterial pressure ratio decrease as an anesthetized patient is placed into the BCP. Systolic blood pressure reduction no lower than 90 mmHg and/or systolic blood pressure and mean arterial pressure reduction no greater than 20% of baseline is typically recommended to maintain adequate cerebral perfusion and prevent catastrophic events such as cerebral ischemia. Studies suggest that patients may be able to safely tolerate a reduction in blood pressure greater than current recommendations. In patients undergoing shoulder surgery under general anesthesia with ISB, BCP was associated with diminished cerebral autoregulation as compared with the lateral decubitus position, but not with a difference in cognitive outcome. While studies have demonstrated the incidence of postoperative neurocognitive deficit is low (overall incidence 0.004%), case reports have described catastrophic neurocognitive complications after shoulder surgery in the BCP. Cerebral oximetry can provide noninvasive, real-time measurement of relative and absolute hemoglobin oxygen saturation in the cerebral cortex. Despite adequate mean arterial pressures, patients under general anesthesia with volatile anesthetics demonstrated substantial cerebral desaturation events, unlike sedated patients with ISB. Thus, the use of ISB along with sedation and spontaneous respiration via a natural airway may reduce the risk of ischemic neurologic injury.

Further Reading

Gillespie R, Shishani Y, Streit J, et al. The safety of controlled hypotension for shoulder arthroscopy in the beach-chair position. *J Bone Joint Surg Am*. 2012;94(14):1284–1290. doi:10.2106/JBJS.J.01550

Koh JL, Levin SD, Chehab EL, Murphy GS. Neer Award 2012: cerebral oxygenation in the beach chair position: a prospective study on the effect of general anesthesia compared with regional anesthesia and sedation. *J Shoulder Elbow Surg*. 2013;22(10):1325–1331. doi:10.1016/j.jse.2013.01.035

Lanier WL. Cerebral perfusion: err on the side of caution. *APSF Newsletter.* 2009. 24:1.

Laflam A, Joshi B, Brady K, et al. Shoulder surgery in the beach chair position is associated with diminished cerebral autoregulation but no differences in postoperative cognition or brain injury biomarker levels compared with supine positioning: the Anesthesia Patient Safety Foundation Beach Chair Study. *Anesth Analg.* 2015;120(1):176–185. doi:10.1213/ANE.0000000000000455

Rohrbaugh M, Kentor ML, Orebaugh SL, Williams B. Outcomes of shoulder surgery in the sitting position with interscalene nerve block: a single-center series. *Reg Anesth Pain Med.* 2013;38(1):28–33. doi:10.1097/AAP.0b013e318277a2eb

Salazar D, Hazel A, Tauchen AJ, Sears BW, Marra G. Neurocognitive deficits and cerebral desaturation during shoulder arthroscopy with patient in beach-chair position: a review of the current literature. *Am J Orthop.* 2016;45(3):E63–E68.

Triplet JJ, Lonetta CM, Everding NG, Moor MA, Levy JC. Association between temporal mean arterial pressure and brachial non-invasive blood pressure during shoulder surgery in the beach chair position during general anesthesia. *J Shoulder Elbow Surg.* 2015;24(1):127–132. doi:10.1016/j.jse.2014.05.011

YaDeau JT, Casciano M, Liu SS, et al. Stroke, regional anesthesia in the sitting position, and hypotension: a review of 4169 ambulatory surgery patients. *Reg Anesth Pain Med.* 2011;36(5):430–435. doi:10.1097/AAP.0b013e318228d54e

3.8. Are there additional cardiac implications of surgical position?

Sudden hypotensive bradycardic events (HBEs) have been reported during shoulder surgery in the sitting position under ISB. The Bezold-Jarish reflex has been one proposed mechanism for the occurrence of HBEs. The reflex originates in cardiac sensory receptors with vagal afferent pathways in the left ventricle. Stimulation of these inhibitory cardiac receptors by stretch, chemical substances, or drugs increases parasympathetic activity and inhibits sympathetic activity. These effects promote reflex bradycardia, vasodilation, and hypotension. Venous pooling in the sitting position with a resultant decreased preload stimulates endogenous catecholamine release and increased cardiac contractility, which may stimulate this reflex. Additionally, exogenous catecholamine sources in this setting include epinephrine added to LA for ISB and irrigation solution. Proposed prophylactic interventions include increasing preload by intravenous fluid administration, beta blockade, and adequate sedation, as a less sedated patient may have more endogenous catecholamines and heightened vagal tone. Additionally, norepinephrine as opposed to epinephrine in the irrigation fluid has been demonstrated to reduce the incidence of HBE while effectively controlling intraoperative bleeding and resultant surgical visualization.

Further Reading

Chierichini A, Frassanito L, Vergari A, et al. The effect of norepinephrine versus epinephrine in irrigation fluid on the incidence of hypotensive/bradycardic events during arthroscopic rotator cuff repair with interscalene block in the sitting position. *Arthroscopy.* 2015;31(5):800–806. doi:10.1016/j.arthro.2015.02.030

D'Alessio JG, Rosenblum M, Shea KP, Freitas DG. A retrospective comparison of interscalene block and general anesthesia for ambulatory surgery shoulder arthroscopy. *Reg Anesth.* 1995;20(1):62–68.

D'Alessio JG, Weller RS, Rosenblum M. Activation of the Bezold-Jarisch reflex in the sitting position for shoulder arthroscopy using interscalene block. *Anesth Analg.* 1995;80(6):1158–1162. doi:10.1016/j.jse.2014.05.011

Liguori GA, Kahn RL, Gordon J, Gordon MA. The use of metoprolol and glycopyrrolate to prevent hypotensive/bradycardic events during shoulder arthroscopy in the sitting position under interscalene block. *Anesth Analg. 1998 Dec;87(6):1320-5.*

4. Postoperative Management: Ambulatory Continuous Perineural Infusions

4.1. What is the ideal infusate for CISB?

Data suggest that ropivacaine, bupivacaine, and levobupivacaine provide similar analgesia. While ropivacaine is more expensive, it has a safer cardiac profile, and it may induce fewer finger paresthesias and less hand weakness than comparable concentrations of bupivacaine. Ropivacaine 0.2% provides more effective analgesia than ropivacaine 0.1% during the first 24 hours for CISB after shoulder surgery. There remains no medications other than LA approved for continuous perineural administration by the US Food and Drug Administration.

Further Reading

Choromanski DW, Patel PS, Frederick JM, Lemos SE, Chidiac EJ. The effect of continuous interscalene brachial plexus block with 0.125% bupivacaine vs 0.2% ropivacaine on pain relief, diaphragmatic motility, and ventilatory function. *J Clin Anesth.* 2015;27(8):619–626. doi:10.1016/j.jclinane.2015.03.006

Ilfeld BM. Continuous peripheral nerve blocks: an update of the published evidence and comparison with novel, alternative analgesic modalities. *Anesth Analg.* 2017;124(1):308–335. doi:10.1213/ANE.0000000000001581

Ilfeld BM. Continuous peripheral nerve blocks: a review of the published evidence. *Anesth Analg.* 2011;113(4):904–925. doi:10.1213/ANE.0b013e3182285e01

Yang CW, Jung SM, Kang PS, et al. A randomized comparison of ropivacaine 0.1% and 0.2% for continuous interscalene block after shoulder surgery.—PubMed—NCBI. *Anesth Analg.* 2013;116(3):730–733. doi:10.1213/ANE.0b013e318280e109

4.2. Are bolus doses better than basal infusions during CISB?

The addition of patient-controlled boluses to CISB may allow for (1) decreasing motor block by decreasing the required basal infusion rate; (2) decreasing the incidence of an insensate extremity; and (3) extending infusion/analgesia duration for outpatients discharged with a fixed LA reservoir volume. At the expense of increasing LA consumption, high basal rate (8 mL/h) ropivacaine 0.2% infusion combined with low-volume, patient-controlled bolus doses (2 mL/h) reduced baseline pain scores, sleep disturbances, and the incidence and severity of breakthrough pain in patients undergoing moderately painful outpatient shoulder surgery with a CISB. An alternative or additional bolus strategy is the addition of a mandatory/automatic bolus dose, in an effort to maximize perineural spread by distributing an equivalent slow basal infusion dose/volume as a bolus. However, in ultrasound-guided CISB after shoulder surgery, automated LA boluses combined with PRN boluses did not reduce LA consumption or rescue analgesia, compared with basal infusion combined with PRN boluses.

Further Reading

Byeon GJ, Shin SW, Yoon JU, Kim EJ, Baek SH, Ri HS. Infusion methods for continuous interscalene brachial plexus block for postoperative pain control after arthroscopic rotator cuff repair. *Korean J Pain.* 2015;28(3):210–216. doi:10.3344/kjp.2015.28.3.210

Fredrickson MJ, Abeysekera A, Price DJ, Wong AC. Patient-initiated mandatory boluses for ambulatory continuous interscalene analgesia: an effective strategy for optimizing analgesia and minimizing side-effects. *Br J Anaesth.* 2011;106(2):239–245. doi:10.1093/bja/aeq320

Hamdani M, Chassot O, Fournier R. Ultrasound-guided continuous interscalene block: the influence of local anesthetic background delivery method on postoperative analgesia after shoulder surgery: a randomized trial. *Reg Anesth Pain Med.* 2014;39(5):387–393. doi:10.1097/AAP.0000000000000112

Hashimoto A, Ito H, Sato Y, Fujiwara Y: Automated intermittent bolus infusion for continuous sciatic nerve block: a case report. *Masui* 2011;60:873–875.

Ilfeld BM, Morey TE, Wright TW, Chidgey LK, Enneking FK: Interscalene perineural ropivacaine infusion: a comparison of two dosing regimens for postoperative analgesia. *Reg Anesth Pain Med.* 2004;29:9–16.

4.3. What are the benefits of CISB?

Ambulatory perineural infusions are a critical component to efficacious multimodal postoperative analgesia following shoulder surgery in the outpatient setting. Implementation is indeed challenging, and there is often a perception that CISB and ambulatory perineural infusions are only feasible in an academic setting. However, following RCR in a multiprovider private practice setting, CISB was associated with reduced total opioid and antiemetic consumption, and occurred without a significant increase in the monetary cost.

Evidence suggests that poorly treated acute postoperative pain and acute postoperative opioid use can lead to nociception-induced central sensitization and opioid-induced secondary hyperalgesia, respectively. Both mechanisms may be involved in the pathogenesis of persistent postsurgical pain, an entity that can occur following rotator cuff surgery. CISB may play a part in efforts to reduce these mechanisms. In patients undergoing RCR, CISB has demonstrated improved analgesia and reduced opioid requirements compared with single-injection ISB up to 7 postoperative days. A pilot study found that CISB was associated with lower average/dynamic pain scores, decreased opioid requirements, fewer awakenings from pain, and improved shoulder range of motion up to 12 weeks after shoulder adhesive capsulitis manipulation.

Further Reading

Angst MS, Clark JD: Opioid-induced hyperalgesia: a qualitative systematic review. *Anesthesiology* 2006;104:570–587

Borgeat A, Schappi B, Biasca N, Gerber C. Patient-controlled analgesia after major shoulder surgery: patient-controlled interscalene analgesia versus patient-controlled analgesia. *Anesthesiology*. 1997;87(6):1343–1347.

Fredrickson MJ. Orthopedic anesthesia subspecialization: the way forward to increase utilization of perineural infusions? *Reg Anesth Pain Med*. 2012;37(3):359–360; author reply 360.

Fredrickson MJ, Stewart AW. Continuous interscalene analgesia for rotator cuff repair: a retrospective comparison of effectiveness and cost in 205 patients from a multi-provider private practice setting. *Anaesth Intensive Care*. 2008;36(6):786–791.

Ilfeld BM, Morey TE, Wright TW, Chidgey LK. Continuous interscalene brachial plexus block for postoperative pain control at home: a randomized, double-blinded, placebo-controlled study. *Anesth Analg. 2003 Apr;96(4):1089-95.*

Kehlet H, Jensen TS, Woolf CJ. Persistent postsurgical pain: risk factors and prevention. *Lancet*. 2006;367(9522):1618–1625.

Klein SM, Steele SM, Nielsen KC, et al. The difficulties of ambulatory interscalene and intra-articular infusions for rotator cuff surgery: a preliminary report. *Can J Anaesth*. 2003;50(3):265–269.

Malhotra N, Madison SJ, Ward SR, Mariano ER, Loland VJ, Ilfeld BM. Continuous interscalene nerve block following adhesive capsulitis manipulation. *Reg Anesth Pain Med*. 2013;38(2):171–172. doi:10.1097/AAP.0b013e318283475b

Salviz EA, Xu D, Frulla A, et al. Continuous interscalene block in patients having outpatient rotator cuff repair surgery: a prospective randomized trial. *Anesth Analg*. 2013;117(6):1485–1492. doi:10.1213/01.ane.0000436607.40643.0a

4.4. What items should be discussed with patients, and accompanying caretakers, prior to discharge home with perineural infusions?

It is essential to have specific written instructions discussed with both the patient and his or her accompanying caregiver prior to discharge. It is not recommended that ambulatory perineural infusions be used for any patient unless physician/nurse consultation is immediately available 24/7. Pain team contact numbers (daytime and after hours) should be printed on the instruction form. Instructions should include the following:

1. The expected transition time from surgical block with initial bolus to analgesic block with perineural infusion and signs of surgical block resolution;
2. Review of oral multimodal analgesic regimen;
3. The location of the catheter (interscalene);
4. The infusion system used;
5. The specific LA, including basal rate per hour (if applicable) and bolus dose with lockout interval (if applicable);
6. The expected duration of the infusion;
7. Caution as to protection of the insensate part of the body and care in ambulation;

8. Potential for leakage at catheter insertion site;
9. Instructions to discontinue the system and call the contact anesthesiologist immediately if patient develops skin rash, hives, other allergic responses, ringing in the ears, tingling of the mouth or tongue, or other signs/symptoms of LA toxicity;
10. Instructions for physician/nurse contact if patient develops fever, pain at the catheter insertion site, increased extremity numbness or weakness, inadequate pain control, or problems with the infusion system (malfunction, leakage, disconnection, etc.); and
11. Instructions for removal of catheter.

Further Reading

Greengrass RA, Nielsen KC. Management of peripheral nerve block catheters at home. *Int Anesthesiol Clin*. 2005;43(3):79–87.

4.5. What are causes for PONS, and how can they be managed?

Postoperative neurologic symptoms must be identified and addressed by the surgeon and anesthesiologist. New onset of PONS such as numbness, tingling, and/or weakness in the surgical extremity may occur after surgery, with or without ISB. Marecek describes complications in shoulder arthroscopy: nerve damage after shoulder arthroscopy is fortunately rare, with reported rates of ≤3%, with larger series reporting rates <0.2%; paresthesias have been reported in 10% to 30% of cases; injuries to the median, axillary, musculocutaneous, medial antebrachial cutaneous, radial, ulnar, medial pectoral, and anterior interosseous nerves, as well as cutaneous hypoesthesias, have all been reported. These injuries are generally transient, although permanent damage requiring tendon transfers has been described. Positioning, traction, joint distention and fluid extravasation, and direct injury from portal placement have all been implicated in postoperative nerve injuries. Sulcus ulnaris syndrome, carpal tunnel syndrome, and the development of complex regional pain syndrome are additional potential etiologies. By obtaining a detailed history and report of signs/symptoms, serious etiologies can often be excluded, and patient reassurance about the transient nature of such symptoms is the only necessary intervention. While transient numbness/tingling of the extremity is not uncommon, motor weakness after block resolution is more alarming and requires immediate evaluation. Early involvement of neurology for baseline electrophysiologic studies must be considered. Additionally, neurology and/or chronic pain specialists can be utilized to evaluate and manage neuropathic pain and/or symptoms that interfere with activities of daily living. In cases of persistent phrenic nerve paresis, pulmonology should be involved.

Further Reading

Borgeat A, Ekatodramis G, Kalberer F, Benz C. Acute and nonacute complications associated with interscalene block and shoulder surgery: a prospective study. *Anesthesiology*. 2001;95:875–880.

Marecek GS, Saltzman MD. Complications in shoulder arthroscopy. *Orthopedics*. 2010;33(7):492–497.

Neal JM, Barrington MJ, Brull R, et al. The Second ASRA Practice Advisory on Neurologic Complications Associated With Regional Anesthesia and Pain Medicine: Executive Summary 2015. Reg Anesth Pain Med. 2015 Sep-Oct;40(5):401-430.

Painful arthroscopic shoulder surgery and RCR are almost exclusively performed on an outpatient basis. Patient-specific and surgery-specific considerations must be evaluated when making decisions for intraoperative anesthesia and postoperative analgesia. ISB is the most commonly performed PNB for shoulder surgery, although side effects associated with its use has spurred investigation into alternative techniques and combinations therein. The safety and efficacy of adjuvants to extend LA duration achieved with single-injection PNBs are still under investigation. As such, extended postoperative analgesia relies on continuous catheter techniques. Appropriate dosing regimens must be employed for both single-injection ISB and CISB to optimize intraoperative anesthesia and postoperative analgesia. A protocol must be in place for the safe and effective discharge and follow-up of patients going home with continuous perineural infusions.

6

Total Knee Arthroplasty

Rishi Chokshi and Nabil Elkassabany

Case Scenario

A 78-year-old man with a history of coronary artery disease, mild dementia, hyperlipidemia, and obesity presents for a left total knee arthroplasty (TKA). You see the patient in the preoperative holding area and go over different options for anesthesia and the plan for postoperative analgesia. The family expresses concerns about the effects of general anesthesia on his mental state and mentions to you that he underwent general anesthesia for hernia repair 5 years ago, explaining that he was very confused after surgery and took 5 days to return to his "normal self." The patient's daughter thinks the pain medication was, in part, responsible for his confusion after surgery.

1. Patient Factors

1.1 Pain assessment in the elderly population

1.1.1. Do elderly patients report pain differently than their younger counterparts? If so, what are these differences?

The geriatric patient population presenting for surgery is quickly growing, with an estimated 20% of the US population composed of individuals over the age of 65 by the year 2030. Assessment of pain in elderly individuals must take into account the potential for cognitive decline, Alzheimer's disease and dementia, hearing impairment, visual impairment, delirium, speech impediment, and any underlying history of depression. These factors are prevalent in the elderly population and may complicate the proper assessment of pain in the perioperative period, potentially leading to underestimation of the underlying pain.

Further Reading

Booker SS, Pasero C, Herr KA. Practice recommendations for pain assessment by self-report with African American older adults. *Geriatr Nurs*. 2015;36:67–74.

Falzone E, Hoffmann C, Keita H. Postoperative analgesia in elderly patients. *Drugs Aging*. 2013;30:81–90.

Knickman JR, Snell EK. The 2030 problem: caring for aging baby boomers. *Health Serv Res*. 2002;37:849–884.

Ngu SS, Tan MP, Subramanian P, Abdul Rahman R, Kamaruzzaman S, Chin AV, et al. Pain assessment using self-reported, nurse-reported, and observational pain assessment tools among older individuals with cognitive impairment. *Pain Manag Nurs*. 2015;16:595–601.

1.1.2. What are unidimensional pain rating scales?

Unidimensional pain rating scales are used to provide a linear assessment of pain experienced by the patient and primarily focus on pain intensity. The Numerical Rating Scale is most commonly used. Patients grade pain on a scale of 0 (no pain) to 10 (severe pain). The Verbal Descriptor Scale is another unidimensional tool that simply asks the patient to describe the pain as mild, moderate, or severe. The Visual Analog Scale is often used for patients who are unable to communicate their pain description verbally; it is a graded line from 0 to 10 with illustrated markings describing varying degrees of distress. The patient is able to point to the description that best matches his or her pain level. Other pain scales may use illustrations of a human face showing different levels of distress; with these, the patient may point to the face that best matches his or her subjective experience of pain. It is important to note that elderly patients are more susceptible to the side effects of opioid medication and that the initial baseline pain rating of the elderly patient may be abnormal even prior to surgery. Thus, unidimensional pain rating scales should be used as a supplement to guide the care provider in choosing an appropriate pain management strategy rather than as the primary tool of pain assessment.

Further Reading

Gordon DB. Acute pain assessment tools: let us move beyond simple pain ratings. *Curr Opin Anaesthesiol.* 2015;28:565–569.

1.1.3. What are multidimensional pain rating scales? How are they different from conventional pain scales?

Multidimensional pain rating scales aim to incorporate the psychosocial component of pain and assess its impact on function, emotion, sleep, and overall wellness. There are several multidimensional rating scales available for use and others that are either new or in development. Some of these tools may be proprietary and require a fee for usage. One multidimensional pain rating scale is the Department of Defense Veteran Pain Scale, which includes a series of questions to elucidate the impact of pain on areas such as mood, sleep, and activity. Another is the Patient-Reported Outcomes Measurement Information System tool, or PROMIS, which provides a snapshot of a patient's global health based on the components of physical, social, and mental health. It is important to consider that many of these multidimensional pain rating scales may take several minutes to complete. Thus, they may have a limited role in the quick assessment and treatment of acute pain following surgery. The Revised American Pain Society Patient Outcome Questionnaire was published in 2010 to assess the quality of pain management in hospitalized adults. The instrument assesses the quality of postoperative pain management in 5 domains: (1) pain severity and sleep interference, (2) interference with activity, (3) severity of adverse effects, (4) affective subscale, and (5) patient perception of and satisfaction with care.

Further Reading

Cook KF, Buckenmaier C III, Gershon RC. PASTOR/PROMIS (R) pain outcomes system: what does it mean to pain specialists? *Pain Manag.* 2014;4:277–283.

Gordon DB. Acute pain assessment tools: let us move beyond simple pain ratings. *Curr Opin Anaesthesiol.* 2015;28:565–569.

Gordon DB, Polomano RC, Pellino TA, et al. Revised American Pain Society Patient Outcome Questionnaire (APS-POQ-R) for quality improvement of pain management in hospitalized adults: preliminary psychometric evaluation. *J Pain.* 2010;11:1172–1186.

Polomano RC, Galloway KT, Kent ML, et al. Psychometric testing of the Defense and Veterans Pain Rating Scale (DVPRS): a new pain scale for military population. *Pain Med.* 2016;17:1505–1519.

1.2. Preoperative assessment

1.2.1. Can patients on therapeutic anticoagulation receive a peripheral nerve block?

Currently, the American Society of Regional Anesthesia and Pain Medicine evidence-based guidelines do not provide definitive recommendations for peripheral nerve and plexus blockade in anticoagulated patients due to the lack of sufficient data involving hemorrhagic complications. However, existing case reports suggest that most complications are related to blood loss from anticoagulation rather than neurological trauma resulting from peripheral nerve block (PNB). Furthermore, the principal issue regarding anticoagulation and nerve blockade is bleeding following accidental needle puncture of the surrounding blood vessels. In the event of bleeding following a PNB, most superficial sites are amenable to external pressure by the anesthesiologist because they are easily accessible. This maneuver provides a tamponade effect to control bleeding, and holding pressure for several minutes allows the coagulation cascade to create a clot at the area of the punctured vessel. This is contrary to deep peripheral and neuraxial blockade, in which the area of bleeding is an enclosed space and therefore cannot be externally compressed by the operator. The decision to avoid PNB on an elderly patient on anticoagulation medication must take into consideration the adverse effects of alternative choices. Systemic opioid medications may cause sedation and delirium in elderly patients, whereas a PNB may reduce overall opioid consumption over the course of hospitalization. The anesthesiologist must weigh these choices in discussion with the patient to provide the best, mutually agreed-upon outcome.

Further Reading

Horlocker TT, Wedel DJ, Rowlingson JC, et al. Regional anesthesia in the patient receiving antithrombotic or thrombolytic therapy: American Society of Regional Anesthesia and Pain Medicine Evidence-Based Guidelines (Third Edition). *Reg Anesth Pain Med.* 2010;35:64–101.

2. Surgical and Regional Anesthesia Factors

2.1. Innervation of the knee joint

2.1.1. What nerves supply sensation to the knee joint?

The cutaneous innervation of the knee joint primarily arises from branches of the sciatic and femoral nerves. For simplicity, the innervation of the knee can be divided into a medial component and lateral component. Branches of the femoral nerve include the medial femoral cutaneous nerve and saphenous nerve, which provide sensation to the medial portion of the knee. The saphenous nerve has infrapatellar cutaneous branches, which supply the medial portion of the knee before going on to supply the lower leg. The sciatic nerve gives rise to the common peroneal nerve, which provides cutaneous innervation to the lateral knee via the articular branches. The superior lateral genicular nerve is a branch of the sciatic nerve and provides innervation to the lateral knee. The posterior aspect of the knee is innervated by the branches of the obturator nerve as well as posterior articular branches of the tibial nerve and branches of the sciatic nerve.

Further Reading

Franco CD, Buvanendran A, Petersohn JD, Menzies RD, Menzies LP. Innervation of the anterior capsule of the human knee: implications for radiofrequency ablation. *Reg Anesth Pain Med.* 2015;40:363–368.

Horner G, Dellon AL. Innervation of the human knee joint and implications for surgery. *Clin Orthop Relat Res.* 1994 Apr;301:221–6.

Saleh HA, El-fark MM, Abdel-Hamid GA. Anatomical variation of sciatic nerve division in the popliteal fossa and its implication in popliteal nerve blockade. *Folia Morphol (Warsz).* 2009;68:256–259.

2.1.2. What are the important vascular structures in the knee?

The popliteal fossa contains the major vascular structures that pass through the knee joint. These include the popliteal artery and popliteal vein, which are contained in a tissue sheath separate from the sciatic nerve. Although this separation decreases the likelihood of injury to the vessels during a nerve block, proper aspiration of the needle must still be performed to rule out intravascular injection.

Further Reading

Horner G, Dellon AL. Innervation of the human knee joint and implications for surgery. *Clin Orthop Relat Res.* 1994 Apr;(301):221–6.

2.2. Regional anesthetic concerns

2.2.1. Describe the advantages and disadvantages of a femoral nerve block

The femoral nerve block (FNB) is a widely used means of regional anesthesia for postoperative analgesia for patients undergoing total knee arthroplasty (TKA) and has relatively few complications. The landmarks for performing the block are easy to recognize, and the procedure can quickly and effectively be learned by even the novice operator. Advantages of FNB include better postoperative pain control, decreased opioid requirements, and better functional outcomes after TKA. One disadvantage of the FNB is weakness of the quadriceps muscle. This weakness can inhibit early ambulation and increase the fall risk for patients undergoing TKA and has been implicated as a risk factor for falls after TKA. Nerve injury is still a concern after FNB as well as for other nerve blocks, as the use of ultrasound-guided technique over the past decade did not decrease the rate of nerve injury compared with landmark-based technique. It is debatable whether the use of continuous catheter increases the incidence of nerve injury or not.

Further Reading

Capdevila X, Pirat P, Bringuier S, et al. Continuous PNBs in hospital wards after orthopedic surgery: a multicenter prospective analysis of the quality of postoperative analgesia and complications in 1,416 patients. *Anesthesiology*. 2005;103:1035–1045.

Chan EY, Fransen M, Parker DA, Assam PN, Chua N. Femoral nerve blocks for acute postoperative pain after knee replacement surgery. *Cochrane Database Syst Rev*. 2014:CD009941.

Ilfeld BM, Duke KB, Donohue MC. The association between lower extremity continuous peripheral nerve blocks and patient falls after knee and hip arthroplasty. *Anesth Analg*. 2010;111:1552–1554.

Neal JM, Barrington MJ, Brull R, et al. The Second ASRA Practice Advisory on Neurologic Complications Associated With Regional Anesthesia and Pain Medicine: Executive Summary 2015. *Reg Anesth Pain Med*. 2015;40:401–430.

Terkawi AS, Mavridis D, Sessler DI, et al. Pain management modalities after total knee arthroplasty: a network meta-analysis of 170 randomized controlled trials. *Anesthesiology*. 2017;126:923–937.

2.2.2. Describe the technique of performing an ultrasound-guided femoral nerve block

The FNB begins by placing the patient in the supine position and exposing the area of the inguinal crease. For obese patients, visualization of this area can be optimized by retracting the redundant abdominal wall away from the field with tape. After skin preparation with a disinfectant solution, the ultrasound transducer should be placed transversely slightly below the inguinal crease. The resulting image should show the neurovascular bundle with the femoral nerve appearing in the short-axis view as a triangular, hyperechoic structure lateral to the femoral artery. The femoral nerve lies under the fascia iliaca and overlies the iliacus muscle. The visualization of the femoral nerve can be adjusted with a slight tilt of the ultrasound probe. Local anesthetic infiltration should be placed about 1 to 2 cm lateral to the transducer. Insert the block needle through the skin wheal in plane with the ultrasound probe and advance lateral to medial until the tip of the needle is visualized adjacent to the nerve. It is important to note that the operator may feel "pops" or fascial clicks while advancing the needle toward the nerve, which signifies passage through the fascia lata and the fascia iliaca. Aspirate the needle to confirm the needle tip is not intravascular. Inject 10 to 20 mL of local anesthetic while watching for circumferential spread around the femoral nerve on the ultrasound image. Typically, higher concentrations of local anesthetics are used for surgical anesthetic blocks, whereas lower concentrations of local anesthetics are used for postoperative analgesia.

Further Reading

Hadzic A, ed. *Hadzic's Textbook of Regional Anesthesia and Acute Pain Management*. 2nd ed. New York, NY: McGraw-Hill Education LLC; 2017. http://hdl.library.upenn.edu/1017.12/1843434.

Hadzic A, ed. *Ultrasound-Guided Femoral Nerve Block [two-dimensional moving image]*. New York, NY: McGraw-Hill Education LLC; 2013. http://hdl.library.upenn.edu/1017.12/1743767.

2.2.3. Describe the advantages and disadvantages of an adductor canal block

The adductor canal block (ACB) is a technique in which local anesthetic is deposited in the middle to lower third of the thigh in the "adductor canal," as suggested by its name. The local anesthetic will anesthetize the saphenous nerve and the medial femoral cutaneous branches, providing postoperative analgesia to the medial portion of the knee. The primary advantage of this block involves sparing the motor branches of the femoral nerve to the quadriceps muscle. This preserves muscle strength following surgery. Several studies have demonstrated similar analgesic efficacy when compared with FNB for TKA, but patients receiving ACBs have the added benefit of preserved quadriceps muscle strength. However, whether this preserved muscle strength translates into a clinical rehabilitative advantage remains to be further studied and is the subject of ongoing debate, as ACB blocks still carry the risk of patient falls. Other authors believe that the analgesic efficacy of the ACB is inferior to that of the FNB. However, in the context of a multimodal analgesic protocol, the contribution of regional block to the overall pain management is questioned. In other words, we may substitute one analgesic block for another if the latter offers better functional outcomes even if the analgesic efficacy of both blocks may not be exactly similar. The final decision regarding block preference depends on both patient factors and surgical practice patterns and preferences.

Further Reading

Boezaart AP, Parvataneni HK. Adductor canal block may just be an (unreliable) indirect femoral nerve block. *Reg Anesth Pain Med.* 2014;39:556.

Elkassabany NM, Antosh S, Ahmed M, et al. The risk of falls after total knee arthroplasty with the use of a femoral nerve block versus an adductor canal block: a double-blinded randomized controlled study. *Anesth Analg.* 2016;122:1696–1703.

Hussain N, Ferreri TG, Prusick PJ, et al. Adductor canal block versus femoral canal block for total knee arthroplasty: a meta-analysis: what does the evidence suggest? *Reg Anesth Pain Med.* 2016;41:314–320.

Kwofie MK, Shastri UD, Gadsden JC, et al. The effects of ultrasound-guided adductor canal block versus femoral nerve block on quadriceps strength and fall risk: a blinded, randomized trial of volunteers. *Reg Anesth Pain Med.* 2013;38:321–325.

Manickam B, Perlas A, Duggan E, Brull R, Chan VW, Ramlogan R. Feasibility and efficacy of ultrasound-guided block of the saphenous nerve in the adductor canal. *Reg Anesth Pain Med.* 2009;34:578–580.

Mariano ER, Perlas A. Adductor canal block for total knee arthroplasty: the perfect recipe or just one ingredient? *Anesthesiology.* 2014;120:530–532.

2.2.4. Describe the technique of performing an ultrasound-guided adductor canal nerve block

The ACB begins by placing the patient in the supine position with the leg externally rotated and flexed in what is known as a "frog leg" position. The skin is prepped and draped, followed by placement of the ultrasound probe in the middle third of the anterior thigh. The adductor canal is located posterior and deep to the sartorius muscle and contains the superficial femoral artery. The saphenous nerve may be difficult to visualize due to its small size. As a result, the needle should be inserted in plane with the ultrasound probe and advanced until the tip is within the adductor canal. After aspiration of the catheter, 10 to 20 mL of local anesthetic is deposited within the adductor canal looking for (mainly lateral) spread around the femoral artery under continuous ultrasound guidance. An important consideration when performing ACB with peripheral catheters is the proximity to the operative site. Catheters placed too close to the surgical field may become dislodged, damaged, or intentionally removed during the procedure. Some practitioners question the risk of placement of the catheter under the pneumatic tourniquet and whether this may contribute to increased incidence of nerve injury. Placement of the adductor canal proximally after the end of the femoral triangle is similar to placement of the block close to the adductor hiatus. Proximal block placement can result in involvement of the nerve to vastus medialis. Many authors believe that the resulting motor weakness of the vastus medialis is still favorable to weakness of all four heads of the quadriceps muscle.

Further Reading

Hadzic A, ed. *Hadzic's Textbook of Regional Anesthesia and Acute Pain Management.* 2nd ed. New York, NY: McGraw-Hill Education LLC; 2017. http://hdl.library.upenn.edu/1017.12/1843434.

Mariano ER, Kim TE, Wagner MJ, et al. A randomized comparison of proximal and distal ultrasound-guided adductor canal catheter insertion sites for knee arthroplasty. *J Ultrasound Med.* 2014;33:1653–1662.

2.2.5. Describe the advantages and disadvantages of a lumbar plexus block

The lumbar plexus block, similar to the psoas compartment block, is a lesser utilized regional block for TKA. The lumbar plexus comprises nerves from L1 to L4 with some input from T12 and L5. The plexus eventually proceeds to form the lateral femoral cutaneous nerve, femoral nerve, and obturator nerve. The three major components provide sensory innervation to the anterior knee to variable degrees. Due to its anatomically deep location, the lumbar plexus block carries many potential risks such as injury to the kidney and retroperitoneal structures, local anesthetic spread into the epidural space, local anesthetic systemic toxicity from large volumes and anatomic vascularity, and hematoma formation that may be difficult or impossible to compress. Few studies compare the analgesic efficacy of lumbar plexus block with FNB. The issue of motor block and quadriceps muscle weakness remains a disadvantage as with FNB. Given these factors, the lumbar plexus block is an advanced block and should only be performed by operators with considerable experience with ultrasound-based regional anesthesia. Most commonly, this block is performed using nerve stimulation technique while eliciting a quadriceps motor response.

Further Reading

Auroy Y, Benhamou D, Bargues L, et al. Major complications of regional anesthesia in France: the SOS Regional Anesthesia Hotline Service. *Anesthesiology.* 2002;97:1274–1280.

Capdevila X, Coimbra C, Choquet O. Approaches to the lumbar plexus: success, risks, and outcome. *Reg Anesth Pain Med.* 2005;30:150–162.

Danninger T, Opperer M, Memtsoudis SG. Perioperative pain control after total knee arthroplasty: an evidence based review of the role of peripheral nerve blocks. *World J Orthop.* 2014;5:225–232.

Njathi CW, Johnson RL, Laughlin RS, Schroeder DR, Jacob AK, Kopp SL. Complications after continuous posterior lumbar plexus blockade for total hip arthroplasty: a retrospective cohort study. *Reg Anesth Pain Med.* 2017;42:446–450.

2.2.6. Describe the technique of performing an ultrasound-guided lumbar plexus block

The lumbar plexus block begins with the patient either in sitting position or lateral decubitus. A curvilinear transducer probe is placed transversely at the midline position at L4. At this junction, the operator should note the spinous process on the ultrasound. The probe is then shifted 2 to 3 cm laterally and away from midline until the erector spinae muscle, transverse process, and psoas muscle come into view. The lumbar plexus lies within the body of the psoas muscle, and the block needle should be advanced in plane with the probe until it reaches the psoas compartment. As a supplement to ultrasound guidance, nerve stimulation can be utilized to confirm proper needle placement by looking for twitches of the quadriceps muscle in response to nerve stimulation. Local anesthetic is then deposited into the fascial plane of the psoas compartment.

Another approach to the lumbar plexus block involves an out-of-plane needle approach. The ultrasound transducer is placed vertical and parallel to and 3 cm lateral from midline in the direction of the intended extremity to be blocked. The initial scan with the ultrasound should move caudally to identify the sacrum and the transverse process of L5. Once this landmark is identified, the transducer is shifted cephalad until the L3-L4 transverse processes are seen on the image. The image created by the shadow of the transverse processes is known as the "trident" sign, and immediately below them lies the psoas muscle and compartment, which contain the roots of the lumbar plexus. The needle is inserted out of plane, and with the assistance of nerve stimulation, local anesthetic is deposited to complete the lumbar plexus block.

Further Reading

Karmakar MK, Ho AM, Li X, Kwok WH, Tsang K, Ngan Kee WD. Ultrasound-guided lumbar plexus block through the acoustic window of the lumbar ultrasound trident. *Br J Anaesth*. 2008;100:533–537.

Karmakar MK, Li JW, Kwok WH, Hadzic A. Ultrasound-guided lumbar plexus block using a transverse scan through the lumbar intertransverse space: a prospective case series. *Reg Anesth Pain Med*. 2015;40:75–81.

Madison SJ, Ilfeld BM, Loland VJ, Mariano ER. Posterior lumbar plexus perineural catheter insertion by ultrasound guidance alone. *Acta Anaesthesiol Scand*. 2011;55:1031–1032.

2.2.7. Describe the role of periarticular local anesthetic infiltration for total knee arthroplasty

Local anesthetic infiltration has been used to provide postoperative analgesia for TKA. It involves the infiltration of local anesthetic along with a combination of additives such as steroids, nonsteroidal anti-inflammatory drugs, epinephrine, and opioids directly into the surgical site by the operating surgeon. The local anesthetic is usually blindly infiltrated into all layers of the knee joint, including the anterior capsule, posterior capsule, and periarticular soft tissue. As with any blind technique, injury to the surrounding vascular structures must be taken into consideration. Some studies have even demonstrated placement of periarticular catheters for continuous infusion of local anesthetic into the postoperative period. The proclaimed benefit of this method is the avoidance of motor blockade to the quadriceps muscle. However, there is much uncertainty as to whether this method of regional anesthesia confers any analgesic or functional benefit, especially when compared with more commonly utilized regional anesthesia techniques. The existing studies provide conflicting results. Furthermore, study results vary regarding volume of local anesthetic used and the components and quantities of additives, making comparison across institutions difficult. It is clear that local infiltration can have a major role in postoperative analgesia after TKA and can complement the role of PNBs. Whether the use of long-acting formulations of local anesthetics offers any advantage over conventional local anesthetic remains unanswered.

Further Reading

Albrecht E, Guyen O, Jacot-Guillarmod A, Kirkham KR. The analgesic efficacy of local infiltration analgesia vs femoral nerve block after total knee arthroplasty: a systematic review and meta-analysis. *Br J Anaesth*. 2016;116:597–609.

Amundson AW, Johnson RL, Abdel MP, et al. A three-arm randomized clinical trial comparing continuous femoral plus single-injection sciatic peripheral nerve blocks versus periarticular injection with ropivacaine or liposomal bupivacaine for patients undergoing total knee arthroplasty. *Anesthesiology*. 126:1139–1150.

McCartney CJ, McLeod GA. Local infiltration analgesia for total knee arthroplasty. *Br J Anaesth*. 2011;107:487–489.

Nader A, Kendall MC, Manning DW, et al. Single-dose adductor canal block with local infiltrative analgesia compared with local infiltrate analgesia after total knee arthroplasty: a randomized, double-blind, placebo-controlled trial. *Reg Anesth Pain Med*. 2016;41:678–684.

2.2.8. Describe the advantages and disadvantages of sciatic nerve blocks

Patients undergoing TKA with FNB may still complain of significant postoperative pain, as the sensory fibers of the sciatic nerve supplying the lateral knee and posterior capsule remain unblocked. As a result, sciatic nerve blocks are commonly performed in conjunction with FNB to provide more comprehensive postoperative analgesia for TKA. Most studies that have compared the combination of femoral and sciatic nerve blocks versus FNB alone have shown that combination blocks resulted in improved analgesia for only the first postoperative day, failing to show any added benefit thereafter. Adding a sciatic nerve block does not seem to confer any rehabilitative advantage or reduction in hospital length of stay. One study compared sciatic nerve block with local infiltration of the posterior capsule of the knee and concluded that the analgesic benefit of sciatic nerve block was limited to the few first hours after surgery. Alternative approaches for analgesia of the posterior capsule of the knee include selective tibial nerve block and ultrasound-guided *injection* of local anesthetic between the *popliteal artery* and posterior *capsule* of the *knee (iPACK block)*. Evidence to support or refute the value of adding the IPACK block to the multimodal analgesia regimen is still preliminary. More studies are needed to document the efficacy of this approach

Further Reading

Abdallah FW, Brull R. Is sciatic nerve block advantageous when combined with femoral nerve block for postoperative analgesia following total knee arthroplasty? A systematic review. *Reg Anesth Pain Med*. 2011;36:493–498.

Abdallah FW, Brull R. Sciatic nerve block for analgesia after total knee arthroplasty: the jury is still out. *Reg Anesth Pain Med*. 2012;37:122–123; author reply 3–4.

Abdallah FW, Madjdpour C, Brull R. Is sciatic nerve block advantageous when combined with femoral nerve block for postoperative analgesia following total knee arthroplasty? A meta-analysis. *Can J Anaesth*. 2016;63:552–568.

Cullom C, Weed JT. Anesthetic and analgesic management for outpatient knee arthroplasty. *Curr Pain Headache Rep*. 2017;21:23.

Safa B, Gollish J, Haslam L, McCartney CJ. Comparing the effects of single shot sciatic nerve block versus posterior capsule local anesthetic infiltration on analgesia and functional outcome after total knee arthroplasty: a prospective, randomized, double-blinded, controlled trial. *J Arthroplasty*. 2014;29:1149–1153.

Sankineani SR, Reddy ARC, Eachempati KK, et al. Comparison of adductor canal block and IPACK block (interspace between the popliteal artery and the capsule of the posterior knee) with adductor canal block alone after total knee arthroplasty: a prospective control trial on pain and knee function in immediate postoperative period. *Eur J Orthop Surg Traumatol*. 2018 Oct;28(7):1391–1395.

Sinha SK, Abrams JH, Arumugam S, et al. Femoral nerve block with selective tibial nerve block provides effective analgesia without foot drop after total knee arthroplasty: a prospective, randomized, observer-blinded study. *Anesth Analg*. 2012;115:202–206.

2.2.9. Describe the technique of an ultrasound-guided sciatic nerve block

Some of the common approaches used to perform an ultrasound-guided sciatic nerve block are (1) anterior approach, (2) transgluteal approach, (3) subgluteal approach, and (4) popliteal-sciatic approach. The anterior approach does not require lateral positioning and is thus beneficial for patients who are in pain or have external hardware. Because sciatic blocks are performed mostly in conjunction with FNB for TKA, the anterior approach may be more practical in terms of patient positioning.

Anterior approach: The sciatic nerve block begins with the patient in the supine position and the knee slightly flexed. One of advantages of the anterior approach is that the patient remains in a supine position without the need to significantly manipulate the lower extremity. After skin preparation and draping, a curvilinear ultrasound probe is placed transversely at the level of the lesser trochanter on the anterior and medial portion of the thigh. The resulting ultrasound image will delineate the femoral artery, femur, and adductor magnus muscle. The sciatic nerve is the hyperechoic, triangular structure posterior to the adductor magnus muscle. The needle is inserted in plane with the ultrasound probe from medial to lateral until the tip reaches the sciatic nerve. After needle aspiration, 15 to 20 mL of local anesthetic is deposited with needle repositioning as needed to allow circumferential spread around the sciatic nerve.

Transgluteal approach: The patient is placed in the lateral decubitus position with knees and hips slightly flexed. The transducer is placed transversely over the gluteus muscle, and the resulting ultrasound image will show the ischial tuberosity and greater trochanter of the femur. Between these structures and deep to the gluteus muscle lies the sciatic nerve. Visualization of the sciatic nerve can be improved with slight tilting of the ultrasound transducer. The needle is inserted in plane with the ultrasound probe from lateral to medial until it reaches the sciatic nerve.

Subgluteal approach: The subgluteal approach involves the same patient positioning as the transgluteal approach. However, the ultrasound probe is placed transversely below the level of the subgluteal crease rather than over the gluteus muscle to avoid the interference of bony prominences on the ultrasound image. Instead, the image will show the sciatic nerve located deep to the long head of the biceps muscle and below the posterior surface of the adductor magnus muscle.

Popliteal-sciatic approach: This approach involves placing the patient either in lateral decubitus or prone position depending on the patient factors. In either case, the block begins by placing the ultrasound probe just above the popliteal crease. The popliteal artery should be visualized along with the biceps femoris muscle laterally and the semitendinosus and semimembranosus muscle medially. At this level, the tibial nerve and common peroneal nerve can be visualized. The ultrasound probe is then shifted cephalad while visualizing the tibial and peroneal nerves merging into a single nerve: the sciatic nerve. Once again, the probe can be tilted for better visualization of the sciatic nerve and the needle is inserted in plane from lateral to medial.

Further Reading

Boezaart AP, ed. *Atlas of Peripheral Nerve Blocks and Anatomy for Orthopaedic Anesthesia.* Philadelphia, PA: Saunders/Elsevier; 2008. http://hdl.library.upenn.edu/1017.12/1337779.

Brown DL, ed. *Atlas of Regional Anesthesia.* 4th ed. Philadelphia, PA: Saunders/Elsevier; 2010:xiv, 40.

Enneking FK, Chan V, Greger J, Hadzic A, Lang SA, Horlocker TT. Lower-extremity peripheral nerve blockade: essentials of our current understanding. *Reg Anesth Pain Med.* 2005;30:4–35.

2.2.10. Discuss the role of continuous nerve blocks in total knee arthroplasty?

Regional anesthetic techniques can involve either a single injection of local anesthetic and additives or placement of a catheter, which will continuously infuse local anesthetic in the area of the nerve to be blocked. Compared with systemic opioids, peripheral nerve catheters provide site-specific pain control and minimize opioid side effects such as nausea, vomiting, and respiratory depression. The decision to place a catheter must be weighed against the possibility of secondary failure of the catheter, infectious complications, and potentially increased risk of nerve injury. Secondary block failure is defined as catheter migration away from its original intended location and failure to provide any postoperative analgesia due to its distance from the intended nerve. In addition, the process of threading the catheter without visualization of the target can lead to unpredictable catheter direction. The authors recommend either identifying endpoints for catheter insertion in real time or observing the pattern of spread of local anesthetic injected through the catheter. Many operators often provide the initial bolus of local anesthetic via the Tuohy needle followed by catheter insertion to avoid complete block failure. Motor response may provide a valid endpoint for catheter insertion if a stimulating catheter is used.

Further Reading

Boezaart AP, ed. *Atlas of Peripheral Nerve Blocks and Anatomy for Orthopaedic Anesthesia.* Philadelphia, PA: Saunders/Elsevier; 2008:xi, 242

Capdevila X, Pirat P, Bringuier S, et al. Continuous peripheral nerve blocks in hospital wards after orthopedic surgery: a multicenter prospective analysis of the quality of postoperative analgesia and complications in 1,416 patients. *Anesthesiology.* 2005;103:1035–1045.

Salinas FV. Location, location, location: continuous peripheral nerve blocks and stimulating catheters. *Reg Anesth Pain Med.* 2003;28:79–82.

2.3. Surgical technique and impact on planning for perioperative anesthesia and analgesia

2.3.1. What are the different types of knee arthroplasty?

Total knee replacement refers to replacement of both the tibial and femoral components and the patellar surface of the knee joint. Complex or revision arthroplasty often occurs because of loosening of the prosthesis, advanced arthritis, or infection. A good portion of patients with revision arthroplasty are taking opioids for treatment of pain, which may make planning for postoperative analgesia more challenging. Partial or unicompartmental knee arthroplasty can be done in the setting where arthritis of the knee joint involves one compartment and the ligaments of the knee joints are relatively healthy. Partial knee replacement is often less invasive and is offered as an outpatient procedure for younger patients with less advanced arthritis. Details of the surgical techniques are beyond the scope of this chapter.

Further Reading

Borus T, Thornhill T. Unicompartmental knee arthroplasty. *JAAOS.* 2008 Jan;16(1):9–18.

Insall JN, Binazzi R, Soudry M, et al. Total knee arthroplasty. *CORR.* 1985 Jan;192:13–22.

2.3.2. How does the type of knee arthroplasty affect your planning for anesthesia and postoperative analgesia?

Unicompartmental knee arthroplasty is less invasive and often associated with less postoperative pain when compared with TKA. These patients tend to have less arthritis and to be opioid naive. Multimodal analgesia protocols, including a combination of local periarticular infiltration and/or PNBs, are usually effective for postoperative pain control. Planning for anesthesia and postoperative analgesia has to take into account the fact that these procedures are often done as outpatient surgery or in the setting of reduced length of hospital stay. Immediate participation in physical therapy and quick functional recovery are especially important in this setting. Anesthesia and postoperative analgesia plans have to be designed to achieve these goals. On the other hand, most of the studies that address efficacy of different analgesic techniques after TKA would have revision arthroplasty and patients with chronic pain syndromes as exclusion criteria. Few studies have addressed postoperative analgesia in revision arthroplasty. Pain management in patients who have chronic pain and who take opioid medication before surgery can be challenging. Individualized multimodal analgesia protocols designed for these patients, under direction of the acute pain service, can lead to better patient outcomes. Pain medicine plays an integral role in some of the perioperative care models designed to care for these patients, including the perioperative surgical home and the transitional pain service.

Further Reading

Grant AE, Schwenk ES, Torjman MC, et al. Postoperative analgesia in patients undergoing primary or revision knee arthroplasty with adductor canal block. *Anesth Pain Med.* 2017 Apr 17;7(3).

Walters TL, Mariano ER, Clark JD. Perioperative surgical home and the integral role of pain medicine. *Pain Med.* 2015 Sep;16 (9):1666–1672.

3. Postoperative Pain Management

3.1. Multimodal analgesia

3.1.1. What is the mechanism of action of gabapentin?

Gabapentin is a structural derivative of the endogenous GABA neurotransmitter. It acts on voltage-dependent calcium channels in the brain, spinal cord, and periphery, serving to ultimately decrease the release of excitatory neurotransmitters. Gabapentin is available in oral formulation, and its onset of action is 1 to 3 hours upon administration.

Further Reading

Sills GJ. The mechanisms of action of gabapentin and pregabalin. *Curr Opin Pharmacol.* 2006;6:108–113.

3.1.2. What is the role of gabapentin in total knee arthroplasty surgery?

Gabapentin was originally designed as an antiepileptic drug. However, its use has expanded to include treatment for neuropathic pain, fibromyalgia, and more recently acute postsurgical pain following hysterectomy, spinal surgery, joint arthroplasty, and other procedures. As a result of its success, there have been several randomized controlled trials to determine if gabapentin has any role in TKA. It has been shown to decrease opioid consumption and improve pain scores after TKA. It has also been suggested that the use of perioperative gabapentinoids may decrease the incidence of chronic persistent pain after TKA. However, the most recent meta-analysis reviews of these trials have shown no significant difference in pain scores between patients receiving gabapentin perioperatively compared with control groups at any time period for up to 72 hours after surgery. The optimal dosing regimen for perioperative gabapentinoids is still debatable, especially considering discrepancies between typical perioperative dosing regimens and target doses used for chronic pain conditions.

Further Reading

Buvanendran A, Kroin JS. Multimodal analgesia for controlling acute postoperative pain. *Curr Opin Anaesthesiol.* 2009;22:588–593.

Buvanendran A, Kroin JS, Della Valle CJ, Kari M, Moric M, Tuman KJ. Perioperative oral pregabalin reduces chronic pain after total knee arthroplasty: a prospective, randomized, controlled trial. *Anesth Analg.* 2010;110:199–207.

Carroll I, Hah J, Mackey S, et al. Perioperative interventions to reduce chronic postsurgical pain. *J Reconstr Microsurg.* 2013;29:213–222.

Clarke HA, Katz J, McCartney CJ, et al. Perioperative gabapentin reduces 24 h opioid consumption and improves in-hospital rehabilitation but not post-discharge outcomes after total knee arthroplasty with peripheral nerve block. *Br J Anaesth.* 2014;113:855–864.

Hamilton TW, Strickland LH, Pandit HG. A meta-analysis on the use of gabapentinoids for the treatment of acute postoperative pain following total knee arthroplasty. *J Bone Joint Surg Am.* 2016;98:1340–1350.

Schmidt PC, Ruchelli G, Mackey SC, Carroll IR. Perioperative gabapentinoids: choice of agent, dose, timing, and effects on chronic postsurgical pain. *Anesthesiology.* 2013;119:1215–1221.

3.1.3. What other agents are available for analgesia following surgery?

Multimodal analgesia is now the centerpiece of perioperative pain management. The goal is to implement a protocol that involves medications from a variety of drug classes to provide comprehensive pain management after surgery. The American Society of Regional Anesthesia and Pain Medicine, the American Pain Society, the American Association of Physicists in Medicine, the American Society of Anesthesiologists, and other pain medicine societies now recommend the use of multimodal analgesia in the postoperative period whenever feasible. One class of drugs is the nonsteroidal anti-inflammatory drugs, specifically cyclooxygenase-2 (COX-2) specific inhibitors, which are administered before and after surgery. One such drug, celecoxib, inhibits prostaglandin formation and does not interfere with platelet function, unlike nonspecific COX inhibitors. The existing studies have shown promising results with reduction in pain scores, reduced opioid consumption, and improved active range of motion after TKA. It is important to note that COX-2 inhibitors have been associated with an increase in adverse cardiovascular events. However, doses less than 400 mg per day and the short-term use of celecoxib in the setting of TKA have not been associated with increased risk.

Acetaminophen is another drug used in the multimodal analgesia regimen. Its mechanism of action in the setting of surgery is unclear, but it is believed to work on a variety of central nervous system pathways including serotonin. Acetaminophen is typically given in a 1-g dose preoperatively and given every 8 hours after surgery. The Food and Drug Administration issued a black box warning limiting the total daily dose of acetaminophen to 4000 mg. Intravenous formulations are available for use. Some studies suggest better pain control in the setting of TKA when intravenous acetaminophen is used as part of a multimodal analgesia protocol. However, most of the current studies do not show a clear clinical difference between the efficacies of oral versus intravenous administration.

Further Reading

American Society of Anesthesiologists Task Force on Acute Pain Management. Practice guidelines for acute pain management in the perioperative setting: an updated report by the American Society of Anesthesiologists Task Force on Acute Pain Management. *Anesthesiology*. 2012;116:248–273.

Brett CN, Barnett SG, Pearson J. Postoperative plasma paracetamol levels following oral or intravenous paracetamol administration: a double-blind randomised controlled trial. *Anaesth Intensive Care*. 2012;40:166–171.

Buvanendran A, Kroin JS, Tuman KJ, et al. Effects of perioperative administration of a selective cyclooxygenase 2 inhibitor on pain management and recovery of function after knee replacement: a randomized controlled trial. *JAMA*. 2003;290:2411–2418.

Chou R, Gordon DB, de Leon-Casasola OA, et al. Management of postoperative pain: a clinical practice guideline from the American Pain Society, the American Society of Regional Anesthesia and Pain Medicine, and the American Society of Anesthesiologists' Committee on Regional Anesthesia, Executive Committee, and Administrative Council. *J Pain*. 2016;17:131–157.

Gallipani A, Mathis AS, Lee Ghin H, Fahim G. Adverse effect profile comparison of pain regimens with and without intravenous acetaminophen in total hip and knee arthroplasty patients. *SAGE Open Med*. 2017;5:2050312117699146.

Huang YM, Wang CM, Wang CT, Lin WP, Horng LC, Jiang CC. Perioperative celecoxib administration for pain management after total knee arthroplasty: a randomized, controlled study. *BMC Musculoskelet Disord*. 2008;9:77.

Liu SS, Bae JJ, Bieltz M, Ma Y, Memtsoudis S. Association of perioperative use of nonsteroidal anti-inflammatory drugs with postoperative myocardial infarction after total joint replacement. *Reg Anesth Pain Med*. 2012;37:45–50.

Moucha CS, Weiser MC, Levin EJ. Current strategies in anesthesia and analgesia for total knee arthroplasty. *J Am Acad Orthop Surg*. 2016;24:60–73.

Murata-Ooiwa M, Tsukada S, Wakui M. Intravenous acetaminophen in multimodal pain management for patients undergoing total knee arthroplasty: a randomized, double-blind, placebo-controlled trial. *J Arthroplasty*. 2017;32(10):3024–3028.

Politi JR, Davis RL 2nd, Matrka AK. Randomized prospective trial comparing the use of intravenous versus oral acetaminophen in total joint arthroplasty. *J Arthroplasty*. 2017;32:1125–1127.

3.1.4. How can hospitals develop a fall prevention program following surgery?

Geriatric patients are at increased risk for falls due to underlying health issues associated with aging such as osteoarthritis, vision changes, and gait disturbances. Adding the insult of an acute surgery further increases the risk of falls in this patient population. In addition, patients may have received PNBs (single injection or continuous catheter) following surgery that can increase the risk of falls due to compromised quadriceps muscle strength. Patients who sustain falls have a longer hospital stay, could possibly be at higher risk for in-hospital mortality and complications, and incur higher hospital costs. Studies involving inpatients who have had TKA found that nearly all patients who fell had a peripheral nerve catheter at one point in their hospitalization and that 25% had a catheter in place during the time of the actual fall. Patients with femoral nerve catheters seemed to have the greatest increase in the risk of falls. More recently, a population-based study associated falls after TKA with receiving general anesthesia. The same study found no association between administration of PNBs and inpatient falls. Patients who had general anesthesia were more likely to fall in this study. Possible mechanisms of falls after TKA include lingering effects of sedatives and anesthetics, postural hypotension, weak quadriceps muscle, and impaired proprioception in patients receiving PNBs.

Fall reduction programs for surgical patients should involve collaboration by members from multiple disciplines. These strategies may include patient and family education, posted signs, bed alarms, and mandatory assistance with toileting needs. The role of the anesthesiologist in fall prophylaxis may best be defined as educational. These risks may be discussed at the preoperative outpatient visit prior to surgery or on the operative day prior to administration of regional anesthesia. Best practice includes educating both the patient and family members so that all stakeholders are aware of the potential risks. Some practices may provide the patient with written information and guidelines on how to prevent falls in addition to oral instructions. In either case, it is important to assess actual patient understanding of the provided instructions, as patient compliance will ultimately lead to a successful reduction in falls. Educational programs should include teaching physical therapists and nursing staff about mechanisms of fall and the importance of using knee support devices especially in patients with PNBs.

Further Reading

Clarke HD, Timm VL, Goldberg BR, Hattrup SJ. Preoperative patient education reduces in-hospital falls after total knee arthroplasty. *Clin Orthop Relat Res*. 2012;470:244–249.

Ilfeld BM. Single-injection and continuous femoral nerve blocks are associated with different risks of falling. *Anesthesiology*. 2014;121:668–669.

Ilfeld BM, Duke KB, Donohue MC. The association between lower extremity continuous peripheral nerve blocks and patient falls after knee and hip arthroplasty. *Anesth Analg*. 2010;111:1552–1554.

Johnson RL, Duncan CM, Ahn KS, Schroeder DR, Horlocker TT, Kopp SL. Fall-prevention strategies and patient characteristics that impact fall rates after total knee arthroplasty. *Anesth Analg*. 2014;119:1113–1118

Kim TE, Mariano ER. Developing a multidisciplinary fall reduction program for lower-extremity joint arthroplasty patients. *Anesthesiol Clin*. 2014;32:853–864.

Memtsoudis SG, Danninger T, Rasul R, et al. Inpatient falls after total knee arthroplasty: the role of anesthesia type and peripheral nerve blocks. *Anesthesiology*. 2014;120:551–563.

Memtsoudis SG, Dy CJ, Ma Y, Chiu YL, Della Valle AG, Mazumdar M. In-hospital patient falls after total joint arthroplasty: incidence, demographics, and risk factors in the United States. *J Arthroplasty*. 2012;27:823–828.e1.

3.1.5. Can enhanced recovery after surgery protocols and outpatient total knee arthroplasty programs be applied to certain patients?

Enhanced recovery after surgery (ERAS) protocols have been a core focus of researchers, clinicians, and hospital administrators. Benefits of early discharge from the hospital include reducing the chance of nosocomial infection and completion of physical and occupational therapy at the patient's home or local environment. As the volume of patients undergoing TKA increases, there has been much interest in reducing hospital length of stay and expediting recovery and rehabilitation to maintain optimal cost-effectiveness. Thus, ERAS protocols are increasingly being used for TKA patients. The exact protocol may vary among institutions, but the main features remain in place. Patient selection, including familial support, is a key component to the success of these protocols. Involving all the stakeholders and defining a priori measurable outcomes are also integral to success. Elements of the enhanced recovery protocols include patient education, instructions on fluid management, postoperative nausea and vomiting prophylaxis, regional anesthesia, and medication management. The decision to use an ERAS protocol on a patient remains at the discretion of the perioperative team, as certain patients may not benefit. For example, patients on long-acting chronic pain medications or patients who present for revision procedures may benefit from a customized perioperative plan rather than a generalized ERAS protocol. Performing primary TKA as an ambulatory procedure, in select groups of patients, is the natural evolution of these ERAS protocols. Outpatient TKA can be less expensive than TKA requiring multiple days of hospitalization. Some studies have concluded inpatient TKA and outpatient TKA lead to similar outcomes and postoperative complications. Thus, outpatient TKA may be a more cost-effective choice. Physicians must select patients with care, also taking into account the ability to manage any complications in settings with fewer resources.

Further Reading

Auyong DB, Allen CJ, Pahang JA, Clabeaux JJ, MacDonald KM, Hanson NA. Reduced length of hospitalization in primary total knee arthroplasty patients using an updated enhanced recovery after orthopedic surgery (ERAS) pathway. *J Arthroplasty*. 2015;30:1705–1709.

Bovonratwet P, Ondeck NT, Nelson SJ, Cui JJ, Webb ML, Grauer JN. Comparison of outpatient vs inpatient total knee arthroplasty: an ACS-NSQIP analysis. *J Arthroplasty*. 2017;32:1773–1778.

Courtney PM, Boniello AJ, Berger RA. Complications following outpatient total joint arthroplasty: an analysis of a national database. *J Arthroplasty*. 2017;32:1426–1430.

Huang A, Ryu JJ, Dervin G. Cost savings of outpatient versus standard inpatient total knee arthroplasty. *Can J Surg*. 2017;60:57–62.

Total Hip Arthroplasty

Sydney E. Rose and Julio A. Gonzalez-Sotomayor

7

Case Scenario

A 75-year-old woman with osteoarthritis presents for elective right total hip arthroplasty. She has a history of hypertension, myasthenia gravis, and gastrointestinal reflux disease. Her past surgical history includes a transcervical thymectomy 10 years ago. The patient reports progressively worsening, chronic hip pain over the past 2 years. On a 0–10 level of pain severity, she reports a baseline pain level of 6/10. She takes hydrocodone/acetaminophen 10 mg/325 mg every 6 to 8 hours while she is awake. She reports that over the last 3 months she has had very little to no improvement in pain. Additional medications include lisinopril 5 mg daily, pyridostigmine 60 mg 4 times daily, and omeprazole 20 mg daily. Her preoperative vital signs are HR = 70, BP = 130/60 mmHg, SpO_2 = 98% on room air, and a temperature of 36.4°C

1. Patient Factors

1.1. Postoperative opioid metabolism

1.1.1. What opioids are commonly used for postoperative pain control in orthopedic surgeries?

The most commonly used opioids in this setting are short-acting PO opioid medications such as oxycodone, oxycodone/acetaminophen, hydrocodone/acetaminophen, hydromorphone, morphine, and tramadol.

1.1.2. What is the mechanism of action of opioids?

Opioids are drugs that are derived directly from or are synthetically similar to those medications derived from the opium poppy plant. Opioids bind to certain receptors that are expressed in pain-modulating descending pathways throughout the brain, brainstem, spinal cord, and peripheral nervous system. These receptors are referred to as *opioid receptors* and have multiple types and subtypes. Classic opioid receptor types are the mu (μ), kappa (κ), and delta (δ) receptors. Analgesia that results from exogenous opioids is primarily through action at the μ receptor. Opioid receptors are G1-protein-coupled receptors, and for the most part the action of opioids at these receptors is inhibitory. Binding of opioid ligands to opioid receptor propagates intracellular pathways that inhibit N-type voltage-operated calcium channels from opening (preventing $Ca2^+$ entry) and stimulate potassium channels promoting K^+ efflux from the cell. This results in hyperpolarization of the neuronal membrane and a reduction in neuronal excitability. Binding of opioids also leads to inhibition of adenylyl cyclase and therefore a decrease in intracellular cAMP, interfering with the release of nociceptive neurotransmitters (e.g., acetylcholine, dopamine, norepinephrine, and substance P).

Further Reading

McDonald J, Lambert DG. Opioid receptors. *BJA Education*. 2015 Oct;15(1):219–224.

1.1.3. How are opioids metabolized?

Individual opioids are metabolized differently, and patients have differing abilities to metabolize specific opioids as well. Opioids are lipophilic, in varying degrees, and once they reach the systemic circulation, they passively cross cell membranes or target tissues. The liver is the main site of biotransformation to active or inactive metabolites. Most opioids undergo first-pass metabolism, and much of the parent drug is limited from reaching the systemic circulation, reducing the bioavailability of the drug. In the liver, 2 phases of metabolism occur. Phase 1 entails oxidation (most common) or reduction and hydrolysis to introduce a polar functional group to the lipophilic molecule and increase water solubility so that the product can be easily excreted and/or conjugated and then excreted. The cytochrome P450 enzymatic system catalyzes the oxidation of many opioid drugs. Phase 2 entails conjugating a molecule with a hydrophilic endogenous substance such as glucuronic acid, sulfate, or glycine, creating more polar molecules that can be readily excreted in urine or bile. Glucuronidation is an enzymatic reaction catalyzed by uridine diphosphate glucuronsyltransferase (UGT) and is essential to producing hydrophilic molecules. Opioids undergo varying degrees of phase 1 and/or phase 2 metabolism. Some undergo phase 1 metabolism only, others undergo phase 1 followed by phase 2 metabolism, and others undergo phase 2 metabolism only. Fentanyl, tramadol, and methadone are examples of opioids that undergo phase 1 metabolism. Hydrocodone and oxycodone undergo phase 1 and produce metabolites that undergo phase 2 metabolism as well. Morphine, hydromorphone, and oxymorphone undergo phase 2 metabolism only. Note that both phases can produce active or inactive metabolites, depending on the original parent drug being metabolized. Ultimately, the opioid being metabolized is converted to a more soluble hydrophilic molecule that can be excreted from the body.

1.1.4. What factors influence opioid metabolism?

Many opioids undergoing phase 1 metabolism are involved in reactions with enzymes CYP3A4 and CYP2D6. CYP3A4 is a primary drug-metabolizing enzyme and is involved in the metabolization of more than 50% of all drugs. Thus, any opioid that is metabolized by CYP3A4 has a high risk of interacting with other drugs metabolized by this enzyme. Likewise, any drugs or genetic factors influencing the CYP2D6 enzyme will influence the metabolism of opioids also metabolized by this pathway. Opioids metabolized by phase 2 metabolism are less affected by other drugs' metabolism. They may, however, be subjected to any factors that influence the UGT enzyme, and significant gene variability exists.

Further Reading

Smith HS. Opioid metabolism. *Mayo Clin Proc.* 2009 Jul; 84(7):613–624.

1.1.5. What are the recommended starting doses for commonly used opioids in opioid-naive patients undergoing a total hip arthroplasty?

The intensity and duration of pain after surgery are influenced by a variety of factors including diagnosis, the surgical procedure, patient's demographics, cultural/ethnic factors, history of alcohol, illicit drug, or prescription drug consumption, and psychological factors like anxiety and depression. Therefore, it is challenging to predict optimal dosing of postoperative opioids. In general, surgeries involving bones and joints tend to be more painful than those involving soft tissue only. Taking individual patient factors at the time of opioid prescription, at our institution, the starting doses for opioid-naive patients are as follows:

- Oxycodone 5 mg PO 1 to 2 tablets every 3 to 4 hours as needed
- Hydrocodone/acetaminophen 5 mg/325 mg PO 1 to 2 tablets every 3 to 4 hours as needed
- Hydromorphone 2 mg PO 1 to 2 tablets every 3 to 4 hours as needed

1.1.6. How might chronic opioid exposure influence this patient's postoperative course?

Chronic opioid exposure puts a patient at risk for inadequate pain control postoperatively. Elevated levels of postoperative pain can have negative cardiovascular and pulmonary implications. Poor pain control is the most common reason for delayed discharge from the postanesthesia care unit (PACU) and the most common reason for admission to the hospital after ambulatory surgery. Poorly controlled pain can also lead to a prolonged recovery after inpatient surgery.

1.1.7. What are the causes of increased postoperative pain and opioid consumption in patients on chronic opioids?

There are a multiple reasons why a patient chronically using opioid medication (COOM) might experience exaggerated amounts of postoperative pain and require increasing doses of opioids. First, the surgical site should always be examined for bleeding, infection, or wound dehiscence when a patient is having increased pain and requiring escalating doses of opioids. Another possible cause of increased postoperative pain in COOM patients is opioid-induced hyperalgesia (OIH). Regular exposure to opioids can induce an increased sensitivity to nociceptive stimulation. When this occurs, a COOM patient tends to experience more pain from a given nociceptive stimulus than a non-opioid-exposed patient. The development of tolerance is also a common cause that contributes to increased requirements of opioids. COOM patients typically require increasing doses of opioid medication to achieve adequate postoperative analgesia. Other independent factors associated with increased postoperative pain and increasing analgesic requirements include preexisting pain conditions, anxiety, depression, gender, and age. Any of these factors confounded with a COOM patient add to the risk of increased pain and escalating opioid consumption.

1.1.8. How does a patient's chronic opioid therapy affect your postoperative pain control strategy?

Postoperative pain management for opioid-tolerant patients can be challenging. It is important to identify a COOM patient preoperatively so that an appropriate postoperative strategy for pain can be executed. Prejudices and misconceptions surrounding opioid usage must be recognized to avoid inadequate analgesia. Goals for treating acute surgical pain in a COOM patient are to provide adequate pain control, avoid adverse effects, and prevent withdrawal.

Steps to devise a postoperative pain management plan for an opioid-tolerant patient include the following:

1. Discuss the patient's opioid regimen during the preoperative interview.
2. Calculate the patient's baseline 24-hour opioid requirements. This serves as the patient's baseline requirement before any surgery is done.
3. An equianalgesic chart can be used to convert the patient's home regimen to an oral morphine equivalent daily dose (MEDD). (Table 7.1) Equianalgesic charts help to compare different opioids and calculate equivalent doses in oral, intravenous, and transdermal forms. One such example is listed below.
4. If possible, it is easiest to continue the patient's preoperative opioid to manage the acute pain as one can escalate the dose from the baseline and there is less concern about potential adverse effects from a new agent. If changing from the patient's preoperative opioid to a different one, reduce the new opioid daily baseline dose by 25% to 40% to account for cross-tolerance.
5. If the patient is unable to take PO, or there is a potential problem with absorption, use the oral MEDD to convert to a parenteral drug that could be administered via a patient-controlled analgesia (PCA) pump or as intermittent scheduled IV doses. PCA pumps are ideal for patients who are alert and have the capacity to press the button to deliver additional needed doses for acute pain control.
6. If opioid is delivered orally, reassess the patient in 1 hour. If delivered intravenously, reassessment should occur within 15 to 30 minutes. If the patient's pain becomes tolerable, continue the preceding regimen, increasing the administration interval or decreasing dose amount as appropriate with recovery.
7. Aggressive multimodal analgesia should be utilized in almost all cases. Using adjuvants such as nonsteroidal anti-inflammatory drugs (NSAIDs), acetaminophen, and calcium channel modulators (gabapentin, pregabalin) can improve pain control, reduce adverse effects, and decrease the risk of hyperalgesia and increasing tolerance.

Table 7.1:
Equianalgesic doses of commonly used opioid medications

Opioid Medication	Oral (mg)	Parenteral (mg)
Morphine	30	10
Hydromorphone	7.5	1.5
Oxycodone	20	n/a
Hydrocodone	30	n/a
Methadone*	3–30	3–10
Fentanyl	n/a	0.1
Meperidine	300	100
Codeine	200	n/a
Tramadol	100	n/a

*Typical doses of methadone are 15 to 40 mg/d, given in divide doses. The relative potency of methadone to morphine increases considerably as MEDD increase due to its accumulation and excretion into the circulation from the liver.

Further Reading

Carroll IR, Angst MS, Clark JD. Management of perioperative pain in patients chronically consuming opioids. *Reg Anesth Pain Med.* 2004 Nov–Dec;29(6):576–591.

Case Scenario

The patient continues her physostigmine through the day of surgery. She was unable to wean herself off of hydrocodone/acetaminophen and was taking it up to 8 times daily immediately prior to surgery. She undergoes an uneventful intraoperative procedure after the placement of a lumbar plexus catheter. The patient received dexamethasone 10 mg intravenously prior to induction. In addition to her lumbar plexus catheter, the patient's postoperative pain regimen consists of hydrocodone/acetaminophen 10/325 mg every 6 hours, celecoxib 400 mg daily, and as needed IV hydromorphone. The patient reports good pain control but has progressively worsening tachycardia and hypertension.

2. Surgical Factors

2.1. Anatomy of the hip

2.1.1. What bones make up the hip joint?

i. The hip joint or acetabulofemoral joint is the synovial articulation between the head of the femur and the acetabulum of the pelvis. In adults, 3 pelvic bones, that is, ilium, ischium, and pubis, are fused to form the acetabulum. With a cuplike shape, the acetabulum contains about half of the femoral head. The grip is increased by the acetabular labrum, a ring-shaped fibrocartilage that extends the joint past the head equator. The femoral neck connects the head to the shaft of the femur. A strong but loose fibrous capsule covers the joint by attaching to the acetabulum and to the femoral neck. Three extracapsular ligaments, that is, iliofemoral, ischiofemoral, and pubofemoral, add stability to the joint. A fourth ligament, the ligamentum teres, is an intracapsular ligament that contains a small artery that may play a major role in maintaining blood supply to the femoral head in some cases of fractures of the femoral neck.
ii. The proximal end of the femoral shaft contains 2 protuberances, the greater and lesser trochanters, which play a major role in muscle attachment.

2.1.2. What are the surface landmarks of the hip?

i. The pelvic bone is formed by the fusion of the ilium, the ischium, and the pubic bones. The hip bone has 3 articulations, that is, posteriorly the sacroiliac joint to articulate with the sacrum, anteriorly the pubic symphysis to articulate with the other pelvic bone, and laterally the hip joint to articulate with the femur.
ii. The upper edge of the ilium is called the iliac crest and can be palpated in the flank area. The iliac crest extends, front to back, from the anterior superior iliac spine (ASIS) to the posterior superior iliac spine (PSIS).
iii. The ASIS provides attachment to the inguinal ligament and the sartorius muscle and is easy to palpate in most individuals.
iv. The PSIS is at the level of the second sacral spinal process or midportion of the sacroiliac joint. Most individuals have recognizable dimples at the skin covering the PSIS.
v. The pubic tubercle is just lateral to the pubic symphysis and provides attachment to the medial end of the inguinal ligament. The pubic tubercle can be palpated as a small eminence next to midline at the lowest part of the anterior abdomen. Halfway along the inguinal ligament, between the ASIS and the pubic tubercle, the femoral artery can be palpated as well.
vi. The ischial tuberosity is the lowest portion of the ischium and bears the weight of the trunk in a sitting position. It can be palpated when the hip is flexed just above the gluteal fold.
vii. The greater trochanter is a palpable bony protuberance located laterally in the upper part of the lower extremity and a few inches below the midpoint of the iliac crest.

2.1.3. Describe the main vasculature supply hip

i. Arteries supplying the hip region are branches arising from the internal iliac artery or from the femoral artery. Branches of the internal iliac artery include the iliolumbar, obturator, superior gluteal (SGA), inferior gluteal (IGA), and internal pudendal arteries. Branches of the femoral artery include the medial femoral circumflex (MFCA) and lateral femoral circumflex (LFCA) arteries.
ii. Acetabulum
   1. The main sources of arterial supply of the acetabulum are branches from the obturator artery, the SGA, and the IGA.
   2. Branches of the SGA supply the superior rim of the acetabulum. Branches of the IGA supply mostly the inferior and posterior region of the acetabulum.
   3. The obturator artery supplies the pelvic surface of the acetabulum. Its posterior branch gives origin to the acetabular artery and anastomoses with the IGA to complete the periacetabular vascular circle. Also, a branch of the obturator artery enters the acetabular fossa.
iii. Femur
   1. The femoral head receives blood supply from retinacular vessels, arising from (1) the MFCA and the LFCA, both arising from the profunda femoris artery in most individuals; (2) terminal branches of the medullary artery from the shaft of the femur; and (3) the posterior division of the obturator artery through the artery of the ligamentum teres.
   2. The IGA contributes to the blood supply of the femoral head as well. It anastomoses with the MFCA through its piriformis branch.

Further Reading

Itokazu M, Takahashi K, Matsunaga T, Hayakawa D, et al. A study of the arterial supply of the human acetabulum using a corrosion casting method. *Clini Anat.* 1977;10:77–81.

Seeley MA, Georgiadis AG, Sankar WN. Hip vascularity: a review of the anatomy and clinical implications. *J Am Acad Orthop Surg.* 2016;24:515–526.

2.1.4. What are the main muscles that act on the hip joint?

i. The muscles that provide movement and stability to the hip joint can be divided in different groups as follows:
   1. The gluteal group includes the gluteus maximus, medius, and minimus muscles and the tensor fasciae latae. The gluteus maximus originates on the ilium and sacrum and inserts on the posterior aspect of the femur as well as on the iliotibial tract. The gluteus medius and minimus also originate on the ilium, and both insert on the greater trochanter of the femur. Similar to the gluteus maximus, the tensor fasciae latae runs from the ilium to the iliotibial tract. The gluteus maximus is the main hip extensor and assists with hip abduction when the hip is in extension. The gluteus medius is a strong hip abductor. The gluteus minimus and tensor fascia latae are abductors when the hip is flexed.
   2. The iliopsoas group includes the psoas major and the iliacus muscles. The psoas major originates from the lumbar spine and the iliacus on the iliac fossa of the ilium. Both muscles then connect and insert on the lesser trochanter of the femur. The iliopsoas muscle, as this is commonly called, is a major hip flexor.
   3. The lateral rotator group includes the externus and internus obturators, the piriformis, the superior and inferior gemelli, and the quadratus femoris. These 6 muscles originate at the lower portion of the pelvic bone and insert on or near the greater trochanter of the femur. Their main function is as external rotators of the hip.
   4. The adductor group includes the adductor brevis, longus, and magnus, the pectineus, and the gracilis muscles. The adductor muscles and the pectineus originate on the pubis and insert on the posteromedial aspect of the femur. The gracilis runs from the pubis to the medial condyle of the tibia. This group of muscles participates in adduction and flexion of the hip.

ii. Other muscles contributing to movements of the hip joint are the rectus femoris, the sartorius, and the hamstrings. The rectus femoris is part of the quadriceps muscle and runs from the anterior inferior iliac spine to the upper tibia. It is an important hip flexor and a knee extensor as well. The sartorius originates at the ASIS and on the medial aspect of the upper tibia. It is a hip flexor and external rotator. The semitendinosus, semimembranosus, and the long head of the biceps femoris originate at the ischial tuberosity and insert on the medial upper tibia (semitendinosus and semimembranosus) and the head of the fibula (biceps). They are hip extensors, as well as knee flexors.

2.1.5. Describe the nerve innervation of the hip joint

i. The nerves that serve the hip joint originate at the lumbosacral plexus, which is formed by the ventral rami of T12 to S3. The main nerves covering the hip joint are the femoral, the lateral femoral cutaneous (LFCN), the obturator, the superior and the inferior gluteal, and the sciatic nerves.

ii. The skin covering the hip joint is innervated as follows:
   1. Anteriorly by branches of the ilioinguinal and genitofemoral nerves.
   2. Laterally by the LFCN and a lateral cutaneous branch of the subcostal nerve.
   3. Posteriorly by a lateral cutaneous branch of the iliohypogastric nerve, the superior and medial cluneal nerves, and the posterior cutaneous nerve of the thigh.

iii. In terms of muscular innervation:
   1. The femoral nerve innervates the sartorius, pectineus, and quadriceps muscles.
   2. The obturator nerve innervates the obturator externus, gracilis, and adductor muscles.
   3. The superior gluteal nerve innervates the gluteus medius and minimus and the tensor fasciae latae.
   4. The inferior gluteal nerve innervates the gluteus maximus.
   5. The sciatic nerve innervates the hamstrings.

iv. In terms of capsular and bone innervation:
   1. Branches from the femoral and the obturator nerves provide innervation to the anterior aspect of the hip capsule, anterior portion of the femoral head and neck, and acetabulum. Contributions from the accessory obturator nerve are less consistent. The posterior aspect of these structures is mainly innervated by branches arising from the sciatic nerve or directly from the sacral plexus.
   2. The greater trochanter is innervated by the sciatic and the femoral nerves. The obturator nerve covers the lesser trochanter.

Further Reading

Bonica JJ. Applied anatomy relevant to pain. In: Loeser JD, ed. *Bonica's Management of Pain*. 3rd ed. Philadelphia, PA: Lippincott, Williams and Wilkins; 2001:202–203.

Short AJ, Barnett JJG, Gofeld M, Baig E, et al. Anatomic study of innervation of the anterior hip capsule: implication for image-guided intervention. *Reg Anesth Pain Med*. 2018 Feb;43(2):186–192.

3. Regional Anesthesia Factors

This section describes regional anesthesia options for THA, which include neuraxial anesthesia, fascia iliaca block, lumbar plexus block, and local anesthetic infiltration. These blocks are often part of a multimodal approach to perioperative pain management.

There has been ongoing debate regarding the advantages of neuraxial anesthesia versus general anesthesia in orthopedic surgery. Domains of concern include morbidity, mortality, postoperative pain control, opioid consumption and adverse effects, time to PACU discharge, length of hospital stay, postoperative nausea, and patient satisfaction. A recent systematic review included randomized controlled trials and prospective observational studies comparing neuraxial (spinal and epidural) anesthesia with general anesthesia for THA, total knee arthroplasty, or both. After 126 studies were reviewed, 29 studies involving a total of 10,488 patients met inclusion criteria. Outcomes evaluated were mortality, major morbidity defined as vascular events (deep venous thrombosis, cerebrovascular accidents, and myocardial infarctions), infection, nerve injury, postoperative nausea and vomiting, postoperative pain persisting beyond 3 months, changes in mental status, length of hospital stay, duration of surgery, and anesthetic cost. Results suggested that, when compared with general anesthesia, neuraxial anesthesia was associated with shorter length of hospital stay. There was no statistical difference between the 2 groups in terms of mortality, surgical site or chest infection, nerve palsy, postoperative nausea and vomiting, length of surgery, or thromboembolic disease when antithrombotic prophylaxis was used. This analysis suggests that neuraxial anesthesia is a viable alternative to general anesthesia for hip surgery.

Further Reading

Johnson RL, Kopp SL, Burkle CM, Duncan CM, et al. Neuraxial vs general anaesthesia for total hip and total knee arthroplasty: a systematic review of comparative effectiveness research. *Br J Anaest*. 2016;116(2):163–176.

3.1. Epidural anesthesia

This type of neuraxial blockade can be used as the primary anesthetic for THA and/or for postoperative pain control. Epidural anesthesia involves placing a lumbar epidural catheter, typically at the L2-L4 level, recognizing that blockade of sensory innervation to the surgical area should cover nerve roots from L1 to S3 levels. When used for analgesia, the epidural catheter is used most commonly to infuse long-acting local anesthetics like bupivacaine or ropivacaine, with typical rates between 4 mL/h and 10 mL/h. Concentrations of 0.05% to 0.1% of bupivacaine or ropivacaine are often preferred to minimize motor blockade and sympathectomy.

Contraindications: Patient refusal, coagulopathy, infection at insertion site, septicemia, severe hypovolemia, severe aortic stenosis, increased intracranial pressures (due to consequences of accidental dural puncture), and precluding spinal deformities.

Advantages:

- Epidural can be used as the primary anesthetic in patients in whom general anesthesia is deemed riskier, for example, patients with severe cardiac or respiratory comorbidities, difficult airway.
- Often provides superior analgesia compared with systemic opioids.
- Helps decrease opioid use in patients at increased risk of respiratory depression, for example, elderly, patients with pulmonary pathology.
- Provides alternative analgesic options in opioid-tolerant patients.
- Better hemodynamic control than spinal block.

Disadvantages:

- Positioning patient for placement may be challenging or not possible in the setting of a hip fracture.
- To decrease risk of epidural hematoma, only limited anticoagulation regimens are acceptable while epidural catheter is in place.
- Most patients will require a Foley catheter until the epidural is stopped.
- Motor blockade of lower extremities could decrease participation in physical therapy.

Further Reading

Guay J. The epidural test dose: a review. *Anesth Analg.* 2006 Mar;102(3):921–929.

3.2. Spinal anesthesia

Spinal anesthesia is often used as the primary anesthetic for hip surgery and could be associated with less postoperative delirium when compared with general anesthesia.

Spinal blockade often involves accessing the intrathecal space at the L2-L4 levels where local anesthetic with or without opioids is injected. A commonly use local anesthetic is bupivacaine, of which options are hyperbaric, isobaric, or hypobaric. There is some evidence showing that both hyperbaric and isobaric bupivacaine provide effective anesthesia albeit in the setting of cesarean sections, with no difference in failure rates or adverse effects. Hypobaric spinal anesthesia for hip surgery has been shown to provide better hemodynamic stability during surgery, when compared with general anesthesia.

Contraindications: Similar to epidural anesthesia.

Advantages:

- Possibly associated with lower postoperative pain scores and less opioid consumption than general anesthesia.
- Associated with less postoperative nausea than general anesthesia.
- As with epidural anesthesia, it can be used in patients with comorbidities, which put them at high risk for general anesthesia, for example, cardiac comorbidities and difficult airway.
- Associated with shorter hospital stay.

Disadvantages:

- Patient positioning in the setting of hip injury could be difficult.
- Could be technically difficult in patients with spinal deformities.
- Often contraindicated in patients with coagulopathies associated with increased bleeding.
- Contraindicated in severe cardiac valve diseases like severe aortic stenosis.
- Could lead to increased risk of perioperative hypothermia.
- Might be associated with increased risk of venous thromboembolism.
- Risk for post dural puncture headache.

Further Reading

Bapat V, Vishwasrao S. Spinal anaesthesia with midline and paramedian technique in elderly patients. *Indian J Appl Res.* 2015:5:2249–2555.

Haghighi M, Sedighinejad A, Nabi BN, Mardani-Kivi M, et al. Is spinal anesthesia with low dose lidocaine better than Sevoflorane anesthesia in patients undergoing hip fracture surgery. *Arch Bone Jt Surg.* 2017 Jul;5(4):226–230.

Khraise WN, Allouh MZ, El-Radaideh KM, Said RS, et al. Assessment of risk factors for postdural puncture headache in women undergoing cesarean delivery in Jordan: a retrospective analytical study. *Local Reg Anesth.* 2017;10:9–13.

Meuret P, Bouvet L, Villet B, Hafez M, et al. Hypobaric unilateral spinal anaesthesia versus general anaesthesia in elderly patients undergoing hip fracture surgical repair: a prospective randomised open trial. *Turk J Anaesthesiol Reanim*. 2018 Apr; 46(2):121–130. doi:10.5152/TJAR.2018.90699. Epub 2018 Apr 1.

Nakamura M, Kamei M, Bito S, Migita K, et al. Spinal anesthesia increases the risk of venous thromboembolism in total arthroplasty: secondary analysis of a J-PSVT cohort study on anesthesia. *Medicine (Baltimore)*. 2017 May;96(18):e6748.

Perlas A, Chan VW, Beattie S. Anesthesia technique and mortality after total hip or knee arthroplasty: a retrospective, propensity score–matched cohort study. *Anesthesiology*. 2016 Oct;125(4):724–731.

Scholten R, Leijtens B, Kremers K, Snoeck M, et al. The incidence of mild hypothermia after total knee or hip arthroplasty: a study of 2600 patients. *J Orthop*. 2018 Mar 17;15(2):408–411. doi:10.1016/j.jor.2018.03.014

Uppal V, Retter S, Shanthanna H, Prabhakar C, et al. Hyperbaric versus isobaric bupivacaine for spinal anesthesia: systematic review and meta-analysis for adult patients undergoing noncesarean delivery surgery. *Anesth Analg*. 2017 Nov;125(5):1627–1637.

Xu H, Liu Y, Song W, Kan S, Liu F, et al. Comparison of cutting and pencil-point spinal needle in spinal anesthesia regarding postdural puncture headache: a meta-analysis. *Medicine (Baltimore)*. 2017 Apr; 96(14):e6527.

3.3. Local anesthetic infiltration

An option for postoperative pain control is local anesthetic infiltration, which is usually done by the surgeon during the procedure. One common choice is the infiltration of bupivacaine with or without epinephrine. Liposomal bupivacaine consists of molecules of bupivacaine encapsulated in lipid layers, which allows for prolonged release of the drug. In THA, when compared with regular bupivacaine, liposomal bupivacaine showed superior pain control at 24 hours with shorter hospital stay. However, it did not show any difference in pain intensity scores after 48 hours.

Contraindications: Allergy to local anesthetic.

Advantages:

- Cost-effective.
- Technically easier to perform than neuraxial and peripheral nerve blocks.
- An option for patients who cannot receive peripheral nerve blocks or neuraxial procedures.
- Could decrease opioid consumption.
- Less motor blockade than with neuraxial or peripheral blocks, which could enable early participation in physical therapy and rehabilitation.

Disadvantages:

- Short duration of analgesia.
- High volume of local anesthetic often needed, which puts the patient at increased risk for local anesthetic toxicity.
- Inadequate analgesia in areas not properly infiltrated.
- High dose of local anesthetic given could preclude use of other nerve blocks.
- Local anesthetic could be toxic to cartilage.

Further Reading

Chahar P, Cummings KC. Liposomal bupivacaine: a review of a new bupivacaine formulation. *J Pain Res*. 2012;5:257–264.

Gulihar A, Robati S, Twaij H, Salih A, et al. Articular cartilage and local anaesthetic: a systematic review of the current literature. *J Orthop*. 2015 Dec; 12(suppl 2):S200–S210.

Ma TT, Wang YH, Jiang YF, Peng CB, et al. Liposomal bupivacaine versus traditional bupivacaine for pain control after total hip arthroplasty. *Medicine (Baltimore)*. 2017 Jun;96(25):e7190.

Zhang X, Yang Q, Zhang Z. The efficiency and safety of local liposomal bupivacaine infiltration for pain control in total hip arthroplasty: a systematic review and meta-analysis. *Medicine (Baltimore)*. 2017 Dec;96(49):e8433.

3.4. Fascia Iliaca Block

This is often considered a field block where local anesthetic is infiltrated under the iliacus muscle fascia to spread medial to the femoral nerve and lateral to the LFCN. Proximal spread to the lumbar plexus is also possible, but it is often not the case. The femoral nerve contributes to the innervation of the hip and femoral neck while the lateral femoral cutaneous nerve contributes to the cutaneous innervation of the lateral hip and thigh. Both of these nerves provide some but not all the innervation to the surgical area involved in THA.

Contraindications: Patient refusal, allergy to local anesthetic, infection at site of needle entry.

Advantages:

- An alternative for patients with coagulopathy who are not candidates for lumbar plexus blocks or neuraxial anesthesia.
- Potential reduction in opioid consumption.
- Block is done farther away from neurovascular structures and hence might have a safer profile.

Disadvantages:

- Does not reliably cover parts of the hip joint and skin not innervated by the femoral nerve and lateral femoral cutaneous nerve.
- High doses of local anesthetic put patient at risk for local anesthetic systemic toxicity.
- Short duration of pain control compared with neuraxial catheter or lumbar plexus catheter technique.

3.5. Lumbar plexus block

This block, also known as the psoas compartment block, is often used for hip, anterior thigh, and knee surgery or injuries. The major nerves blocked with this technique are iliohypogastric, ilioinguinal, genitofemoral, LFCN, femoral, and obturator, all arising from T12-L4 nerve roots. A lumbar plexus block will not block nerves to the hip joint arising from the sacral plexus.

Contraindications: Patient refusal, coagulopathy, infection at sight of injection, severe hypovolemia (risk for epidural distribution), allergy to local anesthetic.

Advantages:

- Might be a safer alternative to neuraxial anesthesia when neuraxial anesthesia is contraindicated.
- Unilateral motor blockade could prevent patient from being completely bed bound.
- Possible reduction of opioid consumption.
- Catheter can provide continuous analgesia for multiple days after procedure.
- When used as the primary anesthetic combined with sciatic nerve block, it provides more hemodynamic stability.

Disadvantages:

- High catheter failure rate (up to 40%).
- Risk of epidural or spinal spread of local anesthetic.
- Risk of neurovascular injury from bleeding, infection, or direct trauma during block placement.
- Motor blockade of ipsilateral extremity and hence decreasing ability to participate in physical therapy.
- Risk of renal puncture during block placement.
- Risk of hemodynamic instability.

Further Reading

Alzaharani A, Bali K, Gudena R, Railton P, et al. The innervation of the human acetabular labrum and hip joint: an anatomic study. *BMC Musculoskelet Disord.* 2014;15:41.

deVisme V, Picart F, Le Jouan R, Legrand A, et al. Combined lumbar and sacral plexus block compared with plain bupivacaine spinal anesthesia for hip fractures in the elderly. *Reg Anesth Pain Med.* 2000;25:158–162.

Salinas FV. Location, location, location: continuous peripheral nerve blocks and stimulating catheters. *Reg Anesth Pain Med.* 2003;28:79–82.

Case Scenario

The patient undergoes an uneventful intraoperative procedure after the placement of a lumbar plexus catheter. The patient received dexamethasone 10 mg prior to induction. The postoperative pain regimen consists of hydrocodone/acetaminophen, celecoxib, and as needed IV hydromorphone. The patient continues to report no pain benefit despite increasing her dose of hydrocodone/acetaminophen.

4. Postoperative Pain Management

4.1. How do glucocorticoids affect postoperative pain control?

The perioperative use of glucocorticoids has been associated with better analgesia and decreased use of opioids. The mechanisms of action could be related to their anti-inflammatory and immunosuppressive properties. They block eicosanoid production and inhibit multiple leukocyte inflammatory events (e.g., epithelial adhesion, emigration, chemotaxis, phagocytosis, and respiratory burst). Corticosteroids were also found to suppress transmission in thin unmyelinated C-fibers, which are involved in nociceptive signaling. In a meta-analysis of randomized clinical trials, De Oliveira et al. showed that dexamethasone at doses >0.1 mg/kg IV reduced postoperative pain and opioid consumption when compared with placebo. Specific to THA, a single preoperative dose of dexamethasone 40 mg IV resulted in less dynamic pain at 24 hours. However, specific dosing recommendations are unclear at present. Also, in a randomized, double-blind, placebo-controlled trial, methylprednisolone 125 mg IV before elective, unilateral primary THA decreased pain at 24 hours after surgery as well.

Further Reading

De Oliveira GS Jr, Almeida MD, Benzon HT, McCarthy RJ. Perioperative single dose systemic dexamethasone for postoperative pain: a meta-analysis of randomized controlled trials. *Anesthesiology*. 2011 Sep;115(3):575–588.

Johansson A, Hao J, Sjolund B. Local corticosteroid application blocks transmission in normal nociceptive C-fibers. *Acta Anaesthesiol Scand*. 1990 Jul;34(5):335–338.

Kardash KJ, Sarrazin F, Tessler MJ, Velly AM. Single-dose dexamethasone reduces dynamic pain after total hip arthroplasty. *Anesth Analg*. 2008;106:1253–1257.

Lunn TH, Andersen LØ, Kristensen BB, Husted H, et al. Effect of high-dose preoperative methylprednisolone on recovery after total hip arthroplasty: a randomized, double blind, placebo-controlled trial. *Br J Anaesth*. 2013;110(1):66–73.

4.2. What is perineural dexamethasone?

Dexamethasone has also been evaluated as an adjunct in regional anesthesia in an attempt to prolong the effect of local anesthetics. The perineural injection of a solution containing dexamethasone and local anesthetic has shown faster onset of action and increased duration of analgesia and motor blockade when compared with a solution containing only local anesthetic.

Further Reading

Albrecht E, Kern C, Kirkham KR. A systematic review and meta-analysis of perineural dexamethasone for peripheral nerve blocks. *Anaesthesia*. 2015;70:71–83.

Huynh TM, Marret E, Bonnet F. Combination of dexamethasone and local anaesthetic solution in peripheral nerve blocks: a meta-analysis of randomised controlled trials. *Eur J Anaesthesiol*. 2015 Nov;32(11):751–758.

4.3. Is perineural dexamethasone superior to IV?

Whether or not perineural dexamethasone provides analgesia that is clinically superior to that with IV dexamethasone remains unclear. Recent systematic reviews and meta-analyses show that perineural dexamethasone slightly prolongs the duration of analgesia, but conclusions are based on trials of moderate or low overall quality and high heterogeneity. The current consensus seems to be that the injection of perineural dexamethasone should be evaluated with caution, considering its off-label use as well.

Further Reading

Baeriswyl M, Kirkham KR, Jacot-Guillarmod A, Albrecht E. Efficacy of perineural vs systemic dexamethasone to prolong analgesia after peripheral nerve block: a systematic review and meta-analysis. *Br J Anaesth.* 2017 Aug 1;119(2):183–191.

Heesen M, et al. Co-administration of dexamethasone with peripheral nerve block: intravenous vs perineural application: systematic review, meta-analysis, meta-regression and trial-sequential analysis. *Br J Anaesth.* 2018;120(2):212–227.

Hussain N, Van den Langenbergh T, Sermer C, Fontes ML, et al. Equivalent analgesic effectiveness between perineural and intravenous dexamethasone as adjuvants for peripheral nerve blockade: a systematic review and meta-analysis. *Can J Anaesth.* 2018 Feb;65(2):194–206.

Zhao WL, Ou XF, Liu J, Zhang WS. Perineural versus intravenous dexamethasone as an adjuvant in regional anesthesia: a systematic review and meta-analysis. *J Pain Res.* 2017 Jul 4;10:1529–1543.

Zorrilla-Vaca A, Jinlei Li J. Dexamethasone injected perineurally is more effective than administered intravenously for peripheral nerve blocks: a meta-analysis of randomized controlled trials. *Clin J Pain.* 2018;34:276–284.

8

Ankle Arthrodesis

Jill Berlin and Thomas Halaszynski

Case Scenario

A 55-year-old woman with a history of hypertension and numerous ankle surgeries now presents for a left ankle arthrodesis. She has a significant history of long-term opioid use for her ankle pain and has been transitioned to oral buprenorphine/naloxone by her primary care provider. Her medical history is significant for atrial fibrillation (paroxysmal) and low back pain. Her surgical history includes an L3-S1 fusion 3 years ago and right rotator cuff repair 7 years ago. Additional medications include dabigatran and a daily baby aspirin. Vital signs show atrial fibrillation with a ventricular rate of 82 and blood pressure of 125/65 mmHg.

Case Scenario

The patient stopped her buprenorphine/naloxone 3 days prior to the surgery. She received a sciatic perineural catheter and a single- injection saphenous nerve block. She was discharged home on postoperative day 1 with an elastomeric pump intended for a 3-day perineural infusion time. One week following surgery, she returns to the hospital complaining of the inability to dorsiflex her foot.

1. Patient Factors

1.1. What are the perioperative considerations for the patient on buprenorphine/naloxone?

Buprenorphine is used in the management of chronic pain and opioid use disorders. It is a semisynthetic partial opioid agonist at the mu opioid receptor (has an affinity higher than that of a full agonist at the mu receptor) and an antagonist of the kappa opioid receptor. The attraction of this methadone alternative is its increased safety profile and the convenience of use for both the patient and the physician provider; in addition, the US formulation, known as Suboxone, has properties to discourage abuse. It has lower efficacy, slower offset, and a ceiling effect, making surgical analgesia difficult to control for those on maintenance therapy.

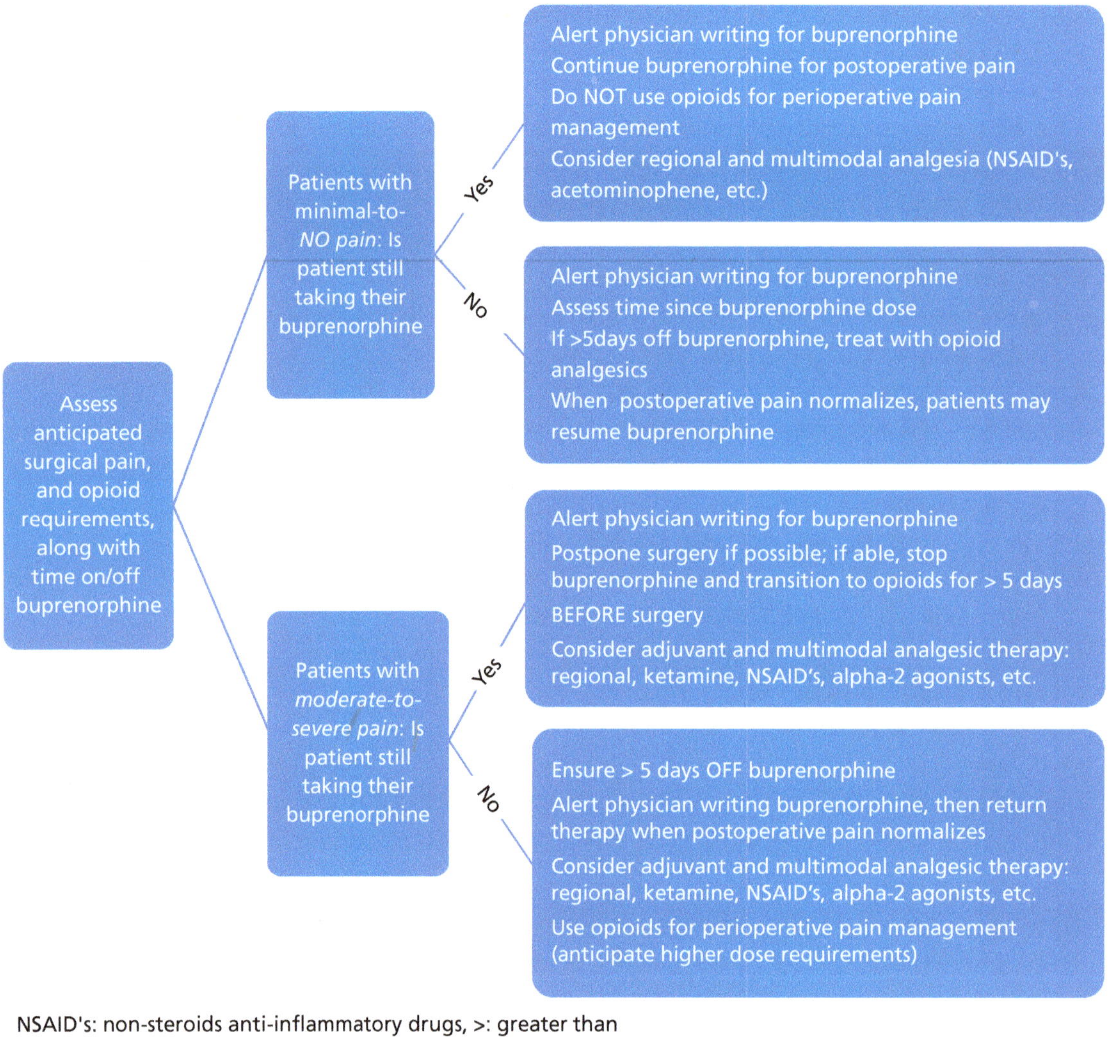

Figure 8.1 Management of buprenorphine in the acute perioperative setting.

Macintyre PE, Russell RA, Usher KA, Gaughwin M, Huxtable CA. Pain relief and opioid requirements in the first 24 hours after surgery in patients taking buprenorphine and methadone opioid substitution therapy. *Anaesthes Intensive Care* 2013;41(2):222–230.

In the clinical setting, many opinions and theories have been discussed in the approach to managing perioperative pain for patients on buprenorphine (Figure 8.1). Multimodal perioperative approaches should be utilized, including ketamine (NMDA antagonist; opioid alternative), infiltration of local anesthesia (peripheral nerve blockade [PNB] with indwelling catheters when possible), as well as use of nonopioid adjuncts such as nonsteroidal anti-inflammatory drugs (NSAIDs), acetaminophen, COX-2 inhibitors (Celebrex), and gabapentin. Consulting the patient's pain specialist and the facility's pain specialist/pain management team is recommended.

Further Reading

Chiang CN, Hawks RL. Pharmacokinetics of the combination tablet of buprenorphine and naloxone. *Drug Alcohol Depend.* 2003;702:S39–S47.

Cowan A, Lewis JW, Macfarlane IR. Agonist and antagonist properties of buprenorphine, a new antinociceptive agent. *Br J Pharmacol.* 1977;60:537–545.

2. Preoperative Evaluation and Preparation

2.1. Should the diagnosis of atrial fibrillation be addressed prior to surgery and how?

In patients with a history of atrial fibrillation, inquiries should be focused on asking the following (prior to surgery): Do they know when their last episode of atrial fibrillation occurred and if they had any symptoms when it was occurring? Are they rate controlled, or were they ever prescribed medications for rate control? And have they ever had a cardioversion or cardiac ablation? Because many of these patients could also have preexisting cardiac disease, a preoperative transthoracic echocardiogram (nonemergent cases) may be helpful in evaluating either/both cardiac and valve function, especially if they describe symptoms. In non-rate-controlled patients, a beta blocker or calcium channel blocker could be considered as tolerated by their blood pressure. In addition and prior to surgery, a discussion with the surgical team about any plans related to the possible perioperative use of anticoagulation should be made in conjunction with inquiring about the patient's last dabigatran (Pradaxa) administration.

Further Reading

Cornia P, Wong C, eds. *The Perioperative Medicine Consult Handbook*. New York, NY: Springer; 2013:57–66.

Lee SI, Sayers M, Lip GY, Lane DA. Use of non–vitamin K antagonist oral anticoagulants in atrial fibrillation patients: insights from a specialist atrial fibrillation clinic. *Int J Clin Pract*. 2015;69(11):1341–1348.

2.2. What is dabigatran (Pradaxa)? Is it a reversible anticoagulant? How are its clinical effects measured? Do anticoagulation issues need to be addressed prior to surgery, and if so, how? Should it be discontinued prior to surgery, and if so, for how long?

Dabigatran etexilate (Pradaxa; anticoagulant to reduce risk of stroke in patients with atrial fibrillation) is a direct thrombin inhibitor (factor IIa) that is among a group of newer oral anticoagulants (NOACs; novel oral anticoagulants). This medication is generally easier to manage than warfarin, does not require laboratory monitoring, and now has a reversal agent, idarucizumab, which can be utilized in the following scenarios:

- Emergency surgery/urgent procedures
- Life-threatening or uncontrolled bleeding

Hemodialysis can remove dabigatran (experience as a treatment for bleeding is limited); administration of prothrombin complex concentrates, recombinant factor VIIa (has not been evaluated), or platelet concentrates may be considered for reversal as well. Protamine sulfate and vitamin K are not expected to affect dabigatran activity. Hemoclot direct thrombin inhibitor assay, Ecarin clotting time, and Ecarin chromogenic assay all serve as quantitative testing of dabigatran activity; a normal activated partial thromboplastin time and thrombin time would suggest lack of significant dabigatran activity.

Dabigatran (prodrug hydrolyzed by serum esterases to its active form) inhibits free and clot-bound thrombin with 80% of the medication excreted unchanged through the kidneys. Peak plasma level occurs within 1.5 to 3 hours of administration with a half-life of 14 to 17 hours in healthy patients, but up to 28 hours in those with end-stage renal disease. In patients with normal renal function, the medication should be stopped 24 hours prior to low-risk surgery and 48 hours prior to high-risk surgery, but administration should be stopped up to 4 times longer depending on degree of renal impairment. In patients not at high risk for thrombosis along with a normal creatinine clearance, it is appropriate to wait 4 to 6 half-life intervals (70–100 hours) from discontinuing the medication prior to neuraxial injection (or removal of epidural catheters).

Following an assessment of a patient's current medical status and prior medical history, an anesthetic plan of general, regional, or neuraxial anesthesia can be considered for ankle arthrodesis surgery. If the patient's atrial fibrillation is stable along with preserved cardiac function and does not have any renal insufficiency, surgery can proceed within 24 to 48 hours of stopping the medication. However, if choosing an anesthetic plan of neuraxial anesthesia or one involving deep regional blockade, it would be preferable to wait 3 to 5 days (4 to 6 dabigatran half-life intervals).

Further Reading

Benzon HT, Avram MJ, Green D, et al. New oral anticoagulants and regional anaesthesia. *Br J Anaesth.* 2013;111(suppl 1):i96–i113.

Fawole A, Daw HA, Crowther MA. Practical management of bleeding due to the anticoagulants dabigatran, rivaroxaban, and apixaban. *Cleve Clin J Med.* 2013;80:443–451.

Schiele F, Ryn van J, Canada K, et al. A specific antidote to dabigatran: functional and structural characterization. *Blood.* 2013;121(18):3554–3562.

Tran H, Joseph J, Young L, McRae S, Curnow J, Nandurkar H, Wood P, McLintock C. New oral anticoagulants: a practical guide on prescription, laboratory testing and peri-procedural/bleeding management. *Intern Med J.* 2014;44(6):525–536.

2.3. Are there any concerns about performing neuraxial blockade in patients with prior lumbar spine surgery? Are there any concerns about neuraxial anesthesia in patients taking dabigatran?

Lumbar neuraxial blockade (spinal/epidural) can be considered, but with caution in the patient with a history of lumbar fusion surgery (confirm the level that the patient reports). Ultrasound guidance can be helpful in determining the best lumbar interspace, correct level, and midline and to estimate epidural space depth. Neuraxial anesthesia could be challenging in such a patient population due to presence of hardware and bone grafts, abnormalities of the typical landmarks, scar formation, higher risk for false loss of resistance, inability to access the epidural or subarachnoid space, patchy and failed blocks, unintentional dural puncture, and traumatic needle placement and may require multiple attempts (increasing morbidity).

An anesthetic plan of neuraxial blockade can be considered after assessing a patient's medical status and medical history. In those with no history of renal insufficiency and taking dabigatran (half-life is 14 to 17 hours), neuraxial anesthesia could still be considered. However, it would be preferable to wait 3 to 5 days (4 to 6 half-life intervals) following dabigatran discontinuation before proceeding with neuraxial blockade.

Further Reading

Hebl JR, Herlocker TT, Kopp SL, et al. Neuraxial blockade in patients with preexisting spinal stenosis, lumbar disk disease, or prior spine surgery: efficacy and neurologic complications. *Anesth Analg.* 2010;111(6):1511–1519.

Vercauteren M, Heytens L. Anaesthetic considerations for patients with a pre-existing neurological deficit: are neuraxial techniques safe? *Acta Anaesthesiol Scand.* 2007;51(7):831–838.

Vercauteren M, Waets P, Pitkanen M, et al. Neuraxfal techniques in patients with pre-existing back impairment or prior spine interventions: a topical review with special reference to obstetrics. *Acta Anaesthesia Scand.* 2011;55:910–917.

3. Intraoperative Medicine and Surgical/Regional Anesthesia Factors

3.1. Innervation of the ankle joint

3.1.1. What is the nerve innervation of the ankle joint? What nerve(s) innervate the lateral, medial, and posterior aspects of the ankle and leg below the knee?

The lower extremity, from below the knee to the foot and ankle, is innervated by the common peroneal nerve laterally with tibial nerve innervating the posterior aspect, while the saphenous nerve provides innervation (sensory only) to the medial aspect (generally to the medial malleolus) of the lower extremity. Dorsal aspect of the foot is innervated by the superficial peroneal nerve with the deep peroneal nerve innervating the deep dorsal structures of the foot and web space between the first and second toes. The lateral foot is innervated by the sural nerve, and medial innervation is derived from the saphenous nerve. The plantar aspect of the foot is supplied by the calcaneal and medial plantar nerves that branch from the tibial nerve.

Further Reading

Brown D, ed. *Atlas of Regional Anesthesia.* 4th ed. Philadelphia, PA: Saunders/Elsevier; 2010:89–96.

Miller, RD, ed. *Miller's Anesthesia.* 8th ed. Philadelphia, PA: Elsevier Churchill Livingstone; 2015:1721–1751.

3.1.2. What nerve(s)/nerve plexus(es) need to be anesthetized for this patient? What roots make up the nerve plexus?

Both lumbar and lumbosacral nerve plexus innervate the lower extremities and would need to be anesthetized at a location along their anatomic distribution from the central neuraxis (neuraxial blockade; spinal or epidural) to the ankle for a patient who is scheduled for ankle arthrodesis surgery. Therefore, to provide effective surgical anesthesia, both the medial and the lateral aspects of the ankle would need to be anesthetized to include the tibial, common peroneal, and saphenous nerves(branch of the femoral nerve) that originate from the lumbar and the lumbosacral nerve plexus.

The lumbar plexus innervates the ventral aspect of the lower extremity consisting of ventral rami of L2-L3 and part of L4 nerve roots along with potential contributions from ventral rami of the L1 and T12 nerve roots. The lumbar plexus originates/forms within the psoas muscle, anterior to the transverse processes, of the lumbar vertebral column and gives off the iliohypogastric (T12-Ll), ilioinguinal (L1), genitofemoral (L1-L2), lateral femoral cutaneous (L2-L3), femoral (L2-L4), and obturator nerves (L2-L4).

The lumbosacral trunk innervates the dorsal aspect of the lower extremity and is formed from ventral rami of L4, L5, and S1, while the sacral plexus consists of the union of the lumbosacral trunk in addition to S1-S3 and occasionally S4. The sciatic nerve (from lumbosacral trunk) contains the tibial nerve (made up of anterior divisions of the ventral rami of L4, L5, and S1-S3) and the common peroneal nerve (made of dorsal branches of L4, L5, and S1-S3). The sciatic nerve splits into tibial and common peroneal nerves usually within the popliteal fossa. The common peroneal nerve then branches into the superficial and deep peroneal nerves while the tibial nerve branches into the medial/lateral plantar nerves, calcaneal, and sural (with contribution from communicating superficial peroneal branches) nerves. Other nerves from the lumbosacral plexus include the superior gluteal (L4-S1), inferior gluteal (L5-S2), posterior femoral cutaneous (S1-S3), piriformis (S1-S2), obturator internus (L5, S1-S2), and quadratus femoris (L4-L5, S1).

Further Reading

Brown D, ed. *Atlas of Regional Anesthesia.* 4th ed. Philadelphia, PA: Saunders/Elsevier; 2010:89–96.

Hadzic, A, ed. *Hadzic's Peripheral Nerve Blocks and Anatomy for Ultrasound-Guided Regional Anesthesia.* 2nd ed. New York, NY: McGraw-Hill Professional; 2012: 217–248.

Miller, RD, ed. *Miller's Anesthesia.* 8th ed. Philadelphia, PA: Elsevier Churchill Livingstone; 2015: 1721–1751

Narouze SN, ed. *Atlas of Ultrasound-Guided Procedures in Interventional Pain Management.* New York: Springer; 2011:240–258.

3.1.3. What are the nerves that branch from the nerve plexus innervating the foot and ankle? What peripheral nerves need to be blocked for ankle arthrodesis surgery?

Nerves innervating the foot and ankle originating from the lumbar and lumbosacral plexus give rise to the femoral (L2-L4) and sciatic (L4-L5 and S1-3; gives rise to tibial and common peroneal nerves in the popliteal fossa) nerves, respectively. The common peroneal nerve further branches into the superficial and deep peroneal nerves. The tibial nerve branches into the medial plantar, calcaneal, and sural (in combination with superficial peroneal branches) nerves.

For ankle arthrodesis surgery, in order to provide surgical anesthesia and perioperative analgesia, the tibial and common peroneal nerves along with the saphenous nerve branch of the femoral nerve would require blockade.

Further Reading

Brown D, ed. *Atlas of Regional Anesthesia*. 4th ed. Philadelphia, PA: Saunders/Elsevier; 2010:135–138.

Hadzic, A, ed. *Hadzic's Peripheral Nerve Blocks and Anatomy for Ultrasound-Guided Regional Anesthesia*. 2nd ed. New York, NY: McGraw-Hill Professional; 2012:217–248.

Miller, RD, ed. *Miller's Anesthesia*. 8th ed. Philadelphia, PA: Elsevier Churchill Livingstone; 2015:1721–1751.

3.1.4. What nerves should be anesthetized during an ankle block? Would you perform an ankle block for ankle arthrodesis surgery?

During an ankle block, the posterior tibial, deep and superficial peroneal, sural, and saphenous nerves require blockade. An ankle block is performed at the medial and lateral malleoli. The posterior tibial nerve is blocked along the medial aspect of the Achilles tendon at the level of the medial malleolus, and local anesthetic is deposited superficial to the periosteum. At the ankle, the deep peroneal nerve lies deep between the tendons of the tibialis anterior and the extensor halluces longis. These tendons can be identified by dorsiflexion of the ankle and big toe, respectively. Local anesthetic is deposited superficial to the periosteum at this point. To block the branches of the superficial peroneal and the saphenous nerves, a subcutaneous ring of local anesthetic is deposited across the dorsum of the foot. The sural nerve can be blocked by inserting a needle lateral to the Achilles tendon at the level of the lateral malleolus, and local anesthetic is deposited superficial to the periosteum. An example of local anesthetic volume used during an ankle block is presented in Table 8.1.

An ankle block would not cover any portion of the lower extremity cephalad to the malleoli. An ankle block would not provide for adequate anesthesia should a tourniquet (thigh or calf) be necessary during surgery. Such an approach could limit surgical anesthesia duration (especially compared with a more cephalad nerve block approach) and would not provide extended postoperative analgesia following ankle arthrodesis surgery. Therefore, appropriate risks and benefits along with limitations of an "ankle block" as the primary anesthetic need to be considered for ankle arthrodesis surgery.

Further Reading

Brown D, ed. *Atlas of Regional Anesthesia*. 4th ed. Philadelphia, PA: Saunders/Elsevier; 2010:89–96.

Hadzic, A, ed. *Hadzic's Peripheral Nerve Blocks and Anatomy for Ultrasound-Guided Regional Anesthesia*. 2nd ed. New York, NY: McGraw-Hill Professional; 2012:217–248.

Miller, RD, ed. *Miller's Anesthesia*. 8th ed. Philadelphia, PA: Elsevier Churchill Livingstone; 2015:1721–1751.

Table 8.1:
Nerve(s) and local anesthetic used during an ankle block

Nerve	Local Anesthetic
Posterior tibial nerve	3–5 mL of local superficial to the periosteum
Deep peroneal nerve	2–3 mL of local superficial to the periosteum
Branches of the superficial peroneal nerve and saphenous nerve	Subcutaneous ring across the dorsum of the foot using 3–5 mL of local anesthetic
Sural nerve	3–5 mL of local anesthetic superficial to the periosteum

3.2. Regional anesthetic concerns

3.2.1. What are the approaches to saphenous nerve blockade? Is it necessary to block the saphenous nerve for ankle arthrodesis surgery, and if so, what approach could be chosen?

To provide anesthesia distal to the knee, both the saphenous (sensory branch of the femoral nerve) and the sciatic nerves should be blocked. Traditionally, the saphenous nerve was blocked by creating a subcutaneous wheel of local anesthetics from the anteromedial aspect of the tibial tuberosity to the anterior aspect of the tibia just below the knee. However, evidence has shown that various ultrasound-guided, more cephalad, approaches can lead to more effective and longer duration blockade of the saphenous nerve.

Studies have proven ultrasound techniques to be effective in blocking this nerve, as the saphenous nerve emerges from the adductor canal. The saphenous nerve lies lateral to the femoral artery while exiting the femoral triangle and then crosses over the roof of the adductor canal (subsartorial canal) and lays medial to the artery at the distal aspect of the adductor canal (canal bound anterolaterally by the vastus medialis muscle, anteromedially by the sartorius muscle, and posteromedially by the adductor magnus muscle). The goal is to place the block needle medial to the femoral artery below the sartorius muscle, depositing 5 to 10 mL of local anesthetic around the artery.

The saphenous nerve emerges from the adductor canal with the saphenous branch of the descending genicular artery, then divides into the infrapatellar and sartorial branches. The sartorial branch courses through the fascia between the sartorius and gracilis muscles and emerges subcutaneously below the knee. Just above the level of the knee, the nerve can be blocked between the sartorius and gracilis muscles in close proximity to the saphenous branch of the descending genicular artery. However, using a more proximal location such as the adductor canal, where the femoral artery is a highly visible landmark, can help better identify the sartorius muscle and the saphenous nerve.

The saphenous nerve can also be blocked about 5 to 7 cm proximal to the popliteal crease, in the vastoadductor membrane (facial plane adjacent to the vastus medialis) deep to the sartorius muscle. Blocking the saphenous nerve more proximally can be achieved in the distal adductor canal deep to the sartorius and anteromedial to the femoral artery.

Further Reading

Horn JL, Pitsch T, Salinas F, et al. Anatomic basis to the ultrasound-guided approach for saphenous nerve blockade. *Reg Anesth Pain Med.* 2009;34(5):486–489.

Miller RD, ed. *Miller's Anesthesia.* 8th ed. Philadelphia, PA: Elsevier Churchill Livingstone; 2015:1751–1766.

Saranteas T, Anagnostis G, Paraskeuopoulos T, et al. Anatomy and clinical implications of the ultrasound-guided subsartorial saphenous nerve block. *Reg Anesth Pain Med.* 2011; 36(4): 399–402.

3.2.2. If a lumbar plexus blockade (also known as a psoas compartment block) is chosen to block the saphenous nerve, describe the landmark/nerve stimulation technique

A lumbar plexus blockade involves injecting local anesthetic (20–40 mL) at the posterior lumbar paravertebral level with the patient in a lateral decubitus position. The original approach used a paresthesia technique that was first described by Winnie et al. This then evolved into using a nerve stimulator technique at the level of L4 with needle insertion at the intersection of 2 lines: (1) the intercristal line joining the 2 iliac crests and (2) a caudad-cephalad line 5 cm parallel to the midline spinous processes passing to the posterior superior iliac spine. If there is difficulty identifying the lumbar plexus, the needle can be directed medially; however, no more than 15 degrees should be used to reduce the risk of bilateral spread (Mannion et al.). Another approach to perform this block (described by Capdevila et al.) directs the block needle to be inserted at a lateral two-thirds distance between the spinous process and the posterior superior iliac spine and 1 cm above the intercristal line. The needle should enter at a perpendicular angle toward the L4 transverse process and then directed caudally until a quadriceps femoris twitch is obtained using stimulation of 0.5 to 1.0 mA. Using lower currents could potentially result in inadvertent epidural or spinal spread of local anesthetic. Use of ultrasound for this block has not gained popularity due to the deep nature of the target structures, frequency of obese patients, and need for a curved low-frequency ultrasound transducer.

Further Reading

Capdevila X, Macaire P, Dadure C, et al. Continuous psoas compartment block for postoperative analgesia after total hip arthroplasty: new landmarks, technical guidelines, and clinical evaluation. *Anesth Analg.* 2002;94:1606–1613.

Capdevila X, Coimbra C, Choquet O. Approaches to the lumbar plexus: success, risks, and outcome. *Reg Anesth Pain Med.* 2005;30(2):150–162.

Mannion S, O'Callaghan S, Walsh M, et al. In with the new, out with the old? Comparison of two approaches for psoas compartment block. *Anesth Analg.* 2005;101:259–264.

Miller RD, ed. *Miller's Anesthesia.* 8th ed. Philadelphia, PA: Elsevier Churchill Livingstone; 2015:1737–1739.

Winnie AP, Ramamurthy S, Durrani Z, et al. Plexus blocks for lower extremity surgery: new answers to old problems. *Anesthesiol Rev.* 1974;1:11–16.

3.2.3. The surgeon plans on placing a thigh tourniquet for surgery expected to last 4 hours. Should the anticipated pain caused from the tourniquet (midthigh) influence the type of regional technique(s) to use for ankle arthrodesis surgery?

A thigh tourniquet, used to decrease intraoperative blood loss at the surgical site, can also cause ischemic pain within the thigh. This unintended ischemic or "dull" pain can often remain detectable to the patient, even if the appropriate and effective PNB coverage has been performed. Pain from a midthigh tourniquet is due to pressure that transmits signals involving unmyelinated C-fibers and myelinated A-fibers affecting both the femoral and sciatic nerves. Therefore, it is important to block these nerves at an anatomic site more proximal than the adductor canal (saphenous/femoral coverage) or popliteal fossa (tibial and common peroneal/sciatic coverage) areas to help reduce ischemic pain intensity.

Further Reading

Hadzic A, ed. *Hadzic's Peripheral Nerve Blocks and Anatomy for Ultrasound-Guided Regional Anesthesia.* 2nd ed. New York, NY: McGraw-Hill Professional; 2012:229–248.

Miller RD, ed. *Miller's Anesthesia.* 8th ed. Philadelphia, PA: Elsevier Churchill Livingstone; 2015:1721–1751.

3.2.4. What are the blockade technique options that can be used to block the sciatic nerve?

Blockade of the sciatic nerve along with the saphenous nerve will provide analgesia for surgical procedures below the knee, such as ankle arthrodesis surgery, which can be accomplished with neuraxial blockade. Providing anesthesia/analgesia independently to the sciatic nerve can be accomplished with a transgluteal or subgluteal approach as 2 common techniques. Another PNB approach to the sciatic nerve can be targeted within the popliteal fossa, which is advantageous for distal surgery of the lower extremity while also preserving quadriceps muscle integrity and thus reducing the potential for patient falls.

The transgluteal landmark technique involves the patient being positioned in a lateral decubitus orientation with the leg to be blocked uppermost and flexed at the hip and the knee. Using the center points of the palpable greater trochanter and posterior superior iliac spine as landmarks (straight line connecting these 2 points), the midpoint between the two is identified and measured perpendicular 4 cm caudal to this point marking the site of block needle insertion. The regional block needle is inserted through the skin at a 90-degree angle to this surface landmark. Muscle twitches of the gluteal muscles followed by hamstring or calf muscles are often seen when using a nerve stimulator; however, with the nerve stimulator reduced to 0.2 to 0.5 mA along with foot and/or ankle, a twitch indicates appropriate placement of the needle tip to the appropriate target site. Local anesthetic (20–30 mL) can be injected once negative aspiration has been confirmed and delivered in 3- to 5-mL increments being paused with intermittent aspiration.

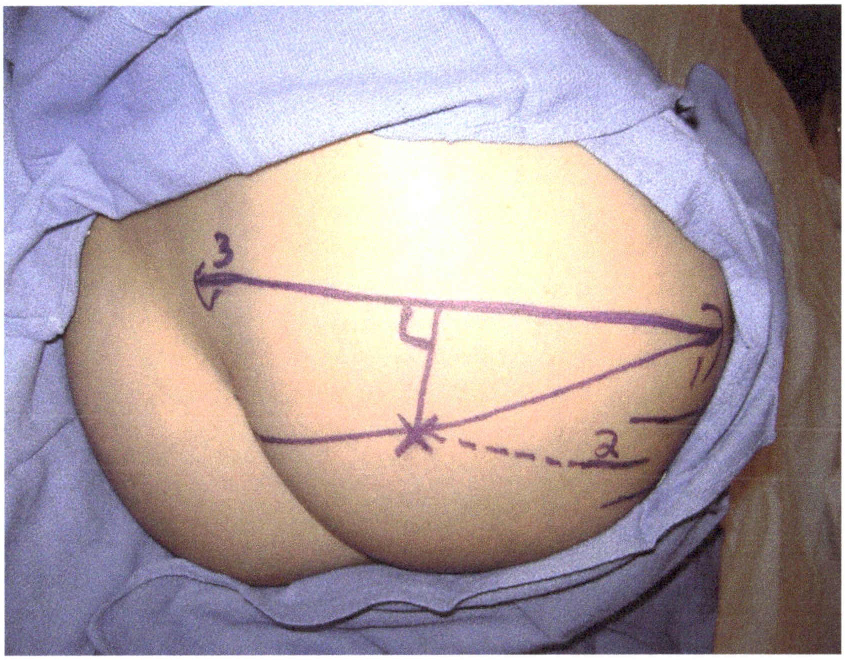

Use of an ultrasound-guided transgluteal approach is not usually performed on a routine basis secondary to depth of the target structure and lack of consistently identifiable surrounding structures (i.e., blood vessels) to assist with block needle guidance.

The subgluteal approach involves similar patient positioning as described earlier for the transgluteal technique or with the patient assuming a prone position. Different from the transgluteal approach, the subgluteal technique for sciatic nerve blockade is more amendable to using ultrasound as a tool to assist in achieving block success.

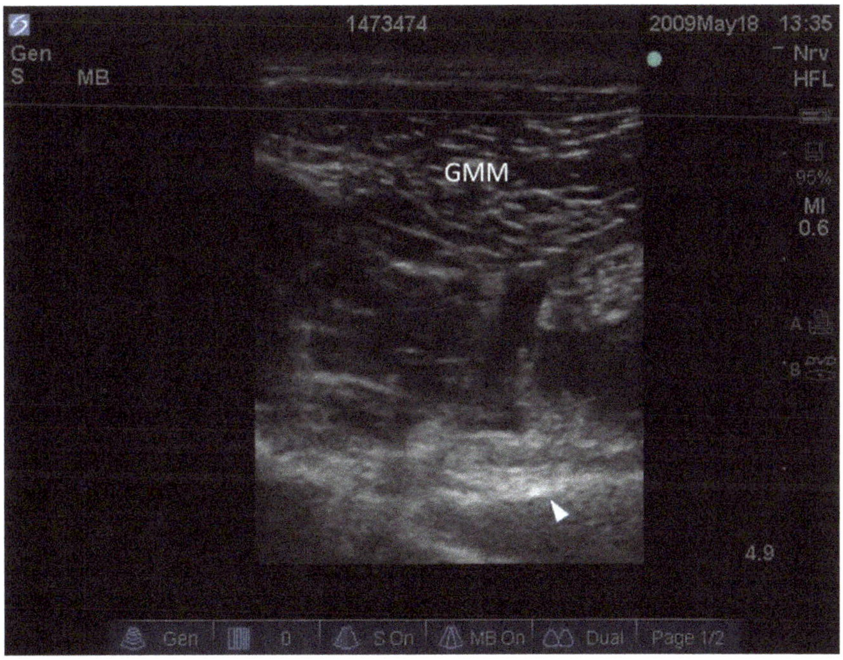

The sciatic nerve is visualized just distal to the gluteal cleft, midway between the line connecting the palpable ischial tuberosity and greater trochanter. The nerve will be hyperechoic, and needle placement can be achieved in an in- or out-of-plane technique. Using a landmark method, the sciatic nerve can be found perpendicular to a line drawn between the above 2 osseous structures.

In the popliteal fossa, an ultrasound technique to sciatic nerve blockade has a great success rate, is efficient to perform, and is usually recommended to target this nerve at the position of branching due to the variability of location of division of the nerve into the common peroneal and tibial nerve branches.

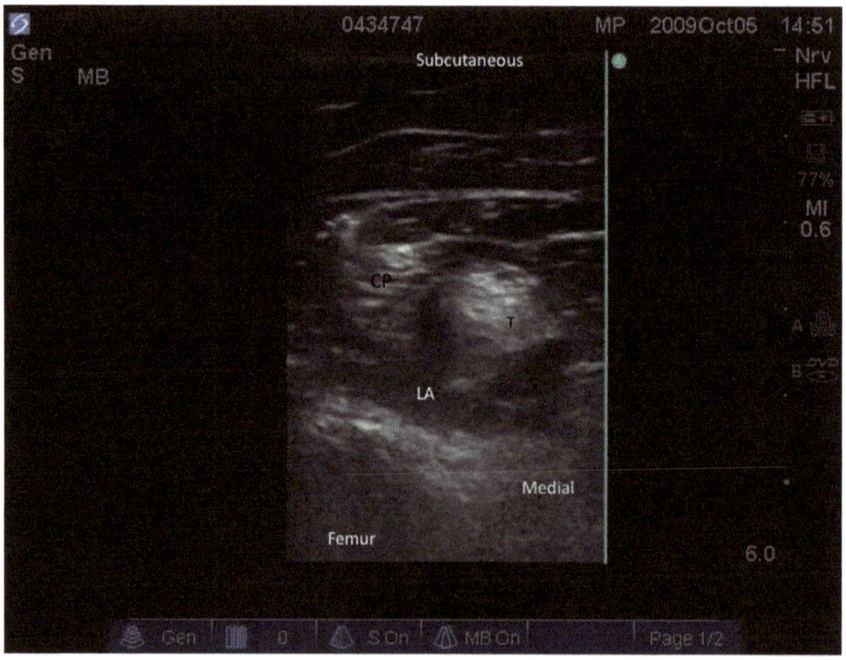

This block can be achieved with local anesthetic injected within the connective tissue (Vloka's) sheath that envelops the common peroneal and tibial nerve branches (usually located lateral and superficial to the popliteal vasculature).

Further Reading

Hadzic A, ed. *Hadzic's Peripheral Nerve Blocks and Anatomy for Ultrasound-Guided Regional Anesthesia.* 2nd ed. New York, NY: McGraw-Hill Professional; 2012:229–248.

Miller RD, ed. *Miller's Anesthesia.* 8th ed. Philadelphia, PA: Elsevier Churchill Livingstone; 2015:1721–1751.

3.2.5. Which peripheral nerve block approach, ultrasound or landmark/nerve stimulation technique, should be used for ankle arthrodesis surgery? What are some advantages and disadvantages to each technique?

During ankle arthrodesis surgery, PNB performed with either landmark or ultrasound technique can be used. Some benefits of an ultrasound-guided approach include direct/real-time visualization of bony and surrounding vascular landmarks (often used for identification of the various nerve target structures), reduced likelihood of accidental vascular puncture, visualization of local anesthetic spread around target nerve structures, reduced likelihood of "incomplete" or "partial" blockade success as aberrant anatomy can often be recognized and targeted, and higher overall PNB success rates; in addition, ultrasound guidance is theorized to reduce nerve injury that may be caused by the regional block needle. In addition, the use of ultrasound guidance can often result in lowering the local anesthetic volume requirements to achieve blockade success along with some study evidence reporting more efficient blockade performance and faster blockade onset when a PNB is performed with the guidance of ultrasound.

One advantage of a landmark/stimulator regional technique when compared with ultrasound-guided PNB entails a lower cost as ultrasound equipment purchasing and maintenance is not needed. In addition, another cost associated with ultrasound regional patient care when compared with landmark/nerve stimulation techniques is the continuing cost of compliance mandates and technical/medical record-keeping requirements of performing ultrasound approaches.

Notably, an important consideration is the potential value added of using both ultrasound-guided and nerve stimulation techniques together with the anticipation of improving patient safety when using regional anesthesia/analgesia. For example, ultrasound guidance can often more accurately direct the practitioner to the appropriate anatomic nerve target, and using nerve stimulation prior to local anesthetic injection may also reduce the chance of nerve injury.

Historically, a stimulation current of no more than 0.5 mA was regarded as safe in avoiding nerve injury while also delivering an adequate stimulus to provoke a motor response. However, there was no evidence of a consistent level of safely determining stimulating threshold that would reliably indicate intraneural placement of the regional block needle. Within limitations, studies (with the use of ultrasound) have shown that a stimulation current of 0.2 mA or less is reliable in detecting intraneural placement of the block needle. However, stimulation currents of more than 0.2 mA and no more than 0.5 mA could not always rule out intraneural needle tip positioning.

Further Reading

Antonakakis JG, et al. Ultrasound-Guided Regional Anesthesia for Peripheral Nerve Blocks: An Evidence Based Outcome Review. *Anesthesiol Clin*. 2011 Jun;29(2):179–191.

Barash P, et al. *Clinical Anesthesia*. 6th ed. Philadelphia, PA: Lippincott Williams & Wilkins; 2009:521–548.

Bigeleisen PE, Moayeri N, Groen GJ. Extraneural versus intraneural stimulation thresholds during ultrasound-guided supraclavicular block. *Anesthesiology*. 2009;110(6):1235–1243.

Kay J, Delmonte RJ, Greenberg PM. Chapter 39. Ankle Block. In: Hadzic A. eds. NYSORA Textbook of Regional Anesthesia and Acute Pain Management New York, NY: McGraw-Hill; 2007. http://accessanesthesiology.mhmedical.com/content.aspx?bookid=413&sectionid=39828190. Accessed December 18, 2018.

Miller RD, ed. *Miller's Anesthesia*. 8th ed. Philadelphia, PA. Elsevier Churchill Livingstone; 2015:1721–1751.

3.2.6. Does perioperative regional anesthesia/analgesia contribute to postoperative care?

Successful preoperative implementation of perioperative regional anesthesia can positively influence and potentially attenuate the negative endocrine, psychosocial, metabolic, and inflammatory responses to surgery. Reducing or eliminating these deleterious physical and psychological response impact(s) of interventional patient care can decrease morbidity and hospitalization (need for, duration of, readmission, etc.) rate parameters. Regional anesthesia techniques (neuraxial and peripheral nerve/nerve plexus blockade) can often allow for the complete avoidance of general anesthesia and/or minimize intraoperative inhalational agent requirements, muscle relaxants, and rescue opioid needs, leading to faster postoperative mobilization and reduced acuity of immediate postoperative recovery following surgery.

Regional anesthesia/analgesia techniques can also improve upon a patient's perioperative pain medicine experience, decrease postoperative gastrointestinal dysfunction (i.e., nausea/vomiting, secondary to lowering of opioid administration along with reduced interventional stress responses) along with elimination or reductions of immediate postoperative shivering, earlier return of bowel function, decreased incidence of deep venous thrombosis, shorter stays in the postanesthesia care unit, improved overall patient satisfaction with their interventional procedure, reduced or eliminated hospital admissions, reduced or eliminated postoperative emergency room and/or surgeon office visits, reduced need for prolonged narcotic requirements, and reduced patient/physician fears of narcotic addiction.

Regional analgesia can facilitate fast-track postoperative patient care. These fast-track programs are implemented to assist in reducing morbidity by decreasing perioperative hospitalization requirements. Both neuraxial and peripheral nerve blockade can be utilized as an effective modality in fast-track programs. Specifically, for lower extremity surgery, regional anesthesia can improve patient satisfaction and decrease time to postanesthesia care unit and home readiness from the hospital, opioid rescue requirements, pain scores, and time to ambulation along with immediate postoperative physical therapy.

Prolonged regional anesthesia using peripheral nerve/nerve plexus catheters infusing local anesthetics are another proven method for prolonging postoperative pain control. Perineural catheters infusing local anesthetics alone can decrease intravenous and/or oral narcotic requirements and also decrease or eliminate opioid-related side effects. Postoperative pain medicine using regional anesthesia peripheral nerve/nerve plexus catheter techniques provide patients with autonomy and the ability to control their own postoperative pain management. When compared with single-injection regional anesthesia, implementing a catheter technique provides for analgesia beyond the anticipated 16 to 24 hours (limited duration of single-shot regional blockade) of postoperative analgesia.

Further Reading

Carli F, Kehlet H, Baldini G, et al. Evidence basis for regional anesthesia in multidisciplinary fast-track surgical care pathways. *Reg Anesth Pain Med.* 2011;36(1):63–72.

Kaye AD, Helander EM, Vadivelu N, et al. Consensus Statement for Clinical Pathway Development for Perioperative Pain Management and Care Transitions. *Pain Ther.* 2017;6(2):129–141.

3.2.7. Would the addition of a steroid to the local, use of an indwelling perineural catheter, or injection of liposomal bupivacaine provide any advantage over long-acting local anesthetics?

Addition of a steroid (e.g., dexamethasone) to the local anesthetic mixture can often increase the duration of effect from PNB. Adding dexamethasone to bupivacaine or ropivacaine can increase sensory analgesia from 12 to 24 hours up to 24 to 36 hours. Prolongation of postoperative analgesia achieved with implementing regional techniques has been shown to decrease postoperative opioid use/requirements. It has also been shown that giving an equivalent dose of intravenous dexamethasone may prolong the duration of sensory nerve blockade beyond that expected from a single-shot PNB alone.

Use of an indwelling perineural catheter permits for a more prolonged postoperative pain management experience. In addition to prolonging postoperative pain control, perineural catheter insertion will often decrease the need for other intravenous medications and/or rescue opioid analgesics. Indwelling nerve/nerve plexus catheters permit patients to control their own postoperative pain management with the addition of patient control devices to the preset continuous perineural infusion rate administration. Catheter placement at the time of performing regional techniques can provide postoperative analgesia beyond 24 hours after surgery in contrast to long-acting single-shot local anesthetics alone. However, caution must be exercised; limitations with catheter use include risk of infection, damage/dysfunction to surrounding structures and nerve tissue, accidental intravascular catheter placement or migration of the catheter, and added technical challenges with catheter placement and catheter management.

Similar to the addition of a steroid to the local anesthetic mixture, liposomal bupivacaine use during perioperative regional anesthesia/analgesia has not received Food and Drug Administration (FDA) approval for routine use and is not the standard of care during PNB procedures. Liposomal bupivacaine, however, is a slow-release form of bupivacaine HCl in which liposomes release encapsulated bupivacaine HCl over an extended period (up to 96 hours) and can prolong analgesia. At the current time, this agent has been approved by the FDA for local infiltration and transversus abdominis plane blockade. Liposomal bupivacaine has been shown to provide prolongation of analgesic effect compared with bupivacaine HCl when administered alone. If the safety and efficacy of this medication are proven, it may be used to prolong neuraxial and peripheral nerve block duration and potentially replace neuraxial and peripheral catheters.

Further Reading

De Oliveira GS Jr, Castro Alves LJ, Nader A, et al. Perineural dexamethasone to improve postoperative analgesia with peripheral nerve blocks: a meta-analysis of randomized control trials. *Pain Res Treat.* 2014;2014:179029.

Desmet M, Braems H, Reynvoet M, et al. I.V. and perineural dexamethasone are equivalent in increasing the analgesic duration of a single-shot interscalene block with ropivacaine for shoulder surgery: a prospective, randomized, placebo-controlled study. *Br J Anaesth.* 2013;111(3):445–452.

Ilfeld B. Liposome bupivacaine in peripheral nerve blocks and epidural injections to manage postoperative pain. *Expert Opin Pharmacother.* 2013;14(17):2421–2431.

Merritt CK, Mariano ER, Kaye AD, et al. Peripheral nerve catheters and local anesthetic infiltration in perioperative analgesia. *Best Pract Res Clin Anaesthesiol.* 2014;28(1):41–57.

Skolnik A, Gan T. New formulation of bupivacaine for the treatment of postoperative pain: liposomal bupivacaine and SABER-Bupivacaine. *Expert Opin Pharmacother.* 2014;15(11):1535–1542.

3.2.8. Which local anesthetics can be used, and what are the maximum doses?

Parameters of local anesthetic choice and dose of administration used during performance of regional anesthesia and PNB depend on the desired duration of analgesia when a single-shot technique is being implemented, anatomic location of local anesthetic injection, admixture of additives such as epinephrine to the mixture, and patient weight. Longer-acting anesthetics such as ropivacaine and bupivacaine provide analgesia up to 24 hours. Intermediate, shorter-acting local anesthetics (lidocaine or mepivacaine) can be considered for ambulatory surgery or to limit concern of motor blockade to the limb being blocked. Vasoconstrictors such as epinephrine can be added to local anesthetics to slow medication uptake and to prolong both sensory analgesia and motor blockade. A concentration of 1:100,00 to 1:200,000 epinephrine is most often administered. Whichever local anesthetic agent is used, the total maximum dose injected for each patient should be calculated on a milligram-per-kilogram basis of reference to reduce the incidence of local anesthetic toxicity (Table 8.2).

Table 8.2:
Recommended local anesthetic dosing and onset/duration characteristics

Drug	Usual Concentration (%)	Total Maximum Dose (mg) Without/With Epinephrine	Onset (min)	Duration (h)
Lidocaine	1–2	350/500	10–20	2–4
Mepivacaine	1–1.5	350/500	10–20	3–5
Prilocaine	1–2	400/600	10–20	3–5
Bupivacaine	0.25–0.5	175/225	20–30	6–12
Levobupivacaine	0.25–0.5	200/225	20–30	6–12
Ropivacaine	0.2–0.5	200/250	20–30	6–12

Further Reading

Miller RD, ed. *Miller's Anesthesia*. 8th ed. Philadelphia, PA: Elsevier Churchill Livingstone; 2015:1721–1751.
Barash P, et al. *Clinical Anesthesia*. 6th ed. Philadelphia, PA: Lippincott Williams & Wilkins; 2009:521–548.

4. Postoperative Pain Management

4.1. Postoperative/postblock nerve injury

4.1.1. What steps can be taken to mitigate risk of nerve injury during regional blockade techniques?

- Application of a proper understanding of peripheral neural and surrounding anatomy.
- Skin-cleansing aseptic solutions and technique (i.e., to reduce infection and neurotoxicity).
- Regional block needles of appropriate length and blunt-tipped/short-bevel needles.
- Slow and deliberate block needle advancement and avoid excessive needle passes.
- Fractionated injection of local (3–5 mL) with intermittent aspiration.
- Avoid forceful and fast medication injections.
- Avoid high injection pressures.
- Exercise caution when choosing off-label use of adjuvants with local anesthetics.
- STOP injecting when pain is reported.
- PNBs in anesthetized, heavily sedated patients or performing lower extremity PNB with residual neuraxial anesthesia should only be practiced with extreme caution.
- Use caution when repeating a PNB following a failed or partially effective PNB.

Published data suggest neurologic complications of PNBs are rare (the main inciting mechanism of injury appears to be intrafascicular or intraneural injection); however, potential severity of consequences and lack of "prevention" strategies remain a source of concern. Therefore, coupling the relatively low incidence of complications together with speculation regarding the actual mechanism(s) of injury can be further minimized with improved objective documentation and more precise monitoring of *all* events related to the administration of PNBs.

Historically, the objective during PNB procedures has been to deposit local anesthetic around and in close proximity to, but not within, the substance of the nerve target. Evidence from more than 30 years ago has revealed deleterious effects being caused by intraneural injection(s). In addition, the increasing use of ultrasound guidance during regional techniques has resulted in an increased recognition that inadvertent intraneural injections have most likely occurred. However, this convention has been challenged with publications suggesting that intraneural needle placement, and even injection of local anesthetic, may not necessarily result in detectable clinical nerve injury. Nevertheless, data suggest performing PNBs without the benefit of ultrasound visualization has an increased likelihood of resulting in an intra-epineural injection that may increase the incidence of neuropathy.

There are currently no assurances of preventing nerve injury during performance of regional anesthesia. However, several techniques have been advocated toward enhancing the safety profile during performance of PNBs: (1) Despite being difficult to evaluate, pain on injection is traditionally taught to be an indicator and to potentially guard against intraneural injection. Therefore, despite a "pressure paresthesia," any patient complaint of pain on injection should dictate that additional injection should be stopped, followed by an assessment and consideration of the merits of block needle tip repositioning. (2) Electrical nerve stimulation is used to locate nerves but may also be used to rule out an inadvertent intraneural location of the block needle. It is suggested that, although neurostimulation may not be highly *sensitive* in detecting intraneural needle position (i.e., high current intensities may still be required to elicit motor responses even with intra-epineural needle placement), neurostimulation has a high *specificity* for identifying (evidence of a motor response at ≤0.2 mA) intraneural needle tip placement. (3) Clinical and experimental evidence indicates that injection pressure can be useful in detecting needle-nerve contact such that PNBs associated with high injection pressure have been reported to result in neurologic injury. A syringe-hand-feel subjective technique or objective monitoring of injection pressure using commercially available inline devices (highly sensitive but lacks specificity) can measure the resistance to injection that may have clinical merit.

Further Reading

Bigeleisen PE, Moayeri N, Groen GJ. Extraneural versus intraneural stimulation thresholds during ultrasound-guided supraclavicular block. *Anesthesiology*. 2009;110(6):1235–1243.

Claudio R, Hadzic A, Shih H, Vloka JD, Castro J, Koscielniak-Nielsen Z, Thys DM, Santos AC. Injection pressures by anesthesiologists during simulated peripheral nerve block. *Reg Anesth Pain Med*. 2004;29(3):201–205.

Klein SM, Melton MS, Grill WM, Nielsen KC. Peripheral nerve stimulation in regional anesthesia. *Reg Anesth Pain Med*. 2012;37(4):383–392.

Robards C, Hadzic A, Somasundaram L, Iwata T, Gadsden J, Xu D, Sala-Blanch X. Intraneural injection with low-current stimulation during popliteal sciatic nerve block. *Anesth Analg*. 2009;109(2):673–677.

Selander D, Brattsand R, Lundborg G, Nordborg C, Olsson Y. Local anesthetics: importance of mode of application, concentration and adrenaline for the appearance of nerve lesions. An experimental study of axonal degeneration and barrier damage after intrafascicular injection or topical application of bupivacaine (Marcain). *Acta Anaesthesiol Scand*. 1979;23(2):127–136.

4.1.2. What are the mechanism(s) and incidence of nerve injury following regional blockade?

Mechanical

Surgical factors
Laceration (iatrogenic)
Stretch (patient position)
Intraneural injection

- Needle design and direct needle trauma
- Intraneural injection and its prevention
  - Pain on injection (cardinal sign?)
  - Pain versus pressure-paresthesia
  - Stimulating current (1.0–0.1 mA?)
  - Injection resistance "syringe feel" (>20 psi)
  - Ultrasound (image resolution)

Vascular

Acute ischemia, neural ischemia, and hemorrhage

- Lack of blood flow to primary afferent neuron (metabolic stress)
- Function can return within 6 hours if ischemic times <2 hours- Ischemic periods >6 hours may produce permanent structural changes (edema and fiber degeneration/regeneration, oxidative injury, initiating apoptosis)

- Perineurium: an injection here or in a fascicle can cause increase in endoneurial pressure exceeding capillary perfusion pressure resulting in endoneurial ischemia
- Addition of vasoconstricting agents can enhance ischemia (e.g., epinephrine)

Pressure

Extraneural (carpal tunnel), intraneural (capillary occlusion), and compartment syndrome

- Tourniquet neuropathy (150 mmHg >SBP, tourniquet rest every 90–120 minutes)
- Compression hematoma (risk-benefit for patients prescribed anticoagulants)

Chemical

Injection of neurotoxic solutions

- Toxicity of injected solutions
  - Local anesthetic (cytotoxic effects vary, mitochondrial degradation)
  - Additives (e.g., epinephrine)
  - "Double-crush"

Nerve injury and permanent disability along with other devastating neurologic complications are potentially possible following PNB procedures. Published studies suggest that the incidence of neurologic symptoms (which varies depending on the anatomic location) following PNBs can range from 0.03% for supraclavicular blocks to 0.3% for femoral blocks and up to 3% for interscalene blocks. However, most of these neurologic issues/neuropathies are fortunately temporary rather than permanent, and most resolve over the following weeks to months. In most circumstances, the exact etiology of neurologic injury related to PNB remains unclear. Suggested causes can include direct mechanical trauma from the block needle, nerve edema and/or hematoma, pressure effects from the injected local anesthetic, neurotoxicity of the local anesthetic solutions, and adjuvants being administered (i.e., steroids, epinephrine). In addition, several other confounding factors can play a role and must be considered, including iatrogenic surgical manipulation/trauma or compression from postoperative casting/splinting, prolonged tourniquet pressure, and preexisting nerve injuries or neuropathies (e.g., diabetes mellitus).

Typically, the objective during PNB procedures has been to deposit local anesthetic in the vicinity of, but not within, the substance of the nerve. During PNB techniques, an intentional intraneural injection should be avoided as it is well established that direct injection into peripheral nerves can result in nerve injury. However, data also exist suggesting that intraneural injections are not always associated with nerve injury compared with the more likely incidence of a neuropathy from an intrafascicular injection as depicted in Figure 8.2.

Further Reading

Borgeat A, Blumenthal S. Nerve injury and regional anaesthesia. *Curr Opin Anaesthesiol.* 2004;17(5):417–421.

Brull R, McCartney CJ, Chan VW, El-Beheiry H. Neurological complications after regional anesthesia: contemporary estimates of risk. *Anesth Analg.* 2007;104(4):965–974.

Clark K, Williams PE Jr, Willis W, McGavran WL III. Injection injury of the sciatic nerve. *Clin Neurosurg.* 1970;17:111–125.

Hogan QH. Pathophysiology of peripheral nerve injury during regional anesthesia. *Reg Anesth Pain Med.* 2008;33(5):435–441.

Sorenson EJ. Neurological injuries associated with regional anesthesia. *Reg Anesth Pain Med.* 2008;33(5):442–448.

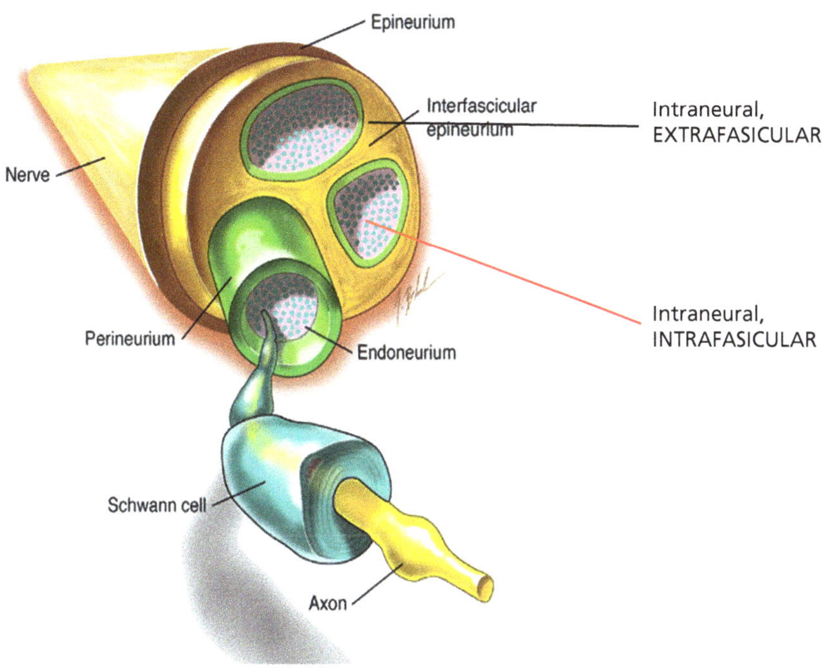

Figure 8.2 Intraneural needle tip placement (mechanical needle trauma).

4.1.3. How should one address the workup and follow-up of patients with suspected peripheral nerve injury?

Inclusive documentation of block placement remains important if sensory and/or motor function is depressed beyond the expected duration of action of administered local anesthetics for diagnostic and therapeutic purposes. It also remains important to note that most causes of nerve injury are unrelated to the performance of the regional techniques, and that neurologic deficits may be related to vascular injuries, compression injuries, local anesthetic action, and/or traumatic nerve injury. However, recognition, diagnosis, a plan for management, and proper treatment of peripheral nerve injuries with *early* intervention can help reduce the long-term sequelae associated with nerve injuries from PNBs. An understanding of any long-term prognosis, importance of neurology consultations, and familiarity with appropriate diagnostic tests remain essential for intervention and proper management of patients with neurologic injury. Symptoms of nerve injury usually resolve within 4 to 6 weeks in >95% of patients and in 99% of patients within the first year.

PEHE Peripheral Nerve Injury After Peripheral Nerve Blockade

- Mechanisms of injury and symptoms (e.g., depressed sensory and/or motor function) compression, vascular, traumatic and toxic
- Magnitude of neural injury neurapraxia, axonotmesis, and neurotmesis

Patient Evaluation and Physical Examination

- Symptoms of nerve injury
- Vascular mediated
- Neurologically mediated

Diagnostic Tests

- Electrophysiology testing: nerve conduction studies and electromyography
- Doppler ultrasound/high-frequency ultrasound
- Magnetic resonance imaging/magnetic resonance neurography

Symptoms of a nerve lesion following regional anesthesia usually manifest after the block has receded (within 48 hours). Physical examination should focus on an assessment of vascular integrity, sensory/motor function, and reflexes. Physical examination of findings/abnormalities may be acute or may not become clinically apparent for several days to several weeks and may range from mild to severe (dyesthesia, paresthesia, numbness, weakness, and pain). Intensity and duration of symptoms also vary with the severity of the injury, perception of symptoms influenced by origin of the nerve lesion, and other factors, and some injuries can evolve into a causalgia or reflex sympathetic dystrophy.

Vascular injuries can include injury to arteries or veins, formation of deep venous thrombosis, or a combination that may result in vascular compromise. Vascular injury associated with ischemia should be immediately evaluated, including assessment of venous and arterial circulation, pain at the surgical/block site, skin color changes, hematoma, and presence of engorgement or edema. For example, if a vascular injury is suspected, the surgical team should be immediately consulted (e.g., patients with lower extremity joint surgeries prone to deep venous thrombosis may be completely asymptomatic or complain of limb pain or limb swelling). With arterial compromise, patients often complain of intense pain, paresthesia, and cold extremity with an onset that is usually rapid. A common diagnostic test to aid in this emergency situation would be a Doppler/vascular study (arterial occlusion/compromise requires emergent surgical intervention).

When a physical examination identifies intact circulation in patients with suspected nerve injury, a neurologic examination (clinical exam to evaluate the degree of deficit and to determine what further diagnostic tests are indicated) should be initiated. This includes motor and sensory exams as well as assessment of the reflexes. Almost all mild symptoms such as dysesthesia, mild paresthesia or numbness, or mild pain usually resolve within the first few days to weeks of the insult, and additional diagnostic testing is not indicated. However, an evaluation by a neurologist may be warranted if neurologic deficits persist or are more severe in nature (moderate to severe numbness, weakness, and/or pain). Both the magnitude and the rate of progression of symptoms influence the urgency of the neurology consultation and subsequent examination.

Diagnostic testing for the detection of nerve injury often depends on the injury and patient characteristics surrounding the injury (from placement of a nerve block, nerve compression, traction, laceration, etc.). Electrophysiology testing involves (1) nerve conduction study (NCS) to detect the presence of a nerve lesion (can be performed within days of injury) and (2) electromyography (EMG) with the purpose to localize the lesion (tool for evaluating the *etiology* of a nerve lesion). An NCSs can detect a lesion within 1 to 2 days of an injury. If an initial study is normal, the patient probably has a neurapraxia (which should resolve with time) and should be followed for improvement of symptoms (if symptoms persist or worsen, the NCS should be repeated 46 weeks later). If the initial NCS identifies an abnormality, the lesion within a nerve or plexus needs to be localized with an EMG. Following nerve injury, muscle fibers are no longer controlled by the nerve and can result in spontaneous muscle discharge. An EMG can record abnormal muscle depolarization (there should be no spontaneous depolarization in normal muscle) and is usually performed 2 to 4 weeks following a suspected nerve injury (may perform EMG at the time of initial NCS to determine if nerve damage existed prior to surgery). If EMG is delayed beyond 4 weeks, re-innervation could appear and complicate the evaluation.

High-frequency Doppler ultrasound provides structural information about the scanned image and is an effective modality for identifying morphologic changes within peripheral nerves. This diagnostic imaging can be used as a tool for initial imaging of a suspected peripheral nerve injury or for follow-up imaging. It can localize the nerve lesion and is faster and more cost-effective than magnetic resonance imaging (MRI). It can be used to evaluate nerve rupture, nerve inflammatory processes, and compressive syndromes within peripheral nerves. However, there are limitations in that the test is operator-dependent and limited to nerves within 2 cm of the skin surface. At greater depths, a coarser-quality nerve image is obtained that can be difficult to distinguish from other tissues.

MRI, or more specifically magnetic resonance neurography, is an imaging technique of peripheral nerves that provides information about nerve compression, nerve inflammation, nerve trauma, systemic neuropathies, and recovery of nerves from pathologic states. Direct nerve imaging can demonstrate nerve continuity, distinguish intraneural from perineural masses, and localize nerve compressions prior to initiating surgical exploration. Similar to ultrasound, its indication is in localizing a nerve lesion from an acute peripheral nerve injury. The MRI signal alterations have been shown to occur within 24 hours following an axonal nerve lesion.

Further Reading

Bendszus M, Wessig C, Solymosi L, et al. MRI of peripheral nerve degeneration and regeneration: correlation with electrophysiology and histology. *Exp Neurol.* 2004;188:171–177.

Borgeat A, Ekatodramis G, Kalberer F, Benz C. Acute and nonacute complications associated with interscalene block and shoulder surgery: a prospective study. *Anesthesiology.* 2001;95:875–880.

Burns T. Mechanisms of acute and chronic compression neuropathy. In: Dyck P, Thomas P, eds. *Peripheral Neuropathy.* 4th ed. Elsevier-Saunders; 2005:1391–1402.

Silvestri E, Martinoli C, Derchi L, et al. Echotexture of peripheral nerves: correlation between US and histological findings to differentiate tendons. *Radiology.* 1995;197:291–296.

4.1.4. What are treatment options secondary to peripheral nerve injury/pathology?

Treatment Options for Peripheral Nerve Injury

- Minor deficits: Reassurance to relieve the anxiety and diagnostic testing or therapy is usually not indicated.
- Major deficits: Early neurologic and/or neurosurgery consultation is advisable; if surgery is not indicated, physical therapy/occupational therapy/social services consults should obtained as needed.
- The more commonly prescribed medication therapy includes tricyclic antidepressants, serotonin reuptake inhibitors, anticonvulsants, opioids, and capsaicin cream.

Treatment of the patient with a nerve injury depends on the severity of the injury (Figure 8.3). Patients with nerve injuries (most of which resolve with time) can be divided into 2 groups: (1) patients with minor deficits and (2) those with major deficits. Multiple drugs or multimodal therapy can be effective in treating neurally mediated pain. These medications should be administered by a chronic pain specialist or neurologist who has evaluated the patient and has the capacity to perform ongoing evaluations. Regardless of the type of injury, all patients should be evaluated to determine that a more serious injury or correctable contributing condition is not overlooked.

Further Reading

McCarson KE, Ralya A, Reisman SA, Enna SJ. Amitriptyline prevents thermal hyperalgesia and modifications in rat spinal cord GABA(B) receptor expression and function in an animal model of neuropathic pain. *Biochem Pharmacol.* 2005;71:196–202.

Rogawski M, Loscher W. The neurobiology of antiepileptic drugs. *Nat Rev Neurosci.* 2004;10:685–692.

Rowbotham M. Mechanisms and pharmacologic management of neuropathic pain. In: Dyck P, Thomas P. eds. *Peripheral Neuropathy.* 4th ed. Pennsylvania, PA: Elsevier; 2005:2637–2652.

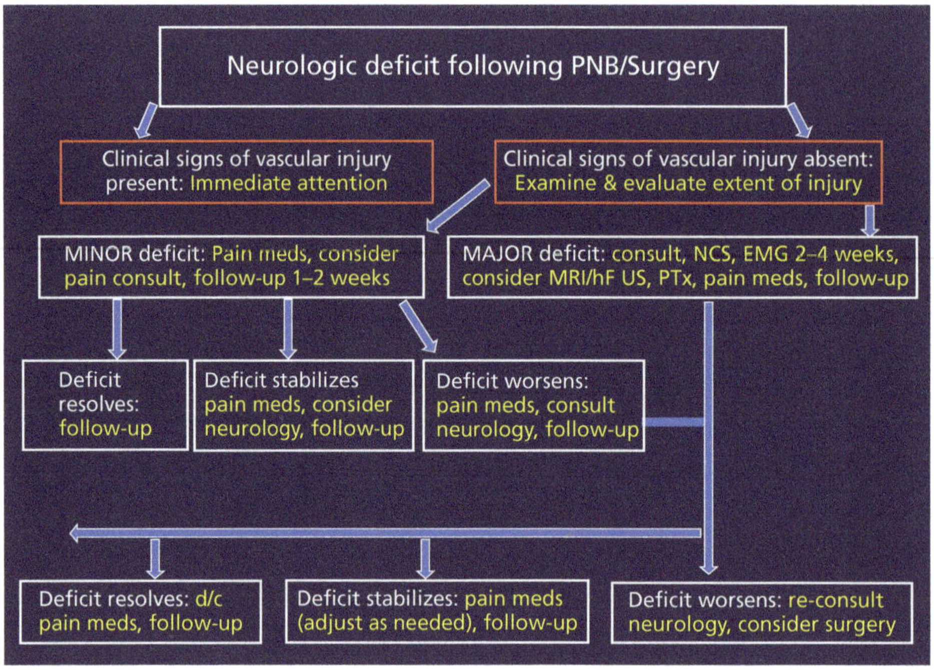

Figure 8.3 Approach to management of the patient with neurologic deficit(s).

Legend: med: medication(s); NCS: nerve conduction study; EMG: electromyography; MRI/hF US: magnetic resonance imaging/high-frequency ultrasound; d/c: discontinue.

4.2. What are the advantages of regional anesthesia/analgesia?

Surgical candidates and various surgical specialties could realize "value-added" perioperative management when incorporating regional programs into systems/protocols of patient care. For example, "fast-track" regional postoperative care is used to decrease perioperative hospitalization parameters, minimize or eliminate rescue opioid requirements, improve patient pain management experiences, improve patient perioperative satisfaction, decrease time to discharge readiness, and help to decrease morbidity. Regional anesthesia/acute pain medicine incorporating perineural blockade as part of multimodal anesthesia care can attenuate endocrine and metabolic responses to surgical stress and inflammation associated with surgical insult that can decrease perioperative side effects/complications. Regional techniques can be used to minimize intraoperative inhalational agent requirements (they temper the shivering response and could reduce postanesthetic care unit stay), need for muscle relaxants, and intraoperative opioids that could result in earlier awakening from general anesthesia (complete avoidance of general in many situations). In addition, there is often a decrease in postoperative nausea and vomiting with earlier return of bowel function, reduced perioperative transfusion requirements, and a decreased risk of deep vein thrombosis.

Further Reading

Carli F, Kehlet H, Baldini G, et al. Evidence basis for regional anesthesia in multidisciplinary fast-track surgical care pathways. *Reg Anesth Pain Med.* 2011;36(1):63–72.

Kranke P, Redel A, Schuster F, Muellenbach R, Eberhart LH. Pharmacological interventions and concepts of fast-track perioperative medical care for enhanced recovery programs. *Expert Opin Pharmacother.* 2008;9(9):1541–1564.

Arthroscopic Knee Surgery

James Flaherty, Clint Elliott, and Richa Wardhan

9

Case Scenario

A 45-year-old man ruptured his right anterior cruciate ligament (ACL) while walking down a staircase at his home. He presents to an ambulatory surgical center for arthroscopic repair of his ACL. He is obese (BMI 40), with a history of asthma, obstructive sleep apnea, and hypertension. He is noncompliant with his home CPAP and takes lisinopril for his hypertension.

1. Acetaminophen Pharmacology and Its Efficacy as a Multimodal Analgesic

1.1. Describe the mechanism of acetaminophen

The precise mechanism of acetaminophen remains unclear, but several pathways are known to be impacted by its use. A long-held belief is that its effect may be mediated by the inhibition of a cyclooxygenase (COX-2), thereby decreasing inflammatory prostaglandin synthesis. Animal research suggests that a centrally active COX isoenzyme, COX-3, may mediate its analgesic effects, but the existence of this isoform has been refuted in humans. Acetaminophen administration has also been shown to activate descending serotonergic pathways with a resultant reduction in pain signaling. Additional proposed mechanisms include inhibition of nitric oxide formation via the L-arginine pathway and indirect activation of the cannabinoid system. The majority of the analgesic effect of acetaminophen is most likely centrally mediated.

Further Reading

Bannwarth B, Netter P, Lapicque F, et al. Plasma and Cerebrospinal Fluid Concentrations of Paracetamol After a Single Intravenous Dose of Propacetamol. *Br J Clin Pharmacol.* 1992 Jul;34(1):79–81.

Hinz B, Cheremina O, Brune K. Acetaminophen (Paracetamol) Is a Selective Cyclooxygenase-2 Inhibitor in Man. *FASEB J.* 2008 Feb;22(2):383–390.

Jóźwiak-Bebenista M, Nowak JZ. Paracetamol: Mechanism of Action, Applications, and Safety Concern. *Acta Pol Pharm.* 2014 Jan–Feb;71(1):11–23.

Langford RA, Hogg M, Dip G, et al. Comparative Plasma and Cerebrospinal Fluid Pharmacokinetics of Paracetamol After Intravenous and Oral Administration. *Anesth Analg.* 2016 Sep;123(3):610–615.

Moriarity C, Carroll W. Paracetamol: Pharmacology, Prescribing and Controversies. *Arch Dis Child Educ Pract Ed.* 2016 Dec;101(6):331–334.

Pickering G, Loriot MA, Libert F, Eschalier A, Beaune P, Dubray C. Analgesic Effect of Acetaminophen in Humans: First Evidence of a Central Serotonergic Mechanism. *Clin Pharmacol Ther.* 2006 Apr;79(4):371–378.

Smith HS. Potential Analgesic Mechanisms of Acetaminophen. *Pain Physician.* 2009 Jan–Feb;12(1):269–280.

1.2. As a COX-2 inhibitor, does acetaminophen have anti-inflammatory effects?

Despite its function as a COX-2 inhibitor, acetaminophen only has weak anti-inflammatory effects. While not effective in reducing inflammation in rheumatoid arthritis, acetaminophen has been shown to reduce swelling following oral surgery. High concentrations of peroxides at areas of inflammation limit the ability of acetaminophen to inhibit COX-2. Unlike coxibs, acetaminophen does not inhibit platelet aggregation, lead to gastric ulcer formation, or have deleterious cardiovascular effects when used at therapeutic doses.

Further Reading

Jóźwiak-Bebenista M, Nowak JZ. Paracetamol: Mechanism of Action, Applications, and Safety Concern. *Acta Pol Pharm.* 2014 Jan–Feb;71(1):11–23.

Birmingham B, Buvanendran A. Nonsteroidal Anti-inflammatory Drugs, Acetaminophen, and COX-2 Inhibitors. In: Benzon H, Rathmell J, Wu CL, Turk D, Argoff C, Hurley R, eds. *Practical Management of Pain.* 5th ed. Philadelphia, PA: Mosby; 2014:553–567.

1.3. Describe the relative bioavailability of oral and rectal acetaminophen

The bioavailability of oral acetaminophen varies with dose. The bioavailability of a 500-mg dose is reported as 63%, 650 mg as 79%, and 1000 mg as 89%. A 650-mg elixir of acetaminophen has been shown to have a bioavailability as high as 87%. The absorption of acetaminophen is dependent on gastric emptying as it is absorbed within the small intestine. Therefore, factors that may delay gastric emptying, such as pain and anxiety, may affect its absorption. The relative bioavailability of rectal acetaminophen, compared with oral acetaminophen, has been reported as 52% (range 24%98%) in children but in excess of 80% in adults.

Further Reading

Ameer B, Divoll M, Abernethy DR, Greenblatt D, Shargel L. Absolute and Relative Bioavailability of Oral Acetaminophen Preparations. *J Pharm Sci.* 1983 Aug;72(8):955–958.

Anderson BJ, Holford NH. Rectal Acetaminophen Pharmacokinetics. *Anesthesiology.* 1998 Apr;88(4):1131–1133.

Anderson BJ, Holford NH, Woollard GA, Kanagasundarum S, Mahadevan M. Perioperative Pharmacodynamics of Acetaminophen Analgesia in Children. *Anesthesiology.* 1999 Feb;90(2):411–421.

Blume H, Ali SL, Elze M, Krämer J, Wendt G, Scholz ME. Relative Bioavailability of Paracetamol in Suppositories Preparations in Comparison to Tablets. *Arzneimittelforschung.* 1994 Dec;44(12):1333–1338.

Langford RA, Hogg M, Dip G, et al. Comparative Plasma and Cerebrospinal Fluid Pharmacokinetics of Paracetamol After Intravenous and Oral Administration. *Anesth Analg.* 2016 Sep;123(3):610–615.

Rawlins MD, Henderson DB, Hijab AR. Pharmacokinetics of Paracetamol (Acetaminophen) After Intravenous and Oral Administration. *Eur J Clin Pharmacol.* 1977 Apr 20;11(4):283–286.

1.4. What is the pharmacokinetic advantage of the intravenous form of acetaminophen?

The onset of analgesia with intravenous (IV) acetaminophen is rapid, occurring within 3 minutes of a bolus or 5 minutes into a 15-minute infusion, compared with 11 minutes for oral acetaminophen. The peak plasma concentration of IV acetaminophen occurs at the conclusion of a 15-minute infusion, in contrast to approximately 45 to 120 minutes for the pill form. Further, the peak plasma concentrations of IV acetaminophen may be as much as 75% greater than equivalent doses of oral acetaminophen. However, the area under the curve (AUC) of concentration versus time does not vary significantly between the 2 formulations. Whether the relatively rapid achievement of peak plasma levels with IV acetaminophen correlates to significant analgesic benefit is not well established. IV acetaminophen does appear to be associated with less interindividual variability in plasma concentrations than oral acetaminophen and may be more likely to reach a therapeutic maximum concentration.

While data regarding the relative cerebrospinal fluid (CSF) pharmacokinetic profile are less robust, the available literature suggests that CSF pharmacokinetics reflect that of plasma. Acetaminophen is more rapidly detectable and achieves a higher peak concentration in the CSF when given intravenously.

Further Reading

Bannwarth B, Netter P, Lapicque F, et al. Plasma and Cerebrospinal Fluid Concentrations of Paracetamol After a Single Intravenous Dose of Propacetamol. *Br J Clin Pharmacol.* 1992 Jul;34(1):79–81.

Brett CN, Barnett SG, Pearson J. Postoperative Plasma Paracetamol Levels Following Oral or Intravenous Paracetamol Administration: A Double-Blind Randomised Controlled Trial. *Anaesth Intensive Care.* 2012 Jan;40(1):166–171.

Fenlon S, Collyer J, Giles J, et al. Oral vs Intravenous Paracetamol for Lower Third Molar Extractions Under General Anaesthesia: Is Oral Administration Inferior? *Br J Anaesth.* 2013 Mar;110(3):432–437.

Holmér Pettersson P, Owall A, Jakobsson J. Early Bioavailability of Paracetamol After Oral or Intravenous Administration. *Acta Anaesthesiol Scand.* 2004 Aug;48(7):867–870.

Jibril F, Sharaby S, Mohamed A, Wilby K. Intravenous Versus Oral Acetaminophen for Pain: Systematic Review of Current Evidence to Support Clinical Decision-Making. *Can J Hosp Pharm.* 2015 May–Jun;68(3):238–247.

Koh W, Nguyen KP, Jahr JS. Intravenous Non-opioid Analgesia for Peri- and Postoperative Pain Management: A Scientific Review of Intravenous Acetaminophen and Ibuprofen. *Korean J Anesthesiol.* 2015 Feb;68(1):3–12.

Langford RA, Hogg M, Dip G, et al. Comparative Plasma and Cerebrospinal Fluid Pharmacokinetics of Paracetamol After Intravenous and Oral Administration. *Anesth Analg.* 2016 Sep;123(3):610–615.

Moller PL, Sindet-Pedersen S, Petersen CT, Juhl GI, Dillenschneider A, Skoglund LA. Onset of Acetaminophen Analgesia: Comparison of Oral and Intravenous Routes After Third Molar Surgery. *Br J Anaesth.* 2005 May;94(5):642–648.

Singla NK, Parulan C, Samson R, et al. Plasma and Cerebrospinal Fluid Pharmacokinetic Parameters After Single-Dose Administration of Intravenous, Oral, or Rectal Acetaminophen. *Pain Pract.* 2012 Sep;12(7):523–532.

1.5. What is the appropriate regimen for one-time administration and for chronic dosing? Should the dose be reduced in patients with liver disease?

A single 1000-mg dose of acetaminophen provides superior analgesia to smaller doses and is noninferior to a dose of 2000 mg. The safety of the original Food and Drug Administration recommendation of a daily 4000-mg limit not to exceed 10 days has been supported by numerous clinical trials, with long-term safety data showing no adverse effects when used up to 1 year. However, findings that 4000 mg daily use may lead to alanine aminotransferase elevation in as many as 44% of healthy volunteers prompted some experts to make more conservative recommendations. The American Liver Foundation recommends that patients not exceed 3000 mg daily.

In patients with liver disease, there is concern that reduced glutathione stores may lead to impaired conjugation of acetaminophen with the subsequent accumulation of toxic metabolites. Acetaminophen clearance is in fact delayed in patients with chronic liver disease. However, neither an accumulation of thiol metabolites nor evidence of increased susceptibility to liver toxicity has been observed in these patients.

Further Reading

Birmingham B, Buvanendran A. Nonsteroidal Anti-inflammatory Drugs, Acetaminophen, and COX-2 Inhibitors. In: Benzon H, Rathmell J, Wu CL, Turk D, Argoff C, Hurley R, eds. *Practical Management of Pain.* 5th ed. Philadelphia, PA: Mosby; 2014:553–567.

Hayward KL, Powell EE, Irvine KM, Martin JH. Can Paracetamol (Acetaminophen) Be Administered to Patients With Liver Impairment? *Br J Clin Pharmacol.* 2016 Feb;81(2):210–222.

Kuffner EK, Temple AR, Cooper KM, Baggish JS, Parenti DL. Retrospective Analysis of Transient Elevations in Alanine Aminotransferase During Long-Term Treatment With Acetaminophen in Osteoarthritis Clinical Trials. *Curr Med Res Opin.* 2006;22:2137–2148.

Pogatzki-Zahn E, Chandrasena C, Schug SA. Nonopioid Analgesics for Postoperative Pain Management. *Curr Opin Anaesthesiol.* 2014 Oct;27(5):513–519.

Watkins PB, Kaplowitz N, Slattery JT, et al. Aminotransferase Elevations in Healthy Adults Receiving 4 Grams of Acetaminophen Daily: A Randomized Controlled Trial. *JAMA.* 2006 Jul 5;296(1):87–93.

Zapater P, Lasso de la Vega MC, Horga JF, et al. Pharmacokinetic Variations of Acetaminophen According to Liver Dysfunction and Portal Hypertension Status. *Aliment Pharmacol Ther.* 2004 Jul 1;20(1):29–36.

1.6. Describe the metabolism of acetaminophen and how it relates to acetaminophen-mediated liver toxicity

Acetaminophen is metabolized in the liver via sulfation, oxidation, and glucuronidation. Less than 10% is excreted by the kidneys unchanged. Glucoronide and sulfide metabolites are pharmacologically inactive and excreted primarily by the kidneys. Cytochrome P450–based oxidation produces the potentially hepatotoxic metabolite N-acetyl-p-benzoquinone imine (NAPQI). Normally, NAPQI then undergoes phase 2 conjugation with glutathione to produce harmless metabolites that are excreted by the kidneys as mercapturic acid. Glutathione depletion, in the setting of heavy alcohol consumption or acetaminophen overdose, creates susceptibility to the accumulation of NAPQI, which untreated can lead to fulminant liver failure and death. N-acetylcysteine, a glutathione precursor, is the primary treatment for patients with acetaminophen hepatotoxicity.

Further Reading

Hayward KL, Powell EE, Irvine KM, Martin JH. Can Paracetamol (Acetaminophen) Be Administered to Patients With Liver Impairment? *Br J Clin Pharmacol.* 2016 Feb;81(2):210–222.

Jóźwiak-Bebenista M, Nowak JZ. Paracetamol: Mechanism of Action, Applications, and Safety Concern. *Acta Pol Pharm.* 2014 Jan–Feb;71(1):11–23.

Koh W, Nguyen KP, Jahr JS. Intravenous Non-opioid Analgesia for Peri- and Postoperative Pain Management: A Scientific Review of Intravenous Acetaminophen and Ibuprofen. *Korean J Anesthesiol.* 2015 Feb;68(1):3–12.

1.7. Is acetaminophen safe to use in pregnancy?

Acetaminophen falls within pregnancy category C, though it is generally considered a safer over-the-counter analgesic for pregnant women than ibuprofen. Retrospective studies have recently linked maternal acetaminophen use to attention deficit and hyperkinetic disorders in children. While these studies adjusted for confounding variables, randomized trials are still needed to support this association. Another concern is an association between maternal acetaminophen use and childhood asthma. Acetaminophen is hypothesized to deplete lung glutathione stores and therefore increase oxidative damage to the lungs, and a recent review of population data concluded that there is "reasonably compelling evidence" to link prenatal exposure to acetaminophen to childhood asthma. However, randomized prospective data are lacking. The results of a trial in asthmatic children aged 12 to 59 months randomized to receive acetaminophen or ibuprofen as needed for pain or fever over a 48-week course are encouraging. This study found no association of acetaminophen use with asthma exacerbations.

Further Reading

Henderson AJ, Shaheen SO. Acetaminophen and Asthma. *Paediatr Respir Rev.* 2013 Mar;14(1):9–15; quiz 16.

Liew Z, Ritz B, Rebordosa C, Lee P, Olsen J. Acetaminophen Use During Pregnancy, Behavioral Problems, and Hyperkinetic Disorders. *JAMA Pediatr.* 2014 Apr;168(4):313–320.

Sheehan WJ, Mauger DT, Paul IM, et al. Acetaminophen Versus Ibuprofen in Young Children With Mild Persistent Asthma. *N Engl J Med*. 2016 Aug 18;375(7):619–630.

Thompson JM, Waldie KE, Wall CR, Murphy R, Mitchell E. Associations Between Acetaminophen Use During Pregnancy and ADHD Symptoms Measured at Ages 7 and 11 Years. *PLoS One*. 2014 Sep 24;9(9):e108210.

1.8. What is the incidence of intravenous opioid-related side effects in the perioperative period?

Wheeler et al. systematically reviewed the side effects of perioperative opioid use, inclusive of all randomized trials conducted between 1990 and 2000. Overall, central nervous system side effects (somnolence, dizziness, psychoses, adverse cognitive effects) were most common, occurring in 75.9% of patients. Gastrointestinal side effects (nausea, vomiting, constipation) were reported in 28.2% of patients, 4.1% of patients developed urinary retention, and 2.4% of patients experienced respiratory events.

Further Reading

Wheeler M, Oderda GM, Ashburn MA, Lipman A. Adverse Events Associated With Postoperative Opioid Analgesia: A Systematic Review. *J Pain*. 2002 Jun;3(3):159–180.

1.9. What is the value of acetaminophen when included as part of a multimodal analgesic regimen?

Henrik Kehlet first proposed multimodal analgesia as a strategy to improve pain control through analgesic synergy while aiming to reduce adverse effects from a single analgesic class, namely, opioids. While the ability of acetaminophen to accomplish this is supported by meta-analyses, the effect is modest, and data from individual studies are conflicting. Acetaminophen use has been reported to reduce morphine requirements, postoperative nausea and vomiting, sedation, pruritis, costs, and hospital length of stay. Some of these benefits may be limited to the IV form of acetaminophen. A large retrospective study by Apfel et al. did not show a reduction in the incidence of respiratory or cardiovascular events in patients taking acetaminophen after total joint replacement.

Further Reading

Apfel C, Jahr JR, Kelly CL, Ang RY, Oderda GM. Effect of I.V. Acetaminophen on Total Hip or Knee Replacement Surgery: A Case-Matched Evaluation of a National Patient Database. *Am J Health Syst Pharm*. 2015 Nov 15;72(22):1961–1968.

Apfel CC, Turan A, Souza K, Pergolizzi J, Hornuss C. Intravenous Acetaminophen Reduces Postoperative Nausea and Vomiting: A Systematic Review and Meta-analysis. *Pain*. 2013 May;154(5):677–689.

Doleman B, Read D, Lund JN, Williams JP. Preventive Acetaminophen Reduces Postoperative Opioid Consumption, Vomiting, and Pain Scores After Surgery: Systematic Review and Meta-analysis. *Reg Anesth Pain Med*. 2015 Nov–Dec;40(6):706–712.

Elia N, Lysakowski C, Tramèr MR. Does Multimodal Analgesia With Acetaminophen, Nonsteroidal Antiinflammatory Drugs, or Selective Cyclooxygenase-2 Inhibitors and Patient-Controlled Analgesia Morphine Offer Advantages Over Morphine Alone? Meta-analyses of Randomized Trials. *Anesthesiology*. 2005 Dec;103(6):1296–1304.

Herring BO, Ader S, Maldonado A, Hawkins C, Kearson M, Camejo M. Impact of Intravenous Acetaminophen on Reducing Opioid Use After Hysterectomy. *Pharmacotherapy*. 2014 Dec;34(suppl 1):27S–33S.

Jahr JS, Filocamo P, Singh S. Intravenous Acetaminophen: A Review of Pharmacoeconomic Science for Perioperative Use. *Am J Ther*. 2013 Mar–Apr;20(2):189–199.

Kehlet H, Dahl JB. The Value of "Multimodal" or "Balanced Analgesia" in Postoperative Pain Treatment. *Anesth Analg*. 1993 Nov;77(5):1048–1056.

Remy C, Marret E, Bonnet F. Effects of Acetaminophen on Morphine Side-Effects and Consumption After Major Surgery: Meta-analysis of Randomized Controlled Trials. *Br J Anaesth.* 2005 Apr;94(4):505–513.

1.10. Is there an optimal time for acetaminophen administration in the perioperative period?

Data regarding the optimal time of administration are limited. However, administration prior to the onset of pain appears to be more effective in reducing the incidence of postoperative nausea and vomiting compared with dosing at the onset of pain.

Further Reading

Apfel C, Jahr JR, Kelly CL, Ang RY, Oderda GM. Effect of I.V. Acetaminophen on Total Hip or Knee Replacement Surgery: A Case-Matched Evaluation of a National Patient Database. *Am J Health Syst Pharm.* 2015 Nov 15;72(22):1961–1968.

1.11. How does the benefit of acetaminophen compare with that obtained with nonsteroidal anti-inflammatory drugs?

Overall, the analgesic effect of acetaminophen as a multimodal analgesic is weak when compared with nonsteroidal anti-inflammatory drugs (NSAIDs). The number needed to treat for a 1000-mg dose of acetaminophen is 3.5, compared with values reported between 1.7 and 2.7 for therapeutic doses of various NSAIDs. The efficacy of co-administering acetaminophen and NSAIDs has repeatedly been proven to be greater than the efficacy of either medication given alone.

Further Reading

Daniels SE, Goulder MA, Aspley S, Reader S. A Randomised, Five-Parallel-Group, Placebo-Controlled Trial Comparing the Efficacy and Tolerability of Analgesic Combinations Including a Novel Single-Tablet Combination of Ibuprofen/Paracetamol for Postoperative Dental Pain. *Pain.* 2011 Mar;152(3):632–642.

Derry CJ, Derry S, Moore RA. Single Dose Oral Ibuprofen Plus Paracetamol (Acetaminophen) for Acute Postoperative Pain. *Cochrane Database Syst Rev.* 2013 Jun 24(6):CD010210.

Gilron I, Tu D, Dumerton-Shore D, et al. The Effect of Triple vs. Double Nonopioid Therapy on Postoperative Pain and Functional Outcome After Abdominal Hysterectomy: A Randomised Double-Blind Control Trial. *Eur J Anaesthesiol.* 2015 Apr;32(4):269–276.

Issioui T, Klein KW, White PF, et al. Cost-Efficacy of Rofecoxib Versus Acetaminophen for Preventing Pain After Ambulatory Surgery. *Anesthesiology.* 2002 Oct;97(4):931–937.

Mehlisch DR, Aspley S, Daniels SE, Bandy DP. Comparison of the Analgesic Efficacy of Concurrent Ibuprofen and Paracetamol With Ibuprofen or Paracetamol Alone in the Management of Moderate to Severe Acute Postoperative Dental Pain in Adolescents and Adults: A Randomized, Double-Blind, Placebo-Controlled, Parallel-Group, Single-Dose, Two-Center, Modified Factorial Study. *Clin Ther.* 2010 May;32(5):882–895.

Mehlisch DR, Aspley S, Daniels SE, Southerden KA, Christensen KS. A Single-Tablet Fixed-Dose Combination of Racemic Ibuprofen/Paracetamol in the Management of Moderate to Severe Postoperative Dental Pain in Adult and Adolescent Patients: A Multicenter, Two-Stage, Randomized, Double-Blind, Parallel-Group, Placebo-Controlled, Factorial Study. *Clin Ther.* 2010 Jun;32(6):1033–1049.

Moore RA, Derry S, Aldington D, Wiffen PJ. Single Dose Oral Analgesics for Acute Postoperative Pain in Adults: An Overview of Cochrane Reviews. *Cochrane Database Syst Rev.* 2015 Sep 28;(9):CD008659.

Moore RA, Straube S, Paine J, Derry S, McQuay HJ. Single Dose Oral Analgesics for Acute Postoperative Pain in Adults. *Cochrane Database Syst Rev.* 2011 Sep 7;(9):CD008659.

Pogatzki-Zahn E, Chandrasena C, Schug SA. Nonopioid Analgesics for Postoperative Pain Management. *Curr Opin Anaesthesiol.* 2014 Oct;27(5):513–519.

2. Surgical/Regional Anesthetic Considerations

2.1. What are surgical considerations during ACL repair?

ACL reconstruction is commonly carried out either by a hamstring graft, which involves making a small incision inferiorly and medially to the tibial tubercle to harvest the semintendinosus and gracilis tendons, or via a midline incision below the patella to harvest a section of the patellar tendon to replace the anterior cruciate ligament. Reconstruction may also be performed with a cadaver graft. In either approach, blockade of femoral dermatomes is necessary to provide adequate pain relief.

Further Reading

Kim, S., J. et al. A Modified Arthroscopic Anterior Cruciate Ligament Double-Bundle Reconstruction Technique With Autogenous Quadriceps Tendon Graft: Remnant-Preserving Technique. *Arch Orthop Trauma Surg.* 2009 Mar;129(3):403–407.

2.2. What is the utility of regional anesthesia in the perioperative pain management of an ACL repair?

The majority of all arthroscopic knee surgeries are now performed on a same-day discharge basis. Optimal analgesia without delaying timely discharge is critical in this ambulatory surgical population. Multimodal pharmacologic agents such as gabapentanoids and NSAIDS have been shown to decrease postoperative opioid consumption in this population. While these pharmacologic agents offer benefit in the immediate postoperative setting, no long-term benefit has been documented in patients undergoing ACL repair. Additionally, therapies such as cryotherapy (particularly continuous flow and compression) as well as early mobilization have demonstrated some benefit in pain scores in both the immediate and subacute postoperative periods.

While analgesia for arthroscopic knee procedures can be obtained through such pharmacologic and conservative therapies, interventional modalities such as perineural blockade (PNB) and intra-articular injection (IA) have shown to be most effective in achieving adequate pain control in this patient population. Both PNB and IA have demonstrated significant benefits by reducing both pain intensity scores and opioid use in the immediate postoperative setting.

Further Reading

Roseaeg OP, et al. Effect of Preemptive Multimodal Analgesia for Arthroscopic knee Ligament Repair. *Reg Anesth Pain Med.* Mar–Apr 26(2):125–130.

Secrust ES, et al. Pain Management After Outpatient Anterior Cruciate Ligament Reconstruction: A Systematic Review of Randomized Controlled Trials. *Am J Sports Med.* 2016 Sep;44(9):2435–2447.

2.3. Discuss the efficacy of intra-articular injections when compared with femoral nerve blocks in patients having arthroscopic knee surgery

Femoral nerve block (FNB), single-injection or continuous infusion, provides superior analgesia as compared with intra-articular injections. Most prospective trials have demonstrated the superiority of FMB as judged by morphine consumption and pain intensity scores. In one such prospective trial, children received combined single-injection femoral and sciatic nerve blocks and were found to have significantly lower opioid consumption in both the immediate and late postoperative course compared with children who received intra-articular medications. In a separate study in patients undergoing ACL repair, the analgesic duration was longer in the FNB group versus the intra-articular group providing better analgesia and demonstrating a significant morphine-sparing effect.

Further Reading

Dauri M, et al. Continuous Femoral Nerve Block Provides Superior Analgesia Compared With Continuous Intra-articular and Wound Infusion After Anterior Cruciate Ligament Reconstruction. *Reg Anesth Pain Med.* 2009 Mar–Apr;34(2):95–99. ISSN 1532-8651.

Iskandar H, et al. Femoral Block Provides Superior Analgesia Compared With Intra-articular Ropivacaine After Anterior Cruciate Ligament Reconstruction. *Reg Anesth Pain Med.* 2003 Jan–Feb;28(1):29–32. ISSN 1098-7339.

Lefevre N, et al. Peri-articular Local Infiltration Analgesia Versus Femoral Nerve Block for Postoperative Pain Control Following Anterior Cruciate Ligament Reconstruction: Prospective, Comparative, Non-inferiority Study. *Orthop Traumatol Surg Res.* 2016 Nov;102(7):873–877. ISSN 1877-0568.

Tran KM, et al. Intraarticular Bupivacaine-Clonidine-Morphine Versus Femoral-Sciatic Nerve Block in Pediatric Patients Undergoing Anterior Cruciate Ligament Reconstruction. *Anesth Analg.* 2005 Nov;101(5):1304–1310. ISSN 0003-2999.

2.4. Do femoral nerve blocks have long-term ill effects on muscle strength in patients receiving ACL repair? Can ACL repair lead to nerve injury?

In some studies, concerns have been raised regarding the long-term effects of FNBs on functional outcome in patients undergoing ACL repair. Retrospective studies have suggested that FNB results in persistent quadriceps weakness; however, recent prospective evidence suggests that while some quadriceps weakness is noted weeks after surgery, this weakness resolves by 6 months. In another electrophysiological study involving femoral nerve catheters following ACL repair, no functional limitations (e.g., active flexion, distance walked, quadriceps strength) or electrophysiologic signs of vastus medialis denervation or femoral nerve injury were found at 4 weeks.

Aside from the concerns of perineural injury due to FNB, perineural injury may also occur due to surgical causes. During arthroscopic ACL repair, the infrapatellar branch of the saphenous nerve is the most commonly injured nerve resulting in loss of sensation along the anterolateral aspect of the knee.

Further Reading

Krych A, et al. Adverse Effect of Femoral Nerve Blockade on Quadriceps Strength and Function After ACL Reconstruction. *J Knee Surg.* 2015 Feb;28(1):83–88. ISSN 1938-2480.

Magnussen RA, et al. Femoral Nerve Block After Anterior Cruciate Ligament Reconstruction. 2017 May;30(4):323-328.

Stebler K, et al. Electrophysiological Study of Femoral Nerve Function After a Continuous Femoral Nerve Block for Anterior Cruciate Ligament Reconstruction: A Randomized, Controlled Single-Blind Trial. *Am J Sports Med.* 2017 Mar;45(3):578-583

Walshaw T, Karuppiah SV, Stewart I. The Course and Distribution of the Infrapatellar Nerve in Relation to ACL Reconstruction. *Knee.* 2015 Oct;22(5):384–388. ISSN 1873-5800.

2.5. What role do adductor canal/saphenous nerve blocks play in the management of postoperative pain resulting from arthroscopic surgery?

In light of the association of persistent quadriceps weakness and FNB, the adductor canal nerve block (ACB) has emerged as an alternative analgesic option following ACL reconstruction. This is largely due to the significant preservation of quadriceps function following adductor canal blockade compared with FNB. However, further research comparing FNB with ACB in the setting of arthroscopic surgery is needed. A recent prospective randomized trial comparing the 2 techniques in a larger patient population has found that compared with FNB, ACB preserves quadriceps strength and provides equivalent postoperative analgesia to patients undergoing anterior cruciate ligament reconstruction. However, a previous double-blind prospective study comparing pain scores only found that adductor canal blocks provided no additional benefit in a patient receiving multimodal analgesia alone.

Further Reading

Abdallah FW, et al. Adductor Canal Block Provides Noninferior Analgesia and Superior Quadriceps Strength Compared With Femoral Nerve Block in Anterior Cruciate Ligament Reconstruction. Anesthesiology. 2016 May;124(5):1053-64.

El Ahl MS. Femoral Nerve Block Versus Adductor Canal Block for Postoperative Pain Control After Anterior Cruciate Ligament Reconstruction: A Randomized Double Blind Study. *Saudi J Anaesth.* 2015 Jul–Sep;9(3):279–282.

Espelund M, et al. Analgesic Efficacy of Ultrasound-Guided Adductor Canal Blockade After Arthroscopic Anterior Cruciate Ligament Reconstruction: A Randomised Controlled Trial. *Eur J Anaesthesiol.* 2013 Jul;30(7):422–428. ISSN 1365-2346.

Case Scenario

The surgery is done. While the patient is in the recovery room, he complains of pain in the back of the knee.

2.6. What are etiologies of posterior knee pain following ACL reconstruction? What are possible treatment strategies?

Often patients undergoing arthroscopic knee procedures will report posterior pain in the presence of a femoral block/catheter. In the setting of hamstring autografts, the etiology is largely related to the sciatic innervation of the graft site. However, posterior knee pain is also reported in ACL repairs with cadaver allografting. The mechanism of this pain stems from articular branches arising from both the tibial (sensory afferents of the posterior knee) and the common peroneal (sensory afferents to both anterior/posterior knee). Indeed, numerous studies have demonstrated improved analgesia and decreased opioid consumption with the addition of sciatic nerve block to the FMB for ACL reconstruction.

Further Reading

Abdallah FW, Brull R. Is Sciatic Nerve Block Advantageous When Combined With Femoral Nerve Block for Postoperative Analgesia Following Total Knee Arthroplasty? A Systematic Review. *Reg Anesth Pain Med.* 2011 Sep–Oct;36(5):493–498. ISSN 1532-8651.

Abdallah FW, et al. The Analgesic Effects of Proximal, Distal, or No Sciatic Nerve Block on Posterior Knee Pain After Total Knee Arthroplasty: A Double-Blind Placebo-Controlled Randomized Trial. *Anesthesiology.* 2014 Dec;121(6):1302–10.

Harbell MW, et al. Combined Preoperative Femoral and Sciatic Nerve Blockade Improves Analgesia After Anterior Cruciate Ligament Reconstruction: A Randomized Controlled Clinical Trial. *J Clin Anesth.* 2016 Sep;33:68–74. ISSN 1873-4529.

2.7. What is liposomal bupivacaine? Discuss its efficacy for intra-articular injections

Liposomal bupivacaine combines bupivacaine within a multivesicular lipid-based delivery platform (DepoFoam, Pacira Pharmaceuticals) that allows the release of the anesthetic agent over an extended period. With its theoretical prolonged duration of action, the periarticular injection of liposomal bupivacaine has been evaluated in patients undergoing ACL repair. However, a recent randomized controlled trial comparing infiltration with plain bupivacaine with liposomal bupivacaine found lower efficacy in the liposomal bupivacaine group at a 200-fold cost. When compared with FNB with regular bupivacaine, patients receiving FNB reported superior pain intensity scores postoperatively but only in the acute postoperative period (5–8 hours).

Further Reading

Okoroha KR, et al. Liposomal Bupivacaine Versus Femoral Nerve Block for Pain Control After Anterior Cruciate Ligament Reconstruction: A Prospective Randomized Trial. *Arthroscopy.* 2016 Sep;32(9):1838–1845. ISSN 1526-3231.

Premkumar A, et al. Liposomal Bupivacaine for Pain Control After Anterior Cruciate Ligament Reconstruction: A Prospective, Double-Blinded, Randomized, Positive-Controlled Trial. *Am J Sports Med.* 2016 Jul;44(7):1680–1686. ISSN 1552-3365.

3. Questions Pertaining to Pharmacogenomics and the Epigenetics of Acute Pain Management

3.1. Define pharmacogenomics and describe broadly how it may impact acute pain management

Pharmacogenomics refers to the study of how the human genome affects drug responsiveness. It is concerned with the development and/or tailoring of therapies based on an individual's genetic makeup. At this time, the field aims to identify frequently occurring genetic polymorphisms that may cause interindividual variability in the metabolism, receptor profile, or transportation and uptake of a medication. This genetic variability may contribute to differences in each patient's response to local anesthetics, opioids, tricyclic antidepressants, and NSAIDs. Further, pharmacogenomics may reveal genetic differences in the way individuals experience pain. Many genetic polymorphisms have been discovered that may affect acute pain management; the most rigorously defined traits are described in the following sections.

Further Reading

Argoff CE. An Introduction to Pharmacogenomics in Pain Management. In: Benzon H, Rathmell J, Wu CL, Turk D, Argoff C, Hurley R, eds. *Practical Management of Pain.* 5th ed. Philadelphia, PA: Mosby; 2014:132–136.

Janicki PK. Pharmacogenomics of Pain Management. In: Deer T, Leong MS, Buvanendran A, Gordin V, Kim P, Panchal SJ, Ray AL, eds. *Comprehensive Treatment of Chronic Pain by Medical, Interventional, and Integrative Approaches: The American Academy of Pain Medicine Textbook on Patient Management.* New York, NY: Springer Publishing Company; 2013:23–33.

3.2. Describe how codeine metabolism affects its analgesic efficacy

Codeine is a prodrug that undergoes conversion to morphine via cytochrome P450 2D6 to provide analgesia. More than 70 polymorphisms of CYP2D6 have been identified. An individual's alleles determine whether they are poor, intermediate, extensive, or ultra-rapid metabolizers of codeine. Between 10% and 21% of whites possess an inactive CYP2D6 enzyme and experience a poor analgesia response to codeine, whereas about 3% of whites are rapid metabolizers and may be more likely to experience typical opioid-related side effects. This genetic profile varies considerably between ethnicities: as many of 50% of Chinese patients have reduced CYP2D6 activity; in contrast, activity is increased in as many 29% of Ethiopian and Saudi Arabian patients. CYP2D6 is also involved in the metabolism of tramadol and oxycodone; allelic differences appear to impact the efficacy of tramadol, but metabolic variability does not seem to produce clinically relevant differences in oxycodone analgesia.

Further Reading

Argoff CE. An Introduction to Pharmacogenomics in Pain Management. In: Benzon H, Rathmell J, Wu CL, Turk D, Argoff C, Hurley R, eds. *Practical Management of Pain.* 5th ed. Philadelphia, PA: Mosby; 2014:132–136.

Cregg R, Russo G, Gubbay A, Branford R, Sato H. Pharmacogenetics of Analgesic Drugs. *Br J Pain.* 2013 Nov;7(4):189–208.

Janicki, PK. Pharmacogenomics of Pain Management. In: Deer T, Leong MS, Buvanendran A, Gordin V, Kim P, Panchal SJ, Ray AL eds. *Comprehensive Treatment of Chronic Pain by Medical, Interventional, and Integrative Approaches: The American Academy of Pain Medicine Textbook on Patient Management.* New York, NY: Springer Publishing Company; 2013:23–33.

3.3. Discuss the impact of opioid receptor gene OPRM1 polymorphisms on opioid analgesia

The OPRM1 gene codes for one opioid receptor type responsible for binding both endogenous and synthetic opioids. OPRM1 mutations impacting a patient's response to opioid analgesics. The substitution of guanine in place of adenine at position 118 (A118G) decreases receptor expression and may increase a patient's opioid requirements. This substitution is found in 10% to 30% of whites. Patients with the homozygous AA genotype have exhibited reduced pain scores and opioid requirements compared with the heterozygous AG (G→ A118G) phenotype or GG homozygotes in some studies. However, others have failed to find a clear link between the polymorphism and opioid requirements, and its absolute effect remains unclear.

Further Reading

Allegri M, De Gregori M, Niebel T, et al. Pharmacogenetics and Postoperative Pain: A New Approach to Improve Acute Pain Management. *Minerva Anestesiol.* 2010 Nov;76(11):937–944.

Argoff, CE. An Introduction to Pharmacogenomics in Pain Management. In: Benzon H, Rathmell J, Wu CL, Turk D, Argoff C, Hurley R, eds. *Practical Management of Pain.* 5th ed. Philadelphia, PA: Mosby; 2014:132–136.

Janicki, PK. Pharmacogenomics of Pain Management. In: Deer T, Leong MS, Buvanendran A, Gordin V, Kim P, Panchal SJ, Ray AL, eds. *Comprehensive Treatment of Chronic Pain by Medical, Interventional, and Integrative Approaches: The American Academy of Pain Medicine Textbook on Patient Management.* New York, NY: Springer Publishing Company; 2013:23–33.

3.4. How do CYP2C9 polymorphisms impact treatment with nonsteroidal anti-inflammatory drugs?

Genetic differences may explain some of the variability in the response and side effect profile of NSAID treatment between individuals. A polymorphism within CYP2C9 has been identified that decreases the rate of clearance of ibuprofen and celecoxib. Patients with this inactive enzyme are at higher risk of gastroduodenal bleeding with NSAID use. Whether these patients experience superior analgesia from NSAIDs compared with the general population is unclear.

Further Reading

Argoff, CE. An Introduction to Pharmacogenomics in Pain Management. In: Benzon H, Rathmell J, Wu CL, Turk D, Argoff C, Hurley R, eds. *Practical Management of Pain.* 5th ed. Philadelphia, PA: Mosby; 2014:132–136.

Janicki, PK. Pharmacogenomics of Pain Management. In: Deer T, Leong MS, Buvanendran A, Gordin V, Kim P, Panchal SJ, Ray AL, eds.. *Comprehensive Treatment of Chronic Pain by Medical, Interventional, and Integrative Approaches: The American Academy of Pain Medicine Textbook on Patient Management.* New York, NY: Springer Publishing Company; 2013:23–33.

Kirchheiner J, Störmer E, Meisel C, Steinbach N, Roots I, Brockmöller J. Influence of CYP2C9 Genetic Polymorphisms on Pharmacokinetics of Celecoxib and Its Metabolites. *Pharmacogenetics.* 2003 Aug;13(8):473–480.

Kirchheiner J, Meineke I, Freytag G, Meisel C, Roots I, Brockmöller J. Enantiospecific Effects of Cytochrome P450 2C9 Amino Acid Variants on Ibuprofen Pharmacokinetics and on the Inhibition of Cyclooxygenases 1 and 2. *Clin Pharmacol Ther.* 2002 Jul;72(1):62–75.

3.5. What is the effect of the COMT variant Val158Met on pain sensitivity and opioid response?

COMT serves as an essential enzyme in the metabolism of dopamine and other adrenergic neurotransmitters and has been linked to both pain sensitivity and opioid treatment response. One of the most common polymorphisms occurs when a valine is substituted for a methionine at codon 158 (Val158Met). Patients may be either heterozygous or homozygous for these alleles. Such polymorphisms are characterized by significantly decreased enzymatic activity resulting in higher adrenergic levels which have been linked to heightened pain sensitivity.

However, patients homozygous for the Val158Met allele are also characterized by a notable increase in central mu receptors. Among cancer patients containing the Val158Met allele, while the reported higher pain sensitivity, they required significantly less morphine equivalents. Numerous additional COMT polymorphisms have been identified and linked to interindividual variability in pain perception. Future work regarding the stratification of individual patients depending on their allelic content will hopefully aid in tailored acute pain regimens.

Further Reading

Allegri M, De Gregori M, Niebel T, et al. Pharmacogenetics and Postoperative Pain: A New Approach to Improve Acute Pain Management. *Minerva Anestesiol.* 2010 Nov;76(11):937–944.

Argoff, CE. An Introduction to Pharmacogenomics in Pain Management. In: Benzon H, Rathmell J, Wu CL, Turk D, Argoff C, Hurley R, eds. *Practical Management of Pain.* 5th ed. Philadelphia, PA: Mosby; 2014:132–136.

Janicki, PK. Pharmacogenomics of Pain Management. In: Deer T, Leong MS, Buvanendran A, Gordin V, Kim P, Panchal SJ, Ray AL, eds. *Comprehensive Treatment of Chronic Pain by Medical, Interventional, and Integrative Approaches: The American Academy of Pain Medicine Textbook on Patient Management.* New York, NY: Springer Publishing Company; 2013:23–33.

3.6. Define epigenetics and how it may affect pain management

Epigenetics differs from pharmacogenetics in that rather than describing changes occurring to the genome itself, epigenetics describes DNA modifications leading to expression and phenotypic changes without altering the genetic sequence. These changes are primarily the result of histone modification and DNA methylation. Epigenetic changes are thought to occur in response to environmental influence and as a result of an individual's experiences.

Epigenetic changes may contribute to individual variability in acute pain sensitivity, chronic pain severity, and even the transition from acute to chronic pain. Proof of these concepts remains investigational, with a need for confirmatory studies. Some interesting findings include a link between methylation of the TRPA-1 ion channel to heat pain sensitivity, a correlation between leukocyte DNA methylation with the severity of chronic pain in long-term opioid users, and decreased signs of opioid-induced hypersensitivity through the inhibition of histone acetyltransferase.

Further Reading

Géranton SM, Tochiki KK. Regulation of Gene Expression and Pain States by Epigenetic Mechanisms. *Prog Mol Biol Transl Sci.* 2015;131:147–183.

Lirk P, Fiegl H, Weber NC, Hollmann MW. Epigenetics in the Perioperative Period. *Br J Pharmacol.* 2015 Jun;172(11):2748–2755.

10

Pain Management for Whipple Surgery

Linh T. Nguyen and Jose M. Soliz

Case Scenario

A 65-year-old man with pancreatic adenocarcinoma is scheduled for a pancreaticoduodenectomy (Whipple procedure). The patient has a history of mild cirrhosis linked to hepatitis C, chronic kidney disease with a baseline creatinine of 1.2 mg/dL, and atrial fibrillation. His home medicines include metoprolol, Coumadin, and ranitidine.

1. Anatomic Considerations

1.1. What is the innervation of the abdominal wall?

The thoracolumbar nerves from the T6-L1 spinal roots provide sensory innervation to the anterolateral abdominal wall. The anterior cutaneous branches run in the neurovascular plane between the internal oblique and transversus abdominis muscles before entering the rectus abdominis muscle, providing sensory innervation of the anterior abdominal wall. The lateral cutaneous branches provide sensory innervation of the lateral portion of the abdominal wall.

1.2. What is the innervation of the viscera?

Visceral components of the abdomen are supplied by the sympathetic and parasympathetic nervous systems. Sympathetic fibers originating from the seventh thoracic through second lumbar nerves form the greater, lesser, least, and lumbar splanchnic nerves. The parasympathetic supply originates from the right and left vagus nerves as well as the pelvic splanchnic nerves.

2. Transversus Abdominis Plane Block

2.1. What is a transversus abdominis plane TAP block?

The transversus abdominis plane (TAP) block is a peripheral abdominal wall block first described in 2001 by Rafi. This block, known now as the posterior TAP block, involves the injection of local anesthetic between the internal oblique and transverse abdominis muscle, where the thoracolumbar nerves are located. The resulting blockade has been shown to consistently provide analgesia in the T10-L1 abdominal dermatome distributions and is commonly used for analgesia involving surgery of the lower abdomen.

The subcostal approach to the TAP involves the injection of local anesthetic inferior to the costal margin. With the subcostal approach, sensory blockade of the abdominal wall may extend up to T7, providing improved analgesia for upper abdominal surgery over the posterior TAP block. The 4-quadrant (or 4-point) TAP block is a newer approach to providing analgesia for major abdominal surgery. This approach, combining the injections of the posterior TAP block and the subcostal TAP block, may provide a more extensive sensory blockade and improved analgesia than either approach alone for major abdominal surgery.

2.2. How is a TAP block performed?

You may perform posterior, lateral, and subcostal approaches to the TAP block in an anesthetized or an awake patient. You may place the patient in the supine position to perform the block. If the posterior or lateral approach is required, the arms are extended laterally. The posterior TAP block is performed within the triangle of Petit, and the patient may need to be turned slightly laterally for adequate ultrasonography. The anatomic landmarks for this triangle include the iliac crest at the base and the external oblique muscle and the latissimus dorsi on the sides. The lateral TAP block is performed at the midaxillary line. Catheters may be threaded in place to extend the block for a longer postoperative use.

Before the widespread use of routine ultrasound-guided regional anesthesia, physicians performed the posterior TAP block blindly with blunt-tip needles. Using this method, as you insert the needle, you feel the first pop as the needle penetrates the external oblique fascia, and the second pop as the needle penetrates the internal oblique muscle. After the second pop, local anesthetic is deposited. Blind insertion of needles may increase the risk of peritoneal injury or visceral puncture. Hepatic injury is possible with right-sided TAP blocks.

However, the ease and precision of injection with the use of ultrasound have increased the use of the ultrasound-guided TAP block. A 5 to 15 MHz linear array ultrasound probe is typically used with a small-bore blunt-end needle. The use of sharp-ended needles should be avoided, as this may increase the risk of peritoneal or inadvertent visceral puncture. Echogenic regional anesthesia needles may also be used for improved visualization during ultrasonography. You should insert the needle in plane, observing it carefully and continuously as you advance it into the TAP. Once the TAP is entered, you can confirm needle placement using preservative-free normal saline or injection of small amounts of local anesthetic. You can achieve adequate sensory blockade by using larger volumes of local anesthetic (15–20 mL per injection site). The spreading of the transverse abdominis and internal oblique muscles, viewed on ultrasound image, will confirm correct local anesthetic deposition. The sensory blockage from a lateral TAP block will cover dermatomes T10-L1. You should pay careful attention to injecting less than the maximum recommended dose of the local anesthetic, as large volumes of local anesthetic are required for this block. Though clinically relevant toxicity is rare, plasma concentrations of local anesthetics can reach toxic levels after a TAP block even at recommended dosing.

2.3. What are the contraindications to TAP block?

Localized infection and patient refusal are contraindications to TAP blocks. Allergies to specific types of local anesthetics, while rare (amide or ester), may preclude patients from receiving this block. Caution is noted in patients receiving local anesthetic infusions via other administered routes (peripheral nerve blocks) as the total dose administered can reach toxic levels.

2.4. What are the possible complications of a TAP block?

Complications with the ultrasound-guided TAP block are rare. However, intraperitoneal injection, liver laceration, vascular injury, and bowel perforation are rare but possible complications. Prior abdominal surgery, abdominal hernia, subcutaneous air in tissue after laparoscopy, and extreme body habitus contributing to the distortion of anatomy can make the TAP ultrasonography challenging. Risk factors for specific TAP block–related complications have not been extensively studied. Staying within the maximum recommended local anesthetic dosing range is of the utmost importance, as the high volumes used for these blocks have rare but potentially toxic side effects. Likewise, the use of continuous infusions after bolus injection of local anesthetics for TAP blocks may result in high plasma concentrations.

3. Epidural Analgesia

3.1. What analgesic (sensory and visceral) coverage does an epidural provide?

For patients undergoing a pancreaticoduodenectomy, visceral pain occurs with transection of the pancreas, proximal jejunum, stomach, and duodenum. Thus, an epidural has the benefit over abdominal wall blocks as it blocks both the sensory nerves of the abdomen and the sympathetic innervation of the viscera. Epidural catheters are placed approximately at the T8 to T9 interspace to provide adequate blockade.

3.2. What are the contraindications to epidural placement?

Localized infection, sepsis, coagulopathy, and patient refusal are all contraindications to epidural placement. The American Society of Regional Anesthesia publishes guidelines for the placement of regional anesthesia in patients on thromboprophylaxis. These guidelines are a resource when determining if a patient on antithrombotic therapy can be considered for epidural placement. In the patient with known liver cirrhosis, coagulopathy and a low platelet count are a possibility. Normal coagulation and platelet profiles are confirmed prior to epidural needle insertion. Likewise, normal coagulation is confirmed prior to epidural catheter removal.

3.3. How does a TAP block compare with an epidural in terms of postoperative pain control?

The current literature comparing TAP block and epidural analgesia for abdominal surgery is inconsistent. A relatively small number of studies have shown that the analgesia via TAP catheter is comparable to epidural analgesia when used as part of a multimodal analgesia regimen.

Although the TAP block does not reliably cover above the T10 dermatome, the addition of the subcostal approach in the 4-quadrant TAP block may provide additional benefits in analgesic coverage. The TAP block provides analgesia for somatic pain only and does not cover visceral pain. Therefore, the addition of intravenous opioids and adjuvants is often required to provide adequate pain relief after surgery. Compared with epidurals, patients receiving TAP blocks require more postoperative opioids.

The TAP block is a viable alternative to epidural analgesia for abdominal surgery. Compared with intravenous patient-controlled analgesia alone, TAP blocks have been shown to reduce the amount of opioids required; however, it is unclear whether it has a clinical impact in terms of lowering opioid side effects, such as nausea and vomiting, pruritis, or return of bowel function.

3.4. What are the advantages of a TAP block compared with an epidural?

While epidural analgesia has been considered the standard after abdominal surgery, the use of epidural analgesia requires 24-hour-a-day in-house availability of physicians to troubleshoot and assess the epidural. The in-house management of epidural analgesia alone highlights the infeasibility of this block in many cases. The TAP block may provide some advantages over epidural analgesia. In one study, TAP blocks were associated with less use of intraoperative vasopressors and fewer intraoperative blood pressure changes. In addition, the TAP block may be used when epidural analgesia is contraindicated, such as in cases of localized infection, the inability to position the patient for epidural, or in cases of coagulopathy. Another advantage is that the TAP block is not generally associated with lower-extremity weakness. However, there is a rare possibility of the local anesthetic from a TAP block tracking down the fascia iliaca, resulting in femoral nerve blockade.

3.5. In addition to epidural and TAP block, what other regional options are available for truncal block?

Portable ultrasound machines have revolutionized the practice of regional anesthesia, shifting it from landmark-based techniques to ultrasound-guided blocks. Rather than identifying the nerve plexus, a large amount of local anesthetic is deposited in a plane and spread to the intended nerves. Many of the new blocks are currently in the research phase, without clearly defined clinical applications.

Truncal blocks are divided into abdominal wall and chest wall blocks. In addition to epidurals and TAP blocks, other abdominal wall blocks include the rectus sheath, quadratus lumborum, and paravertebral blocks. Rectus sheath block coverage is limited to the midline and is useful for umbilical hernia repair. With the increasing use of ultrasound-guided TAP blocks, the rectus sheath block, which provides only midline abdominal analgesia and requires multiple injections, is less clinically popular. The quadratus lumborum block, considered a "posterior TAP block" with visceral pain coverage, has been used for nephrectomies. In a systematic review by El Boghdadly, paravertebral blocks for abdominal surgery resulted in less opioid use and improved early postoperative pain when compared with intravenous analgesia.

Further Reading

Barrington MJ, Ivanusic JJ, Rozen WM, Hebbard P. Spread of injectate after ultrasound-guided subcostal transversus abdominis plane block: a cadaveric study. *Anaesthesia*. 2009;64:745–750.

Bhatia N, Arora S, Jyotsna W, Kaur G. Comparison of posterior and subcostal approaches to ultrasound-guided transverse abdominis plane block for postoperative analgesia in laparoscopic cholecystectomy. *J Clin Anesth*. 2014;26:294–299.

Chakraborty A, Khemka R, Datta T. Ultrasound-guided truncal blocks: a new frontier in regional anesthesia. *Indian J Anaesth*. 2016;60:703–711.

Charlton S, Cyna AM, Middleton P, et al. Perioperative transversus abdominis plane (TAP) block for analgesia after abdominal surgery. *Cochrane Database Syst Rev*. 2010;CD007705.

El Boghdadly K, Madjdpour C, Chin KJ. Thoracic paravertebral blocks in abdominal surgery: a systematic review of randomized controlled trials. *Br J Anaesth.* 2016;117:297–308.

Furuya A, Ikemoto K, Asano N, et al. [Assessment of intraoperative hemodynamics, infusion volume, urinary output and dose of circulatory drugs in general anesthesia with transversus abdominis plane block for cholecystectomy]. *Masui.* 2013;62:1106–1111.

Ganapathy S, Sondekoppam R, Terlecki M, et al. Comparison of efficacy and safety of lateral-to-medial continuous transversus abdominis plane block with thoracic epidural analgesia in patients undergoing abdominal surgery. *Eur J Anaesthesiol.* 2015;32:797–804.

Griffiths JD, Barron FA, Grant S et al. Plasma ropivacaine concentrations after ultrasound-guided transversus abdominis plane block. *Br J Anaesth.* 2010;105:853–856.

Hessian EC, Evans BE, Woods JA et al. Plasma ropivacaine concentrations during bilateral transversus abdominis plane infusions. *Br J Anaesth.* 2013;111:488–495.

Horlocker TT, Wedel DJ, Rowlingson JC, et al. Regional anesthesia in the patient receiving antithrombotic or thrombolytic therapy: American Society of Regional Anesthesia and Pain Medicine Evidence-Based Guidelines (Third Edition). *Reg Anesth Pain Med.* 2010;35:64–101.

Lee TH, Barrington MJ, Tran TM, et al. Comparison of extent of sensory block following posterior and subcostal approaches to ultrasound-guided transversus abdominis plane block. *Anaesth Intensive Care.* 2010;38:452–460.

Lissauer J, Mancuso K, Merritt C, et al. Evolution of the transversus abdominis plane block and its role in postoperative analgesia. *Best Pract Res Clin Anaesthesiol.* 2014;28:117–126.

McDonnell J, O'Donnell B, Curley G, et al. The analgesic efficacy of transversus abdominis plane block after abdominal surgery: a prospective randomized controlled trial. *Anesth Analg.* 2007;104:193–197.

Mukherjee A, Guhabiswas R, Kshirsagar S, Rupert E. Ultrasound-guided oblique subcostal transversus abdominis plane block: an observational study on a new and promising analgesic technique. *Indian J Anaesth.* 2016;60:284–286.

Murouchi T, Yamauchi M, Gi E, et al. [Ultrasound-guided subcostal and mid-axillary transversus abdominis plane block: a cadaveric study of the spread of injectate]. *Masui.* 2013;62:60–63.

Niraj G, Kelkar A, Jeyapalan I, et al. Comparison of analgesic efficacy of subcostal transversus abdominis plane blocks with epidural analgesia following upper abdominal surgery. *Anaesthesia.* 2011;66:465–471.

Niraj G, Kelkar A, Hart E, et al. Comparison of analgesic efficacy of four-quadrant transversus abdominis plane (TAP) block and continuous posterior TAP analgesia with epidural analgesia in patients undergoing laparoscopic colorectal surgery: an open-label, randomized, non-inferiority trial. *Anaesthesia.* 2014;69:348–355.

Niraj G, Kelkar A, Hart E, et al. Four quadrant transversus abdominis plane block and continuous transversus abdominis plane analgesia: a 3-year prospective audit in 124 patients. *J Clin Anesth.* 2015;27:579–584.

Petersen PL, Mathiesen O, Torup H, et al. The transversus abdominis plane block: a valuable option for postoperative analgesia? A topical review. *Acta Anaesthesiol Scand.* 2010;54:529–535.

Rafi AN. Abdominal field block: a new approach via the lumbar triangle. *Anaesthesia.* 2001;56:1024–1026.

Rawal N. Epidural technique for postoperative pain: gold standard no more? *Reg Anesth Pain Med.* 2012;37:310–317.

Wildsmith JA. Continuous thoracic epidural block for surgery: gold standard or debased currency? *Br J Anaesth.* 2012;109:9–12.

Wu Y, Liu F, Tang H, et al. The analgesic efficacy of subcostal transversus abdominis plane block compared with thoracic epidural analgesia and intravenous opioid analgesia after radical gastrectomy. *Anesth Analg.* 2013;117:507–513.

Young MJ, Gorlin AW, Modest VE, Quraishi SA. Clinical implications of the transversus abdominis plane block in adults. *Anesthesiol Res Pract.* 2012;2012:731645.

Yu N, Long X, Lujan-Hernandez JR, et al. Transversus abdominis-plane block versus local anesthetic wound infiltration in lower abdominal surgery: a systematic review and meta-analysis of randomized controlled trials. *BMC Anesthesiol.* 2014;14:121.

4. Renal and Hepatic Considerations in Analgesia

4.1. What are the prevalence and risk factors for chronic kidney disease?

It is estimated that the prevalence of chronic kidney disease (CKD) in the American population is 13.1%, and it affects 10% to 16% of people worldwide. Common risk factors for CKD include hypertension, obesity, diabetes, peripheral vascular disease, smoking, autoimmune diseases, the use of nephrotoxins, and advanced age.

4.2. How is CKD diagnosed and classified?

The following tests are used in the diagnosis of CKD: complete blood count electrolytes, creatinine, glomerular filtration rate (GFR), albumin, urea, urine albumin:creatinine ratio, fasting lipids and glucose, urine microscopy and culture, renal ultrasound, and biopsy. Additional diagnostic tests are indicated when infectious or autoimmune-related causes are suspected.

Serum creatinine is used to calculate GFR; however, a number of factors may affect the creatinine value such as fluid overload, muscle mass, and diuretics. For example, in the elderly with reduced muscle mass and protein intake, the GFR is overestimated. Cystatin C is a low-molecular-weight protein and biomarker that may also be used to estimate GFR. Its level is not affected by changes in muscle mass. In the lower ranges of GFR, cystatin C in combination with creatinine may improve estimates of GFR when evaluating patients with CKD.

CKD is classified into stages 1 through 5 depending on GFR. Stage 1 is described as kidney damage with normal or increased GFR (≥90 mL/min). Stage 2 is described as kidney damage with mildly decreased GFR (60–89 mL/min). Moderate kidney damage with GFR in the range of 30 to 59 mL/min is categorized as stage 3 CKD. Severely decreased GFR (15–29 mL/min) is categorized as stage 4 CKD. Stage 5 is end-stage kidney disease, with GFR <15 mL/min, and requires dialysis.

4.3. How does chronic renal insufficiency affect the choice of medication used in pain management?

Most opioids are renally excreted, and dosing is based on GFR. In renally impaired patients, a lower drug dosage and longer intervals are required.

Morphine is not recommended in severe renal failure due to the accumulation of active metabolites. The liver metabolizes morphine to morphine-3-glucuronide (M3G), morphine-6-glucuronide (M6G), and normorphine. The metabolites are then excreted by the kidneys. The accumulation of M6G leads to narcosis, respiratory depression, and agitation. M3G accumulation is associated with hyperalgesia and seizures. Codeine is metabolized by the liver into morphine, M3G, and M6G and is not recommended in severe renal failure for the reasons listed earlier.

Hydromorphone, a morphine analog, is metabolized to hydromorphone-3-glucoronide (H3G) by the liver. Like M3G, H3G is also neurotoxic, and hydromorphone dosing should be adjusted with low GFR. Hydromorphone does not have a 6-glucuronide metabolite (which causes respiratory depression) and is considered safer than morphine in patients with renal insufficiency.

Meperidine should be avoided due to the accumulation of normeperidine in patients with impaired renal function. The accumulation of normeperidine increases the risk of seizures and respiratory depression. The regular use of meperidine is contraindicated in patients with renal failure.

Fentanyl is metabolized by the liver and displays a favorable safety profile in patients with CKD. Repeated dosing or continuous infusion may result in plasma accumulation, and caution is warranted.

A multimodal pain management approach using acetaminophen and gabapentinoids is preferable to decrease opioid requirements and opioid-related side effects. Neuraxial analgesia, peripheral nerve blocks, and local anesthetic surgical site infiltration are also good options for decreasing opioid requirements. However, patients on dialysis may have abnormal platelet counts and function, requiring careful consideration before neuraxial block placement. In addition, acidosis lowers the threshold of the central nervous system to local anesthetic toxicity, therefore necessitating a 25% dose reduction.

An important caveat about neuraxial blocks is that the resultant sympathectomy can worsen perioperative hypotension due to large fluid shifts, blood loss, and third spacing. The resulting pre-renal oliguric state may predispose patients with CKD to postoperative renal failure.

The use of acetaminophen is generally considered safe in patients with CKD.

Use of nonsteroidal anti-inflammatory drugs (NSAIDs) in patients with CKD requires careful consideration, as NSAIDs may worsen renal function due to the inhibition of prostaglandin biosynthesis. Prostaglandins are important mediators of the compensatory vasodilation of the glomerular afferent arterioles in response to hypovolemia and hypotension. NSAIDs should be limited to short-term use in patients with stage 1 or 2 CKD and should be avoided in patients with stage 3 or 4 CKD.

The selective COX-2 inhibitors, initially thought to be devoid of the renal side effects, may also cause worsening kidney function, as COX-2 metabolites may be involved in the maintenance of renal blood flow.

To prevent toxicity, gabapentinoid dosing should be lowered based on creatinine clearance.

Further Reading

Chou R, Gordon DB, de Leon-Casasola OA, et al. Management of postoperative pain: a clinical practice guideline from the American Pain Society, the American Society of Regional Anesthesia and Pain Medicine, and the American Society of Anesthesiologists' Committee on Regional Anesthesia, Executive Committee, and Administrative Council. *J Pain.* 2016;17:131–157.

Douglas C, Murtagh FEM, Chambers EJ, Howse M, Ellershaw J. Symptom management for the adult patient dying with advanced chronic kidney disease: a review of the literature and development of evidence-based guidelines by a United Kingdom Expert Consensus Group. *Palliat Med.* 2009;23:103–110.

Harris RC, Bryer MD. Update on cyclooxygenase-2 inhibitors. *Clin J Am Soc Nephrol.* 2006;1:236–245.

Kazancioglu R. Risk factors for chronic kidney disease: an update. *Kidney Int.* 2013;3:368–371.

Kohler M, Chiu F, Gelber KM, Webb CA, Weyker PD. Pain management in critically ill patients: a review of multimodal treatment options. *Pain Manag.* 2016;6:591–602.

Launay-Vacher V, Karie S, Fau JB, et al. Treatment of pain in patients with renal insufficiency: the World Health Organization three-step ladder adapted. *J Pain.* 2005;6:137–148.

Levey AS, Coresh J, Balk E, et al. National Kidney Foundation practice guidelines for chronic kidney disease: evaluation, classification, and stratification. *Ann Intern Med.* 2003;139:137–147.

Mazer M, Perrone J. Acetaminophen-induced nephrotoxicity: pathophysiology, clinical manifestations, and management. *J Med Toxicol.* 2008;4:2–6.

Meersch M, Schmidt C, Zarbock A. Patient with chronic renal failure undergoing surgery. *Curr Opin Anesthesiol.* 2016;29:413–420.

Parmar MS, Parmar KS. Management of acute and post-operative pain in chronic kidney disease. *F1000Res.* 2013;2:28.

Tawfic QA, Bellingham G. Postoperative pain management in patients with chronic kidney disease. *J Anaesthesiol Clin Pharmacol.* 2015;31:6–13.

Webster AC, Nagler EV, Morton RL, Masson P. Chronic kidney disease. *Lancet.* 2017;389:1238–1252.

4.4. How does liver cirrhosis impact postoperative pain management?

Pain management in patients with liver impairment is challenging, as the liver metabolizes most analgesic medications. Liver metabolism of drugs occurs via 3 mechanisms. The first mechanism is via the cytochrome P450 (CYP) enzymes. The

CYPP450 3A pathway is involved in the metabolism of approximately 50% of all drugs. While genetic polymorphisms can occur in both CYPP450 3A4 and 3A5 enzymes, both enzymes can compensate for the other in the metabolism of opioids. The CYPP450 2D6 pathway is also involved in the metabolism of a number of opioids. Defects in this enzyme may result in poor metabolism of opioids that have active metabolites. Hence, those with the poor metabolizer phenotypes of the CYPP450 2D6 enzyme can have poor analgesia despite taking routine doses of opioids. It is estimated that 10% of whites are poor metabolizers. The second mechanism is by conjugation to glucuronic acid, and the third mechanism is through biliary excretion. Cirrhosis alters the metabolism of analgesic medications. In addition, the patient's nutritional status and liver synthetic status need to be taken into consideration. Hypoalbuminemia results in less drug being bound and a higher concentration of active drugs.

Most patients with liver cirrhosis have renal impairment, although the serum creatinine level may be normal. This can be secondary to malnutrition, decreased muscle mass, and lower creatinine production. Adjustments, such as lower dosing and less frequent administration, are necessary.

Due to the lack of understanding of acetaminophen liver metabolism, many clinicians are reluctant to prescribe acetaminophen to patients with liver cirrhosis for fear of causing acute liver decompensation, hepatic encephalopathy, or hepatorenal syndrome. Several studies, however, have demonstrated the safety of acetaminophen in reduced dosing in patients with liver cirrhosis. The Food and Drug Administration and hepatologists recommend limiting the maximum dose to 2 to 3 g daily. Medical professionals and patients should be aware that acetaminophen-containing analgesics such as hydrocodone/acetaminophen or oxycodone/acetaminophen are frequently prescribed, and it is crucial to stay within the total maximum allowable daily dose of acetaminophen.

Nonselective NSAIDs block both cyclooxygenase isoforms, COX-1 and COX-2. Prostaglandins play a role in protecting the gastric mucosa. COX-1 inhibition leads to lower prostaglandin production and therefore should be avoided due to the risks of gastrointestinal bleeds in liver patients with thrombocytopenia and coagulopathy.

Selective COX-2 inhibitors have a better safety profile in terms of gastrointestinal ulcer bleeding. Strategies to lower NSAID-associated gastric ulcer bleeding risks include the eradication of *Helicobacter pylori* in infected patients and the concomitant use of proton pump inhibitors and histamine-2 receptor antagonists. All NSAIDs, with the possible exception of naproxen, are associated with increased cardiovascular thromboembolic risks, including myocardial infarction and stroke, thereby limiting their usefulness.

Gabapentin and pregabalin are excellent choices for neuropathic pain as they do not undergo hepatic metabolism and are well tolerated in patients with cirrhosis. Decreased dosing is required with renal insufficiency. The use of these drugs may be limited by their side effect profile, which includes sedation and dizziness.

All opioids need dose adjustment in patients with liver impairment. Opioids should be prescribed with laxatives to avoid constipation and encephalopathy. Opioids are metabolized via the CYP450 enzymes and are affected by liver disease. Immediate-release forms should be used rather than controlled release as their half-life is already increased. Fentanyl and methadone require lower dosing in patients with hypoalbuminemia. Demerol and morphine are best avoided as both are dependent on liver metabolism and both have central nervous system–toxic metabolites that accumulate in the setting of renal insufficiency.

Serum drug levels are affected not only by liver disease but also by genetics; therefore, an understanding of the hepatic cytochrome P450 polymorphism and its clinical significance is crucial. The CYP superfamily consists of 57 genes. Enzymes in the CYP 1, 2, and 3 families are involved in the metabolism of therapeutic drugs such as antiemetics, antihistamines, antipsychotics, centrally acting cholinesterase inhibitors, and opioids.

Codeine, for example, is a prodrug that is metabolized to morphine by CYP2D6 and norcodeine by CYP3A4. Polymorphisms and mutations of these genes explain the differences in analgesic efficacy and drug toxicity. It is estimated that up to 10% of Caucasians have 2 nonfunctional CYP2D6 alleles and are poor metabolizers. Between 1% and 7% of Caucasians are ultrarapid metabolizers due to the amplification or duplication of the CYP2D6 genes. Ultrarapid metabolizers may have life-threatening side effects from standard doses of codeine.

Further Reading

Chandok N, Watt KD. Pain management in the cirrhotic patient: the clinical challenge. *Mayo Clin Proc.* 2010;85:451–448.

Cregg R, Russo G, Gubbay A, Branford R, Sato H. Pharmacogenetics of analgesic drugs. *Br J Pain.* 2013;7:189–208.

Gasche Y, Daali Y, Fathi M, et al. Codeine intoxication associated with ultrarapid CYP2D6 metabolism. *N Engl J Med.* 2004;351:2827–2831.

Imani F, Motavaf M, Safari S, et al. The therapeutic use of analgesics in patients with liver cirrhosis: a literature review and evidence-based recommendations. *Hepat Mon.* 2014;14:e23539.

Lanza FL, Chan FKL, Quickley EMM, et al. Guidelines for prevention of NSAIDs-related ulcer complications. *Am J Gastroenterol.* 2009;104:728–738.

Lee YC, Chang CH, Lin JW, et al. Non-steroidal anti-inflammatory drugs use and risk of upper gastrointestinal adverse events in cirrhotic patients. *Liver Int.* 2012;32:859–866.

Rostom A, Muir K, Dube C, et al. Gastrointestinal safety of cyclooxygenase-2 inhibitors: a Cochrane collaboration systematic review. *Clin Gastroenterol Hepatol.* 2007;5:818–828.

Saab S, Konyn PG, Viramontes MR, et al. Limited knowledge of acetaminophen in patients with liver disease. *J Clin Transl Hepatol.* 2016;4:281–287.

Zhou SF, Liu JP, Chowbay B. Polymorphism of human cytochrome P450 enzymes and its clinical impact. *Drug Metab Rev.* 2009;41:89–295.

5. Systems-Level Considerations for Analgesia

5.1. What is step-down analgesia?

The World Health Organization published cancer pain relief guidelines in 1986, with updates in 1996. It devised a ladder comprising 3 analgesic steps. Nonnarcotics, which form the basis of the first step, are used to treat mild pain. Weak narcotics are used in the second step for moderate pain management. Step 3 includes strong narcotics to treat severe pain. Adjuvant drugs are recommended with all 3 steps.

Adjuvant drugs, which include corticosteroids, antidepressants, and anticonvulsants, are used to treat nausea, anxiety, insomnia, and neuropathic pain.

The ladder may be used in both directions. If the pain is poorly controlled, one can ascend to the next step. Likewise, once the pain is controlled, stepping down the ladder to the lower step is recommended.

The WHO ladder serves as a simple guideline for physicians worldwide and has legitimized the use of opioids for relief of cancer pain. Critics cite several weaknesses of the WHO ladder, including the emphasis on pain intensity without consideration for function, and the omission of preemptive pain management strategies. A fourth step has been suggested to include interventional pain management procedures such as epidural steroid injections, medullary and peripheral nerve stimulators, and neurolytic blocks. Furthermore, updates are needed to include newer drug formulations and methods of administrations that were unavailable 20 years ago.

Pain control after pancreatic surgery is important in the prevention of postoperative complications. Adequate pain control is necessary for patients to participate in respiratory exercises such as incentive spirometry, cough, and deep breathing and for the ability to ambulate. Postoperatively, once a patient is able to tolerate an oral diet, he or she is transitioned off of the epidural analgesia and/or intravenous medications and given oral analgesic medications per the WHO ladder. The use of enhanced recovery protocols for pancreatic surgery may also decrease opioid use while improving patient outcomes.

Further References

Dobosz T, Kaczor M, Stefaniak T. Pain in pancreatic cancer: review of medical and surgical remedies. *ANZ J Surg.* 2016;86:756–761.

do Nascimento Junior P, Modolo NS, Andrade S, et al. Incentive spirometry for prevention of postoperative pulmonary complications in upper abdominal surgery. *Cochrane Database Syst Rev.* 2014;CD006058.

Kagedan DJ, Ahmed M, Devitt KS, Wei AC. Enhanced recovery after pancreatic surgery: a systematic review of the evidence. *HPB (Oxford)*. 2015;17:11–16.

Miguel R. Interventional treatment of cancer pain: the fourth step in the World Health Organization analgesic ladder? *Cancer Control*. 2000;7:149–156.

Vargas-Schaffer G. Is the WHO analgesic ladder still valid? *Can Fam Physician*. 2010;56:514–517.

World Health Organization. Cancer pain relief. http://apps.who.int/iris/bitstream/handle/10665/37896/9241544821.pdf?sequence=1&isAllowed=y. Accessed June 15, 2018.

11

Breast Surgery

Richa Wardhan and Roy Greengrass

Case Scenario

A 45-year-old woman with a recent diagnosis of breast adenocarcinoma but no other significant past medical history presents for left mastectomy. Surgical history includes laparoscopic cholecystectomy complicated by intractable nausea and vomiting. The Patient is interested in utilizing regional anesthesia for the surgery to avoid nausea and vomiting and general anesthesia. The patient presents to the pre-preoperative area and is interested in knowing more about various regional anesthesia techniques and options.

1. Anatomic Considerations to Analgesia for Breast Surgery

1.1. What innervates the breast and the pectoral muscles?

Thoracic intercostal nerves T3-T6 primarily innervate the breast. Most complete mastectomies involve resection into the axilla, and many are associated with sentinel node biopsy and possible axillary dissection. Blockade ofT1-T2 nerves, which innervate the axilla, is therefore often required in addition to the previously mentioned intercostal nerves.

The pectoral muscle is innervated by the lateral pectoral nerve (C5-C7) and medial pectoral nerve (C8-T1), both of which arise from the brachial plexus. The lateral pectoral nerve supplies the pectoralis major (PMm) and runs between it and the pectoralis minor (Pmm) close to the pectoral branch of the thoracoacromial artery. The medial pectoral nerve runs under the PMm. It crosses the muscle and pierces the clavipectoral fascia to reach the lower third of the PMm muscle.

The thoracodorsal and the long thoracic nerves also supply the axillary area. The thoracodorsal nerve supplies the latissimus dorsi muscle. The long thoracic nerve supplies the serratus anterior muscle. Both are important nerves, as the serratus is often dissected along with both pectoralis muscles to make a pocket for breast expanders, whereas the thoracodorsal nerve is important when the latissimus dorsi flap is used for reconstruction.

Further Reading

Blanco R, Fajardo M, Parras Maldonado T. Ultrasound description of Pecs II (modified Pecs I): a novel approach to breast surgery. *Rev Esp Anestesiol Reanim.* 2012;59:470–475.

2. Regional Anesthetic Techniques for Breast Surgery

2.1. What techniques are available to provide anesthesia and postoperative analgesia for mastectomy reconstruction and implants?

The following regional nerve block procedures can be utilized for achieving surgical anesthesia and postoperative pain management.

1. Thoracic epidural block
2. Thoracic paravertebral block
3. Interfascial plane blocks, namely, Pecs I and II, serratus anterior plane blocks

Thoracic epidural block and paravertebral block (PVB) are frequently used for bilateral mastectomy and immediate reconstruction. The use of thoracic epidural for surgery involving the pectoralis muscles would require a level of C5, which would result in hypotension and bradycardia in many patients due to bilateral block of the cardioacceleratory fibers (T1-T4). Thus, a lower-level epidural is usually combined with general anesthesia when surgery involving the pectoralis muscles is required.

Bilateral mastectomy usually involves mastectomy with sentinel node biopsy and possible axillary dissection on the cancer side with prophylactic mastectomy on the noncancer side. Thus PVB from T1 to T6 is performed on the cancer side and from T3 to T6 on the prophylactic side. When reconstruction and insertion of implants is considered, a bilateral pectoral nerve (PEC) block is also performed.

Ultrasound-guided PEC 1 and 2 blocks were first described by Blanco et al. in 2011. PEC block is an interfascial plane block in which local anesthetic is deposited between the PMm and the Pmm (PEC I block) or above the serratus anterior muscle at the third rib (PEC II block). This innovative technique is an effort to block the pectoral, intercostobrachial, intercostal 3–6, and long thoracic nerves.

In addition to the PEC block, serratus anterior plane (SAP) block, as described by Blanco et al. in 2013, aims to block the intercostal nerves and to provide analgesia of the lateral part of the thorax. This may be a viable alternative to paravertebral nerve blockade and thoracic epidural analgesia in this patient population. SAP block involves depositing local anesthetic between serratus anterior and latissimus dorsi muscles in the midaxillary line.

Further Reading

Bashandy GM, Abbas DN. Pectoral nerves I and II blocks in multimodal analgesia for breast cancer surgery: a randomized clinical trial. *Reg Anesth Pain Med.* 2015;40:68–74.

Blanco R. The "pecs block": a novel technique for providing analgesia after breast surgery. *Anaesthesia.* 2011;66:847–848.

Blanco R, Fajardo M, Parras Maldonado T. Ultrasound description of Pecs II (modified Pecs I): a novel approach to breast surgery. *Rev Esp Anestesiol Reanim.* 2012;59:470–475.

Blanco R, Parras T, McDonnell JG, Prats-Galino A. Serratus plane block: a novel ultrasound-guided thoracic wall nerve block. *Anaesthesia.* 2013;68:1107–1113.

Zocca JA, Chen GH, Puttanniah VG, Hung JC, Gulati A. Ultrasound-guided serratus plane block for treatment of postmastectomy pain syndromes in breast cancer patients: a case series. *Pain Pract.* 2017;17:141–146.

2.2. What is a paravertebral block, and how do you perform it?

A PVB is a block of the mixed nerve root that is performed near the location at which the nerve root exits the intervertebral foramen. The paravertebral space that contains the nerve is a triangular space bounded superiorly by the superior costotransverse ligament, anterolaterally by the pleura, and medially by the central neuraxial skeleton. Local anesthetic placed into the paravertebral space produces a profound somatic and sympathetic block. Increased volume of local anesthetic leads to segmental spread along the paravertebral space, but this is unpredictable.

To perform a PVB, the spinous processes of the appropriate dermatomes in the surgical field are located and marked. A mark is made from the midpoint of the spinous process 2.5 cm laterally. From this mark the needle is inserted at a perpendicular angle to contact the transverse process. The needle is then reinserted to walk off the transverse process 1 to 1.5 cm caudally to pierce the superior costotransverse ligament, after which local anesthetic is incrementally injected. Subsequent levels are similarly blocked.

Further Reading

Greengrass R, Buckenmaier CC III. Paravertebral anaesthesia/analgesia for ambulatory surgery. *Best Pract Res Clin Anaesthesiol.* 2002;16:271–283.

Greengrass RA, Duclas R, Paravertebral blocks. *Int Anesthesiol Clin.* 2012; 50:56–73.

2.3. What are pectoralis serratus anterior plane blocks, and how do you perform them?

A PEC block is a block between the PMm and Pmm muscles where the lateral and medial pectoral nerves are located. To perform a PEC block, the same image acquired for performance of an infraclavicular block is obtained. A needle is then inserted from the lateral part of the probe perpendicular and slightly medial to lie between the PMm and Pmm fascia, after which local anesthetic is incrementally injected.

To perform a SAP block, patients are placed in the lateral decubitus position with the affected side facing up, or in the prone position with the affected side facing the operator. After sterile preparation, a linear ultrasound probe is utilized to identify the latissimus dorsi and serratus anterior muscles in a sagittal plane. The plane superficial to the serratus anterior muscle and below the latissimus dorsi muscle is identified. Using an in-plane or out-of-plane approach, a 25-gauge 1.5-cm needle is used to inject local anesthetic under direct ultrasound visualization.

Although PVBs and PEC/SAP blocks can be used as primary anesthetic for bilateral mastectomies and reconstruction, the patient usually requires supplemental anesthesia because of the prolonged surgical time.

Further Reading

Blanco R. The "pecs block": a novel technique for providing analgesia after breast surgery. *Anaesthesia.* 2011;66:847–848.

Zocca JA, Chen GH, Puttanniah VG, Hung JC, Gulati A. Ultrasound-guided serratus plane block for treatment of postmastectomy pain syndromes in breast cancer patients: a case series. *Pain Pract.* 2017;17:141–146.

Table 11.1:
Risks and benefits of PEC/SAP blocks and PBVs

PVB	PEC/SAP
Insertion site completely removed from the surgical site	Close to the surgical site
No risk of cross-infection	Possible risk of cross-infection
Can leave a continuous nerve catheter inserted	Can leave a catheter inserted, however cumbersome
May not cover serratus and latissimus muscle spasms well	Covers muscle spasms well
High skill level required to place the block	Relatively easier to place the block
Can be performed using landmark approach	Ultrasound preferred
Risk of pneumothorax	Fewer side effects

Case Scenario

The patient needs help in deciding between paravertebral blocks and interfascial plane blocks. She would like more information on the advantages and disadvantages of both.

2.4. How do you choose between pectoralis nerve/serratus anterior plane blocks and paravertebral blocks?

Both techniques have advantages and disadvantages. Many of the particulars may relate to localized practice patterns and, more important, patient preferences following review of relevant risks and benefits of each option. Table 11.1 describes some of these risks and benefits.

2.5. What are the advantages of paravertebral block in this patient population?

Patients undergoing mastectomy are at high risk for postoperative nausea and vomiting. Studies have demonstrated a significant reduction in nausea and vomiting when PVB is the primary anesthetic. Similarly, PVB has been determined to significantly reduce pain. PVB with multimodal anesthesia can eliminate the need for opioids. This effect continues into the postoperative period, where it is demonstrated that paravertebral infusions are unnecessary for further pain reduction. PVB has been demonstrated to significantly decrease chronic postmastectomy pain 1 year after surgery. This effect may be due in part to the profound effect of PVB on acute pain. Significant acute pain has been associated with an increased incidence of chronic pain.

Further Reading

Buckenmaier CC III, Kwon KH, Howard RS, et al. Double-blinded, placebo-controlled, prospective randomized trial evaluating the efficacy of paravertebral block with and without continuous paravertebral block analgesia in outpatient breast cancer surgery. *Pain Med.* 2010;11:790–799.

Coveney E, Weltz CR, Greengrass R, et al. Use of paravertebral block anesthesia in the surgical management of breast cancer: experience in 156 cases. *Ann Surg.* 1998;227:496–501.

Kairaluoma PM, Bachmann MS, Rosenberg PH, Pere PJ. Preincisional paravertebral block reduces the prevalence of chronic pain after breast surgery. *Anesth Analg.* 2006;103:703–708.

> **Case Scenario**
>
> The patient's surgery proceeds as planned under left-sided paravertebral blocks. She is now recovering. Do any of the previously mentioned techniques affect cancer metastasis and survival?

3. Analgesia and Cancer Mechanisms

3.1. Can paravertebral block impact cancer metastasis and survival?

There is a heightened interest in the association between choice of anesthetic technique and cancer survival and spread of metastasis. Some retrospective trials have shown regional anesthesia like PVBs to decrease rates of cancer recurrence and metastasis compared with general anesthesia. However, establishing a causal relationship is difficult due to the retrospective nature of these studies. Nevertheless, this topic has intrigued researchers, as several laboratory studies have shown the benefit of local anesthetic on cancer cells. Blood samples from patients who received propofol/paravertebral anesthesia showed inhibited cellular proliferation compared with a sevoflurane/opioid group. High cellular proliferation rate is associated with worse prognosis in untreated patients. Both volatile anesthetics and opioids have been associated with decreased cancer survival rates. Stimulation of mu opioid receptors has been demonstrated to promote metastatic spread in various tumor models.

It remains conjectural whether the salutary effects of PVBs on decreasing metastasis and enhancing survival are caused by a specific benefit of the block and local anesthetic or by avoidance of the known deleterious effects of volatile agents and opioids.

Further Reading

Colozza M, Azambuja E, Cardoso F, Sotiriou C, Larsimont D, Piccart MJ. Proliferative markers as prognostic and predictive tools in early breast cancer: where are we now? *Ann Oncol.* 2005;16:1723–1739.

Exadaktylos AK, Buggy DJ, Moriarty DC, Mascha E, Sessler DI. Can anesthetic technique for primary breast cancer surgery affect recurrence or metastasis? *Anesthesiology.* 2006;105:660–664.

Lennon FE, Mirzapoiazova T, Mambetsariev B, Salgia R, Moss J, Singleton PA. Overexpression of the mu-opioid receptor in human non-small cell lung cancer promotes Akt and mTOR activation, tumor growth, and metastasis. *Anesthesiology.* 2012;116:857–867.

Wigmore TJ, Mohammed K, Jhanji S. Long-term survival for patients undergoing volatile versus IV anesthesia for cancer surgery: a retrospective analysis. *Anesthesiology.* 2016;124:69–79.

Xuan W, Hankin J, Zhao H, Yao S, Ma D. The potential benefits of the use of regional anesthesia in cancer patients. *Int J Cancer.* 2015;137:2774–2784.

Colorectal Surgery

Aaron Persinger and Jeffrey Gonzales

12

Case Scenario

A 55-year-old woman presents for a laparoscopic colectomy. She recently was diagnosed with adenocarcinoma following a routine screening colonoscopy. She has a history of obesity and poorly controlled diabetes (insulin dependent) with concurrent gastroparesis and peripheral neuropathy.

1. Overview of Enhanced Recovery After Surgery

1.1. Summarize the history of enhanced recovery principles in colorectal surgery, discussing how and why they were developed

Enhanced recovery protocols (such as enhanced recovery after surgery [ERAS]) are a multifaceted, protocolized attempt to reduce the surgical stress response in each organ system in an effort to speed up recovery and improve outcomes after major surgery. The development of modern-day enhanced recovery protocols dates back more than 25 years, when Henrik Kehlet and colleagues first proposed that the body's "stress response" to surgical trauma has several downstream effects that have a negative impact on a patient's recovery in the postoperative phase. At that time, the average length of stay (LOS) in the hospital after open colorectal surgery was 8 to 10 days. Reasons for this recovery time included pain, delayed mobility, fatigue, decreased functional status, postoperative nausea and vomiting (PONV), paralytic ileus, infections, thromboembolism, and central nervous system, pulmonary, and cardiac complications. Kehlet et al. posited that the majority of these adverse outcomes were due to organ system dysfunction from the surgical stress response. He and other investigators began to develop perioperative protocols to reduce this stress and hasten recovery. In 1995, Liu and colleagues used epidural analgesia in the context of a multimodal recovery program, which resulted in the earlier return of bowel function and patients meeting discharge criteria 1.5 days earlier. The same year, Bardram et al. attempted to provide "stress-free" anesthesia for 8 patients undergoing colon resection. They used a combination of a laparoscopic approach, epidural analgesia, early oral intake, and early mobilization. They were able to reduce hospital stay to 2 days, with less nausea, ileus, and impairment in functional capacity. Moiniche et al. similarly demonstrated faster recovery with earlier feeding and mobilization, which was facilitated by balanced (epidural) analgesia. Earlier oral intake appeared to reduce morbidity, without a negative impact on colonic anastomoses. On the basis of these and similar studies, perioperative protocols continued to develop, with additional interventions such as preoperative education and counseling, alcohol and tobacco cessation, PONV prophylaxis, antimicrobial prophylaxis, and a more minimally invasive surgical approach. Early in the first decade of the 2000s, Fearon and Ljungqvist assembled the ERAS study group to build upon the foundations set by Kehlet in the 1990s. This group eventually grew into the ERAS Society, which published its first consensus guidelines in 2005, with subsequent updates in 2009 and 2012.

Further Reading

Bardram L, Funch-Jensen P, Jensen P, Crawford ME, Kehlet H. Recovery after laparoscopic colonic surgery with epidural analgesia, and early oral nutrition and mobilisation. *Lancet*. 1995;345:763–764.

Christensen T, Kehlet H. Postoperative fatigue. *World J Surg*. 1993;17:220–225.

ERAS Society. ERAS Society history. http://erassociety.org/about/history/. Accessed May 22, 2017.

Kehlet H. The surgical stress response: should it be prevented? *Can J Surg*. 1991;34:565–567.

Kehlet H. Multimodal approach to control postoperative pathophysiology and rehabilitation. *Br J Anaesth*. 1997;78:606–617.

Liu S, Carpenter RL, Neal JM. Epidural anesthesia and analgesia: their role in postoperative outcome. *Anesthesiology*. 1995;82:1474–1506.

Ljungqvist O, Scott M, Fearon KC. Enhanced Recovery After Surgery: A Review. *JAMA Surg*. 2017;152(3):292–298. doi:10.1001/jamasurg.2016.4952

Moiniche S, Bulow S, Hesselfeldt P, Hestbaek A, Kehlet H. Convalescence and hospital stay after colonic surgery with balanced analgesia, early oral feeding, and enforced mobilisation. *Eur J Surgery*. 1995;161:283–288.

1.2. Describe the components of enhanced recovery practice for patients undergoing abdominal surgery

Modern enhanced recovery protocols can be divided into preoperative, intraoperative, and postoperative phases, each with several evidence-based interventions. The following suggestions for interventions at each perioperative stage are summarized from the most recent ERAS guidelines, authored by Gustaffson et al.

The preoperative phase consists of preoperative physical conditioning ("prehab"), preoperative education and counseling, alcohol cessation, smoking cessation, avoidance of bowel preparation, correction of anemia, allowance of a clear-liquid carbohydrate drink, premedication, and venous thromboembolism (VTE) prophylaxis. The ERAS Society suggests there may be some benefit to preoperative optimization with dedicated education and counseling in addition to alcohol and smoking cessation. There was not enough evidence at the time of the most recent ERAS Society guidelines to recommend prehabilitation. It was found, however, that routine mechanical bowel preparation before surgery should be avoided. Clear fluids may be allowed up to 2 hours, and solids allowed up to 6 hours, prior to the induction of anesthesia, with some consideration given to a preoperative oral carbohydrate drink. Long-acting premedications are best avoided, and short-acting premedications used only when necessary to avoid a delay in immediate postoperative recovery. For VTE prophylaxis, compression stockings, pneumatic compression devices, and pharmacologic prophylaxis with low-molecular-weight-heparin are recommended.

For the intraoperative phase, antibiotic prophylaxis should be given 30 to 60 minutes prior to incision and should be redosed, if necessary, based on half-life. For maintenance of anesthesia, a technique that allows for control of fluid therapy, analgesia, hemodynamics, and blunting of the surgical stress response, while still allowing for a rapid wake-up, should be chosen. For open surgeries, a thoracic epidural is considered a gold standard for analgesia. For laparoscopic procedures, epidural analgesia may still be considered; however, intrathecal morphine, truncal blocks such as transverse abdominis plane (TAP), rectus sheath, or quadratus lumborum also work well, as could intravenous patient-controlled analgesia (PCA). In addition to this, multimodal PONV prophylaxis should be employed for any patients with more than 2 risk factors. Completing procedures laparoscopically, if the expertise is available, does shorten hospital stay. Nasogastric tubes inserted during surgery should be removed before emergence from anesthesia, if possible. A concerted effort to achieve normothermia (36–37°C) should be pursued as well. Routine bladder drainage with bladder catheterization is acceptable in abdominal surgeries, provided there are attempts to discontinue it as soon as possible postoperatively.

Several recommendations can also be made for patients postoperatively. Paralytic ileus appears to be best prevented by utilization of thoracic epidural analgesia (TEA) for open surgeries and a laparoscopic approach when possible. Opioids should be minimized with a multimodal approach to pain management, fluid overload and unnecessary or prolonged gastric drainage should be avoided, and chewing gum can be recommended post-operatively. Foley catheters should be discontinued on postoperative day 1 or 2 whenever possible. Nutritional support should be continued in the postoperative period, with avoidance of hyperglycemia. Although evidence directly supporting early mobilization is somewhat lacking, it is well established that prolonged immobilization increases the risk of pneumonia, VTE, insulin resistance, and muscle weakness and atrophy.

Further Reading

Gustafsson UO, Scott MJ, Schwenk W, et al. Guidelines for perioperative care in elective colonic surgery: Enhanced Recovery After Surgery (ERAS®) Society recommendations. *World J Surg*. 2013;37:259–284.

Kehlet H. Multimodal approach to control postoperative pathophysiology and rehabilitation. *Br J Anaesth*. 1997;78:606–617.

1.3. What patient factors are present in this case that will need to be addressed perioperatively?

This patient has multiple comorbidities that may affect her intraoperative course, recovery, and outcome. As summarized by Samuels and Yao, obesity and its associated conditions increase morbidity with anesthesia and surgery. In these patients, there is an increased incidence of difficult mask ventilation, as well as difficult intubation. Because of reduced functional residual capacity and increased oxygen consumption, they are susceptible to rapid oxygen desaturation. Lung compliance is reduced, and airway resistance may be increased. Severe obesity is a significant risk factor for obstructive sleep apnea. Up to 70% of people presenting for bariatric surgery carry this diagnosis. Anesthesia concerns for this population include a decreased apneic threshold to analgesics, hypnotics, and volatile agents, prolonged emergence, resedation after anesthesia, V/Q mismatch, restrictive and/or obstructive lung disease, pulmonary hypertension, and right heart failure. From a cardiovascular standpoint, autonomic tone can be altered from chronic hypoxia, predisposing patients to bradycardia and arrhythmias during periods of hypoxia. Additionally, myocardial function can be decreased in the case of obesity-related cardiomyopathy. Hypertension is of course common in this population. Aspiration precautions may need to be taken due to increased gastric volume, decreased gastric pH, increased incidence of gastroesophageal reflux disease and hiatal hernia, abnormal lower esophageal sphincter function, and increased intra-abdominal pressure. Hepatic steatosis may be found in up 75% of morbidly obese patients. There is an increase in infection risk and also several types of cancers associated with obesity as well. The volume of distribution and metabolism of drugs would also likely be abnormal in this patient.

Poorly controlled diabetes will make careful perioperative management of this patient's glucose level challenging. It is known that the stress response associated with surgery induces a state of insulin resistance; the degree of insulin resistance correlates with the severity of the injury. Elevated glucose levels intra- and postoperatively are associated with increased morbidity and mortality. Indeed, patients with elevated preoperative hemoglobin A1C levels have an increased complication rate, and reductions in A1C appear to reduce that complication rate. This would suggest that having this patient preoperatively address her glycemic control would confer postoperative benefits. Additionally, many enhanced recovery interventions reduce surgical stress and therefore could lead to better glycemic control.

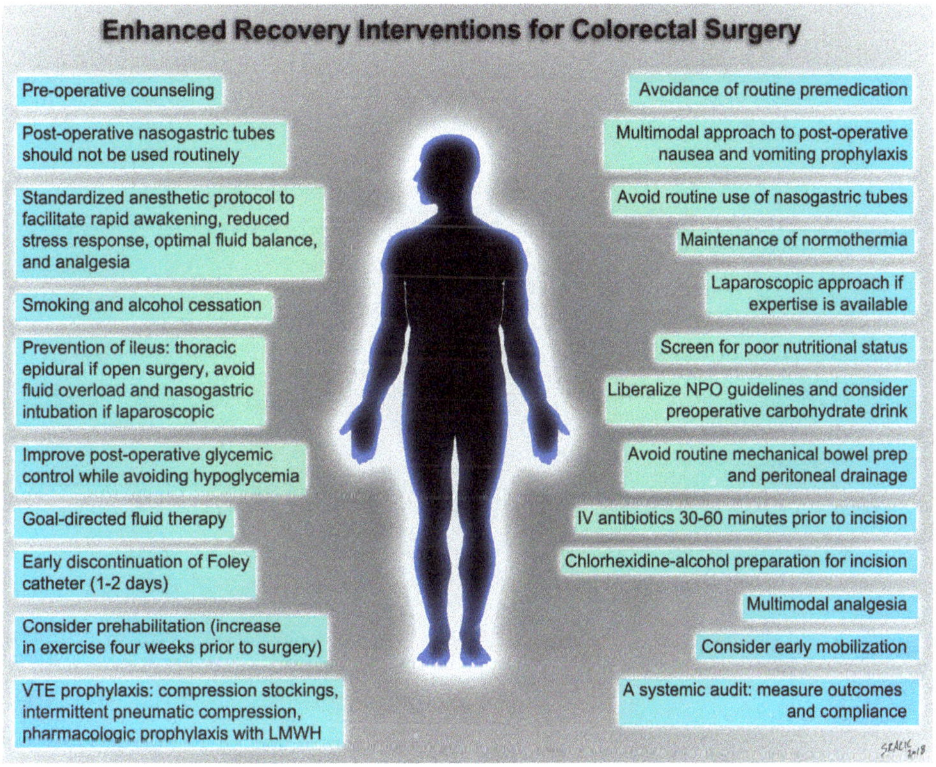

Figure 12.1 Essential interventions in enhanced recovery programs for colorectal surgery.

Finally, the effect of this patient's presenting diagnosis of colon adenocarcinoma should not be overlooked. The incidence of deep vein thrombosis in patients presenting for colorectal surgery without prophylaxis is approximately 30%, with the incidence of fatal pulmonary embolism being as high as 1%. This patient should receive well-fitting compression stockings, pneumatic compression devices, and VTE prophylaxis with low-molecular-weight heparin or unfractionated heparin. In addition to this, her nutrition status should be assessed, as well as her gastrointestinal function. Signs and symptoms suggestive of decreased bowel motility or bowel obstruction may necessitate rapid sequence induction of anesthesia. Some degree of liver dysfunction from hepatic steatosis may also be present.

Further Reading

Blixt C, Ahlstedt C, Ljungqvist O, Isaksson B, Kalman S, Rooyackers O. The effect of perioperative glucose control on postoperative insulin resistance. *Clin Nutr.* 2012;31:676–681.

Endara M, Masden D, Goldstein J, Gondek S, Steinberg J, Attinger C. The role of chronic and perioperative glucose management in high-risk surgical closures: a case for tighter glycemic control. *Plastic Reconstr Surg.* 2013;132:996–1004.

Gustafsson UO, Scott MJ, Schwenk W, et al. Guidelines for perioperative care in elective colonic surgery: Enhanced Recovery After Surgery (ERAS®) Society recommendations. *World J Surg.* 2013;37:259–284.

Krinsley JS. Effect of an intensive glucose management protocol on the mortality of critically ill adult patients. *Mayo Clin Proc.* 2004;79:992–1000.

Lazar HL, McDonnell M, Chipkin SR, et al. The Society of Thoracic Surgeons practice guideline series: blood glucose management during adult cardiac surgery. *Ann Thorac Surg.* 2009;87:663–669.

Ljungqvist O. Insulin resistance and outcomes in surgery. *J Clin Endocrinol Metab.* 2010;95:4217–4219.

Samuels J, Yao FSF. Morbid obesity and obstructive sleep apnea. In: FSF Y, ed. *Yao & Artusio's Problem-Oriented Patient Management.* 7th ed. Philadelphia, PA: Lippincott Williams & Wilkins; 2012.

Sato H, Carvalho G, Sato T, Lattermann R, Matsukawa T, Schricker T. The association of preoperative glycemic control, intraoperative insulin sensitivity, and outcomes after cardiac surgery. *J Clin Endocrinol Metabol.* 2010;95:4338–4344.

Thorell A, Nygren J, Ljungqvist O. Insulin resistance: a marker of surgical stress. *Curr Opin Clin Nutr Metab Care.* 1999;2:69–78.

Van den Berghe G, Schetz M, Vlasselaers D, et al. Clinical review: intensive insulin therapy in critically ill patients: NICE-SUGAR or Leuven blood glucose target? *J Clin Endocrinol Metab.* 2009;94:3163–3170.

1.4. What part might preoperative analgesia management play in optimizing recovery?

Given that many patients today still do not receive any specific analgesic intervention prior to entering the operating room, it is interesting to remind ourselves that the first physician to observe that a preoperative analgesic intervention may have postoperative pain benefit wrote about this phenomenon in the *Lancet* in 1913. Woolf and Wall then conducted work in the 1980s and 1990s that led to the term *preemptive analgesia.* They suggested that giving opioids and/or a local anesthetic before surgical incision would reduce the development of spinal hyperexcitability and "pain behaviours." These abnormalities in the pain-signaling cascade may be driven by peripheral and central sensitization of neurons caused by the noxious stimulation of surgical trauma. Because of these observations, there have been many trials examining the potential benefit of preemptive analgesia. The oral analgesics that have been considered and studied are acetaminophen, nonsteroidal anti-inflammatory drugs (NSAIDs), and gabapentinoids. N-methyl-D-aspartate (NMDA) antagonists, local anesthetics, and epidural analgesia have been studied as well. Unfortunately, a great deal of controversy surrounds these clinical studies, yielding mixed results.

With regard to preoperative acetaminophen, a 2013 randomized controlled trial (RCT) showed that a 15-mg/kg dose of intravenous acetaminophen given 30 minutes before surgery reduced pain scores from a verbal rating scale of 4.48 to 2.72 (p = .001) 6 hours postoperatively, and reduced meperidine consumption from an average of 42 to 23 mg (p = .003). Doleman et al. also conducted a meta-analysis including 544 patients that showed a reduction in pain scores at 1 and 2 hours postoperatively, lower opioid consumption, and less PONV in patients who had received preoperative acetaminophen. Similar results have also been seen with NSAIDs. Although both cyclooxygenase (COX) isoforms COX1 and COX2 can be inhibited by this class of medications, COX2 inhibitors have been more recently used to limit gastrointestinal side effects. Clinical trials of COX2 inhibitors used for 2 weeks perioperatively in patients undergoing both minimally invasive and major surgery have demonstrated improved analgesic outcome. A review by Ong et al. in 2005 found that preemptive NSAID administration reduced postoperative analgesic consumption and time to first rescue analgesic request, although not postoperative pain scores.

A class of oral medications that perhaps has more consistently positive findings are the gabapentinoids. In 2007, Gilron reviewed the available RCTs in the literature and found that gabapentin was superior to placebo for analgesic efficacy in 19 of the 27 published RCTs and opioid sparing in 21 of the 27 RCTs. Gabapentin and pregabalin reduce movement-evoked pain, which can lead to enhanced functional postoperative recovery.

Controversy regarding these and other similar studies in the literature is likely due to the difficulty in studying the effect of a single agent with short duration given preoperatively, and separating that effect out from other confounding factors. Indeed, Katz and McCartney point out in their review of this topic that only 41.7% of preemptive analgesia studies have shown a positive benefit, making the overall level of support for simply giving a preincision medication fairly equivocal. However, when looking at *preventive analgesia,* which refers to instances where a reduction in pain scores or opioid consumption outlasted the expected pharmacologic duration of the intervention, 60% of studies found evidence of benefit. This alternative way of examining the value and timing of both opioid and nonopioid analgesics commands further study in this area to help us identify which enhanced recovery interventions are most effective and efficient at reducing postoperative pain and aiding recovery. Rather than considering only how the timing of the analgesic intervention relates to incision, the authors point out that there are times when the analgesic benefit seems to last longer than the pharmacologic duration of the medication employed (indicating that a reduction of the central sensitization of neurons may be playing a role). Preventive analgesia likely has a role in enhanced recovery protocols. It would likely benefit this patient's recovery by virtue of being opioid sparing, thereby reducing the side effects from opioids and other medications, improving pain control, and facilitating mobility.

Further Reading

Benzon H, Rathmell JP, Wu CL, Turk DC, Argoff CE, Hurley RW. *Practical Management of Pain*. 5th ed. Philadelphia, PA: Elsevier Health Sciences; 2013.

Chou R, Gordon DB, de Leon-Casasola OA, et al. Management of postoperative pain: a clinical practice guideline from the American Pain Society, the American Society of Regional Anesthesia and Pain Medicine, and the American Society of Anesthesiologists' Committee on Regional Anesthesia, Executive Committee, and Administrative Council. *J Pain*. 2016;17:131–157.

Doleman B, Read D, Lund JN, Williams JP. Preventive acetaminophen reduces postoperative opioid consumption, vomiting, and pain scores after surgery: systematic review and meta-analysis. *Reg Anesth Pain Med*. 2015;40:706–712.

Gilron I. Gabapentin and pregabalin for chronic neuropathic and early postsurgical pain: current evidence and future directions. *Curr Opin Anaesthesiol*. 2007;20:456–472.

Hurley RW, Cohen SP, Williams KA, Rowlingson AJ, Wu CL. The analgesic effects of perioperative gabapentin on postoperative pain: a meta-analysis. *Reg Anesth Pain Med*. 2006;31:237–247.

Katz J. George Washington Crile, anoci-association, and pre-emptive analgesia. *Pain*. 1993;53:243–245.

Katz J, McCartney CJ. Current status of preemptive analgesia. *Curr Opin Anaesthesiol*. 2002;15:435–441.

Khalili G, Janghorbani M, Saryazdi H, Emaminejad A. Effect of preemptive and preventive acetaminophen on postoperative pain score: a randomized, double-blind trial of patients undergoing lower extremity surgery. *J Clin Anesth*. 2013;25:188–192.

Ong CK, Lirk P, Seymour RA, Jenkins BJ. The efficacy of preemptive analgesia for acute postoperative pain management: a meta-analysis. *Anesth Analg*. 2005;100:757–773.

Ong CK, Seymour RA, Lirk P, Merry AF. Combining paracetamol (acetaminophen) with nonsteroidal antiinflammatory drugs: a qualitative systematic review of analgesic efficacy for acute postoperative pain. *Anesth Analg*. 2010;110:1170–1179

Woolf CJ. Central mechanisms of acute pain. In: Bold MR, Charlton JE, Woolf CJ, eds. *Proceedings of the VIth World Congress on Pain*. Amsterdam: Elsevier, 1991: 25–34.

Woolf CJ, Wall PD: Morphine-sensitive and morphine-insensitive actions of C-fibre input on the rat spinal cord. Neurosci Lett 1986; 64: 221–5

1.5. Describe multimodal analgesia management and its potential benefits over a traditional narcotic-based approach

In comparison to unimodal analgesia where opioids are the sole or primary form of pain relief, multimodal analgesia can be defined as the use of more than one type of analgesic agent for the purposes of achieving both pain control and a reduction in opioid side effects. Because inadequately controlled pain and opioid side effects delay recovery from surgery, multimodal analgesia is a major part of fast-track recovery programs. Many pharmacologic and nonpharmacologic techniques have been studied with varying levels of efficacy. These include neuraxial blockade, peripheral nerve blockade, systemic local anesthetics, opioids, NMDA antagonists, alpha-2 agonists, beta blockers, acetaminophen, NSAIDs, anticonvulsants, glucocorticoids, and capsaicin. Nonpharmaceutical options are acupuncture, massage therapy, music therapy, and transcutaneous electric nerve stimulation. Many of these interventions have been used in enhanced recovery pathways for a variety of surgery types, colorectal surgery included. Multimodal pain protocols have resulted in reduced LOS, lower average pain score, lower incidence of urinary tract infection, and lower readmission rates.

Further Reading

Kehlet H, Dahl JB. The value of "multimodal" or "balanced analgesia" in postoperative pain treatment. *Anesth Analgesia.* 1993;77:1048–1056.

Khan SK, Malviya A, Muller SD, et al. Reduced short-term complications and mortality following enhanced recovery primary hip and knee arthroplasty: results from 6,000 consecutive procedures. *Acta Orthopaed.* 2014;85:26–31.

Miller TE, Thacker JK, White WD, et al. Reduced length of hospital stay in colorectal surgery after implementation of an enhanced recovery protocol. *Anesth Analg.* 2014;118:1052–1061.

Tan M, Law LS, Gan TJ. Optimizing pain management to facilitate enhanced recovery after surgery pathways. *Can J Anaesth.* 2015;62:203–218.

2. Chronic Pain

2.1. What are the risk factors associated with the development of chronic postsurgical pain for this patient?

The majority of patients recover from surgery without long-term pain sequelae. However, a report by Katz and Seltzer examining the epidemiology of chronic postsurgical pain (CPSP) showed that 5% to 36% of patients may still have CPSP 1 year later, depending on surgery type. Some factors have been identified that may cause increased risk for the development of CPSP; these risks can be categorized based on pre-, intra-, and postoperative factors.

From a preoperative standpoint, the single greatest risk factor for CPSP is the presence of preexisting pain. This seems to be true regardless of type, severity, and/or duration of pain, and across different surgery types. Other preoperative risk factors include patient factors such as preoperative anxiety, fear of surgery, introverted personality, young age, female sex, and/or a psychological phenomenon known as catastrophizing, characterized as a mental construct where there is the unrealistic belief that the current situation is going to lead to the worst possible pain outcome.

The intraoperative factors that have been found to be associated with a higher incidence of CPSP have been thought to be related to the surgery itself. These include the type of surgery (laparoscopic vs. open), increased duration of surgery, and the extent of intraoperative nerve injury. The amount of tissue injury produced intraoperatively that is sensed by the peripheral and central nervous system seems to have an effect on postoperative neuropathic pain and its development into a chronic state. In the patient in question, a laparotomy incision may increase the risk for the development of CPSP versus a successful laparoscopic approach.

Postoperative factors that contribute to CPSP include the effectiveness of postoperative analgesia, the presence of surgical complications, the level of social support, and again, psychosocial factors such as fear, anxiety, and catastrophizing.

Further Reading

Bruce J, Thornton AJ, Scott NW, et al. Chronic preoperative pain and psychological robustness predict acute postoperative pain outcomes after surgery for breast cancer. *Br J Cancer.* 2012;107:937–946.

Harden RN, Bruehl S, Stanos S, et al. Prospective examination of pain-related and psychological predictors of CRPS-like phenomena following total knee arthroplasty: a preliminary study. *Pain.* 2003;106:393–400.

Katz J, Seltzer Z. Transition from acute to chronic postsurgical pain: risk factors and protective factors. *Expert Rev Neurotherapeut.* 2009;9:723–744.

Liem MS, van Duyn EB, van der Graaf Y, van Vroonhoven TJ. Recurrences after conventional anterior and laparoscopic inguinal hernia repair: a randomized comparison. *Ann Surg.* 2003;237:136–141.

Peters ML, Sommer M, de Rijke JM, et al. Somatic and psychologic predictors of long-term unfavorable outcome after surgical intervention. *Ann Surg.* 2007;245:487–494.

Wall PD, Waxman S, Basbaum AI. Ongoing activity in peripheral nerve: injury discharge. *Exp Neurol.* 1974;45:576–589.

2.3. How would you manage this patient if she was already taking oral opioids prior to surgery?

Effective pain management for patients who are already using oral opioids on a daily basis can be challenging. Prolonged use of oral opioids promotes the down-regulation of opioid receptors, requiring increased doses to achieve the same analgesic effect. This concept is known as *tolerance*. This should be distinguished from opioid-induced hyperalgesia, where increasing doses of opioids can cause a reduction of nociceptive threshold such that pain is produced at a lower level of stimulation. The mechanism behind the latter phenomenon is multifactorial and likely includes "central sensitization" of the central nervous system such that cellular signaling pathways involving NMDA, cAMP, CGRP, substance P, serotonin, and other receptors become abnormal. This may render even large doses of perioperative opioids less effective and lead to poor outcomes and increased risk of postoperative complications.

Preoperatively, if this patient has been using opioids for an extended period because of chronic pain, there may be benefit to working with her and her prescribing physician toward weaning her completely off or at least trying to significantly reduce her consumption of opioids prior to surgery. This may help to effect receptor down-regulation and allow for any necessary preoperative opioids to have a more significant analgesic effect, as well as avoiding any potential hyperalgesia. It may also be prudent to determine if this patient would benefit from psychological support. If it is an emergent or urgent surgery, or if a patient's pain is related to cancer, it may be impossible to wean a patient off his or her opioid regimen. In such a case, it is necessary to consider the length of the surgery, the surgical approach (laparoscopic vs. open), and postoperative plans. A well-designed and well-communicated multimodal analgesic management plan should be instituted. If this patient was not weaned from opioids and was thought to be opioid dependent, there would be concern of opioid withdrawal in the perioperative period if an attempt was made to completely eliminate opioids form her care regimen. Regional techniques (epidural, TAP block, quadratus lumborum block), ketamine, and lidocaine infusions have each shown benefit in various surgical procedures in attempting to reduce opioid consumption, minimizing elevation of inflammatory cytokine response, promoting a faster return to bowel movement, and decreasing CPSP in non-opioid-dependent patients. In summary, a preoperative pain management plan is ideal for this patient, with each additional nonopioid therapy representing the potential to improve pain control without increasing adverse drug effects from opioids.

Further Reading

Harvey KP, Adair JD, Isho M, Robinson R. Can intravenous lidocaine decrease postsurgical ileus and shorten hospital stay in elective bowel surgery? A pilot study and literature review. *Am J Surg*. 2009;198:231–236.

Kuo CP, Jao SW, Chen KM, et al. Comparison of the effects of thoracic epidural analgesia and i.v. infusion with lidocaine on cytokine response, postoperative pain and bowel function in patients undergoing colonic surgery. *Br J Anaesth*. 2006;97:640–646.

Pivec R, Issa K, Naziri Q, Kapadia BH, Bonutti PM, Mont MA. Opioid use prior to total hip arthroplasty leads to worse clinical outcomes. *Int Orthopaed*. 2014;38:1159–1165.

Remerand F, Le Tendre C, Baud A, et al. The early and delayed analgesic effects of ketamine after total hip arthroplasty: a prospective, randomized, controlled, double-blind study. *Anesth Anal*. 2009;109:1963–1971.

Streltzer J. Pain management in the opioid-dependent patient. *Curr Psychiatr Rep*. 2001;3:489–496.

3. Perioperative Surgical Home

3.1. What are some of the preoperative components of patient optimization for abdominal cancer surgery?

The components involved in optimizing patients for surgery with the goal of also optimizing recovery fall under the title of *prehabilitation*, or trying to produce the ideal physical, mental, and emotional state for patients before undergoing the trauma of surgery. The components of this include but are not limited to nutrition, exercise, carbohydrate loading, starting multimodal analgesic and preemptive analgesic pathways, pulmonary care, oral care, smoking and alcohol cessation, antibiotic timing, and patient education/counseling. The setting of preoperative expectations with the patient can also be useful to maximizing patient understanding of his or her recovery and may also increase patient satisfaction and help with decreasing hospital LOS. Some of these components may also oppose traditional medicine. These include the minimization of preoperative fasting, the avoidance of mechanical bowel preparations, and preprocedural fluid intake with a carbohydrate load.

Further Reading

Gustafsson UO, Scott MJ, Schwenk W, et al. Guidelines for perioperative care in elective colonic surgery: Enhanced Recovery After Surgery (ERAS®) Society recommendations. *World J Surg*. 2013;37:259–284.

Kehlet H. Multimodal approach to control postoperative pathophysiology and rehabilitation. *Br J Anaesth*. 1997;78:606–617.

Wind J, Polle SW, Fung Kon Jin PH, et al. Systematic review of enhanced recovery programmes in colonic surgery. *Br J Surg*. 2006;93:800–809.

3.2. Define the ideals of the perioperative surgical home and the Strong for Surgery initiative

First, ERAS involves a series of well-timed and well-implemented pathways that will hopefully help to optimize patient outcomes after surgery by promoting practices that work toward reducing the incidence of complications in the surgical patient population. Both ERAS and the perioperative surgical home (PSH) are quality improvement initiatives that have similar goals and ideals regarding the surgical population. The PSH, promoted by the American Society of Anesthesiology, seems to operate on a larger foundation of clinical coordination and sets the time scale from when the decision is made to operate until 30 days after surgery. Although ERAS and the PSH may be complementary, have the same goals, and even measure similar outcomes, there are differences between them.

Strong for Surgery, promoted by the American College of Surgeons, is another quality improvement initiative that is aimed at identifying and promoting evidence-based practice to encourage patient optimization prior to surgery. The idea is, just as with ERAS and the PSH, that implementing evidence-based pathways prior to surgery will help to minimize negative outcomes for patients. Strong for Surgery promotes a presurgical checklist for surgeons to follow to help with education, communication, and standardization of best practices that improve clinical outcomes. The initiatives in Strong for Surgery focus on preprocedural nutrition, smoking cessation, glycemic control, and medication evaluation.

Further Reading

American College of Surgeons. Strong for Surgery. www.facs.org/quality-programs/strong-for-surgery. May 17, 2017.

Cannesson M, Kain Z. Enhanced recovery after surgery versus perioperative surgical home: is it all in the name? *Anesth Analg*. 2014;118:901–902.

4. Opioid Therapy

4.1. What are the concerns with using opioids for this patient undergoing abdominal surgery?

Although opioids are useful for acute pain, they are also associated with myriad side effects that adversely affect recovery. Opioid use prolongs hospital LOS secondary to side effects such as sedation, respiratory depression, PONV, ileus, and urinary retention. The most common complications from opioid therapy are constipation and nausea. These side effects are obviously disadvantages in a person undergoing abdominal surgery where recovery of bowel function is an important milestone for hospital discharge. This patient's risk of impaired bowel function would likely be increased even further given her baseline abnormal gastric emptying from diabetic gastroparesis. Sedation and respiratory depression are also real concerns in this case, given that her obesity is a major risk factor for obstructive sleep apnea. Indeed, 30% of all patients on morphine PCA have clinically significant hypoventilation (respiratory rate <8 breaths/min), and 0.5% of patients receiving opioids have respiratory depression significant enough to require reversal with naloxone. A less common but still pertinent effect of opioid medication would be the adverse effect on the immune system. The function of certain immune system cells such as natural killer (NK) cells is known to be impaired by opioids, and some have suggested that mu receptor agonism may cause proliferation of cancer cells. This is obviously not a desirable effect in a patient presenting for resection of a colorectal cancer; therefore, reduction of opioid doses where possible has sound physiologic basis.

Further Reading

Benyamin R, Trescot AM, Datta S, et al. Opioid complications and side effects. *Pain Physician*. 2008;11:S105–S120.

Dahan A, Neisters M, Olofsen E, Smith T, Overdyk F. Opioids. In: Barash P, Cullen BF, Stoelting RK, Cahalan MK, Stock MC, Ortega R, eds. *Clinical Anesthesia*. 7th ed. Philadelphia, PA: Lippincott Williams & Wilkins; 2013.

Lennon FE, Moss J, Singleton PA. The mu-opioid receptor in cancer progression: is there a direct effect? *Anesthesiology*. 2012;116:940–945.

Oderda GM, Evans RS, Lloyd J, et al. Cost of opioid-related adverse drug events in surgical patients. *J Pain Symptom Manage*. 2003;25:276–283.

4.2. Explain the effect of opioids on the patient's immune system

Opioids can have significant direct and indirect effects on the way the immune system functions, which in turn may have ramifications for infection and cancer outcomes. Acute and chronic opioid administration can inhibit antibody and cellular immune responses, NK cell activity, cytokine expression, and phagocytosis. Mu-opioid receptor stimulation decreases NK cell activity, macrophage phagocytosis, and nitric oxide release and inhibits T cell proliferation. Kappa-opioid receptor activation can cause the suppression of humoral immunity. Evidence that these in vitro findings result in a clinically important increase in perioperative infections does not yet exist, although adequately designed and powered trials to detect this have not been performed. In contrast to this, it is also known that uncontrolled, severe pain negatively affects the hypothalamic-pituitary axis and may also cause depression of NK cell function. The optimal technique to preserve the immune system requires a balance of good pain control while reducing doses of opioid where possible.

Patients who receive general anesthesia with opioids have a greater rate of cancer recurrence than do patients who receive local or regional anesthesia. Gottschalk et al. reviewed the literature on the effect of the type of anesthesia on cancer outcomes and found that the use of both volatile anesthetics and opioids (morphine, in particular) could decrease the body's ability to provide surveillance of dormant cancer, possibly leading to recurrence. The use of nonopioid medications such as propofol, NSAIDs, and local anesthetics may counterbalance the negative effects that opioids and volatile anesthetics may have on the immune system's regulation of cancer cells. Some of this effect may be through preservation of the normal functioning of the hypothalamic-pituitary axis. Another mechanism may be by reducing morphine angiogenesis.

Further Reading

Benyamin R, Trescot AM, Datta S, et al. Opioid complications and side effects. *Pain Physician*. 2008;11:S105–S120.

Bovill JG. Surgery for cancer: does anesthesia matter? *Anesth Analg*. 2010;110:1524–1526.

Gottschalk A, Sharma S, Ford J, Durieux ME, Tiouririne M. The role of the perioperative period in recurrence after cancer surgery. *Anesth Analg*. 2010;110:1636–1643.

Gupta K, Kshirsagar S, Chang L, et al. Morphine stimulates angiogenesis by activating proangiogenic and survival-promoting signaling and promotes breast tumor growth. *Cancer Res*. 2002;62:4491–4498.

Rittner HL, Roewer N, Brack A. The clinical (ir)relevance of opioid-induced immune suppression. *Curr Opinion Anaesthesiol*. 2010;23:588–592.

4.3. What role might cytokines and the inflammatory process have in this patient's proposed surgery, and how might that affect recovery? Is there a benefit of considering preemptive or preventive analgesia?

Many previous studies have tried to characterize measurable adverse physiologic responses to surgical trauma. It has been well demonstrated that inflammatory cytokines such as interleukin-1 and interleukin-6 (IL-6) rise in response to surgical incision, and that the degree of their increase correlates with the magnitude and duration of surgery. C-reactive protein is slow to increase after surgery; however, levels of IL-6 and C-reactive protein can approach those of patients with sepsis after major surgery. Tumor necrosis factor levels do not seem to increase as reliably. IL-6 may be the most reliable early marker of tissue injury. Both preoperative TEA and intravenous lidocaine infusion are associated with decreased levels of these inflammatory cytokines.

Further Reading

Cruickshank AM, Fraser WD, Burns HJ, Van Damme J, Shenkin A. Response of serum interleukin-6 in patients undergoing elective surgery of varying severity. *Clin Sci (London)*. 1990;79:161–165.

Kragsbjerg P, Holmberg H, Vikerfors T. Serum concentrations of interleukin-6, tumour necrosis factor-alpha, and C-reactive protein in patients undergoing major operations. *Eur J Surg*. 1995;161:17–22.

Kuo CP, Jao SW, Chen KM, et al. Comparison of the effects of thoracic epidural analgesia and i.v. infusion with lidocaine on cytokine response, postoperative pain and bowel function in patients undergoing colonic surgery. *Br J Anaesth*. 2006;97:640–646.

Shenkin A, Fraser WD, Series J, et al. The serum interleukin 6 response to elective surgery. *Lymphokine Res*. 1989;8:123–127.

5. Anatomy and Physiology of Abdominal Surgery Pain

5.1. Briefly describe the innervation of the abdominal wall and viscera

The abdomen is innervated by the anterior branches of spinal nerves T7 through L1. The anterior rami of T7 through T9 innervates the skin and abdominal wall above the umbilicus, T10 innervates the area surrounding the umbilicus, and T11 through L1 innervates below the umbilicus. L1 is unique in that it branches into 2 peripheral nerves, the iliohypogastric and the ilioinguinal. These nerves run in the plane around the abdomen and toward the midline, between the transversus abdominis muscle and the internal oblique. This is known as the TAP plane. The fascial layers of the transversus abdominis and internal oblique are normally tightly adherent to one another; however, they can be spread apart by the injection of fluid, making this a potential space to deposit local anesthetic. It should be realized, however, that these nerves transmit somatic pain signals from the skin, abdominal wall, and parietal peritoneum. These nerves are not a target to address visceral pain.

Further Reading

Hadzic A. *Hadzic's Peripheral Nerve Blocks: And Anatomy for Ultrasound-Guided Regional Anesthesia*. 2nd ed. New York, NY: McGraw-Hill; 2012.

Moore K, Dalley AF. *Clinically Oriented Anatomy*. 5th ed. Philadelphia, PA: Lippincott Williams & Williams; 1999.

Mukhtar K. Transversus abdominis plane (TAP) block. *J NY School Reg Anest*. 2009;12:28–33.

5.2. What are the different components of pain that need to be considered (i.e., somatic, visceral)?

Somatic pain is typically perceived as well-localized, sharp, aching, or throbbing pain. In the patient in question, the somatic pain of interest would be from the skin incision and from trauma to the abdominal wall. This type of pain does lend itself to peripheral nerve blockade (such as a TAP or quadratus lumborum block), but blocking these somatic signals does not address any visceral pain originating from the abdominal organs. Visceral pain is poorly localized and usually experienced as vague, dull, aching, squeezing, or pressure-like. The origin of pain could be from irritation, stretching, traction, or ischemia to the smooth muscle surrounding hollow organs or the capsule surrounding solid organs. These visceral afferents travel to the central nervous system by way of the vagus nerve and spinal nerves that run with the sympathetic fibers supplying the abdomen. Visceral pain can be blocked to some degree with spinal and epidural anesthesia, as seen during the first stage of labor; however, noxious visceral stimuli can still cause hemodynamic and autonomic responses even in the face of otherwise effective anesthesia and analgesia.

Further Reading

Benzon H, Rathmell JP, Wu CL, Turk DC, Argoff CE, Hurley RW. *Practical Management of Pain*. 5th ed. Philadelphia, PA: Elsevier Health Sciences; 2013.

5.3. What regional techniques might be chosen for analgesia in this patient? Which techniques might you consider for a laparotomy incision versus low anterior resection versus purely robotic/laparoscopic?

Opioid monotherapy is a poor choice for most surgical approaches involving anything more than mild postoperative pain. It can be associated with suboptimal pain management, morbidity from opioid-mediated side effects (sedation, itching, nausea, vomiting, constipation, respiratory complications, etc.), prolonged recovery, and reduced patient satisfaction. For open abdominal surgeries, epidural analgesia is considered the gold standard and is associated with better pain control, reduced ileus, and reduced hospital LOS. These outcomes seem to be more consistent for incisions extending above the umbilicus. Although epidural analgesia would be an excellent choice for open low-anterior resection, urinary retention and motor weakness of the legs complicate postoperative management and recovery. While it is possible to titrate down local anesthetic concentration and effective rate to reduce or eliminate the problem of undesired motor block, it may still be wise for patients to ambulate with assistance or supervision such as a bedside nurse or physical therapist. Low thoracic and lumbar epidural blockade has also been thought to be a risk factor for urinary retention, although other factors contribute to this, and at least one study has demonstrated that urinary catheters can be removed before epidural catheters, with acceptably low rates of urinary retention, as well as decreased urinary tract infection. As for laparoscopic procedures, these and other minimally invasive techniques are associated with less pain. Although some authors previously demonstrated earlier return of bowel function with epidural analgesia in laparoscopic surgery, a trend toward earlier discharge in these laparoscopic cases may be expanding the number of cases where alternative analgesic therapies could be considered. TAP or quadratus lumborum block, intrathecal morphine (if the patient is staying overnight), intravenous lidocaine infusion, and subanesthetic ketamine in the setting of multimodal analgesia are alternative considerations; however, none of them offers the benefit of reducing sympathetic outflow to the gut that epidural analgesia offers.

Further Reading

Apfelbaum JL, Chen C, Mehta SS, Gan TJ. Postoperative pain experience: results from a national survey suggest postoperative pain continues to be undermanaged. *Anesth Analg* 2003;97:534–540.

Baldini G, Bagry H, Aprikian A, Carli F. Postoperative urinary retention: anesthetic and perioperative considerations. *Anesthesiology*. 2009;110:1139–1157.

Basse L, Werner M, Kehlet H. Is urinary drainage necessary during continuous epidural analgesia after colonic resection? *Reg Anesth Pain Med*. 2000;25:498–501.

Bardram L, Funch-Jensen P, Jensen P, Crawford ME, Kehlet H. Recovery after laparoscopic colonic surgery with epidural analgesia, and early oral nutrition and mobilisation. *Lancet (London)*. 1995;345:763–764.

Benoist S, Panis Y, Denet C, Mauvais F, Mariani P, Valleur P. Optimal duration of urinary drainage after rectal resection: a randomized controlled trial. *Surgery*. 1999;125:135–141.

Grass F, Slieker J, Frauche P, et al. Postoperative urinary retention in colorectal surgery within an enhanced recovery pathway. *J Surg Res*. 2017;207:70–76.

Guay J, Nishimori M, Kopp SL. Epidural local anesthetics versus opioid-based analgesic regimens for postoperative gastrointestinal paralysis, vomiting, and pain after abdominal surgery: a Cochrane Review. *Anesth Analg*. 2016;123:1591–1602.

Gustafsson UO, Scott MJ, Schwenk W, et al. Guidelines for perioperative care in elective colonic surgery: Enhanced Recovery After Surgery (ERAS®) Society recommendations. *J Surg*. 2013;37:259–284.

Levy BF, Scott MJ, Fawcett WJ, Rockall TA. 23-hour-stay laparoscopic colectomy. *Dis Colon Rectum*. 2009;52:1239–1243.

Oderda GM, Evans RS, Lloyd J, et al. Cost of opioid-related adverse drug events in surgical patients. *J Pain Symptom Manage*. 2003;25:276–283.

5.4. How might surgical technique and operating time affect outcomes in patients undergoing abdominal surgery?

Enhanced recovery pathways promote laparoscopic over open procedures when possible to help reduce the risk of postoperative complications and the overall debilitation that a patient might experience. However, this is only one component or "pathway ideal" that quality improvement for the surgical patient can promote. The total duration of a surgical procedure may also have an effect on outcomes, especially LOS. It must be considered that prolonged durations may indicate surgical or anesthetic difficulty. When evaluating factors that can lead to a prolonged LOS in major elective surgery, the duration of the procedure in major bowel surgery is one factor that may be associated with an increased LOS. There are other associated factors that can prolonged LOS and, more important, affect the incidence of postoperative complications. Practitioners must evaluate all factors when trying to promote quality improvement; however, even with a laparoscopic approach, total operative time can negatively impact LOS in an enhanced recovery program, and it appears that times greater than 270 minutes are most consistent with an association with prolonged LOS and complication incidence increases.

Further Reading

Collins TC, Daley J, Henderson WH, Khuri SF. Risk factors for prolonged length of stay after major elective surgery. *Ann Surg*. 1999;230:251–259.

Feroci F, Kroning KC, Lenzi E, Moraldi L, Cantafio S, Scatizzi M. Laparoscopy within a fast-track program enhances the short-term results after elective surgery for resectable colorectal cancer. *Surg Endosc*. 2011;25:2919–2925.

Harrison OJ, Smart NJ, White P, et al. Operative time and outcome of enhanced recovery after surgery after laparoscopic colorectal surgery. *J Soc Laparoendosc Surg*. 2014;18:265–272.

Scheer A, Martel G, Moloo H, et al. Laparoscopic colon surgery: does operative time matter? *Dis Colon Rectum*. 2009;52:1746–1752.

6. Neuraxial and Paravertebral Analgesia

6.1. Explain the benefits of epidural analgesia to abdominal surgery

Abdominal surgery can cause moderate to severe pain that can adversely affect recovery. Because epidural analgesia is effective at both treating this pain and reducing the stress response from surgery, it has several possible benefits to cardiovascular, pulmonary, gastrointestinal, coagulation, metabolic, and immune function. A regional block with local anesthetic may lead to less tachycardia, hypertension, and platelet activation. This, in turn, may lead to fewer cardiovascular complications such as myocardial infarction, deep venous thrombosis, and pulmonary embolism. From a pulmonary standpoint, Ballantyne et al. concluded in a large meta-analysis that compared with intravenous opioids, epidural anesthesia reduced the amount of atelectasis, increased the PaO_2, had a weak tendency to reduce pulmonary infections, and was associated with fewer overall pulmonary complications. Reduced gastrointestinal complications included earlier return of bowel function as evidenced by a shorter amount of time to first flatus and bowel movement as well as earlier oral intake.

A well-documented reduction in serum cortisol and catecholamines during and after major surgery likely plays a role in reduced postoperative insulin resistance and better glycemic control. These effects may translate to reduced perioperative morbidity and mortality after abdominal surgeries such as colectomy for colorectal cancer. As mentioned elsewhere in this chapter, achieving effective pain control with a local anesthetic theoretically better preserves cellular and humoral immunity, specifically NK cell function, as well as helping to avoid an increase in inflammatory cytokines. This not only could result in reduced postoperative infection but also could favorably affect oncologic outcome.

Good pain control is associated with faster recovery, reduced morbidity, and increased patient satisfaction. For open abdominal surgery, epidural blockade has proven superior to opioid therapy for relevant outcomes such as pain scores, PONV, cardiopulmonary complications, and earlier return of bowel function. Given that most patients would rate their postoperative pain control as undermanaged and that epidurals have many other benefits that extend beyond reduced pain scores, this modality is widely considered the gold standard for open abdominal surgery. Although several previous studies have demonstrated more effective postoperative convalescence in laparoscopic surgery, this surgical approach results in significantly less pain, and epidurals are not complication free. More recent studies show that these patients are often ready for discharge as soon as 23 hours after surgery. In these cases, TEA may actually result in a slightly longer hospital stay. Therefore, according to the most recent ERAS guidelines, thoracic epidurals are no longer recommended for laparoscopic surgery. Multimodal options such as lidocaine infusion, subanesthetic ketamine, intrathecal morphine, or truncal block (TAP or quadratus lumborum) may represent better alternatives.

Further Reading

Apfelbaum JL, Chen C, Mehta SS, Gan TJ. Postoperative pain experience: results from a national survey suggest postoperative pain continues to be undermanaged. *Anesth Analg*. 2003;97:534–540.

Ballantyne JC, Carr DB, deFerranti S, et al. The comparative effects of postoperative analgesic therapies on pulmonary outcome: cumulative meta-analyses of randomized, controlled trials. *Anesth Analg*. 1998;86:598–612.

Davies RG, Myles PS, Graham JM. A comparison of the analgesic efficacy and side-effects of paravertebral vs epidural blockade for thoracotomy: a systematic review and meta-analysis of randomized trials. *Br J Anaesth*. 2006;96:418–426.

Ekatodramis G. Regional anesthesia and analgesia: their role in postoperative outcome. *Curr Topic Med Chem*. 2001;1:183–192.

Guay J, Nishimori M, Kopp SL. Epidural local anesthetics versus opioid-based analgesic regimens for postoperative gastrointestinal paralysis, vomiting, and pain after abdominal surgery: a Cochrane Review. *Anesth Analg*. 2016;123:1591–1602.

Gustafsson UO, Scott MJ, Schwenk W, et al. Guidelines for perioperative care in elective colonic surgery: Enhanced Recovery After Surgery (ERAS®) Society recommendations. *World J Surg*. 2013;37:259–284.

Hanna MN, Murphy JD, Kumar K, Wu CL. Regional techniques and outcome: what is the evidence? *Curr Opinion Anaesthesiol*. 2009;22:672–677.

Jackson RS, Amdur RL, White JC, Macsata RA. Hyperglycemia is associated with increased risk of morbidity and mortality after colectomy for cancer. *J Am Coll Surg*. 2012;214:68–80.

Jorgensen H, Wetterslev J, Moiniche S, Dahl JB. Epidural local anaesthetics versus opioid-based analgesic regimens for postoperative gastrointestinal paralysis, PONV, and pain after abdominal surgery. *Cochrane Database Syst Rev*. 2001(4):CD001893.

Kouraklis G, Glinavou A, Raftopoulos L, Alevisou V, Lagos G, Karatzas G. Epidural analgesia attenuates the systemic stress response to upper abdominal surgery: a randomized trial. *Int Surg*. 2000;85:353–357.

Levy BF, Scott MJ, Fawcett W, Fry C, Rockall TA. Randomized clinical trial of epidural, spinal or patient-controlled analgesia for patients undergoing laparoscopic colorectal surgery. *Br J Surg*. 2011;98:1068–1078.

Levy BF, Scott MJ, Fawcett WJ, Rockall TA. 23-hour-stay laparoscopic colectomy. *Dis Colon Rectum*. 2009;52:1239–1243.

Liu S, Carpenter RL, Neal JM. Epidural anesthesia and analgesia: their role in postoperative outcome. *Anesthesiology*. 1995;82:1474–1506.

Mann C, Pouzeratte Y, Boccara G, et al. Comparison of intravenous or epidural patient-controlled analgesia in the elderly after major abdominal surgery. *Anesthesiology*. 2000;92:433–441.

Richardson J, Sabanathan S, Jones J, Shah RD, Cheema S, Mearns AJ. A prospective, randomized comparison of preoperative and continuous balanced epidural or paravertebral bupivacaine on post-thoracotomy pain, pulmonary function and stress responses. *Br J Anaesth*. 1999;83:387–392.

Steinbrook RA. Epidural anesthesia and gastrointestinal motility. *Anesth Analg*. 1998;86:837–844.

Taqi A, Hong X, Mistraletti G, Stein B, Charlebois P, Carli F. Thoracic epidural analgesia facilitates the restoration of bowel function and dietary intake in patients undergoing laparoscopic colon resection using a traditional, nonaccelerated, perioperative care program. *Surg Endosc*. 2007;21:247–252.

Tonnesen E, Wahlgreen C. Influence of extradural and general anaesthesia on natural killer cell activity and lymphocyte subpopulations in patients undergoing hysterectomy. *Br J Anaesth*. 1988;60:500–507.

Uchida I, Asoh T, Shirasaka C, Tsuji H. Effect of epidural analgesia on postoperative insulin resistance as evaluated by insulin clamp technique. *Br J Surg*. 1988;75:557–562.

6.2. What effects does epidural analgesia have on patient outcome?

The preceding section was mentioned that thoracic epidural anesthesia and analgesia has been shown to reduce the incidence of complications in virtually every organ system after major surgery. In 2000, Rodgers et al. conducted a review of 141 trials with more than 9000 patients who were randomized to general anesthesia or neuraxial blockade. They found a 30% reduction in all-cause mortality, a 40% to 50% reduction in VTE events, a 50% reduction in transfusion requirements, and a 39% reduction in pneumonia, as well as fewer myocardial infarctions and infections in the neuraxial group, although the confidence intervals were wider for these last 2 outcomes. It should be noted that some in the neuraxial group received general anesthesia along with epidural blockade and some did not; thus some of these benefits could be due to avoidance of general anesthesia. It should also be realized that anticoagulation protocols for orthopedic surgery have been modernized since this time; however, this review still serves to underscore potential outcome benefits that epidural anesthesia and analgesia may provide. In 2002, Carli et al. compared epidural analgesia to intravenous PCA in an assessment of postoperative recovery after elective colon resection surgery. They found that patients in the epidural group had a significantly smaller decrease in their 6-minute walk test time and their SF-36 physical health component assessment (an objective measurement of physical and mental health performance). This suggests that the patient's functional status immediately following surgery may be better preserved if acute pain signals are blocked with epidural analgesia. Additionally, these patients had better pain control and less fatigue and were able to eat more and mobilize more. Although LOS was not statistically significantly different, the patients in the epidural group were ready for discharge earlier.

In 2006, Guay conducted a meta-analysis of 70 studies that included 5402 patients, about half of whom had epidural analgesia, with attention to perioperative outcomes. This study found that epidural analgesia reduced the incidence of arrhythmia (odds ratio [OR] = 0.59), time to tracheal extubation (OR = −3.90 hours), intensive care unit stay (OR = −2.94 hours), visual analogical pain scores at rest (OR = −0.78) and during movement (OR = −1.28), and maximal blood epinephrine, norepinephrine, cortisol, and glucose concentrations achieved. It also reduced the first 24-hour morphine consumption (OR = −13.62 mg) and improved the forced vital capacity at 24 hours. Finally, a thoracic epidural containing local anesthetic reduced the incidence of renal failure (OR = 0.34). This analysis included cardiac, thoracic, peripheral vascular, general, gynecologic, and orthopedic patients.

Also in 2006 (updated in 2012), Nishimori et al. analyzed outcomes for epidural analgesia in patients presenting for elective abdominal aortic surgery. There were 15 trials involving 1297 patients. The epidural group showed significantly lower pain scores on movement for up to 3 postoperative days. The duration of tracheal intubation and mechanical ventilation also was significantly shorter, by about 48%, in the epidural analgesia group. The overall event rates of myocardial infarction, acute respiratory failure, gastrointestinal complications, and renal complications were significantly lower in the epidural analgesia group. A mortality difference was not found in this review, however.

Because of differences in the effect sizes of various outcomes in these and similar reviews, in 2014 the Cochrane Library did an overview of 9 previous Cochrane Reviews. The authors found that compared with general anesthesia, neuraxial blockade reduced the risk of pneumonia (RR 0.45), and risk of 0- to 30-day mortality (RR 0.71). When epidural blockade was added to general anesthesia, however, the confidence intervals were wider, making the differences not statistically significant. The reviewers did not find a significant difference in myocardial infarction in this report, although they did acknowledge that a larger sample size may be needed to be more definitive about the effect of epidurals on this complication. They concluded that for intermediate- to high-risk surgery (vascular, orthopedic, urologic, intraperitoneal), regional anesthesia with neuraxial blockade would reduce mortality and risk of pneumonia, but that this effect might not be seen when it was simply added to general anesthesia. These results provided some contrast to previous reviews.

This topic was studied further in 2016, with Guay and associates again carrying out a comprehensive review of epidural analgesia on abdominal surgery. They found high-quality evidence that an epidural accelerates the return of the gastrointestinal transit, with a return of flatus 17.5 hours sooner and return of bowel movement 22 hours sooner. A moderate level of evidence was found to support the notion that an epidural with both local anesthetic and an opioid together decreases pain after abdominal surgery. For open surgeries, an epidural anesthetic appeared to reduce hospital stay by about 1 day, although the evidence level for this was rated as low. LOS did not appear to be significantly reduced in abdominal surgeries that are not open and may actually be longer when used in laparoscopic surgery.

Despite a wealth of data supporting the notion that neuraxial blockade leads to earlier return of bowel function, there has been some historical concern about anastomotic breakdown as it relates to the use of epidural analgesia in colorectal surgery. This concern, however, may have grown out of worry that hypotension would adversely affect the sutured colon. Despite this inquiry, evidence has not supported this anxiety. Guay's et al.'s meta-analysis found no difference in the incidence of gastrointestinal anastomotic leak, based on 17 trials, including 848 patients. In fact, others have shown that local anesthetic blockade actually increases blood flow to this area, which may be why epidurals do not appear to cause anastomotic leakage. It is also possible that increased blood flow in the area of sympathetic blockade may have other positive effects. In 2010, a retrospective review of a database of more than 3000 patients revealed that those who underwent joint replacement under general anesthesia had twice the surgical site infection rate as those who had their surgery under regional anesthesia. This twofold reduction in surgical site infection puts this intervention in a similar category as timely antibiotic prophylaxis. In addition to this benefit, reduced sympathetic signal to the gut may push the balance of nerve signals more toward the parasympathetic, which would promote gastrointestinal motility and reduce ileus.

The differences in magnitude of results of the outcome findings in this section may likely be a result of how the regional technique was used, the comorbidities of the patient it was performed on, and specific characteristics about the surgical technique itself. Whether or not the surgery is to be performed open and if the incision will extend above the umbilicus or not can make a substantial difference on the degree of potential benefit. More large, prospective trials specific to surgery type and patient will likely be needed before anything further can be said about individual outcomes relative to specific surgeries. At that point, the value of healthcare delivery that includes neuraxial anesthesia can also be more accurately assessed.

Further Reading

Carli F, Mayo N, Klubien K, Schricker T, Trudel J, Belliveau P. Epidural analgesia enhances functional exercise capacity and health-related quality of life after colonic surgery: results of a randomized trial. *Anesthesiology*. 2002;97:540–549.

Chang CC, Lin HC, Lin HW, Lin HC. Anesthetic management and surgical site infections in total hip or knee replacement: a population-based study. *Anesthesiology*. 2010;113:279–284.

Guay J. The benefits of adding epidural analgesia to general anesthesia: a meta-analysis. *J Anesth*. 2006;20:335–340.

Guay J, Choi P, Suresh S, Albert N, Kopp S, Pace NL. Neuraxial blockade for the prevention of postoperative mortality and major morbidity: an overview of Cochrane systematic reviews. *Cochrane Database Syst Rev*. 2014(1):CD010108.

Guay J, Nishimori M, Kopp SL. Epidural local anesthetics versus opioid-based analgesic regimens for postoperative gastrointestinal paralysis, vomiting, and pain after abdominal surgery: a Cochrane Review. *Anesth Analg.* 2016;123:1591–1602.

Gustafsson UO, Scott MJ, Schwenk W, et al. Guidelines for perioperative care in elective colonic surgery: Enhanced Recovery After Surgery (ERAS®) Society recommendations. *World J Surg.* 2013;37:259–284.

Johansson K, Ahn H, Lindhagen J, Tryselius U. Effect of epidural anaesthesia on intestinal blood flow. *Br J Surg.* 1988;75:73–76.

Kehlet H. Multimodal approach to control postoperative pathophysiology and rehabilitation. *Br J Anaesthes.* 1997;78(5):606–617.

Kehlet H. The surgical stress response: should it be prevented? *Can J Surg.* 1991;34:565–567.

Levy BF, Scott MJ, Fawcett W, Fry C, Rockall TA. Randomized clinical trial of epidural, spinal or patient-controlled analgesia for patients undergoing laparoscopic colorectal surgery. *Br J Surg.* 2011;98:1068–1078.

McIsaac DI, Cole ET, McCartney CJ. Impact of including regional anaesthesia in enhanced recovery protocols: a scoping review. *Br J Anaesth.* 2015;115:ii46–56.

Moiniche S, Bulow S, Hesselfeldt P, Hestbaek A, Kehlet H. Convalescence and hospital stay after colonic surgery with balanced analgesia, early oral feeding, and enforced mobilisation. *Eur J Surg.* 1995;161:283–288.

Nishimori M, Low JH, Zheng H, Ballantyne JC. Epidural pain relief versus systemic opioid-based pain relief for abdominal aortic surgery. *Cochrane Database Syst Rev.* 2012(7):CD005059.

Rodgers A, Walker N, Schug S, et al. Reduction of postoperative mortality and morbidity with epidural or spinal anaesthesia: results from overview of randomised trials. *Br Med J.* 2000;321:1493.

Sessler DI. Neuraxial anesthesia and surgical site infection. *Anesthesiology.* 2010;113:265–267.

6.3. How does neuraxial analgesia affect cancer outcome?

A review of the literature for recent studies regarding epidural analgesia and cancer outcome yielded 11 noteworthy articles. Seven of these were definitively in favor of epidural analgesia improving cancer outcome after surgery, 3 did not find a difference, and 1 found a positive effect only in subgroup analysis. Differences tended to be nonsignificant in prostatectomy for prostate cancer, surgery for ovarian cancer, and a review that included these cancer types along with pancreatic cancer. The differences with regional anesthesia tended to be highly significant, however, in cases of colorectal cancer. A 2008 Veterans Affairs study looked at cancer survival after surgery for colon cancer and found that having an epidural as a part of the anesthetic plan was associated with a survival benefit out to 1.46 years for patients without distant metastasis. This difference may be related to fewer thrombotic, infectious, and pulmonary complications in high-risk patients. Distant metastasis obviated this difference. In 2012, a cohort study also found that epidural use was associated with better survival (66%) in patients with nonmetastatic colon cancer than in patients without an epidural (55%). In 2013, Chen and Miao also hypothesized that epidural use would be associated with better oncologic outcome. After analyzing 14 studies, they concluded that epidural anesthesia and/or analgesia was associated with an improved overall survival (OS), especially in colorectal surgery, when compared with general anesthesia alone. However, they were not able to find a difference in recurrence-free survival (RFS), meaning that although the study supports improved OS, it cannot be used to support the use of epidural for cancer control. Sun and colleagues also found the same association with analysis of 6 different studies, again finding a longer OS but no difference in RFS. Subsequent to these analyses, Zimmitti and associates found that RFS was better with neuraxial analgesia but not OS, and Weng et al. found that both OS and RFS were improved with epidural use. Although the trend with regard to specific outcome varies, the overall results are strongly suggestive that epidural anesthesia and analgesia may have positive effects on cancer outcome. This likely occurs via a reduced stress response, a reduced need for volatile anesthetic and opioids, and reduced perioperative complications such as VTE, infection, pneumonia, and others. Patient selection, cancer type, and surgical technique also likely have a strong influence on these outcomes. Due to our particular patient's combination of obesity, diabetes, and colorectal surgery, an epidural would very likely benefit her from a cancer standpoint. This would need to be balanced against other measures such as epidural-related complications. The availability of technical expertise regarding the safe placement of epidural catheters in the obese population, as well as the infrastructure to safely run these infusions in the intensive care units and wards, would also be an important consideration. It is ideal to have order sets in place, infusions prepared in a sterile fashion by a pharmacist, and nursing education specific to the management of epidurals. It was also mentioned elsewhere in this chapter that a dedicated pain service improves management in these patients.

Further Reading

Capmas P, Billard V, Gouy S, et al. Impact of epidural analgesia on survival in patients undergoing complete cytoreductive surgery for ovarian cancer. *Anticancer Res*. 2012;32:1537–1542.

Chen WK, Miao CH. The effect of anesthetic technique on survival in human cancers: a meta-analysis of retrospective and prospective studies. *PloS One*. 2013;8:e56540.

Christopherson R, James KE, Tableman M, Marshall P, Johnson FE. Long-term survival after colon cancer surgery: a variation associated with choice of anesthesia. *Anesth Analg*. 2008;107:325–332.

Cummings KC III, Xu F, Cummings LC, Cooper GS. A comparison of epidural analgesia and traditional pain management effects on survival and cancer recurrence after colectomy: a population-based study. *Anesthesiology*. 2012;116:797–806.

Myles PS, Peyton P, Silbert B, Hunt J, Rigg JR, Sessler DI. Perioperative epidural analgesia for major abdominal surgery for cancer and recurrence-free survival: randomised trial. *Br* Med J. 2011;342:d1491.

Pei L, Tan G, Wang L, et al. Comparison of combined general-epidural anesthesia with general anesthesia effects on survival and cancer recurrence: a meta-analysis of retrospective and prospective studies. *PloS One*. 2014;9:e114667.

Sun Y, Li T, Gan TJ. The effects of perioperative regional anesthesia and analgesia on cancer recurrence and survival after oncology surgery: a systematic review and meta-analysis. *Reg Anesth Pain Med*. 2015;40:589–598.

Sun X, Yang C, Li K, Ding S. The impact of anesthetic techniques on survival for patients with colorectal cancer: evidence based on six studies. *Hepatogastroenterology*. 2015;62:299–302.

Tsui BC, Rashiq S, Schopflocher D, et al. Epidural anesthesia and cancer recurrence rates after radical prostatectomy. *Can J Anaesth*. 2010;57:107–112.

Weng M, Chen W, Hou W, Li L, Ding M, Miao C. The effect of neuraxial anesthesia on cancer recurrence and survival after cancer surgery: an updated meta-analysis. *Oncotarget*. 2016;7:15262–15273.

Zimmitti G, Soliz J, Aloia TA, et al. Positive impact of epidural analgesia on oncologic outcomes in patients undergoing resection of colorectal liver metastases. *Ann Surgical Oncol*. 2016;23:1003–1011.

6.4. Is there a role for the use of paravertebral nerve block when operating in the abdomen?

There are other alternatives to epidurals emerging for adding regional techniques for surgery of the abdomen. Although epidurals have been the gold standard up to this point, there are now some viable alternatives to epidural use with the acceptance of ultrasound guidance for nerve blocks and infiltration techniques. These include paravertebral blocks (PVBs), ultrasound-guided TAP infiltration, quadratus lumborum injection, and surgical infiltration. PVBs were first performed in 1905, and with the more ubiquitous use of ultrasound for injection, their popularity has once again started to increase. However, the use of bilateral PVBs for midline abdominal surgery is not a universally applied method of care because it may not have any distinct advantage over a continuous thoracic epidural. The advantages of PVB injection can be an analgesic benefit comparable to thoracic epidural; a high success rate; the potential ability to perform safely in patients under general anesthesia; no urinary retention; and less sedation, nausea, vomiting, and constipation compared with opioid-based analgesic techniques, to name a few. The contraindications are similar to those for most neuraxial techniques, including significant coagulopathy, patient refusal, local infection, systemic infection or sepsis, and allergy to local anesthetics.

Further Reading

Gadsden J, Ayad S, Gonzales JJ, Mehta J, Boublik J, Hutchins J. Evolution of transversus abdominis plane infiltration techniques for postsurgical analgesia following abdominal surgeries. *Local Reg Anest*. 2015;8:113–117.

Melnikov AL, Bjoergo S, Kongsgaard UE. Thoracic paravertebral block versus transversus abdominis plane block in major gynecological surgery: a prospective, randomized, controlled, observer-blinded study. *Local Reg Anesth.* 2012;5:55–61.

Niraj G, Kelkar A, Hart E, et al. Comparison of analgesic efficacy of four-quadrant transversus abdominis plane (TAP) block and continuous posterior TAP analgesia with epidural analgesia in patients undergoing laparoscopic colorectal surgery: an open-label, randomised, non-inferiority trial. *Anaesthesia.* 2014;69:348–355.

Richardson J, Lonnqvist PA. Thoracic paravertebral block. *Br J Anaesth.* 1998;81:230–238.

Tighe SQM G, MD, Rajadurai, N. Paravertebral block. *Contin Educ Anaesth Crit Care Pain.* 2010;10:133–137.

7. Regional Anesthesia of the Abdominal Wall

7.1. Discuss the origin and utility of abdominal wall blocks and their role in colorectal surgery

Although there is no substitute for the degree of pain relief that can be achieved with a thoracic epidural for open abdominal surgery, in many other situations the margin between the benefit and risk of this intervention is smaller. This could be true for a more minimally invasive surgical approach such as robotic or laparoscopic, a low-risk patient, expected discharge on postoperative day 0 or 1, or contraindication to neuraxial analgesia. In these situations, alternative regional anesthesia techniques may be attractive. In 2001, Ahmad Rafi described a novel approach to blockade of somatic abdominal nerves as they course together around the lateral aspect of the abdomen, between the costal margin and iliac crest, in the "lumbar triangle of petit." The borders of this triangle are the latissimus dorsi posteriorly, the external oblique anteriorly, and the iliac crest inferiorly. In this anatomic area, the internal oblique makes up the floor of the triangle. The nerves supplying the abdomen (T7-L1) run between the transversus abdominis muscle and the internal oblique. In this technique, the highest point of the iliac crest is palpated and a blunt-tipped needle is inserted perpendicular to the skin and "walked off" the iliac crest until a single pop is felt. At this point, the needle is presumed to be in the fascial plane between the internal oblique and transversus abdominis. After negative aspiration, 20 to 30 mL of appropriately dilute local anesthetic is deposited in this plane. Rafi performed these blocks according to this landmark technique, without ultrasound guidance.

In 2004, McDonnell and co-investigators utilized Rafi's technique, named the regional abdominal field infiltration (R.A.F.I.) technique, as described on unfixed cadaver specimens, and later on healthy volunteers, using methylene blue and radiologic imaging to confirm the spread of local anesthetic, and a T8 to L1 dermatome was reported with the volunteers, thereby establishing the TAP block. In 2007, Hebbard et al. published a description of how to perform this block under ultrasound guidance. This approach overcomes the difficulty with appreciating the "pop" when using the blind landmark technique on obese or elderly populations, and likely increases block success rate.

Although these and other early accounts of TAP blocks describe theoretically or actually blocking a dermatome as wide as T7 to L1, TAP blocks performed on fresh cadavers with aniline dye found staining only of T10 to L1 abdominal nerves. A *subcostal* or *multi-injection* technique may be used to try to reach more cephalad dermatomes, although Barrington's cadaver study revealed staining of T9, T10, and T11. While this issue may still be of some debate, Borglum et al. utilized advanced MRI techniques to reliably demonstrate that the local anesthetic from the classic TAP injection site does not appear to communicate with the local anesthetic deposited in the subcostal area. This would mean that to reliably anesthetize the entire abdominal wall (T6-T12), bilateral injections both at the classic location and in the subcostal area would be necessary. There may be an upper TAP plexus (T6-T9) and a lower TAP plexus (T10-L1), and communication or spread between them should not be assumed to reliably take place. It has also been assumed until recently that the sensory blockade produced with a TAP block is dermatomal. Stoving et al. performed these blocks on healthy volunteers and found that the area of sensory block was in fact patchy and nondermatomal, it spread farther laterally than previously appreciated, its medial spread was far less impressive than previously presumed, and the block did not tend to extend above the umbilicus. They did show, however, that these blocks had a duration of 10 hours (in healthy volunteers not having surgery) and that this technique did provide abdominal wall muscle relaxation.

These limitations of local anesthetic spread should be kept in mind when selecting the anesthetic technique to use for a particular abdominal surgical case. Classic TAP blocks seem to be best for incisions at or below the umbilicus, whereas another set of bilateral injections underneath the costal margin are likely warranted if the incision extends above the umbilicus. Combining the 2 blocks (classic and subcostal) has recently been known as an ultrasound-guided bilateral dual TAP block. The authors favor this block over the classic technique alone for surgeries extending above the umbilicus. If this technique is chosen, a discussion of how much local anesthetic can be safely used is warranted. There is wide variability of regimens used and a paucity of meaningful data; however, it is suggested that 1 to 2.5 mg/kg of bupivacaine or 2 to 3 mg/kg of ropivacaine with epinephrine should be divided among the 4 different injection sites, that lean body mass be used for this calculation, and that this technique not be combined with a lidocaine infusion or other regional techniques simultaneously to avoid potentially toxic serum levels of local anesthetic.

Further Reading

Barrington MJ, Ivanusic JJ, Rozen WM, Hebbard P. Spread of injectate after ultrasound-guided subcostal transversus abdominis plane block: a cadaveric study. *Anaesthesia*. 2009;64:745–750.

Borglum J, Jensen K, Christensen AF, et al. Distribution patterns, dermatomal anesthesia, and ropivacaine serum concentrations after bilateral dual transversus abdominis plane block. *Reg Anesth Pain Med*. 2012;37:294–301.

Chin KM, McDonnell JG, Carvalho B, Sharkey A, Pawa A, Gadsden J. Essentials of our current understanding: abdominal wall blocks. *Reg Anesth Pain Med*. 2017;42:133–183.

Hebbard P, Fujiwara Y, Shibata Y, Royse C. Ultrasound-guided transversus abdominis plane (TAP) block. *Anaesth Intensive Care*. 2007;35:616–617.

Hebbard PD, Barrington MJ, Vasey C. Ultrasound-guided continuous oblique subcostal transversus abdominis plane blockade: description of anatomy and clinical technique. *Reg Anesth Pain Med*. 2010;35:436–441.

McDonnell JG, O'Donnell BD, Tuite D, Farrell T, Power C. The regional abdominal field infiltration technique: computerised tomographic and anatomical identification of a novel approach to the transversus abdominis neurovascular fascial plane. *Anesthesiology*. 2004;101(A899).

McDonnell J, O'Donnell BD, Farrell T, Gough N, Tuite D. Transversus abdominis plane block: a cadaveric and radiological evaluation. *Reg Anesth Pain Med*. 2007;32:399–404.

Rafi AN. Abdominal field block: a new approach via the lumbar triangle. *Anaesthesia*. 2001;56:1024–1026.

Stoving K, Rothe C, Rosenstock CV, Aasvang EK, Lundstrom LH, Lange KH. Cutaneous sensory block area, muscle-relaxing effect, and block duration of the transversus abdominis plane block: a randomized, blinded, and placebo-controlled study in healthy volunteers. *Reg Anesth Pain Med*. 2015;40:355–362.

Tran TM, Ivanusic JJ, Hebbard P, Barrington MJ. Determination of spread of injectate after ultrasound-guided transversus abdominis plane block: a cadaveric study. *Br J Anaesth*. 2009;102:123–127.

7.2. What data are there for truncal blocks in abdominal surgery?

TAP blocks have now been studied extensively for a variety of surgery types and approaches. In fact, at the time of this writing, there are 12 reviews and meta-analyses on the subject, as well as many other studies with diverse and sometimes conflicting results.

One of the earliest clinical studies on TAP blocks was conducted by McDonnell and colleagues in 2007. Patients undergoing large bowel resection were randomized to standard care with morphine PCA or to standard care plus TAP block. The TAP group had reduced pain scores at all time points and reduced 24-hour morphine use.

Of the 12 review articles, a modest reduction in pain scores and reduced morphine use postoperatively were the most consistent findings. One review found a reduction in pain scores at rest but not with movement. Another study found reductions in pain scores at 2 and 6 hours postoperatively but not at 24 hours. A reduction in PONV and other opioid-mediated side effects were found in some studies, but this was less consistent. The magnitude of benefit seems to vary depending on surgery type. Overall, TAP blocks were found to be beneficial in colorectal surgery, cesarean section, cholecystectomy, hysterectomy, appendectomy, donor nephrectomy, retropubic prostatectomy, and bariatric surgery. A 2011 meta-analysis that studied several of these surgery types found the strongest benefit in cesarean section and colon surgery. Interestingly, when TAP blocks were compared with intrathecal morphine injection in cesarean sections, intrathecal morphine outperformed TAP blocks with regard to pain score and postoperative morphine use, although with some increase in itching and nausea. Regarding laparoscopic colorectal surgery, a 2015 study by Smith and colleagues found that there was not a significant reduction in pain scores or morphine consumption; however, a 2014 prospective study with more than 200 cases found that adding a TAP block to an enhanced recovery program facilitated a shorter LOS with low readmission and reoperation rates compared with previous series. The difference in these findings might relate to the degree of invasiveness of surgical approach, the total dose of local anesthetic used, the approach to the TAP plane taken by the regionalist, and patient factors.

In 2015, Jakobssen and colleagues summarized previous reviews with the addition of new data. They found that reduced opioid consumption appears to be the most consistent overall finding, even more than a modest and inconsistent reduction in pain scores. These beneficial effects seemed to be more pronounced with preincision blocks (compared with after surgery), more posterior approaches to the TAP plane, and a higher overall dose of local anesthetic. There were no significant complications in this or any of the other reviews, underscoring the safety of this intervention.

Further Reading

de Oliveira CM, Issy AM, Sakata RK. Intraoperative intravenous lidocaine. *Rev Bras Anestesiol.* 2010;60:325–333.

Jakobsson J, Wickerts L, Forsberg S, Ledin G. Transversus abdominal plane (TAP) block for postoperative pain management: a review. *F1000Res.* 2015 Nov 26;4. pii: F1000 Faculty Rev-1359.

Keller DS, Ermlich BO, Delaney CP. Demonstrating the benefits of transversus abdominis plane blocks on patient outcomes in laparoscopic colorectal surgery: review of 200 consecutive cases. *J Am Coll Surg.* 2014;219:1143–1148.

McDonnell JG, O'Donnell B, Curley G, Heffernan A, Power C, Laffey JG. The analgesic efficacy of transversus abdominis plane block after abdominal surgery: a prospective randomized controlled trial. *Anesth Analg.* 2007;104:193–197.

Mishriky BM, George RB, Habib AS. Transversus abdominis plane block for analgesia after Cesarean delivery: a systematic review and meta-analysis. *Can J Anaesth.* 2012;59:766–778.

Petersen PL, Mathiesen O, Torup H, Dahl JB. The transversus abdominis plane block: a valuable option for postoperative analgesia? A topical review. *Acta Anaesthesiol Scand.* 2010;54:529–535.

Ripolles J, Mezquita SM, Abad A, Calvo J. Analgesic efficacy of the ultrasound-guided blockade of the transversus abdominis plane: a systematic review. *Braz J Anesthesiol.* 2015;65:255–280.

Siddiqui MR, Sajid MS, Uncles DR, Cheek L, Baig MK. A meta-analysis on the clinical effectiveness of transversus abdominis plane block. *J Clin Anesth.* 2011;23:7–14.

Smith SR, Draganic B, Pockney P, et al. Transversus abdominis plane blockade in laparoscopic colorectal surgery: a double-blind randomized clinical trial. *Int J Colorectal Dis.* 2015;30:1237–1245.

Zhao X, Tong Y, Ren H, et al. Transversus abdominis plane block for postoperative analgesia after laparoscopic surgery: a systematic review and meta-analysis. *Int J Clin Exp Med.* 2014;7:2966–2975.

7.3. Discuss the quadratus lumborum block compared with the original approaches to the transversus abdominis plane

Over the course of what is currently a 15-year history with TAP blocks, much debate has occurred regarding the actual dermatomal spread and clinical effectiveness of single-shot TAP blocks, as mentioned earlier in this chapter. The notion that the classic TAP block produces variable results may have been what led Blanco to describe a different ultrasound-guided "no pops" technique in 2007, which many consider to be the origin of the quadratus lumborum block. An MRI contrast study was conducted in healthy volunteers to assess the spread of injectate based on these different approaches to the TAP plane. Carney et al. found that when fluid was injected posteriorly, at the lateral border of the quadratus lumborum muscle, spread along its anterior surface toward the paravertebral space was seen. The craniocaudal spread in this plane was found to reach from T4 to L1. This is in contrast to the midaxillary line approach, where spread was more anterior and seen only from T12 to L2. This prompted Kadam to publish a case report where he administered a block with this technique and obtained T8 to L1 dermatome, as well as very little postoperative pain and opioid use for the first postoperative day. Murouchi, Iwasaki, and Yamakage performed quadratus lumborum block in 11 patients undergoing ovarian surgery with general anesthesia and found that the duration of analgesia from bilateral quadratus lumborum block exceeded 24 hours, which is significantly longer than what is typically observed for TAP blocks. They also found that this block seemed to affect the T7 to T12 dermatome, which would suggest greater spread than classic TAP placement, as well as lower peak ropivacaine serum concentrations compared with a standard TAP block. These authors also proposed that the enhanced spread and duration of blockade may likely be due to local anesthetic spread toward the paravertebral space, perhaps allowing this peripheral nerve block to act as if it were an "indirect paravertebral block." Further confirmation of this mechanism is likely warranted; however, this approach to regional analgesia of the abdominal wall has a significant amount of promise in colorectal surgery.

Further Reading

Blanco R. Tap block under ultrasound guidance: the description of a no pops technique: 271. *Reg Anesth Pain Med.* September–October 2007;32(5):Suppl. 1, p 130.

Carney J, Finnerty O, Rauf J, Bergin D, Laffey JG, McDonnell JG. Studies on the spread of local anaesthetic solution in transversus abdominis plane blocks. *Anaesthesia.* 2011;66:1023–1030.

El-Boghdadly K, Elsharkawy H, Short A, Chin KJ. Quadratus lumborum block nomenclature and anatomical considerations. *Reg Anesth Pain Med.* 2016;41:548–549.

Kadam VR. Ultrasound guided quadratus lumborum block or posterior transversus abdominis plane block catheter infusion as a post-operative analgesic technique for abdominal surgery. *J Anaesthesiol Clin Pharmacol.* 2015;31:130–131.

Murouchi T, Iwasaki S, Yamakage M. Quadratus lumborum block: analgesic effects and chronological ropivacaine concentrations after laparoscopic surgery. *Reg Anesth Pain Med.* 2016;41:146–150.

7.4. Compare the risk versus benefits of the TAP block versus thoracic epidural analgesia

TAP injections and other truncal blocks may work well in ERAS pathways where early ambulation, minimization of catheterization, and minimization of opioid exposure are key metrics. Of course, one must consider the surgical intervention and the patient's coexisting medical problems when evaluating the risks and benefits of either. Any contraindication of a thoracic epidural would allow for discussion concerning truncal injections as an alternative to opioid therapy alone. Single-injection bilateral and multilevel TAP infiltration is better than opioid alone with regard to reducing overall opioid consumption and PONV and the severity of pain after abdominal surgery. When thoracic epidural is compared with continuous wound infiltration in open abdominal surgery, thoracic epidural has shown the benefit of improved VAS scores, improved functional recovery, and a decreased LOS of 1.5 days on average. When thoracic epidurals are compared with opioid therapy in laparoscopic colorectal surgery, epidurals may not show a benefit in reducing LOS, extending return of bowel function, or hastening PO intake. TAP infiltration compared with opioids in laparoscopic colorectal surgery has demonstrated benefits of decreased opioid consumption and shorter hospital LOS. Although TAP blocks may cause less hypotension than epidurals, TEA still offers superior pain control for open surgeries and, in the case of colorectal cancer, may offer a survival benefit. In 2012, a case cohort study of 42,000 patients undergoing resection of colon cancer showed that 5-year survival was greater in those who received epidural analgesia in combination with general anesthesia versus general anesthesia alone (61% vs. 55%). Furthermore, a subgroup analysis of the Veterans Affairs Cooperative Study Number 345 showed that adding epidural analgesia supplementation to general anesthesia in patients having surgery for colorectal cancer was associated with enhanced survival in patients without metastasis through 1.46 years. As expected, patients with metastasis at the time of surgery did worse, and epidural analgesia was not enough to overcome this predictor of poor outcome. Suggested mechanisms of the possible survival benefit include increased splanchnic blood flow via reduced sympathetic tone, preserved immune function, less frequent VTE due to a reduction in the surgical stress response, and reduced surgical site infections.

In summary, it seems prudent to consider developing procedure-specific analgesic pathways with the goals of reducing opioid consumption, providing adequate analgesia, and working toward reducing complications and LOS, while improving patient satisfaction.

Further Reading

Christopherson R, James KE, Tableman M, Marshall P, Johnson FE. Long-term survival after colon cancer surgery: a variation associated with choice of anesthesia. *Anesth Analg.* 2008;107:325–332.

Cummings K, Xu F, Cummings LC, Cooper GS. A comparison of epidural analgesia and traditional pain management effects on survival and cancer recurrence after colectomy: a population-based study. *Anesthesiology.* 2012;116:797–798.

Favuzza J, Brady K, Delaney CP. Transversus abdominis plane blocks and enhanced recovery pathways: making the 23-h hospital stay a realistic goal after laparoscopic colorectal surgery. *Surg Endosc.* 2013;27:2481–2486.

Johns N, O'Neill S, Ventham NT, Barron F, Brady RR, Daniel T. Clinical effectiveness of transversus abdominis plane (TAP) block in abdominal surgery: a systematic review and meta-analysis. *Colorectal Dis.* 2012;14:e635–e642.

Jouve P, Bazin JE, Petit A, et al. Epidural versus continuous preperitoneal analgesia during fast-track open colorectal surgery: a randomized controlled trial. *Anesthesiology.* 2013;118:622–630.

Neudecker J, Schwenk W, Junghans T, Pietsch S, Bohm B, Muller JM. Randomized controlled trial to examine the influence of thoracic epidural analgesia on postoperative ileus after laparoscopic sigmoid resection. *Br J Surg.* 1999;86:1292–1295.

Senagore AJ, Delaney CP, Mekhail N, Dugan A, Fazio VW. Randomized clinical trial comparing epidural anaesthesia and patient-controlled analgesia after laparoscopic segmental colectomy. *Br J Surg.* 2003;90:1195–1199.

8. Other Multimodal Analgesic Interventions

8.1. How might intrathecal morphine be used in abdominal surgery, and how would its benefits compare with those of other analgesic methods?

The mechanism of opioid analgesia can be divided into central and peripheral effects. In the spinal cord, there are several areas where opioid receptors are known to exist. The substantia gelatinosa in the dorsal horn of the spinal cord is the primary area of effect. Here, opioids act on either side of nerve synapses where substance P release from the primary sensory neuron is inhibited by opioids. Other areas of the central nervous system include the amygdala, the mesencephalic reticular formation, the periaqueductal gray, and the rostroventral medulla. The roles that opioids have in these locations are less clear, but they may be summarized by saying that ascending nerve signals are inhibited and descending signals are modulated. Placing opioids intrathecally can reduce local anesthetic–mediated side effects by selectively attenuating dorsal horn nociceptive signaling tracts without affecting motor, proprioceptive, and sympathetic pathways.

For colorectal surgery, intrathecal morphine has been shown to provide improved analgesia compared with intravenous PCA alone. This modality spares the sympathetic blockade and hypotension that can be seen with epidural analgesia but does still come with the risk for pruritus, nausea, sedation, urinary retention, and respiratory depression with an initial peak of 1 hour and a delayed peak of 6 to 12 hours. This last complication is typically monitored with 24 hours of continuous pulse oximetry. Intrathecal morphine is therefore not a good option for patients who may be candidates for same-day discharge. As for assessing what role intrathecal morphine could have in an enhanced recovery for colorectal surgery program, there are few reports in the literature thus far, with the exception of a 2012 study by Wongyingsinn et al., who found that adding a mixture of intrathecal bupivacaine and morphine to an already established enhanced recovery protocol for laparoscopic colorectal surgery improved pain scores but did not significantly reduce other recovery outcomes.

Further Reading

Beaussier M, Weickmans H, Parc Y, et al. Postoperative analgesia and recovery course after major colorectal surgery in elderly patients: a randomized comparison between intrathecal morphine and intravenous PCA morphine. *Reg Anesth Pain Med.* 2006;31:531–538.

Devys JM, Mora A, Plaud B, et al. Intrathecal + PCA morphine improves analgesia during the first 24 hr after major abdominal surgery compared to PCA alone. *Can J Anaesth.* 2003;50:355–361.

Ecoffey C. Spinal opiates. *Middle East J Anaesthesiol.* 1990;10:413–422.

Fukuda K. Opioid analgesics. In: Miller R, ed. *Miller's Anesthesia.* 8th ed. Philadelphia, PA: Elsevier; 2015:864–914.

Wongyingsinn M, Baldini G, Stein B, Charlebois P, Liberman S, Carli F. Spinal analgesia for laparoscopic colonic resection using an enhanced recovery after surgery programme: better analgesia, but no benefits on postoperative recovery: a randomized controlled trial. *Br J Anaesth.* 2012;108:850–856.

8.2. What other multimodal options are available if neuraxial or regional anesthesia is contraindicated?

According to the American Pain Society Guidelines for the Management of Postoperative Pain, there are 32 different recommended pain interventions that can be considered a part of a comprehensive, multimodal approach to managing postoperative acute pain. Half of these are in some way medication related, and the other half are related to education, monitoring, or nonpharmacologic interventions. A summary of possible therapies includes the use of multimodal analgesia, the avoidance of the intramuscular route of delivering of pain medications, giving opioids via the intravenous route, considering intravenous PCA when appropriate, scheduled acetaminophen, the use of NSAIDs if there are no contraindications, adding pregabalin or gabapentin, considering ketamine for adjunctive NMDA receptor antagonism, the consideration of a lidocaine infusion, site-specific peripheral nerve blockade with or without a catheter, local wound infiltration, or neuraxial local anesthetics or opioids. Interestingly, decreasing sympathetic outflow via alpha-2 agonism was not mentioned other than adding clonidine to peripheral nerve blocks to prolong the duration of action, but clonidine or dexmedetomidine could be considered for an opioid-sparing effect as well. In current perioperative practice, a lidocaine infusion, subanesthetic ketamine, gabapentinoids, intravenous or oral acetaminophen, NSAIDs, and dexmedetomidine are all common approaches if central or peripheral nerve blockade is not an option.

Further Reading

Arain SR, Ruehlow RM, Uhrich TD, Ebert TJ. The efficacy of dexmedetomidine versus morphine for postoperative analgesia after major inpatient surgery. *Anesth Analg.* 2004;98:153–158.

Chou R, Gordon DB, de Leon-Casasola OA, et al. Management of postoperative pain: a clinical practice guideline from the American Pain Society, the American Society of Regional Anesthesia and Pain Medicine, and the American Society of Anesthesiologists' Committee on Regional Anesthesia, Executive Committee, and Administrative Council. *J Pain.* 2016;17:131–157.

8.3. Discuss the use of intravenous lidocaine infusions with regard to mechanism of action, pharmacology, side effects, and safety and indications for use; specifically, how they may be beneficial for colorectal surgery. Review some of the available literature on the effectiveness of this intervention

Lidocaine is an amide local anesthetic that interrupts nerve transmission via sodium channel blockade. It is intuitive that this drug tends to have this effect when placed in close proximity to a nerve; however, how it works systemically to achieve analgesia and have an opioid-sparing effect is less clear. Part of its systemic mechanism may still be sodium channel blockade, but others have proposed it may work via a decrease in excitatory amino acids, decreased interleukins, decreased substance P, less proliferation and less activation of new sodium channels, NMDA receptor blockade, decreased central sensitization, sympathetic blockade, and/or a systemic anti-inflammatory effect. Whatever the mechanism, interest in using this infusion perioperatively has increased in recent decades, with many studies reporting reduced pain scores, reduced opioid use, and a pro-motility gastrointestinal effect.

Rimback et al. studied intravenous lidocaine in 30 patients undergoing open cholecystectomy and evaluated postoperative bowel function with radiopaque contrast. The group that received intravenous lidocaine had significantly better bowel function as determined by imaging. These patients also had lower pain scores, lower opioid use, and faster convalescence. The authors proposed the following possible mechanistic reasons for their findings: excitatory effect on gut smooth muscle as a direct effect, and indirect effect via decreased opioid requirements, blockade of sympathetic innervation, decreased catecholamines, and anti-inflammatory effect.

Subsequent to Rimback's study, Groudine and colleagues found increased patient satisfaction and reduced hospital stay in addition to pain and ileus reduction in patients having open prostatectomy. A decade later, Kaba and colleagues added that besides the previously mentioned effects, patients required less volatile anesthetic intraoperatively when anesthetic depth was titrated to processed EEG, and also that pain reduction extended to include dynamic pain (pain while walking and deep coughing), which was noted to improve and enhanced recovery protocol. Another group of investigators also found that these benefits may extend well into the postoperative period. They ran lidocaine until 1 hour after surgery was completed and found that pain with movement and morphine use was less for up to 72 hours after surgery and that these benefits were actually most pronounced on the third day. They hypothesized that this effects may be due to the prevention of the induction of central sensitization and hyperalgesia. In 2015, however, a Cochrane Review was conducted on all lidocaine infusion articles to date and concluded that this intervention has an impact on pain scores in the early (1–4 hours) and intermediate (24 hours) postoperative range but not for the late time range (48 hours). The review also looked at data on other outcomes such as time to first flatus (reduced by 5.49 hours), time to first bowel movement (reduced by 6.12 hours), and risk of ileus (relative risk 0.38). There was also a positive effect on opioid requirements, nausea, and reduced hospital stay.

In 2016, Eipe, Gupta, and Penning reviewed these data and researched the knowledge base that all prescribing clinicians should be familiar with. The most common dosing strategy seems to include a 1- to 2-mg/kg bolus (a maximum of 100 mg) over 1 minute if given in the operating room, or over 4 minutes if given in a less-monitored area such as a surgical floor. The infusion can then proceed at 1 to 2 mg/kg/h. Without the bolus dose, plasma levels do not reach a therapeutic range for 4 to 8 hours. Lidocaine is broken down by the liver, with some metabolites being excreted renally. Therefore, intact hepatic function, hepatic blood flow, and renal function reduce the risk of toxicity, and the converse of these calls for a reduction in dose and increased monitoring. Patients with heart failure or conduction abnormalities such as heart block are also at increased risk. Acidosis, hypoxia, and hypercarbia can also increase the risk of toxicity. However, despite these risks, intravenous lidocaine infusion has appeared to be very safe when dosed correctly. An infusion running for 3 days has a context-sensitive half-life of 20 to 40 minutes. Most cases of toxicity are likely due to error in dose, delivery, programmed infusion delivery, or failure to reduce the dose when premonitory central nervous system toxicity symptoms appear or when the infusion is run at higher doses on high-risk patients. A dose of 1.5 mg/kg/h is likely safe for many patients without significant organ impairment. At the center where this review was conducted, anesthesiologists and pain practitioners were able to run these infusions for several days, even on the surgical floor for American Society of Anesthesiologists (ASA) Physical Status score ASA-1 and ASA-2 patients. They noted a 20% to 25% reduction in opioid requirements within 24 hours of using intravenous lidocaine in this setting. The reader is referred to this review for the exact protocol and further decision-making on the level of care most appropriate for individual patients on lidocaine infusions.

In conclusion, there is a significant amount of evidence to support the outcomes of reduced pain scores both at rest and with movement, reduced opioid and volatile anesthetic consumption, earlier return of bowel function, increased patient satisfaction, and reduced hospital stay when this therapy is used as a part of an enhanced recovery program for abdominal surgery. TEA may still outperform intravenous lidocaine in open surgery, but when epidural analgesia is contraindicated or refused, or when the case is likely to be laparoscopic, intravenous lidocaine should be considered for its anti-inflammatory, antihyperalgesic, and pro-peristaltic properties.

Further Reading

Butterworth J, Mackey DC, Wasnick JD. *Morgan & Mikhail's Clinical Anesthesiology*. 5th ed. New York, NY: McGraw-Hill; 2013:263–276.

de Oliveira CM, Issy AM, Sakata RK. Intraoperative intravenous lidocaine. *Rev Bras Anestesiol.* 2010;60:325–333.

Eipe N, Gupta S, Penning J. Intravenous lidocaine for acute pain: an evidence-based clinical update. *BJA Educ.* 2016;16:292–298.

Groudine SB, Fisher HA, Kaufman RP Jr., et al. Intravenous lidocaine speeds the return of bowel function, decreases postoperative pain, and shortens hospital stay in patients undergoing radical retropubic prostatectomy. *Anesth Analg.* 1998;86:235–239.

Kaba A, Laurent SR, Detroz BJ, et al. Intravenous lidocaine infusion facilitates acute rehabilitation after laparoscopic colectomy. *Anesthesiology*. 2007;106:11–18; discussion 15–16.

Koppert W, Weigand M, Neumann F, et al. Perioperative intravenous lidocaine has preventive effects on postoperative pain and morphine consumption after major abdominal surgery. *Anesth Analg.* 2004;98:1050–1055.

Kranke P, Jokinen J, Pace NL, et al. Continuous intravenous perioperative lidocaine infusion for postoperative pain and recovery. *Cochrane Database Syst Rev.* 2015(7):CD009642.

Rimback G, Cassuto J, Tollesson PO. Treatment of postoperative paralytic ileus by intravenous lidocaine infusion. *Anesth Analg.* 1990;70:414–419.

Sun Y, Li T, Wang N, Yun Y, Gan TJ. Perioperative systemic lidocaine for postoperative analgesia and recovery after abdominal surgery: a meta-analysis of randomized controlled trials. *Dis Colon Rectum.* 2012;55:1183–1194.

8.4. How do lidocaine infusions compare to other techniques?

At the time of this writing, there are two studies known to the authors that compared intravenous lidocaine infusion with TEA. Kuo et al. randomized 60 patients undergoing open colonic surgery to TEA, intravenous lidocaine infusion, or placebo. The amount of lidocaine given in the epidural or in the intravenous infusion was the same. The TEA group experienced better pain control, earlier return of bowel function, and lower levels of inflammatory cytokines than the other 2 groups. Although these results redemonstrate that TEA is the gold standard analgesic method for open surgery, intravenous lidocaine was better than placebo for all of the same outcomes.

The second study that made such a comparison was done in laparoscopic colorectal surgery, with both interventions being done as a part of an enhanced recovery protocol and allowing for morphine PCA as a rescue analgesic method. These investigators did not find a difference in return of bowel function or consumption of diet, although those in the epidural group who had rectal surgery were noted to have better pain control. This work shows that in the case of laparoscopic surgery, similar enhanced recovery outcomes can be achieved with intravenous lidocaine infusion as can be attained with epidural analgesia. This is consistent with current ERAS guidelines suggesting the use of TEA for open abdominal surgeries and recommending against it for laparoscopic surgery.

There was a proposed trial comparing intravenous lidocaine infusion to TAP block described as forthcoming in 2014, but final published results from this early report are not yet available. To our knowledge, as of yet there are no other studies comparing these 2 methods; such prospective comparisons, however, would be clinically useful.

Further Reading

Dewinter G, Van de Velde M, Fieuws S, D'Hoore A, Rex S. Transversus abdominis plane block versus perioperative intravenous lidocaine versus patient-controlled intravenous morphine for postoperative pain control after laparoscopic colorectal surgery: study protocol for a prospective, randomized, double-blind controlled clinical trial. *Trials.* 2014;15:476.

Gustafsson UO, Scott MJ, Schwenk W, et al. Guidelines for perioperative care in elective colonic surgery: Enhanced Recovery After Surgery (ERAS®) Society recommendations. *World J Surg.* 2013;37:259–284.

Kuo CP, Jao SW, Chen KM, et al. Comparison of the effects of thoracic epidural analgesia and i.v. infusion with lidocaine on cytokine response, postoperative pain and bowel function in patients undergoing colonic surgery. *Br J Anaesth.* 2006;97:640–646.

Wongyingsinn M, Baldini G, Charlebois P, Liberman S, Stein B, Carli F. Intravenous lidocaine versus thoracic epidural analgesia: a randomized controlled trial in patients undergoing laparoscopic colorectal surgery using an enhanced recovery program. *Reg Anesth Pain Med.* 2011;36:241–248.

8.5. Can lidocaine infusions be used with another regional technique?

According to a recent *British Journal of Anaesthesia* review article from a center with several years of extensive experience in intravenous lidocaine infusions, it is recommended that any regional anesthesia technique involving a bolus of local anesthetic be temporally separated from intravenous lidocaine infusion by 4 to 8 hours. The authors suggest that if an epidural infusion was previously running and there has not been a bolus or test dose given, an intravenous lidocaine infusion could start sooner than that interval, but with no lidocaine bolus dose given. Recall from the earlier section that plasma steady state of lidocaine will not be reached then for several hours. Local anesthetic systemic toxicity is the obvious concern with using a lidocaine infusion in combination with another technique involving sodium channel blockade. We avoiding the use of another regional technique such as epidural, TAP, quadratus lumborum, or paravertebral block at the beginning or end of a case when a lidocaine infusion can also be used intraoperatively. One technique or the other should be chosen, using the best available data to tailor analgesia specifically to one's patient.

Further Reading

Eipe N, Gupta S, Penning J. Intravenous lidocaine for acute pain: an evidence-based clinical update. *BJA Educ.* 2016;16:292–298.

8.6. Describe how subanesthetic doses of ketamine (bolus vs. infusion) might be used in abdominal surgery

Ketamine is an NMDA receptor antagonist that at subanesthetic doses may have advantages such as analgesia, opioid reduction, and reduction in pro-inflammatory cytokine levels. For decades, evidence has associated both hyperalgesia and opioid tolerance with NMDA receptor activation. Also, ketamine may have an additive effect with opioid analgesia in subanesthetic doses. Because the acute pain that comes with large incisional abdominal surgery, and even smaller laparoscopic incisions, is not well treated with opioids alone, it seems reasonable to use multiple pharmacologic mechanisms to help better manage this acute postoperative pain prior to incisional trauma.

Further Reading

Mao J, Price DD, Mayer DJ. Mechanisms of hyperalgesia and morphine tolerance: a current view of their possible interactions. *Pain.* 1995;62:259–274.

Suzuki M, Tsueda K, Lansing PS, et al. Small-dose ketamine enhances morphine-induced analgesia after outpatient surgery. *Anesth Analg.* 1999;89:98–103.

9. Analgesia Safety Considerations

9.1. What are the financial implications of a single or multiple postoperative complications for patients presenting for surgery?

Inpatient hospitalization accounts for as much as one-third of healthcare expenditures in the United States, with 21% coming from surgical hospital stays. The financial implications of negative postoperative events can be a significant cost to the healthcare system. LOS increases alone can produce a hefty financial burden on payers and hospitals. According to the American Hospital Association, in 2015, the average cost of a hospital day was $2346 for a not-for-profit hospital, $1,798 for a for-profit hospital, and $1,974 for a state/government hospital.

Complications can be stratified by organ system and may include wound (infection), pulmonary (pneumonia/prolonged intubation), cardiac (myocardial infarction), central nervous system (stroke), and urinary (urinary tract infection), to name a few. A study by Boltz et al. reviewed National Surgical Quality Improvement Program data from a major academic institution over a 2-year period to estimate the effect of complications on LOS, as well as the effect on cost for single to multiple complications in general and vascular patients. The study found that the average LOS for surgery patients was 5.5 days, and the average cost was $14,839. For patients with 1 postoperative complication, the LOS was increased by 2.59 days on average, and the cost was increased by an average of $6358. For 2 postoperative complication events, the LOS was increased by 5.18 days, and the average cost increased by $12,082. For 3 or more complications, the average LOS increased by 10.99 days, and the average cost increased by $42,790.

Further Reading

American Hospital Association. 1999–2015 American Hospital Association Annual Survey Database. 2017. www.ahadataviewer.com/additional-data-products/AHA-Survey/. Accessed May 20, 2017.

Boltz MM, Hollenbeak CS, Ortenzi G, Dillon PW. Synergistic implications of multiple postoperative outcomes. *Am J Med Qual.* 2012;27:383–390.

Gonzalez JM. *National Health Care Expenses in the U.S. Civilian Noninstitutionalized Population, 2011.* Rockville, MD: Agency for Healthcare Research and Quality; 2013.

9.2. Describe potential opioid-related adverse events in postoperative pain management. What are the potential costs of any such events?

Opioid-related adverse events (ORAEs) seem to increase in parallel with the total dose of perioperative opioid used. Considerations for the impact this might have on an individual patient should include contexts such as anticipated pain tolerance, comorbidities, ASA physical status, metabolism and clearance as they relate to hepatic and renal function, and genetic and psychosocial factors. Examples of ORAE include respiratory depression/respiratory arrest, ileus, insomnia, hallucinations, constipation, nausea/vomiting, pruritus, urinary retention, and delirium, to name a few—not to mention the risk of future addiction and potential hyperalgesia effects in some patients. Studies around ORAE have examined both incidence and cost. ORAEs in the surgical population have a significant effect on overall cost and LOS. It has also been demonstrated that patients experiencing an ORAE have significantly increased median total hospital costs (7.4% increase) and increased median LOS (0.5 days) versus patients who did not experience an ORAE, with the highest incidence of ORAE occurring in those undergoing general surgery (26%), orthopedics (23%), and gynecologic surgery (22%).

When postoperative ileus and opioid use have been examined, there has been a demonstrable effect on cost and LOS. Patients with ileus receiving opioids had an increased LOS ranging from 4.8 to 5.7 days, a total cost increase from $9945 to $13,055, and a 30-day all-cause readmission rate 2.3% to 5.3% higher compared with patients without ileus.

Further Reading

Gan TJ, Robinson SB, Oderda GM, Scranton R, Pepin J, Ramamoorthy S. Impact of postsurgical opioid use and ileus on economic outcomes in gastrointestinal surgeries. *Curr Med Res Opin.* 2015;31:677–686.

Oderda GM, Said Q, Evans RS, et al. Opioid-related adverse drug events in surgical hospitalizations: impact on costs and length of stay. *Ann Pharmacother.* 2007;41:400–406.

9.3. Describe the incidence of PSP in the United States and its potential financial burden on society

A study by Macrae et al. published in the *British Journal of Anaesthesia* in 2008 compared the incidence of CPSP from a variety of surgeries. It also compared the incidence of CPSP between the United Kingdom and the United States. In that review, surgeries with the highest rates of CPSP were thoracotomy, mastectomy, abdominal surgery (including hernia), amputation, and cardiac surgery, with incidences as high as 50% in some groups.

A more recent review from Simanski et al. in 2014 looked once again retrospectively at the incidence of CPSP. That study found that the most frequently cited pain sites were joint (49.4%), incisional/scar (37.7%), and nerves (33.7%). It seems that CPSP can occur from any type of surgery, although some may have a higher anticipated incidence.

In terms of the financial burden of CPSP, it may be difficult to produce an exact number, although the Centers for Disease Control and Prevention? (CDC) has examined this in some detail. Generally, the costs can be categorized as indirect or incremental costs include the cost of healthcare due to CPSP, and indirect costs include extrapolated costs from decreased productivity associated with lost days and hours of work, as well as lower wages. One article by Gaskin and Richard in the *Journal of Pain* in 2012 suggested that the annual cost of chronic pain in the United States was estimated to be between $560 and $635 billion in 2010.

Further Reading

Gaskin DJ, Richard P. The economic costs of pain in the United States. *J Pain*. 2012;13:715–724.

Macrae WA. Chronic post-surgical pain: 10 years on. *Br J Anaesth*. 2008;101:77–86.

Simanski CJ, Althaus A, Hoederath S, et al. Incidence of chronic postsurgical pain (CPSP) after general surgery. *Pain Med*. 2014;15:1222–1229.

9.4. Compare the incidence of death from prescription opioid abuse versus other illicit drugs

According to the CDC, since 2000, the United States has seen a 137% increase in the rate of deaths due to drug overdoses and a 200% increase in the rate of overdose deaths that involve opioids (prescription opioids and heroin). There are increases not only in drug-related overdose deaths but also specifically in opioid-related overdose deaths. In 2014, a total of 47,055 deaths occurred in the United States that were related to drug overdose. That represented a 6.5% increase from the year prior, to about 14.7 per 100,000 people. In terms of opioid-related deaths, the CDC reported that 61% (28,647) of those drug overdose deaths in 2014 involved some type of opioid, including heroin. Therefore, opioid overdose deaths increased to 9.0 per 100,000 people in 2014, representing a 14% increase from the previous year.

Further Reading

Rudd RA, Aleshire N, Zibbell JE, Gladden RM. Increases in drug and opioid overdose deaths: United States, 2000–2014. *Morbid Mortal Week Rep*. 2016;64:1378–1382.

Thoracic Surgery in the Elderly Patient

Melanie Donnelly and Elizabeth Wilson

13

Case Scenario

An 85-year-old man presents for a left upper lobectomy for mass found to be non-small-cell lung cancer on biopsy. He has a history of chronic obstructive pulmonary disease, chronic renal insufficiency (baseline creatinine 1.4), and chronic low back pain.

The patient received a preoperative epidural that was utilized throughout the case. His postoperative pain regimen consists of a continuous thoracic epidural with 0.0625% bupivacaine + 10 mcg/mL hydromorphone, and PRN oral oxycodone and scheduled acetaminophen.

1. Patient Considerations

1.1. What are the challenges to performing an accurate pain assessment in the elderly?

The approach to pain management in the elderly patients differs from that in younger patients. The challenges to accurate assessment of pain in the elderly include the following:

1. Presence of concurrent illnesses and comorbidities
2. Tendency of the elderly to underreport pain
3. Potential for cognitive impairment impacting perception of pain
4. Ability of the patient to effectively communicate pain symptoms

Differences in reporting pain may be attributable to a range of factors, including cultural or religious beliefs, cognitive impairment, or misbeliefs that pain is something to be endured, that pain is a normal part of aging, or that strong analgesics lead to addiction. Some elderly patients may underreport pain because they believe that complaining about pain is a sign of personal weakness, they think physicians are too busy to hear their complaints, or they do not want to be viewed as "bad" patients.

Effective postoperative pain management begins with a comprehensive assessment using self-reporting as the gold standard. It is important to allow older people sufficient time to process and answer open-ended questions when self-reporting pain. Several tools are available to assist in the assessment. Quantitative assessments of pain include the Visual Analogue Scale (VAS), the Faces Pain Scale (FPS), the Verbal Rating Scale (VRS), and the Numerical Rating Scale (NRS). While all of these scales have been validated for use in the elderly, FPS and VRS have shown good reliability in several studies and may be preferred by elderly patients. Qualitative assessments such as the Brief Pain Inventory (BPI) and the Pain Disability Index (PDI) have also been validated for use in the elderly.

Pasero and McCaffery developed the Hierarchy of Pain Assessment Techniques for patients who are unable to self-report. The recommended stepwise approach includes the following:

1. Attempt self-report
2. Search for potential causes of pain
3. Observe patient behaviors
4. Reporting by proxy
5. Attempt analgesic trial

Self-reporting should be attempted regardless as research has shown that many patients with mild to moderate cognitive impairment are able to report pain. In nonverbal patients, successful communication can possibly be achieved through alternative methods of communication such as hand gestures or eye blinking. Physical exam can be used to search for potential causes of pain such as a decubitus ulcer. With respect to observed behaviors, a prospective observational study revealed that facial grimacing was the highest-frequency behavior observed in both cognitively intact and cognitively impaired older adults. When report by proxy is used, it is important to recognize that several studies have suggested healthcare providers tend to underestimate pain severity, whereas relatives of the patient perceive greater pain severity than reported by the patient. Finally, if all else fails, an analgesic trial with a low-dose analgesic should be attempted. A successful analgesic trial involves understanding that the initial low dose may not be enough to elicit a change in behavior.

Further Reading

Catananti C, Gambassi G. Pain assessment in the elderly. Surgical Oncology. 2010 Sep 30;19(3):140–148.

Herr K. Pain assessment strategies in older patients. Journal of Pain. 2011 Mar 31;12(3):S3–S13.

Herr K, Coyne PJ, Key T, Manworren R, McCaffery M, Merkel S, Pelosi-Kelly J, Wild L. Pain assessment in the nonverbal patient: position statement with clinical practice recommendations. Pain Management Nursing. 2006 Jun 30;7(2):44–52.

Kappesser J, Williams AC. Pain estimation: asking the right questions. Pain. 2010 Feb 1;148(2):184–187.

Pasero C. Challenges in pain assessment. Journal of PeriAnesthesia Nursing. 2009 Feb 28;24(1):50–54.

Pasero, C., & McCaffery, M. Pain assessment and pharmacologic management. St. Louis: Mosby, 2011.

1.2. How do the physiologic changes of aging affect pain management in elderly patients?

There are several changes in the elderly related to physiology, pharmacodynamics, pharmacokinetics, and processing of nociceptive information that may influence the effectiveness of postoperative pain control. In addition, drug-to-drug interactions resulting from polypharmacy and drug-to-disease interactions combine to make elderly patients more sensitive to adverse events associated with medications, all of which must be considered in drug selection.

Table 13.1 highlights the physiologic changes of aging and potential consequences related to anesthesia and analgesia in the perioperative setting.

Further Reading

Atkinson TJ, Fudin J, Pandula A, Mirza M. Medication pain management in the elderly: unique and underutilized analgesic treatment options. Clinical Therapeutics. 2013 Nov 30;35(11):1669–1689.

Hanna MN, Murphy JD, Kumar K, Wu CL. Postoperative pain management in the elderly undergoing thoracic surgery. Thoracic Surgery Clinics. 2009 Aug 31;19(3):353–361.

Jaklitsch M, Billmeier S. Preoperative evaluation and risk assessment for elderly thoracic surgery patients. Thoracic Surgery Clinics. 2009 Aug 31;19(3):301–312.

1.3. Is creatinine a reliable measure of renal function in the elderly?

Renal aging is a multifactorial process where gender, race, genetic background, and several key mediators such as chronic inflammation, oxidative stress, the renin-angiotensin-aldosterone system, impairment in kidney repair capacities, and

Table 13.1:
Physiologic changes in the elderly

System	Changes in Elderly Patients	Anesthetic Implications
Neurologic	↓ Neuronal and neurotransmitter density and activity and in the number of neurotransmitter receptor sites Neuronal loss in the autonomic nervous system (Sympathetic Nervous System and Peripheral Nervous System)	↓ Anesthetic requirements for both regional and general anesthesia Change in all forms of perception ↓ Response to cardiovascular reflexes Possible ↓ in intensity of pain perception (experimental) but ↑ response to higher-intensity noxious stimuli ↑ Incidence of postoperative cognitive dysfunction ↑ Risk for postoperative delirium
Cardiovascular	↓ Arterial compliance ↓ Cardiac output ↓ Myocardial response to catecholamines ↑ Risk of valvular dysfunction and pathology ↓ Cardiac reserve with decreased ability to tolerate perioperative demands	Hypovolemia or decreased sympathetic response following epidural anesthesia ↑ Incidence of ischemia, congestive heart failure, atherosclerotic disease
Gastrointestinal	↓ Decrease in first-pass activity ↓ Liver mass and hepatic perfusion Slower transit time Altered biotransformation and metabolism of drugs	↑ Systemic bioavailability of drugs ↓ Plasma drug clearance ↑ Duration of action for drugs
Immune function	↓ Immune responsiveness	↑ Incidence of perioperative infections
Musculoskeletal Metabolic	↓ Total body water ↓ Lean body mass ↑ Body fat ↓ Body heat production ↓ Thermoregulatory vasoconstriction	Leading to ↓ peak plasma drug concentrations Leading to changes in distribution and redistribution, altering clearance and elimination; fat-soluble drugs like fentanyl have higher volume of distribution whereas water-soluble drugs like morphine have lower volume of distribution
Pulmonary	↓ Chest wall compliance ↓ Pulmonary reserve ↓ Vital capacity ↓ FEV1 ↑ Residual volume Blunted respiratory response to both hypoxic and hypercapnic insults	↑ Incidence of chest wall rigidity ↑ V/Q mismatch with increased respiratory rate ↑ Sensitivity to narcotics, muscle relaxants, and supine positioning ↑ Risk of respiratory infection (due to waning immune responses; risk increases if concurrent tobacco use leading to bronchial mucociliary dysfunction)
Renal	↓ Renal mass ↓ Glomerular filtration rate ↓ Accuracy of calculating GFR ↓ Renal blood flow	↓ Drug excretion ↑ Drug duration of action ↑ Risk of accumulation of toxic substances or active metabolites

background cardiovascular disease play a significant role. Renal function is widely assessed on the basis of the level of serum creatinine, which mainly results from the balance between muscle mass catabolism and renal excretion. Due to the reduction in muscle mass that occurs with normal aging, the rate of creatinine production islower; therefore, the reference range for creatinine considered normal in the general population is inappropriately high in the elderly. Serum values in the upper normal range may underlie early renal dysfunction. At the third decade of life, glomerular filtration rate (GFR) peaks at approximately 140 mL/min/1.73 m^2 and, from then on, progressively declines to an approximate rate of 8 mL/min/1.73 m^2 per decade. This fall in creatinine clearance (Ccr) is accompanied by a decrease in creatinine production (senile sarcopenia), and consequently serum creatinine does not increase with the progressive decrease in GFR. Thus, more reliable GFR estimates should be employed whenever indicated; however, no single method may be satisfactory. For example, timed creatinine clearance, serum creatinine-based equations such as the Modification of Diet in Renal Disease (MDRD) formula, or serum cystatin C can be utilized. The MDRD formulas for GFR estimation, although mathematically complex, are now being readily used by most laboratories. Several variations (aMDRD, MDRD6, and MDRD7) have been developed, with the most precise formulas based on 6 variables: age, gender, BUN, albumin, race, and body surface area (BSA).

MDRD7 formula:

$$\begin{aligned}\text{Estimated GFR (mL/min/1.73 m}^2) = {} & (170 \times [\text{serum creatinine (mg/dL)}] - 0.999 \times [\text{age (years)}] - [0.176 \text{ if woman}] \\ & \times [1.18 \text{ if African American}] \times \text{BUN (mg/dL)}] - 0.170 \\ & \times [\text{albumin (g / dL)}] + 0.318) \text{ to give result in mL / min} \times \text{BSA}/1.73\end{aligned}$$

Chronic kidney disease is defined as either kidney damage or GFR <60 mL/min/1.73 m^2 for greater than 3 months. Kidney damage is defined as pathologic abnormalities or markers of damage, including abnormalities in blood or urine tests or imaging studies.

Further Reading

Bolignano D, Mattace-Raso F, Sijbrands EJ, Zoccali C. The aging kidney revisited: a systematic review. Ageing Research Reviews. 2014 Mar 31;14:65–80.

Cockcroft DW, Gault MH. Prediction of creatinine clearance from serum creatinine. Nephron. 1976 Jul 1;16(1):31–41.

Fliser D. Assessment of renal function in elderly patients. Current Opinion in Nephrology and Hypertension. 2008 Nov 1;17(6):604–608.

Kimmel PL, Lew SQ, Bosch JP. Nutrition, ageing and GFR: is age-associated decline inevitable? Nephrology Dialysis Transplantation. 1996 Jan 1;11(suppl 9):85–88.

Musso CG, Oreopoulos DG. Aging and physiological changes of the kidneys including changes in glomerular filtration rate. Nephron Physiology. 2011 Aug 10;119(suppl. 1):1–5.

Table 13.2:
Stages of Chronic Kidney Disease

Stage	Description	GFR (mL/min/1.73 m^2)
1	Kidney damage with normal or ↑ GFR	≥90
2	Kidney damage with mild ↓ GFR	60–89
3	Moderate ↓ GFR	30–59
4	Severe ↓ GFR	15–29
5	Kidney failure	<15 (or dialysis)

1.4. How does this patient's renal insufficiency impact your decisions regarding what medications to use to treat the patient's pain?

The presence of CKD, with or without dialysis, alters the pharmacokinetics and pharmacodynamics of many analgesics and most opioids and needs to be considered carefully. Caution must be used for pain management in elderly patients with renal dysfunction with respect to NSAIDs or any medications that have reliance on renal clearance and active metabolites. Overall, recommendations for pain management in patients with chronic kidney disease include utilizing lower doses with longer intervals, adjusting based on GFR or creatinine clearance.

A modified version of the World Health Organization analgesic ladder was created for patients with CKD and adapted from Konicicki et al. The following is an example of suggested pain regimens for patients with stage 4 CKD:

Stage 1: For mild pain (a score of 1–3 on the numeric pain scale), recommendations include acetaminophen 650 mg every 6 hours as needed; all other NSAIDs have been removed. While limited trials of NSAIDs for patients on dialysis have been published, NSAIDs should be avoided and in rare cases used with extreme caution for elderly patients or patients with CKD.

Stage 2: For moderate pain (a score of 4–6 on the numeric pain scale), recommendations would be to add a weak opioid such as tramadol 25 mg every 12 hours or low-dose oxycodone 2.5 to 5 mg every 4 to 5 hours as needed. Tramadol has a favorable profile for elderly patients, with lower risk of misuse and addiction.

Stage 3: Severe pain (pain score of 7–10 on the numeric pain scale) includes narcotics such as hydromorphone 1 mg PO every 6 hours or fentanyl patch 12.5 to 25 mcg every 72 hours. It is important to note that the dose titration of a fentanyl patch should not occur prior to 72 hours after initial use. It is equally important to recognize that absorption is limited in patients with low muscle mass. An alternative would be to increase the dose of oxycodone.

Further Reading

Barakzoy AS, Moss AH. Efficacy of the World Health Organization analgesic ladder to treat pain in end-stage renal disease. Journal of the American Society of nephrology. 2006 Nov 1;17(11):3198–3203.

Koncicki HM, Unruh M, Schell JO. Pain management in CKD: a guide for nephrology providers. American Journal of Kidney Diseases. 2017 Mar;69(3):451-460.

1.5. Describe why caution needs to be exercised when using and dosing NSAIDs, benzodiazepines, and opioids in the elderly patient

Use of NSAIDs in the elderly population, beyond that seen in the general population, is complicated by the substantial risks for gastrointestinal bleeding, ulcerations, perforations, nephrotoxicity, and cardiovascular morbidity and mortality. In 2006, the Food and Drug Administration issued a warning concerning the co-administration of aspirin and NSAIDs (both traditional and selective) due to the antiplatelet effect. Evidence of adverse cardiovascular outcomes in a placebo-controlled trial was found with the selective COX-2 inhibitor rofecoxib in 2004, resulting in its withdrawal from the market. More recently, however, the PRECISION trial compared the cardiovascular safety of celecoxib, naproxen, or ibuprofen in patients with arthritis. At moderate doses (200 mg/d), celecoxib was found to be noninferior to ibuprofen or naproxen in regard to cardiovascular safety.

Some researchers have explored the option of topical NSAIDs to avoid the unwanted systemic effects. A Cochrane Systematic Review from 2016 showed that topical diclofenac and topical ketoprofen can provide good levels of pain relief in osteoarthritis for a minority of people, but there is no evidence for other chronic painful conditions.

With respect to benzodiazepines and opioids, it has been shown that elderly patients may be more sensitive to their effects due to a decrease in the number of receptors or affinity of the receptors for neurotransmitters. In addition, physiologic changes of aging (see Table 13.1) such as decreased lean body mass and increased adipose tissue can lead to fat-soluble drugs such as fentanyl or diazepam having a larger volume of distribution, whereas water-soluble drugs such as morphine have a smaller volume of distribution.

Further Reading

Aubrun F, Marmion F. The elderly patient and postoperative pain treatment. Best Practice & Research Clinical Anaesthesiology. 2007 Mar 31;21(1):109–127.

Derry S, Conaghan P, Da Silva JA, Wiffen PJ, Moore RA. Topical NSAIDs for chronic musculoskeletal pain in adults. Cochrane Database Systematic Review. 2016 Apr 22;4:CD007400

Food and Drug Administration. FDA public health advisory: safety of Vioxx. September 30, 2004. www.fda.gov/ Drugs/DrugSafety/ PostmarketDrugSafety InformationforPatientsandProviders/ ucm106274.htm.

Nissen SE, Yeomans ND, Solomon DH, Lüscher TF, Libby P, Husni ME, Graham DY, Borer JS, Wisniewski LM, Wolski KE, Wang Q. Cardiovascular safety of celecoxib, naproxen, or ibuprofen for arthritis. New England Journal of Medicine. 2016 Dec 29;375:2519–2529.

1.6. What specific opioid class medications should be avoided in patients with diminished renal function and why?

In patients with reduced renal function, there is a risk of reduced clearance, prolonged half-life, and potential presence of active metabolites that can accumulate, leading to unwanted effects. Opioids such as codeine, hydrocodone, and tapentadol all have been shown to have reduced clearance and increased half-life in patients with CKD. With respect to active metabolites, morphine and meperidine are well known for adverse outcomes such as central nervous system (CNS) and respiratory depression secondary to an active metabolite. Morphine is metabolized into morphine-6-glucuronide, which has been shown to accumulate in the cerebral spinal fluid of dialysis patients to a level 15 times that of patients with normal kidney function, leading to both CNS and respiratory depression. Normeperidine, the active metabolite of meperidine, has a prolonged half-life in decreased kidney function, with adverse effects such as myoclonus, altered mental status, and seizures.

Further Reading

American Geriatrics Society Panel on the Pharmacological Management of Persistent Pain in Older Persons. Pharmacological management of persistent pain in older persons. Pain Medicine. 2009 Sep 1;10(6):1062–1083.

Aubrun F, Marmion F. The elderly patient and postoperative pain treatment. Best Practice & Research Clinical Anaesthesiology. 2007 Mar 31;21(1):109–127.

Derry S, Conaghan P, Da Silva JA, Wiffen PJ, Moore RA. Topical NSAIDs for chronic musculoskeletal pain in adults. The Cochrane Library. 2016 Apr 22;4:CD007400.

Koncicki HM, Unruh M, Schell JO. Pain management in CKD: a guide for nephrology providers. American Journal of Kidney Diseases. 2017 Mar;69(3):451-460.

1.7. How would you adjust the dosing of oral pain medicines in elderly patients?

Because of pharmacokinetic and pharmacodynamic changes with aging, opioids should be started at the lower dose, about 25% to 20% of the dose given to younger patients. For elderly patients with renal or hepatic dysfunction, dose-escalation percentages should also be reduced. Dose escalation depends on the half-life of medications. In opioid-naive patients, the lowest dose is recommended. It is recommended to "start low and go slow" with titration, monitoring effectiveness of pain control, side effects, and tolerance. In addition, elderly patients are at increased risk for respiratory complications related to opioids due to a blunted response to hypoxia and hypercarbia.

Further Reading

Chau DL, Walker V, Pai L, Cho LM. Opiates and elderly: use and side effects. Clinical Interventions in Aging. 2008 Jan 1;3(2):273.
Clark PM. Pharmacologic pain management on the elderly cancer patient. In 26th Congress of the Oncology Nursing Society. 2001 May 17.

1.8. What additional history would you want to obtain in order to develop an appropriate postoperative pain plan for this patient (e.g., low back pain, narcotics)?

The elderly may be afflicted with a myriad of painful conditions, including osteoarthritis, degenerative joint disease, rheumatoid disorders, cancer, postherpetic neuralgia, fibromyalgia, and diabetic neuropathy. A thorough initial assessment of current pain management issues and concerns should be performed. A detailed history of current and prior analgesic medications use, including prescription, over-the-counter, alternative methods, and/or history of drug or alcohol abuse, in addition to the effectiveness of each medication, is valuable information that is necessary to formulate a successful postoperative pain regimen.

Prior history of opioid drug use for pain control before surgery could result in patients being tolerant before they even arrive in the operating room. As to the development of tolerance to side effects, not all opioid targets develop tolerance at the same rate and to the same degree (i.e., analgesia vs. respiratory depression). The opioid-tolerant patient is at an increased risk for respiratory depression. This *differential tolerance* may put patients at a significant risk.

In addition, recent studies have made it clear that continued exposure to opioids induces more than tolerance. It may also induce a degree of *hyperalgesia*, in which a patient develops increased sensitivity to both pain (hyperalgesia) and nonpainful stimuli (allodynia). Hyperalgesia is thought to be due to toxic metabolites of opioids and activation of NMDA receptors in the CNS. Whereas, in principle, tolerance can be overcome by increasing the opioid dose, hyperalgesia is made worse in the long run by increasing the opioid administration.

Further Reading

Chau DL, Walker V, Pai L, Cho LM. Opiates and elderly: use and side effects. Clinical Interventions in Aging. 2008 Jan 1;3(2):273.
Hayhurst CJ, Durieux ME. Differential opioid tolerance and opioid-induced hyperalgesia: a clinical reality. Anesthesiology. 2016 Feb;124(2):483-8

2. Surgical Factors

2.1. What is chronic postsurgical pain syndrome?

Chronic postsurgical pain syndrome (CPSP) is a condition in which pain attributable to a surgical procedure persists for at least 2 months following surgery, with all other causes having been examined and excluded. Postthoracotomy pain syndrome is the specific type of CPSP referring to pain along a thoracotomy incision site that persists for at least 2 months following surgery.

Some sources extend the time frame that defines CPSP out to 3 months.

Further Reading

Hetmann F, Kongsgaard UE, Sandvik L, Schou-Bredal I. Prevalence and predictors of persistent post-surgical pain 12 months after thoracotomy. Acta Anaethesiologica Scandinavica. 2015;59:740–748.
Shipton EA. The transition of acute postoperative pain to chronic pain: Part 1—Risk factors for the development of postoperative acute persistent pain. Trends in Anesthesia and Critical Care. 2014;4:67–70.

2.2. What factors are known to put patients at higher risk for CPSP?

A multitude of risk factors have been associated with the development of CPSP and are listed in the following table. These risk factors likely represent "vulnerability factors" that increase a person's risk of CPSP but do not predict the

Table 13.3:
Risk Factors for Developing CPSP

Preoperative	Pain condition in either surgical or nonsurgical location Female Younger age Lower education status Lower socioeconomic status
Intraoperative	Longer-duration surgery Site of surgery → increased risk with major limb amputation, thoracotomy, mastectomy, sternotomy Intraoperative nerve damage/resection
Postoperative	Increased severity of acute postoperative pain Unrelieved postoperative pain High postoperative use of analgesics Surgery performed in previously injured area (e.g., surgical procedure, radiation)

occurrence of CPSP in any one individual. Deumens et al. propose that the balance between vulnerability factors and resilience factors influences the impact of surgical intervention on the development of CPSP. They state that vulnerability factors are the risk factors for CPSP that range from patient-specific to surgery-specific factors, as shown in the table. Resilience factors are those that are protective and allow an individual to cope with adversity. These might protect against the development of CPSP. Resilience factors have not been studied extensively, though some literature suggests that dispositional optimism is one psychological trait that may exert some protection against the development of CPSP for patients having hernia surgery.

The factor most consistently associated with increased risk of CPSP is the intensity of acute pain postoperatively.

Further Reading

Deumens R, Steyaert A, Forget P, Schubert M, Lavand'homme P, Hermans E, De Kock M. Prevention of chronic postoperative pain: Cellular, molecular and clinical insights for mechanisms based treatment approaches. Progress in Neurobiology. 2013;104:1–37.

Shipton EA. The transition of acute postoperative pain to chronic pain: Part 1—Risk factors for the development of postoperative acute persistent pain. Trends in Anesthesia and Critical Care. 2014;4:67–70.

2.3. How common is CPSP?

The prevalence of CPSP differs by the location of surgery. It has been found that up to 63% of patients having lower-extremity or hip surgery experience CPSP, while up to 20% of patients having abdominal or pelvic surgery experience CPSP. Postoperative pain can evolve into chronic pain for up to 10% of patients having inguinal repair or cesarean section, for 20% to 30% of those having breast surgery, for 30% to 40% of patients having thoracotomies, and for 30% to 50% of patients having an extremity amputation or coronary artery bypass grafting.

Deumens et al. present data on the prevalence of postoperative pain from a different perspective based on postoperative time frames. For thoracotomy it is estimated that 71% of patients experience subacute pain that lasts for up to 3 months, 41% to 58% of patients experience chronic pain that lasts up to 12 months, and 25% to 33% of patients experience chronic pain that lasts for more than 12 months.

Further Reading

Deumens R, Steyaert A, Forget P, Schubert M, Lavand'homme P, Hermans E, De Kock M. Prevention of chronic postoperative pain: Cellular, molecular and clinical insights for mechanisms based treatment approaches. Progress in Neurobiology. 2013;104:1–37.

Leon-Casasola OL. A review of the literature on multiple factors involved in postoperative pain course and duration. Postgraduate Medicine. 2014;126(4):42–52.

2.4. Is there a genetic component to the development of CPSP?

Genetic alterations likely contribute to the phenotypic variation in the patient's experience of both acute and chronic pain following surgery because not all patients with the same group of classic risk factors develop CPSP. Genetic studies on chronic pain estimate that there may be a 50% heritability in conditions of chronic pain. There are thought to be many genetic variants and environmental factors or triggers that influence the development of chronic pain syndromes. The environment clearly plays a role in the pain phenotype expressed by individuals, as has been demonstrated in studies of monozygotic twins who developed different pain phenotypes. Epigenetics is the study of how environment and genetics interact to produce a certain phenotype. The epigenetic regulation of genes has been demonstrated to play a role in neck pain development in twins and in responses to opioids.

There are ongoing investigations into how genetics and epigenetics play a role in the development of chronic pain syndromes. These include studies examining the disease processes of fibromyalgia, osteoarthritis, and orofacial pain. Some genetic mutations have also been identified for reduction of pain intensity after mastectomy for individuals who carry certain genetic mutations.

Further Reading

Badiola IJ. Can chronic pain be prevented? Anesthesiology Clinics. 2016;34:303–315.

2.5. What are the concepts behind the generation of acute pain with this surgery and its evolution into a chronic pain condition?

Sources of painful stimuli after a thoracotomy include the site of surgical incision, disruption of the intercostal nerves, inflammation of chest wall structures near the incision, pulmonary tissues, and chest tube insertion sites. Somatic pain

Table 13.4:
Important Terms and Definitions

Term	Definition
Peripheral sensitization	Response of nociceptors to the inflammatory cascade, which results in a reduced excitation threshold of primary afferent terminals and increased responsiveness. The result also includes increased expression of substance P and calcitonin gene-related peptide within the superficial distal horn.
Central sensitization	"Afferent barrage" of central nervous system nociceptors from activation in response to surgery results in an alteration of central neurons in the dorsal horn; result includes an enhanced responsiveness to activation, reduced threshold for activation, expanded fields of reception, and spontaneous activity.
Allodynia	A consequence of central sensitization, pain experienced in an area due to a nonpainful stimulus.
Secondary hyperalgesia	A consequence of central sensitization, pain sensitivity extends beyond the area of primary injury to the outlying noninjured areas.
Primary hyperalgesia	Noxious stimuli perceived as more painful.

is mediated by the intercostal nerves; visceral pain from the mediastinum, diaphragm, and pleura via the vagus and phrenic nerves; ipsilateral shoulder pain referred via the phrenic. Damage to tissue of any kind leads to peripheral inflammation and a cascade of inflammatory mediator release. Direct nerve damage, as in the case of intercostal nerves during a thoracotomy, can lead to the development of neural degeneration, axonal sprouting, and formation of a neuromata. This can lead to persistent spontaneous nerve impulse generation, resulting in allodynia and hyperalgesia. The phrenic nerve is also involved in mediation of painful stimuli after chest surgery and has been difficult to mitigate with local anesthetic via epidural use but has been diminished with the use of an interscalene block or direct phrenic nerve block.

Acute pain begins with the transduction of mechanical, thermal, or chemical stimuli detected by peripheral nociceptors. Painful stimulus is detected by the C-fibers and Aδ-fibers. These free nerve endings don't simply receive and transmit this information; rather, the messaging of these nerves is modulated by inflammatory mediators at the site of tissue injury and is impacted by axonal release of substances as well. The inflammatory mediators released by injured tissue include histamine, cytokines, bradykinin, prostaglandins, and many others. As neutrophils and macrophages are attracted to the site of injury, they propagate the inflammatory response and set in place a positive feedback loop for the attraction of additional macrophages to the site of injury. These substances act upon the nociceptors to result in an increase in spontaneous activity, lowered activation threshold, and an increased and longer firing by the primary afferent neurons. The result is allodynia and hyperalgesia in that area of the body. If the painful stimulus is persistent, the Aδ-fibers will become increasingly excitable, resulting in peripheral sensitization. Centrally, there is an exposure to this persistent afferent input of painful stimuli from peripheral neurons resulting in central sensitization. These 2 processes contribute to the postoperative sensitivity state known as *spinal wind-up*. This term describes the condition that is responsible for the resulting decrease in pain threshold at both the site of activity and the surrounding tissue, otherwise known as *primary* and *secondary hyperalgesia*. When the macrophages arrive at the site of injury, early in the process, they can enter the nerve, since the blood-nerve barrier has been disrupted. This can result in sprouting of sympathetic nerve fibers around the dorsal horn, which can lead to neuropathic pain. Other immune cells, microglia, are also attracted to the site of injury and can switch on an "unrestrained gliosis," contributing to central sensitization.

Processes of pain generation are normally self-limited as the afferent inputs lessen, but in the development of CPSP there is a maladaptive state taking place that is not well understood. Persistent pain and inflammation likely play a role in the transition to chronic pain. Other factors that play a role in development of CPSP are related to the state of pain modulatory processes for individuals. Those with poor pain inhibitory systems are more likely to develop CPSP. Additionally, those with more vulnerability factors may also be at higher risk for CPSP.

Further Reading

Badiola, IJ. Can chronic pain be prevented? Anesthesiology Clinics. 2016;34:303–315.

Deumens R, Steyaert A, Forget P, Schubert M, Lavand'homme P, Hermans E, De Kock M. Prevention of chronic postoperative pain: Cellular, molecular and clinical insights for mechanisms based treatment approaches. Progress in Neurobiology. 2013;104:1–37.

Reuben SS, Yalavarthy L. Preventing the development of chronic pain after thoracic surgery. Journal of Cardiovascular and Vascular Analgesia. 2008;22(6):890–903.

Shipton EA. The transition of acute postoperative pain to chronic pain: Part 1—Risk factors for the development of postoperative acute persistent pain. Trends in Anesthesia and Critical Care. 2014;4:67–70.

2.6. What are the proposed mechanisms of action for some of the nonopioid analgesics used when treating patients with acute postsurgical pain, including after a thoracotomy?

Table 13.5:
Non-opioid Analgesic Medications

Medication	Sites of Action
IV nonsteroidal anti-inflammatories	• Reduce COX-mediated production of prostaglandins
Local anesthetics for blocks	• At level of placement, bind receptors in sodium channel, stop depolarization, and interrupt conduction of nerve impulse
Gabapentin/pregabalin	• Agonists for alpha2-delta 1 subunit of presynaptic calcium channels • Bind to the voltage-gated calcium channels and prevent release of pain-inducing neurotransmitters (e.g., glutamate, substance P, noradrenaline)
Ketamine	• Noncompetitive antagonism of NMDA receptors centrally • Activation of descending inhibitor pain pathways • Reduce central sensitization
Acetaminophen	• Works centrally, possibly by reducing central prostaglandin synthesis vs. serotonergic mechanisms vs. COX-3 receptor activity
Glucocorticoids	• Reduce inflammation

2.7. What are some of the negative consequences of inadequately treating postoperative pain after thoracic surgery?

When patients experience severe pain after a thoracotomy, they can also experience complications such as increased pulmonary complications, increased need for reintubation and mechanical ventilation, prolonged intensive care unit duration, extended hospital duration, delayed return of function for activities of daily living, decreased satisfaction, decreased mental and social functioning, and increased risk of developing chronic persistent postsurgical pain (postthoracotomy syndrome). Moderate to severe postoperative pain is believed to play an important role in the development of persisting postoperative pain.

Furthermore, inadequately controlled pain can increase postoperative morbidity as well as reduce quality of life and patient satisfaction.

Further Reading

Hetmann F, Schou-Bredal I, Sandvik L, Kongsgaard UE. Does chronic pre-operative pain predict severe post-operative pain after thoracotomy? A prospective longitudinal study. Acta Anaesthesiologica Scandinavica. 2013 Sep 1;57(8):1065–1072.

Kinney MA, Hooten WM, Cassivi SD, et al: Chronic post-thoracotomy pain and health-related quality of life. Annals of Thoracic Surgery. 2012;93:1242–1247.

Romero A, Enrique J, Garcia EL, Joshi GP. The state of the art in preventing post-thoracotomy pain. Seminars in Thoracic and Cardiovascular Surgery. 2013;25(2):116–124.

2.8. How can healthcare providers help mitigate the risk of CPSP when patient have high-risk procedures or multiple risk factors?

One of the risk factors most clearly associated with the development of CPSP is uncontrolled acute postoperative pain. For this reason, it is reasonable for a provider to aggressively treat acute postoperative pain using multimodal therapies. It is hoped that by disrupting the process of peripheral and central sensitization, and the resulting hyperalgesic states, this risk of CPSP can be lowered. There are not enough consistent data to strongly recommend one specific combination of analgesics, though placement of an epidural is the most consistently endorsed practice in reducing the risk of CPSP for patients having a thoracotomy. An epidural should be part of the patient's pain management plan if there are no contraindications. According to a Cochrane Review performed in 2013, epidural analgesia reduced the risks of persistent pain 6 months after an open thoracotomy, preventing CPSP in 1 in 4 patients treated.

Further Reading

Badiola, IJ. Can chronic pain be prevented? Anesthesiology Clinics 2016;34:303–315.

Maxwell C, Nicoara A. New developments in the treatment of acute pain after thoracic surgery. Current Opinion in Anesthesiology. 2014;27:6–11.

Reddi D. Preventing chronic postoperative pain. Anaesthesia. 2016;71(suppl 1):64–71.

Richardson J, Sabanathan S, Mearns AJ, et al. Post-thoracotomy neuralgia. Pain Clinics 1994;7:87–97.

Romero A, Enrique J, Garcia EL, Joshi GP. The state of the art in preventing post-thoracotomy pain. Seminars in Thoracic and Cardiovascular Surgery. 2013;25(2):116–124.

2.9. Would the addition of ketamine intraoperatively assist in reducing the risk of CPSP in this patient?

Ketamine has demonstrated utility in reducing acute postoperative pain and reducing opioid consumption. Evidence of a benefit in the prevention of CPSP after a thoracotomy is limited and conflicting.

Further Reading

Maxwell C, Nicoara A. New developments in the treatment of acute pain after thoracic surgery. Current Opinion in Anesthesiology. 2014;27(1):6–11.

Romero A, Enrique J, Garcia EL, Joshi GP. The state of the art in preventing post-thoracotomy pain. Seminars in Thoracic and Cardiovascular Surgery. 2013;25(2):116–124.

2.10. Would the addition of gabapentin or pregabalin be useful to reduce this patient's risk of CPSP?

Use of gabapentin and pregabalin has been shown to reduce acute postoperative pain and narcotic consumption, but their use has variable results on the incidence of CPSP. Some studies have shown benefit while others have not, and use of this type of drug has been shown to contribute to sedation postoperatively.

Further Reading

Romero A, Enrique J, Garcia EL, Joshi GP. The state of the art in preventing post-thoracotomy pain. Seminars in Thoracic and Cardiovascular Surgery. 2013;25(2):116–124.

2.11. What is the value of adding acetaminophen to this patient's analgesic regimen?

Acetaminophen has consistently been demonstrated to be a safe and effective analgesic with limited side effects when dosed appropriately. The use of this medication postoperatively has been shown to reduce pain scores and opioid requirements. For thoracic surgery, use of acetaminophen has been shown to reduce ipsilateral shoulder pain but has not demonstrated a reduction in the incidence of chronic pain.

Further Reading

Maxwell C, Nicoara A. New developments in the treatment of acute pain after thoracic surgery. Current Opinion in Anesthesiology. 2014;27:6–11.

Reddi D. Preventing chronic postoperative pain. Anaesthesia 2016;71(suppl 1):64–71.

Richardson J, Sabanathan S, Mearns AJ, et al. Post-thoracotomy neuralgia. Pain Clinics 1994;7:87–97.

Romero A, Enrique J, Garcia EL, Joshi GP. The state of the art in preventing post-thoracotomy pain. Seminars in Thoracic and Cardiovascular Surgery. 2013;25(2):116–124.

2.12. What is the role of regional anesthesia in reducing the risk of CPSP in thoracotomy patients?

While a recent Cochrane Review concludes that epidural analgesia for patients having a thoracotomy likely reduces the risk of chronic pain, the authors provide the caveat that this conclusion was reached with use of heterogeneous data that were not "high caliber." If, however, regional anesthesia does provide some protection from CPSP, how it does so is not clear. Some possible mechanisms include decreased nociceptive nerve impulse activity postoperatively; a reduction of changes in synaptic neuroplasticity in the CNS; and reduction of acute inflammatory mediators leading to less pain sensitization and acute postoperative pain. It is also possible that nerve blocks reduce chronic pain both by controlling pain in the acute postoperative phase (severe or unmanageable pain in this period being a key risk factor for development of CPSP) and by reducing opioid use and opioid-induced hyperalgesia.

Further Reading

Rivat C, Bollag L, Richebe P. Mechanisms of regional anesthesia protection against hyperalgesia and pain chronicization. Current Opinion Anesthesiology. 2013;26:621–625.

3. Regional Anesthesia/Postoperative Pain Management

3.1. How do epidurals versus paravertebral blocks/catheters compare in treating pain after a thoracotomy?

Epidurals have a long track record of being used to treat postthoracotomy pain and have been considered the gold standard analgesic for these types of cases. They provide excellent analgesia postoperatively and, according to a recent Cochrane Review, likely reduce the incidence of chronic postoperative pain as well.

A recent Cochrane Review in 2016 by Yeung et al. compared thoracic epidural blockade and paravertebral blockade in adults undergoing thoracotomy with respect to analgesic efficacy, the incidence of major and minor complications, hospital length of stay, and cost-effectiveness. The review looked at 14 studies with a total of 698 subjects. The results showed that paravertebral blockade reduced the risks of developing minor complications compared with thoracic epidural blockade and that paravertebral blockade was as effective as thoracic epidural in controlling acute pain. There were no differences in 30-day mortality, major complications, or length of hospital stay. There were insufficient data with respect to chronic pain and costs. The authors stress that the results of this review should be interpreted with caution due to the heterogeneity of the studies and lack of reliable evidence.

3.2. Describe the differences in major and minor complications that can be seen when using these 2 techniques

There are some basic differences between these techniques that result in different benefits and drawbacks. Epidurals are generally placed via a loss-of-resistance technique and not under any type of visualization. As such they have up to a 20% failure rate. Paravertebral blocks are considered a peripheral nerve block that may be done either by the surgeon under direct visualization or by an anesthesia provider using a landmark and/or ultrasound-guided percutaneous technique.

Side effects from thoracic epidural analgesia include hypotension, urinary retention, nausea and vomiting, and pruritus. Hypotension can also develop with the use of a thoracic paravertebral block, mainly happening with inadvertent epidural spread (4%–5%). Other side effects or complications that can occur with paravertebral block placement include pneumothorax and injection of local anesthetic intrathecally (larger dose than epidural potentially due to dosing considerations with this type of block).

The most devastating complications of epidural analgesia are epidural hematoma and epidural abscess, which on rare occasion may result in permanent neurologic deficits. Estimates of the incidence of epidural hematoma vary widely. Traditional estimates had been as low as 1 in 150,000 patients after placement of an epidural catheter, but newer evidence has suggested a significantly higher risk in certain populations. A study of 62,450 patients from centers participating in the Multicenter Perioperative Outcomes Group found an incidence of hematoma requiring surgical evacuation in nonobstetric patients of 1 in 8921. Unfortunately, are few investigations have examined the frequency and severity of hemorrhagic complications after peripheral nerve blockade, and none have focused on paravertebral blocks. Some providers treat paravertebral blockade similarly to an epidural in terms of the patient's anticoagulation status due to proximity to the neuraxis.

Further Reading

Bateman BT, Mhyre JM, Ehrenfeld J, et al. The risk and outcomes of epidural hematomas after perioperative and obstetric epidural catheterization: a report from the MultiCenter Perioperative Outcomes Group Research Consortium. Anesthesia and Analgesia. 2013;116:1380–1385.

Maxwell C, Nicoara A. New developments in the treatment of acute pain after thoracic surgery. Current Opinion in Anesthesiology. 2014;27:6–11.

Powell ES, Cook D, Pearce AC, et al. A prospective multicenter, observational cohort study of analgesia and outcome after pneumonectomy. British Journal of Anaesthesia. 2011;106:364–370.

Yeung JH, Gates S, Naidu BV, Wilson MJ, Gao Smith F. Paravertebral block versus thoracic epidural for patients undergoing thoracotomy. Cochrane Database Syst Rev. 2016 Feb 21;2:CD009121.

3.3. What is the benefit of using a paravertebral catheter for patients having thoracic surgery?

Powell et al. examined the use of paravertebral versus epidural catheters for pneumonectomy patients in a prospective, multicenter observational cohort trial. They found an increased incidence of clinically important major postpneumonectomy complications associated with thoracic epidural compared with paravertebral blockade analgesia. These complications included hypotension requiring an inotrope, arrhythmias requiring therapy, and respiratory complications requiring support. Previous reviews came to similar conclusions when comparing epidurals to paravertebral analgesia showing an increase in side effects with epidural analgesia, and that paravertebral analgesia was associated with less postoperative hypotension and fewer pulmonary complications.

While it is not clear in any of these studies why respiratory function appears to be improved with use of paravertebral analgesia versus epidural analgesia, one possible mechanism is the preservation of contralateral intercostal muscle function and decreased need for IV fluid resuscitation due to the lower incidence of hypotension. The Powell study, however, found that there was less IV fluid given to the epidural analgesia group in the first 24 hours when compared with the paravertebral group. Thus, the cause of these findings from these studies remains unknown.

Further Reading

Powell ES, Cook D, Pearce AC, et al. A prospective multicenter, observational cohort study of analgesia and outcome after pneumonectomy. British Journal of Anaesthesia. 2011;106:364–370.

3.4. What are the physiologic changes of aging that affect opioid metabolism?

The physiologic changes with aging related to drug metabolism include slowed gastrointestinal transit time, which can affect the rate of absorption. Changes in body composition, including a decrease in lean body and total body water and an increase in adipose tissue, affect the drug distribution. Lipophilic opioids such as fentanyl tend to have a greater volume of distribution and can take longer to be eliminated in the elderly patient with decreased lean body weight and increased body fat.

In general, opiates are rapidly absorbed in the gut, have a high rate of first-pass metabolism in the liver, are conjugated in the liver, have metabolites, and vary in distribution based on their differing protein affinity. In aging patients, decreased hepatic and renal blood flow can lead to both a slower metabolism and elimination of opioids. Additional impairments can occur with impaired phase I reactions, which include oxidation, hydroxylation, and dealkylation.

Further Reading

Tegeder I, Lotsch J, Geisslinger G. Pharmacokinetics of opioids in liver disease. Clinical Pharmacokinetics. 1999;37:17–40.

3.5. Does the use of a minimally invasive approach to this surgery reduce the risk of CPSP?

Video-assisted thoracic surgery is a minimally invasive approach to chest surgery and avoids the long incision of a thoracotomy. While there are benefits to this approach in terms of length of stay and acute pain, no differences have been observed in the incidence of CPSP in these patients when evaluated prospectively.

Further Reading

Badiola IJ. Can chronic pain be prevented? Anesthesiology Clinics. 2016;34:303–315.

Open Abdominal Aortic Aneurysm Repair

Danielle Cobb, Lori Dangler, and Albert Robinson III

14

Case Scenario

A 74-year-old man presents for a scheduled open abdominal aortic bifemoral bypass. He has hypertension, atrial fibrillation, moderate chronic obstructive pulmonary disease, diabetes, and depression. His current home medications include lisinopril, dabigatran (Pradaxa), metformin, fluticasone (Advair), and albuterol as needed. Due to extensive atherosclerosis, he has complained of increasing circumferential left leg pain over the last 2 months.

1. Medical Disease and Differential Diagnosis

1.1. What is the differential diagnosis of the circumferential left leg pain in this patient?

- Ischemic pain
- Diabetic neuropathy
- Deep vein thrombosis
- Orthopedic injury
- Cramping/muscle spasm
- Arthritis

A more detailed patient history will help refine the differential diagnosis. Questions to ask include: Does the patient have pain at rest? Does the pain get worse with activity and diminish with rest? Is the pain superficial and burning and stocking glove in distribution or deeper? Does the patient have decreased sensation in his lower legs? Given that his symptoms are unilateral and he has known extensive atherosclerosis, this patient is likely having claudication, which is pain caused by inadequate blood flow. Initially, the patient likely had deep pain in one area of the leg that progressed to circumferential pain as the atherosclerotic plaques evolved or ruptured. High blood pressure, smoking, elevated cholesterol, diabetes, and age older than 70 years are all risk factors for claudication. The progression of this patient's peripheral arterial disease will increasingly limit circulation, leading from claudication with activity to developing pain at rest (ischemic rest pain), poor wound healing, and a cool extremity. These symptoms can occur in any patient with lower extremity peripheral arterial occlusive disease, as well as in patients with other vascular conditions such as an atherosclerotic abdominal aortic aneurysm that obstructs blood flow or embolizes thrombotic debris to more distal arteries in the leg. An angiogram and Doppler blood flow studies would reveal the degree of and locations(s) of the arterial blood flow obstruction(s).

Further Reading

Meijer WT, Grobbee DE, Hunink MG, et al. Determinants of peripheral arterial disease in the elderly: the Rotterdam study. *Arch Intern Med*. 2000;160:2934–2938.

1.2. What is the epidemiology and the risk factors for abdominal aortic aneurysms? How do you manage patients presenting with concomitant AAA and arterial aortoiliac disease?

An abdominal aortic aneurysm (AAA) is an enlargement or dilatation of the aorta; it can affect any portion of the aorta but most often starts in the area between the inferior mesenteric artery and the renal arteries. The concern with AAA is that as it enlarges, it becomes potentially life-threatening due to the risk of its rupturing. An abdominal aorta is considered aneurysmal once it is larger than 3.0 cm. The etiology of an AAA is multifactorial. The main risk factors are advanced age, tobacco use, atherosclerosis, male sex, positive family history, and hypertension. The prevalence of AAAs is 4% to 8%. Interestingly, studies have shown that patients with an AAA and diabetes mellitus are believed to have less rapid aneurysm expansion; however, the exact mechanism for this association remains unknown. Data from the Centers for Disease Control and Prevention (CDC) reveal AAA to be the 15th leading cause of death in the 60- to 64-year-old age group based on an AAA rupture rate of 4.2 deaths per 100,000 people.

The clinical presentation of a patient with an AAA is variable. It can range from asymptomatic to acutely symptomatic, with a ruptured AAA requiring emergent intervention. Patients complain of and/or present with abdominal and/or back pain or other clinical manifestations, including fever, fatigue, malaise, and ischemic limb pain. Aortobifemoral bypass grafting is recommended for patients presenting with bilateral aortoiliac disease as it has been shown to be robust and lasting. Because of the proximal location of the occlusive aortoiliac disease and the potential for emboli to migrate distally down the peripheral arterial tree, aortobifemoral graft repair—open or endovascular if anatomically amenable—is indicated. At 5 years, the expected patency rate for aortoiliac disease following an aortobifemoral bypass is 85% to 90%.

Further Reading

Ashton HA, Buxton MJ, Day NE, et al. The Multicentre Aneurysm Screening Study (MASS) into the effect of abdominal aortic aneurysm screening on mortality in men: a randomised controlled trial. *Lancet*. 2002;360:1531–1539.

Ashton HA, Gao L, Kim LG, et al. Fifteen-year follow-up of a randomized clinical trial of ultrasonographic screening for abdominal aortic aneurysms. *Br J Surg*. 2007;94:696–701.

Brady AR, Thompson SG, Fowkes FG, et al. Abdominal aortic aneurysm expansion: risk factors and time intervals for surveillance. *Circulation*. 2004;110:16–21.

Centers for Disease Control and Prevention. Deaths, percent of total deaths, and death rates for the 15 leading causes of death in 5-year age groups, by race, and sex: United States, 2014. www.cdc.gov/nchs/data/dvs/lcwk1_2014.pdf.

Chaikof EL, Brewster DC, Dalman RL, et al. SVS practice guidelines for the care of patients with an abdominal aortic aneurysm: executive summary. *J Vasc Surg*. 2009;50:880–896.

Chaikof EL, Dalman RL, Eskandari MK, et al. The Society for Vascular Surgery practice guidelines on the care of patients with an abdominal aortic aneurysm. *J Vasc Surg*. 2018;67:2–77.e2.

Gerhard-Herman MD, Gornik HL, Barrett C, et al. 2016 AHA/ACC guideline on the management of patients with lower extremity peripheral artery disease: a report of the American College of Cardiology/American Heart Association Task Force on Clinical Practice Guidelines. *Circulation*. 2017;135:e726–e779.

Johnston KW, Rutherford RB, Tilson MD, et al. Suggested standards for reporting on arterial aneurysms: Subcommittee on Reporting Standards for Arterial Aneurysms, Ad Hoc Committee on Reporting Standards, Society for Vascular Surgery and North American Chapter, International Society for Cardiovascular Surgery. *J Vasc Surg*. 1991;13:452–458.

Kent KC, Zwolak RM, Egorova NN, et al. Analysis of risk factors for abdominal aortic aneurysm in a cohort of more than 3 million individuals. *J Vasc Surg*. 2010;52:539–548.

Kuivaniemi H, Elmore JR. Opportunities in abdominal aortic aneurysm research: epidemiology, genetics, and pathophysiology. *Ann Vasc Surg*. 2012;26:862–870.

Lederle FA, Johnson GR, Wilson SE, et al. The aneurysm detection and management study screening program: validation cohort and final results. Aneurysm Detection and Management Veterans Affairs Cooperative Study Investigators. *Arch Intern Med*. 2000;160:1425–1430.

Lederle FA, Wilson SE, Johnson GR, et al. Immediate repair compared with surveillance of small abdominal aortic aneurysms. *N Engl J Med*. 2002;346:1437–1444.

Lillvis JH, Lenk GM, Kuivaniemi H. Genetics of abdominal aortic aneurysms. In: Upchurch GR, Criado E, eds. *Aortic Aneurysms: Pathogenesis and Treatment*. Totowa, NJ: Humana Press; 2009:1–26.

Lindholt JS, Juul S, Fasting H, Henneberg EW. Screening for abdominal aortic aneurysms: single centre randomised controlled trial. *Br Med J*. 2005;330:750.

Moll FL, Powell JT, Fraedrich G, et al. Management of abdominal aortic aneurysms clinical practice guidelines of the European Society for Vascular Surgery. *Eur J Vasc Endovasc Surg*. 2011;41(suppl 1):S1–S58.

Newman AB, Arnold AM, Burke GL, et al. Cardiovascular disease and mortality in older adults with small abdominal aortic aneurysms detected by ultrasonography: The Cardiovascular Health Study. *Ann Intern Med*. 2001;134:182–190.

Norman PE, Jamrozik K, Lawrence-Brown MM, et al. Population based randomised controlled trial on impact of screening on mortality from abdominal aortic aneurysm. *Br Med J*. 2004;329:1259.

Norman PE, Powell JT. Abdominal aortic aneurysm: the prognosis in women is worse than in men. *Circulation*. 2007; 115:2865–2869.

Santilli SM, Littooy FN, Cambria RA, et al. Expansion rates and outcomes for the 3.0-cm to the 3.9-cm infrarenal abdominal aortic aneurysm. *J Vasc Surg*. 2002;35:666–671.

West CA Jr., Johnson LW, Doucet L, et al. A contemporary experience of open aortic reconstruction in patients with chronic atherosclerotic occlusion of the abdominal aorta. *J Vasc Surg*. 2010;52:1164–1172.

Zannetti S, L'Italien GJ, Cambria RP. Functional outcome after surgical treatment for intermittent claudication. *J Vasc Surg*. 1996;24:65–73.

1.3. How is pain differentially classified?

Pain is defined by the International Association for the Study of Pain (IASP) as "an unpleasant sensory and emotional experience associated with actual or potential tissue damage, or described in terms of such damage." Pain can be classified in multiple ways and is often unique to an individual patient. Pain can be also classified as acute versus chronic and as nociceptive versus neuropathic.

Acute versus chronic pain is differentiated based on timelines. Acute pain is typically associated with damage to a specific tissue and is therefore of a limited duration in time (e.g., <30 days), although specific times to classify as acute versus chronic vary. In contrast, chronic pain is continuous. Pain can further be classified as malignant (secondary to cancer) or nonmalignant. Acute pain ends with the resolution of the injury, whereas chronic pain continues beyond the standard healing time of a specific injury. Unfortunately, acute pain sometimes evolves into chronic pain if tissue injury and its accompanying pain are not adequately managed in the acute phase.

A second manner in which to classify pain is nociceptive versus neuropathic. Nociceptive pain stems from the stimulation of peripheral nociceptors and is typically transduced through Aδ-fibers and C-fibers. Nociceptive pain can be further broken down into visceral or somatic pain. Visceral pain is secondary to the insult of a visceral structure and is usually described as intense diffuse and is poorly localized. It may be accompanied by nausea and may cause a referred dermatomal pain. Neuropathic pain is secondary to damage to the nervous system, resulting in a maladaptive pathway. It is typically described as a spontaneous shooting or burning pain and is often associated with hyperalgesia and allodynia.

Further Reading

Carr DB, Goudas LC. Acute pain. *Lancet.* 1999;353:2051–2058.

Loeser, JD, Melzack R. Pain: an overview. *Lancet.* 1999;353:1607–1609.

Miller RD, ed. *Miller's Anesthesia.* Philadelphia, PA: Churchill Livingstone/Elsevier; 2010.

Stoelting RK, Hillier SC, eds. *Pharmacology and Physiology in Anesthetic Practice.* 4th ed. Philadelphia, PA: Lippincott Williams & Wilkins; 2005.

1.4. What is ischemia? What is ischemic pain, and what are the characteristics of ischemic pain?

Ischemia is an inadequate blood supply to an organ or certain part of the body due to an impediment in blood flow. This could be due to diseased arteries or vasospasm. Ischemic pain is the pain that results from ischemia. The most common symptom of peripheral arterial disease is intermittent claudication where patients have symptoms of pain, cramps, and/or fatigue in their lower extremities (calves, thighs, and buttocks) with exercise or walking. The pain is usually worse with activity and is typically relieved by rest; in its more advanced form, ischemic pain can also be present at rest and is frequently described as burning or aching. Often, there are nonhealing wounds present distally that represent insufficient blood supply that is causing the ischemia and ischemic pain. Most patients with peripheral artery disease are asymptomatic. About 10% to 30% present with classic intermittent activity-related claudication, and a minority progress to pain at rest or critical limb ischemia (ischemic ulcers). Critical limb ischemia results when the claudication pain becomes constant and can also result in chronic wounds and gangrene.

In addition to symptoms of ischemic pain, it is important for clinicians to evaluate for signs of ischemia in the lower extremities. Dependent rubor, early pallor on elevation of the extremity, reduced capillary refill, and the presence of wounds all suggest ischemic changes in an extremity.

Two commonly used criteria for classifying ischemia in peripheral arterial disease are the Fontaine Classification and the Rutherford Classification. The Rutherford Classification system describes these criteria in 7 stages:

0 = Asymptomatic
1 = Mild claudication
2 = Moderate claudication
3 = Severe claudication
4 = Rest pain
5 = Minor tissue loss
6 = Severe tissue loss or gangrene

Further Reading

Gerhard-Herman MD, Gornik HL, Barrett C, et al. 2016 AHA/ACC guideline on the management of patients with lower extremity peripheral artery disease: a report of the American College of Cardiology/American Heart Association Task Force on Clinical Practice Guidelines. *Circulation.* 2017;135:e726–e779.

Merriam-Webster Medical Dictionary. (n.d.). Medical terms and abbreviations: retrieved March 05, 2017. www.merriam-webster.com/medical.

Mills JL Sr. Update and validation of the Society for Vascular Surgery wound, ischemia, and foot infection threatened limb classification system. *Semin Vasc Surg*. 2014;27:16–22.

Rutherford RB, Baker JD, Ernst C, et al. Recommended standards for reports dealing with lower extremity ischemia: revised version. *J Vasc Surg*. 1997;26:517–538.

Varu VN, Hogg ME, Kibbe MR. Critical limb ischemia. *J Vasc Surg*. 2010:51:230–241.

1.5. What are the risk factors for developing ischemia and ischemic pain?

Ischemia and ischemic pain result from an inadequate blood supply to distal extremities. This occurs most frequently secondary to vessel narrowing from atherosclerosis. Atherosclerotic disease is characterized by lipid-filled plaques, smooth muscle cells, and inflammatory cells surrounded by a fibrous cap in the vascular system. Aortoiliac occlusive disease occurs when significant plaque builds up enough to block the iliac arteries. Peripheral arterial disease in the distal extremities is a highly prevalent atherosclerotic syndrome that affects approximately 10 million Americans.

Peripheral arterial disease itself is part of a systemic disease process that includes atherosclerosis, vascular inflammation (arteritis), degenerative diseases, dysplastic disorders, and thromboembolism. Additionally, aneurysmal disease and dissection can result in the occlusion of peripheral vessels, causing ischemia distal to the obstruction. Individuals at risk for lower extremity peripheral arterial disease include (1) age greater than 70; (2) age 50 to 69 with a history of diabetes or smoking; (3) age less than 50 with diabetes or one other atherosclerotic risk factor (smoking, hyperlipidemia, or hypertension); (4) known atherosclerotic coronary, carotid, or renal arterial disease; and (5) abnormal lower extremity pulse examination.

Further Reading

Gerhard-Herman MD, Gornik HL, Barrett C, et al. 2016 AHA/ACC guideline on the management of patients with lower extremity peripheral artery disease: a report of the American College of Cardiology/American Heart Association Task Force on Clinical Practice Guidelines. *Circulation*. 2017;135:e726–e779.

Hirsch AT, Hartman L, Town RJ, Virnig BA. National health care costs of peripheral arterial disease in the Medicare population. *Vasc Med*. 2008;13:209–215.

1.6. What is the mechanism of ischemic pain?

When an arterial system has a narrowing, an obstruction, or vascular reactivity resulting in diminished blood flow to the distal tissue and the blood supply cannot meet the metabolic demands of the tissues, it results in ischemia. The main cause of ischemic pain is tissue hypoxia, with the pain serving as a warning signal to alert the central nervous system about imminent tissue damage.

Ischemia results in hypoxic and acidotic tissues that release inflammatory and nociceptive mediators including substance P, bradykinin, histamine, serotonin, adenosine, and potassium. The presence of these mediators is transmitted as pain via the dorsal root ganglion into the central nervous system. This aspect of ischemic pain is classified as nociceptive pain. Chronic ischemia leads to changes in the endothelium that ultimately promote edema, free radical production, leukocyte adhesion, and inappropriate platelet activation. These changes can also promote the development of microthrombi, which further impair distal circulation. Degeneration of nerve endings secondary to ischemia can also then cause neuropathic pain, a second component of ischemic pain.

Further Reading

Baldeschi GC. Spinal cord stimulation in patients suffering from critical lower limb ischemia. International Neuromodulation Society. 2012. www.neuromodulation.com/scs-in-chronic-critical-limb-ischemia.

Gerhard-Herman MD, Gornik HL, Barrett C, et al. 2016 AHA/ACC guideline on the management of patients with lower extremity peripheral artery disease: a report of the American College of Cardiology/American Heart Association Task Force on Clinical Practice Guidelines. *Circulation*. 2017;135:e726–e779.
Vadivelu N, Urman RD, Hines RL, Kunnumpurath S. *Essentials of Pain Management*. New York, New York: Springer; 2011.
Varu VN, Hogg ME, Kibbe MR. Critical limb ischemia. *J Vasc Surg*. 2010:51:230–241.

1.7. What evaluation should be performed on this patient? What physical examination, tests, and/or indices are used to measure ischemia?

A complete medical history and physical examination should be performed when evaluating a patient for aortoiliac occlusive disease. The medical history should seek to obtain symptoms, how often symptoms occur, and risk factors. Cardiopulmonary status should be thoroughly assessed in the patient as at least 10% to 20% of patients with AAA have significant coronary artery disease (CAD) that may need to be addressed prior to an aortobifemoral repair. Physical examination should determine the presence or absence of extremity pulses. The absence of femoral arterial pulses indicates significant lesions in the aortoiliac arterial segment and the existence of a proximal obstruction. Arteriography and Doppler ultrasound of the blood vessels can help to assess the blood flow within the vessels.

The most common measurement used is the ankle-brachial index (ABI), which is a measure of the systolic blood pressure in the dorsalis pedis or posterior tibial artery (measured at the ankle) compared with the brachial artery. The traditional cutoff for "normal" is an ABI >0.9, with normal being 1.0 to 1.1. Ischemic pain or claudication normally occurs at an ABI of 0.5 to 0.8, with critical limb ischemia present at an ABI <0.4.

Systolic load pressure should normally be slightly higher in the ankles than in the arms in a supine patient. This is because the systolic pressure becomes amplified as blood moves distally secondary to retrograde wave reflection, adding to the antegrade wave in the setting of resistance in the distal arterioles. Additionally, the arterioles themselves become more stiff distally secondary to the thickening of the vascular walls from increased hydrostatic pressure associated with standing upright.

Further Reading

Aboyans V, Criqui MH, Abraham P, et al. Measurement and interpretation of the ankle-brachial index. *Circulation*. 2012;126:2890–2909.
Gerhard-Herman MD, Gornik HL, Barrett C, et al. 2016 AHA/ACC guideline on the management of patients with lower extremity peripheral artery disease: a report of the American College of Cardiology/American Heart Association Task Force on Clinical Practice Guidelines. *Circulation*. 2017;135:e726–e779.
Hertzer NR, Beven EG, Young JR, et al. Coronary artery disease in peripheral vascular patients: a classification of 1000 coronary angiograms and results of surgical management. *Ann Surg*. 1984;199:222–233.
Miller RD. *Miller's Anesthesia*. Philadelphia, PA: Churchill Livingstone/Elsevier; 2010.
Santilli JD, Santilli SM. Chronic critical limb ischemia: diagnosis, treatment, and prognosis. *Am Fam Physician*. 1999;59:1899–1908.
Zelenock GB, Huber TS, Messina LM, et al. *Mastery of Vascular and Endovascular Surgery*. Philadelphia, PA: Lippincott Williams & Wilkins; 2006.

1.8. How do you manage aortoiliac occlusive disease?

Aortoiliac occlusive disease management should include lifestyle change modifications to address/reduce modifiable risk factors that contribute to the disease process. It has been shown that there is a clear reduction in the progression of peripheral arterial disease and improved graft patency rates with smoking cessation. Medications such as blood thinners (e.g., aspirin, clopidogrel) should be strongly considered to lower the patient's risk of developing blood clots and to help slow the progression of the disease. Surgery will be necessary for patients who have severe aortoiliac occlusive disease and/or a concomitant disease process of aortoiliac occlusive disease and AAA. Aortobifemoral artery bypass restores blood flow to the legs through a patent Y-shaped synthetic fabric graft. The indications for aortic bifemoral bypass include atherosclerosis of the abdominal aorta or iliac arteries, aortic aneurysms involving the iliac arteries for which aortoiliac bypass cannot be performed, the presence of severe claudication symptoms, nonhealing ulcers in the extremities, and critical limb ischemia. Endovascular treatment for AAA and aortoiliac occlusive disease offers a faster recovery, reduced length of stay, less morbidity, and less postoperative pain.

Further Reading

Ameli FM, Stein M, Provan JL, Prosser R. The effect of postoperative smoking on femoropopliteal bypass grafts. *Ann Vasc Surg.* 1989;3:20–25.

Belch J, Topol EJ, Agnelli G, et al., Prevention of Atherothrombotic Disease Network: critical issues in peripheral arterial disease detection and management. *Arch Intern Med.* 2003;163:884–892.

Cronewett JL, Johnston KW, eds. *Rutherford's Vascular Surgery.* 8th ed. Philadelphia, PA: Saudners; 2014.

Dhaliqal G, Mukjerjee D. Peripheral arterial disease: epidemiology, natural history, diagnosis and treatment. *Int J Angiol.* 2007; 16:36–44.

Girolami B, Bernardi E, Prins MH, et al. Antithrombotic drugs in the primary medical management of intermittent claudication: a meta-analysis. *Thromb Haemost.* 1999;81:715–722.

Tierney S, Fennessy FM, Hayes DB. ABC or arterial and vascular disease: secondary prevention of peripheral vascular disease. *Br Med J.* 2000;320:1262–1265.

Zelenock GB, Huber TS, Messina LM, et al. *Mastery of Vascular and Endovascular Surgery.* Philadelphia, PA: Lippincott Williams & Wilkins; 2006.

2. Anticoagulation Guidelines and Neuraxial/Peripheral Intervention Techniques

2.1. What anesthetic techniques are possible for this open abdominal aortic bifemoral bypass?

Abdominal aortic bifemoral bypasses are typically performed under general anesthesia (with or without an epidural for perioperative analgesia), as these patients often have significant comorbidities regarding coronary artery disease, chronic obstructive pulmonary disease, hypertension, diabetes, and hyperlipidemia, and the surgery itself often results in significant intraoperative blood loss. It is important to recognize that in a patient who is receiving antithrombotic medication (dabigatran) and in whom neuraxial regional analgesia is being considered, the benefits (e.g., postoperative pain relief) and risks (e.g., epidural hematoma) must be carefully weighed.

Endovascular techniques to treat aortoiliac occlusive disease have been performed under local, loco-regional, and neuraxial technique, and early results compared with open repair are promising, but longer-term data are still needed. The data regarding endovascular aortic aneurysm repair for AAA with general, regional, and local/monitored anesthesia care show that patients who receive local/regional anesthesia instead of general anesthesia have lower morbidity and mortality, require less cardiovascular support, and have a shorter length of hospital stay.

Further Reading

Barash PG, Cullen BF, Stoelting RK, et al. *Anesthesia for Vascular Surgery: Clinical Anesthesia.* 7th ed. Philadelphia, PA: Lippincott; 2013.

Cronewett JL, Johnston KW, eds. *Rutherford's Vascular Surgery.* 8th ed. Philadelphia, PA: Saunders; 2014.

Edward MS, Andrews JS, Edwards AF, et al. Results of endovascular aortic aneurysm repair with general, regional, and local/monitored anesthesia care in the American College of Surgeons National Quality Improvement Program database. *J Vasc Surg.* 2011;54:1273–1282.

Kashyap VS, Pavkov ML, Bena JF, et al. The management of severe aortoiliac occlusive disease: endovascular therapy rivals open reconstruction. *J Vasc Surg.* 2008;48:1451–1457.

Munter Sellevold OF, de Hert S, Pelosi P. A major step forward: guidelines for the management of cardiac patients for non-cardiac surgery: the art of anaesthesia. *Eur J Anaesthesiol.* 2010:27:89–91.

Psacharopulo D, Ferrero E, Ferri M, et al. Increasing efficacy of endovascular recanalization with covered stent graft for TransAtlantic Inter-Society Consensus II D aortoiliac complex occlusion. *J Vasc Surg.* 2015;62:1219–1226.

Chaikof EL, Dalman RL, Eskandari MK, et al. Society for Vascular Surgery practice guidelines on the care of patients with an abdominal aortic aneurysm. *J Vasc Surg.* 2018;67:2–77.e2.

2.2. Does the fact that the patient has been on dabigatran at home affect your decision regarding using a neuraxial technique? What about other direct thrombin inhibitors (e.g., argatroban and bivalirudin)? What is the incidence of neurologic complications resulting from epidural bleeding in patients receiving antithrombotic therapy?

This patient has a history of atherosclerosis and atrial fibrillation and is symptomatic for claudication and is at risk for thromboembolism. Thus, he has been receiving dabigatran and is at increased risk for bleeding complications surrounding the abdominal aortic bifemoral bypass operation. It is important to recognize patients who are on medications that affect blood clotting so that timing of any neuraxial needle intervention and discontinuation of any relevant blood thinner(s) can be managed. Dabigatran is a direct thrombin inhibitor because of its mechanism of action that blocks thrombin formation. Only recently has the American Society of Regional Anesthesia and Pain Medicine (ASRA) made recommendations regarding direct thrombin inhibitors, given our limited experience with these drugs. The current recommended time interval before neuraxial needle or catheter placement for dabigatran is 5 days. Dabigatran has a half-life of 8 to 17 hours, and it is rational to delay 5 half-lives prior to spinal or epidural needle placement (5 half-lives is 97% elimination). The American Heart Association (AHA) also recommended a 5-day discontinuation of dabigatran for patients undergoing neuraxial needle catheter placement. Patients who are on these newer direct thrombin inhibitors who also have renal impairment—as is common in the population of patients with an AAA or in older adults—should have a longer time between taking medication and having an epidural or spinal placed. There are different published recommendations regarding the prudent timing between the performance of neuraxial procedures and the discontinuation of an anticoagulant. According to the European guidelines, the recommendation prior to neuraxial block for patients taking rivaroxaban, a factor Xa inhibitor drug, is that the medication should be discontinued 22 to 26 hours prior to placement of an indwelling catheter. The Scandinavian guidelines for rivaroxaban recommend a minimum of 18 hours as the interval between neuraxial procedure and discontinuation of an anticoagulant drug. The goal is to get to a low level of anticoagulant by waiting on the elimination of several drug half-lives in an effort to reduce the risk of bleeding and spinal hematoma. Apixaban, another oral factor Xa inhibitor used to treat nonvalvular atrial fibrillation, should be discontinued a minimum time of 48 hours or 2 days before neuraxial placement.

Direct thrombin inhibitor anticoagulants such as bivalirudin and argatroban are contraindicated and should be avoided while a neuraxial catheter is in place. A patient could receive a neuraxial needle placement after bivalirudin or argatroban discontinuation when a laboratory test confirms his or her activated partial thromboplastin time (aPTT) <40 sec or a direct thrombin inhibitor (DTI) assay is normal. At least 4 hours after the last dose of bivalirudin or argatroban should occur prior to attempting to removal a neuraxial catheter. This is due to the fact that the anticoagulant effect following intravenous administration of thrombin inhibitors may be present for 1 to 3 hours.

There has been an increase in the use of thrombolytic, anticoagulant, and antiplatelet medication therapies for thromboprophylaxis. Tirofiban, eptifibatide, and abciximab are platelet inhibitors that have a mechanism of action that inhibits von Willebrand factor and platelet binding that leads to limited platelet aggregation. For agents used for full systemic anticoagulation such as the glycoprotein IIb/IIIa receptor antagonists, tirofiban or eptifibatide, it has been recommended that at least 8 hours pass between the last dose of medication and any neuraxial technique. A time interval of at least 48 hours should be observed for abciximab before a neuraxial procedure.

The incidence of neurologic complications resulting from bleeding after a neuraxial needle or catheter placement or removal in patients receiving antithrombotic therapy remains unknown. The patient may experience numbness, lower extremity weakness, or complete motor loss due to a bleeding complication. From the literature, it is reported that the incidence of neurologic complications with spinal and epidural anesthetics is 1 in 220,000 and 1 in 150,000, respectively; however, these data are from thromboprophylaxis and antithrombolytic agents that are prior to our common modern drugs. It remains important for the clinician to be vigilant regarding the potential for a bleeding complication. Early detection is essential and helps to improve the possibility of recovery if diagnosis is made early and treatment is started.

Further Reading

Barash PG, Cullen BF, Stoelting RK, et al. *Anesthesia for Vascular Surgery: Clinical Anesthesia.* 7th ed. Philadelphia, PA: Lippincott; 2013.

Benzon HT, Avram MJ, Green D, Bonow RO. New oral anticoagulants and regional anaesthesia. *Br J Anaesth* .2013;111(suppl 1):i96–i113.

Breivik H, Bang U, Jalonen J, Vigfusson G, Alahuhta S, Lagerkranser M. Nordic guidelines for neuraxial blocks in disturbed haemostasis from the Scandinavian Society of Anaesthesiology and Intensive Care Medicine. *Acta Anaesthesiol Scand.* 2010;54:16–41.

Curvers J, Kerekhof D, Stroobants, AK, Dool E, Scharnhorst V. Measuring direct thrombin inhibitors with routing and dedicated coagulation assays: which assay is helpful? *Am J Clin Pathol.* 2012:134:551–558.

Di Nisio M, Middeldorp S, Buller HR. Direct thrombin inhibitors. *N Engl J Med.* 2005;352:1028–1040.

Gogarten W, Vandermeulen E, Van Aken H, et al. Regional anaesthesia and antithrombotic agents: recommendations of the European Society of Anaesthesiology. *Eur J Anaesthesiol.* 2010;27:999–1015.

Horlocher TT, Vandermeuelen E, Kopp SL, Gogarten W, Leffert LR, Benzon HT. Regional anesthesia in the patient receiving antithrombotic or thrombolytic therapy: American Society of Regional Anesthesia and Pain Medicine Evidence-Based Guidelines. (Fourth Edition). *Reg Anesth Pain Med.* 2018;43:263–309.

Eikelboom JW, Hirsh J, Spencer FA, Baglin TP, Weitz JI. Antiplatelet drugs: Antithrombotic Therapy and Prevention of Thrombosis, 9th ed: American College of Chest Physicians Evidence-Based Clinical Practice Guidelines. *Chest.* 2012 Feb;141(2 Suppl):e89S–e119S.

Thakkar RN, Rathbun SW, Wright SM. Role of direct oral anticoagulants in the management of anticoagulation. *South Med J.* 2017;110:293–299.

Tryba M. [Epidural regional anesthesia and low molecular heparin: Pro]. *Anasthesiol Intensivmed Notfallmed Schmerzther.* 1993; 28:179–181.

Wysokinski WE, McBane RD 2nd. Periprocedural bridging management of anticoagulation. *Circulation.* 2012;126:486–490.

2.3. Preoperatively, after the patient's dabigatran was discontinued, he was bridged for 5 days with intravenous unfractionated heparin due to his high risk of thromboembolism. He was brought to the block room for a preinduction epidural, but it was found that the systemic intravenous heparin was still infusing. Would you proceed with the epidural placement? If you delay the case, how long would you wait before you proceeded with placing the neuraxial catheter?

The guidelines for patients on antithrombotic medication presenting for regional anesthesia were published by ASRA. There is an increased risk of epidural hematoma in heparinized patients who have undergone neuraxial procedures. For intravenous therapeutic dosing of unfractionated heparin, a period of 2 to 4 hours since the administration of systemic heparin should pass prior to the needle placement of this patient's epidural. In addition, his partial thromboplastin time (PTT) should be checked and documented as normal (activated PTT <40s) before needle placement. A frank discussion with the patient and the surgeon should occur to detail the specific benefit-to-risk ratio so that all involved understand the potential hazards of proceeding and what steps are being taking to minimize the risks.

Restarting an infusion of intravenous heparin in patients postoperatively while there is an indwelling epidural catheter increases the risk of hematoma formation at the time of catheter removal, and thus it is generally recommended to avoid this while a catheter is in place. It is similarly recommended that heparin be stopped for 2 to 4 hours and activated PTT checked to verify that it is normal prior to removal of a neuraxial catheter.

Regarding patients who have been taking aspirin, the current ASRA guidelines do not recommend stopping aspirin or other nonsteroidal anti-inflammatory drugs (NSAIDs), as there has been no evidence of increased risk of bleeding leading to spinal hematomas.

Further Reading

Barash PG, Cullen BF, Stoelting RK, et al. *Anesthesia for Vascular Surgery: Clinical Anesthesia*. 7th ed. Philadelphia, PA: Lippincott; 2013.

Horlocher TT, Vandermeuelen E, Kopp SL, Gogarten W, Leffert LR, Benzon HT. Regional anesthesia in the patient receiving antithrombotic or thrombolytic therapy: American Society of Regional Anesthesia and Pain Medicine Evidence-Based Guidelines. (Fourth Edition). *Reg Anesth Pain Med*. 2018;43:263–309.

Lee LA, Posner KL, Domino KB, Caplan RA, Cheney FW. Injuries associated with regional anesthesia in the 1980s and 1990s: a closed claims analysis. *Anesthesiology*. 2004;101:143–152.

Moen B, Dahlgren N, Irestedt L. Severe neurological complications after central neuraxial blockades in Sweden 1990–1999. *Anesthesiology*. 2004;101:950–959.

Urmey WR, Rowlingson J. Do antiplatelet agents contribute to the development of perioperative spinal hematoma? *Reg Anesth Pain Med*. 1998;23:146–151.

Vandermeulen EP, Van Aken H, Vermylen J. Anticoagulants and spinal-epidural anesthesia. *Anesth Analg*. 1994;79:1165–1177.

2.4. What are the risk factors for epidural hematoma after neuraxial anesthesia?

The risk factors for epidural hematoma in patients on antithrombotic medications include (1) older age, (2) female sex, (3) timing of the epidural or spinal needle placement in relation to the last dose of antithrombotic drugs, (4) traumatic or difficult placement, and (5) spinal pathology. Although limited evidence exists, traumatic placements or multiple attempts at using a neuraxial technique should prompt discussion with the surgeon regarding subsequent anticoagulation and delaying bolus of intravenous unfractionated heparin within 1 hour of the traumatic placement.

Further Reading

Gogarten W, Vandermeulen E, Van Aken H, et al. Regional anaesthesia and antithrombotic agents: recommendations of the European Society of Anaesthesiology. *Eur J Anaesthesiol*. 2010;27:999–1015.

Moen V, Dahlgren N, Irestedt L. Severe neurological complications after central neuraxial blockades in Sweden 1990–1999. *Anesthesiology*. 2004;101:950–959.

Vandermeulen EP, Van Aken H, Vermylen J. Anticoagulants and spinal-epidural anesthesia. *Anesth Analg*. 1994;79:1165–1177.

2.5. What laboratory test, if any, would you order prior to placement of an epidural catheter?

It is important that the anesthesiologist be familiar with laboratory monitoring of anticoagulants. This patient was receiving dabigatran prior to the planned surgery. Before beginning neuraxial anesthesia, the anesthesiologist must delay 5 elimination half-lives as well as document laboratory monitoring. Dabigatran prolongs activated partial thromboplastin time (aPTT); thus activity can be measured by PTT or a thrombin time. For patients receiving an infusion of unfractionated heparin or a direct thrombin inhibitor (argatroban, bivalirudin, lepirudin), the medication can be stopped and the patient's anticoagulation status followed with aPTT targeting normal value of <40 seconds or normal thrombin time prior to catheter placement.

A patient who has been receiving warfarin should typically have his or her medication discontinued at least 5 days prior and a normalized international normalized ration (INR) <1.5 to show that his or her coagulation status is normal before placing a neuraxial needle or catheter. The INR test measures vitamin K–dependent coagulation factors that are depleted by warfarin because of its anticoagulant effect.

Further Reading

Barash PG, Cullen BF, Stoelting RK, et al. *Anesthesia for Vascular Surgery: Clinical Anesthesia.* 7th ed. Philadelphia, PA: Lippincott; 2013.

Benzon HT, Avram MJ, Green D, Bonow RO. New oral anticoagulants and regional anaesthesia. *Br J Anaesth.* 2013;111(suppl 1): i96–i113.

Curvers J, Kerekhof D, Stroobants AK, Dool E, Scharnhorst V. Measuring direct thrombin inhibitors with routing and dedicated coagulation assays: which assay is helpful? *Am J Clin Pathol.* 2012:134:551–558.

Douketis JD, Berger PB, Dunn AS, et al. The perioperative management of antithrombotic therapy: American College of Chest Physicians evidence-based clinical practice guidelines (eighth ed). *Chest.* 2008;133:299S–339S.

Enneking FK, Benzon H. Oral anticoagulants and regional anesthesia: a perspective. *Reg Anesth Pain Med.* 1998;23:140–145.

Horlocher TT, Vandermeuelen E, Kopp SL, Gogarten W, Leffert LR, Benzon HT. Regional anesthesia in the patient receiving antithrombotic or thrombolytic therapy: American Society of Regional Anesthesia and Pain Medicine Evidence-Based Guidelines. (Fourth Edition). *Reg Anesth Pain Med.* 2018;43:263–309.

2.6. Would your management and timing for needle placement be different if the patient had been taking enoxaparin? What about clopidogrel? What about other factor Xa inhibitors such as fondaparinux?

There are several antithrombotic medications, and the recommendations for the timing of preoperative discontinuation differ by drug, and often even within the same class of drugs. It is critically important to consider the timing and management in patients on low-molecular-weight heparins (LMWHs) such as enoxaparin as there is no laboratory test that reveals the anticoagulant effect. In general, the ASRA recommends that patients receiving multiple antithrombotic drugs (e.g., LMWHs plus aspirin, LMWHs plus antiplatelet drugs, etc.) not receive neuraxial anesthesia because of the increased risk of spinal hematoma. It should be noted that the longer the patient has been on an LMWH, the higher the likelihood of fibrinolysis and anti-Xa activity. Patients receiving subcutaneous prophylactic dosing of LMWHs (30 mg of enoxaparin every 12 hours, 40 mg of enoxaparin once a day, 2500–5000 units of dalteparin daily) should have an interval of at least 10 to 12 hours from the last dose to needle or catheter placement. Higher doses of subcutaneous enoxaparin (1 mg/kg enoxaparin every 12 hours or 1.5 mg/kg/d, or 200 units/kg/d dalteparin), considered therapeutic dosing, warrant delaying the placement of an epidural catheter for a least 24 hours after the last dose. Once the catheter is in place, anticoagulation therapy should not be administered in patients on a twice-daily dosing schedule. It is recommended that the indwelling epidural catheter be removed prior to the first dose of an LMWH. For patients on a once-daily dosing regimen of an LMWH, an indwelling neuraxial catheter can be carefully continued. For patients receiving once-daily dosing, a minimum of 10 to 12 hours after the last dose of an LMWH should occur prior to the removal of a neuraxial catheter.

Clopidogrel is an antiplatelet agent and a P2Y12 receptor blocker. Platelet function returns to normal 7 day after discontinuing clopidogrel. In ticlopidine, another thienopyridine derivative and antiplatelet agent, the mechanism of action occurs due to the inhibition of adenosine diphosphate–induced platelet aggregation, as it does in clopidogrel. It is reasonable to obtain and document a platelet count and/or platelet function test prior to using a neuraxial technique in patients receiving antiplatelet medication. The recommendation is to discontinue clopidogrel 5 to 7 days before neuraxial blockade. For other antiplatelet agents such as ticagrelor, prasugrel, and ticlopidine, it is recommended that the minimum time between the initial catheter placement and the last dose of anticoagulant be 5 to 7 days, 7 to 10 days, and 10 to 14 days, respectively.

The decision to perform a neuraxial block in a patient receiving factor Xa inhibitors such as rivaroxaban ($t_{½}$ = 5–9 hours), apixaban ($t_{½}$ = 6–12 hours), and fondaparinux2 ($t_{½}$ = 17–21 hours) varies due to their half-lives. The minimum times that have been recommended between the initial catheter placement and the time of the last dose of factor Xa inhibitor for rivaroxaban, apixaban, and fondaparinux are 24, 48, and 72 hours, respectively.

Further Reading

Barash PG, Cullen BF, Stoelting RK, et al. *Anesthesia for Vascular Surgery: Clinical Anesthesia*. 7th ed. Philadelphia, PA: Lippincott; 2013.

Benzon HT, Avram MJ, Green D, Bonow RO. New oral anticoagulants and regional anaesthesia. *Br J Anaesth*. 2013;111(suppl 1): i96–i113.

Benzon HT, McCarthy RJ, Benzon HA, et al. Determination of residual activity of clopidogrel before neuraxial injections. *Br J Anaesth*. 2011;107:966–977.

Gogarten W, Vandermeulen E, Van Aken H, et al. Regional anaesthesia and antithrombotic agents: recommendations of the European Society of Anaesthesiology. *Eur J Anaesthesiol*. 2010;27:999–1015.

Horlocher TT, Vandermeuelen E, Kopp SL, Gogarten W, Leffert LR, Benzon HT. Regional anesthesia in the patient receiving antithrombotic or thrombolytic therapy: American Society of Regional Anesthesia and Pain Medicine Evidence-Based Guidelines. (Fourth Edition). *Reg Anesth Pain Med*. 2018;43:263–309.

Lojewski B, Bacher P, Iqbal O, et al. Evaluation of hemostatic and fibrinolytic alterations associated with daily administration of low-molecular-weight heparin for a 12-week period. *Semin Thromb Hemost*. 1995;21:228–239.

Moen V, Dahlgren N, Irestedt L. Severe neurological complications after central neuraxial blockades in Sweden 1990-1999. *Anesthesiology*. 2004;202:950–959.

2.7. Following epidural placement, the surgeon obtains surgical exposure in 50 minutes and requests that you heparinize the patient. What is your action/response?

During this abdominal aortic bifemoral bypass, the surgeon will request the intravenous administration of heparin (5000–10,000 units) prior to aortic cross-clamping. In vascular surgery, it is safe to administer heparin 1 hour after epidural or spinal placement. The relative risk of spinal hematoma following central neuraxial anesthesia has been shown to increase from 2.18 to 25.2 when intravenous heparin is administered less than 1 hour after neuraxial puncture compared with waiting at least 1 hour. It has also been reported that it is possible to give heparin 1 hour before the insertion of an epidural without increasing the risk of hemorrhage. The anesthesiologist should be highly vigilant if the patient is receiving multiple anticoagulants, such as the combined administration of heparin and aspirin, as a multidrug regimen increases the risk of spinal epidural hematoma. Vascular surgical patients are a particularly high-risk patient group for neuraxial hematomas, per American Society of Anesthesiology closed claims analysis.

Further Reading

Gogarten W, Vandermeulen E, Van Aken H, et al. Regional anaesthesia and antithrombotic agents: recommendations of the European Society of Anaesthesiology. *Eur J Anaesthesiol*. 2010;27:999–1015.

Hirsh J, Raschke R, Warkentin TE, Dalen JE, Deykin D, Poller L. Heparin: mechanism of action, pharmacokinetics, dosing considerations, monitoring, efficacy, and safety. *Chest*. 1995;108:258S–275S.

Horlocher TT, Vandermeuelen E, Kopp SL, Gogarten W, Leffert LR, Benzon HT. Regional anesthesia in the patient receiving antithrombotic or thrombolytic therapy: American Society of Regional Anesthesia and Pain Medicine Evidence-Based Guidelines. (Fourth Edition). *Reg Anesth Pain Med*. 2018;43:263–309.

Lee LA, Posner KL, Domino KB, Caplan RA, Cheney FW. Injuries associated with regional anesthesia in the 1980s and 1990s: a closed claims analysis. *Anesthhesiology*. 2004;101:143–152.

Liu SS, Mulroy MF. Neuraxial anesthesia and analgesia in the presence of standard heparin. *Reg Anesth Pain Med*. 1998;23:157–163.

Rao TL, El-Etr AA. Anticoagulation following placement of epidural and subarachnoid catheters: an evaluation of neurologic sequelae. *Anesthesiology*. 1981;55:618–620.

Stafford-Smith M. Impaired haemostasis and regional anaesthesia. *Can J Anaesth*. 1996;43:R129–R141.

2.8. On postoperative day 2, the surgical team is ready to begin thromboprophylaxis and requests that the acute pain service remove the indwelling catheter. Forty-five minutes earlier, the patient received 5000 units of heparin subcutaneously. Should you remove the catheter? What is the recommended time interval before you should remove the epidural catheter?

Ideally, morning doses of heparin should be withheld prior to epidural catheter removal. However, if 5000 units of subcutaneous heparin given twice daily for deep venous thrombosis prophylaxis have been administered, it is safe to remove the catheter with little increased risk of hematoma formation. If total dosing is less than 10,000 units daily, there are no contraindications to a neuraxial procedure. However, the safety profile is not well established for higher or more frequent dosages. Increasing subcutaneous heparin to 7500 units and administering it 3 times per day (increased dose and/or time interval) presumably puts the patient at higher risk for bleeding. Subcutaneous heparin may be resumed 2 hours after catheter removal. The European Society of Anaesthesiology recommends at least 4 to 6 hours between subcutaneous heparin administration and removing a catheter.

Along the same lines as making the decision to place neuraxial catheters in a patient receiving perioperative anticoagulation medication, serious consideration must be given to the timing of restarting these medications after catheter removal. Because this patient had been taking dabigatran prior to any neuraxial procedure, such a medication can be resumed 6 hours after the catheter has been removed. Patients taking warfarin as their thromboprophylaxis may receive their first dose 24 hours prior to the removal of the catheter, but an international normalized ration level <1.5 should be documented before the removal takes place. Alternatively, warfarin may be resumed 2 hours after catheter removal. Other antiplatelet agents such as the glycoprotein IIb/IIIa receptor inhibitors clopidogrel and ticlopidine can be restarted 6 hours after removal of an epidural catheter. Following catheter removal, repeated neurologic assessment is recommended for at least 24 hours.

Based on European Society of Anaesthesiology guidelines and US Food and Drug Administration recommendations to decrease the risk of spinal column bleeding, prophylactic low-molecular-weight heparins should not be dosed for at least 4 hours after neuraxial catheter removal.

Further Reading

Barash PG, Cullen BF, Stoelting RK, et al. *Anesthesia for Vascular Surgery: Clinical Anesthesia*. 7th ed. Philadelphia, PA: Lippincott; 2013.

Collins R, Scrimgeour A, Yusurf S, Peto R. Reduction in fatal pulmonary embolism and venous thrombosis by perioperative administration of subcutaneous heparin: overview of results of randomized trials in general, orthopedic, and urologic surgery. *N Engl J Med*. 1988;318:1162–1173.

Gogarten W, Vandermeulen E, Van Aken H, et al. Regional anaesthesia and antithrombotic agents: recommendations of the European Society of Anaesthesiology. *Eur J Anaesthesiol*. 2010;27:999–1015.

Horlocher TT, Vandermeuelen E, Kopp SL, Gogarten W, Leffert LR, Benzon HT. Regional anesthesia in the patient receiving antithrombotic or thrombolytic therapy: American Society of Regional Anesthesia and Pain Medicine Evidence-Based Guidelines. (Fourth Edition). *Reg Anesth Pain Med*. 2018;43:263–309.

King CS, Holley AB, Jackson JL, et al. Twice vs three times daily heparin dosing for thromboembolism prophylaxis in the general medical population: a meta-analysis. *Chest*. 2007;131:507–516.

Leonardi MJ, McGory ML, Ko CY. The rate of bleeding complications after pharmacologic deep venous thrombosis prophylaxis: a systematic review of 33 randomized controlled trials. *Arch Surg*. 2006;141:790–799.

Liu SS, Mulroy MF. Neuraxial anesthesia and analgesia in the presence of standard heparin. *Reg Anesth Pain Med*. 1998;23:157–163.

US Food and Drug Administration. FDA Drug Safety Communication: Updated recommendations to decrease risk of spinal column bleeding and paralysis in patients on low molecular weight heparins. www.fda.gov/Drugs/DrugSafety/ucm373595.htm.

Wildsmith JA, McClure JH. Anticoagulant drugs and central nerve blockade. *Anaesthesia*. 1991;46:612–614.

2.9. What are the potential major complications of antithrombotic therapy following neuraxial techniques?

Bleeding in the spinal canal, which is a closed space, can lead to an expanding epidural/spinal hematoma, resulting in spinal cord ischemia or infarction. Unfortunately, these complications are not recognized until the patient complains about back pain or has neurologic impairment. Neurologic impairments can present as sensory and/or motor block and bladder/bowel dysfunction. Careful neurologic monitoring should occur, especially in high-risk patients. A thorough clinical assessment, immediate evaluation, and emergent imaging (e.g., MRI) should occur if there is any change in the patient's neurologic status and/or epidural hematoma is suspected. Neurologic outcomes are better if surgical decompression occurs within 8 hours of any change in neurologic status.

Further Reading

Gogarten W, Vandermeulen E, Van Aken H, et al. Regional anaesthesia and antithrombotic agents: recommendations of the European Society of Anaesthesiology. *Eur J Anaesthesiol.* 2010;27:999–1015.

Horlocker TT, Wedel DJ. Neuraxial block and low-molecular-weight heparin: balancing perioperative analgesia and thromboprophylaxis. *Reg Anesth Pain Med.* 1998;23(6 suppl 2):164.

Lee LA, Posner KL, Domino KB, et al. Injuries associated with regional anesthesia in the 1980s and 1990s: a closed claims analysis. *Anesthesiology.* 2004;101:143–152.

Vandermeulen EP, Van Aken H, Vermylen J. Anticoagulants and spinal-epidural anesthesia. *Anesth Analg.* 1994;79:1165–1177.

Case Scenario

The patient received a preoperative thoracic epidural that is being utilized postoperatively for analgesia. The patient was also written a hydromorphone patient-controlled analgesia (PCA) at a 0.2 mg bolus with a 10-minute lockout for breakthrough pain.

3. Strategic PCA Use and Adverse Opioid-Related Concerns

3.1. Discuss perioperative and pain relief goals for this procedure

Open aortic bifemoral bypass surgery is a procedure involving an extensive incision. Challenges for the anesthesiologist are numerous and include managing hemodynamic changes, maintaining perfusion and oxygenation, and attenuating reperfusion injury. A well-thought-out plan for intraoperative and postoperative pain control is imperative.

The overarching goals for acute pain relief are to reduce physiologic and psychological discomfort. This requires tailored management depending on the incision and intervention, comorbidities, age, anticoagulation, and patient choice.

Cardiopulmonary complications are frequent after this procedure, and patients are typically placed in an intensive care or high-acuity area for monitoring and prevention of postoperative complications. Diaphragm dysfunction occurs and lasts about 1 week. Decreases in surfactant, hypoxemia, and upper lobe patchy atelectasis occur. The most common respiratory complication is pneumonia, followed by pneumonitis, bronchitis, pulmonary emboli, and acute respiratory failure.

A meta-analysis of the effects of common analgesic therapies on postoperative pulmonary function found that epidural opioids decreased the incidence of atelectasis and had a weak tendency to reduce the incidence of pulmonary infections and pulmonary complications overall. Epidural local anesthetics increased PaO_2 and decreased the incidence of pulmonary infections and pulmonary complications compared with systemic opioids.

Improved extremity blood flow, anticoagulant properties of local anesthetics, and earlier mobility from better analgesia with epidurals augment the benefits of anticoagulation in preventing clot formation. However, anticoagulation in the setting of epidural catheters remains controversial due to the risk of epidural hematoma. Reports in the late 1990s of epidural hematomas associated with low-molecular-weight heparin use were concerning. Extensive American Society of Regional Anesthesia and Pain Medicine literature reviews note the safe use of both therapeutic anticoagulation (with perioperative Coumadin international normalized ratio >1.5 or intravenous intraoperative heparin) and deep venous thrombosis prophylaxis (unfractionated subcutaneous) when using epidural catheters that are indwelling.

The stress response to surgery initiates a predictable cascade of physiologic and metabolic events through direct activation of the sympathetic system, beginning with the induction of general anesthesia and lasting about 4 days postoperatively. The release of neuroendocrine mediators and cytokines (IL-1, IL-6, TNF-α) produces tachycardia, hypertension, fever, immunosuppression, and protein catabolism.

A catecholamine surge, increasing myocardial oxygen demand, may occur with poor pain control. Attenuation of the stress response through pain management may lessen myocardial risk, improve cardiac function, and shorten the hospital length of stay.

Epidurals can prevent the stimulation of the sympathetic nervous system that is caused by pain. Epidural analgesia with local anesthetics prevents the neuroendocrine and metabolic responses to pelvic and lower limb surgery. Epidural blockade of T4 to S5, established before the start of surgery, prevents increases in cortisol and glucose concentrations in hysterectomies. Both afferent input from the operative site to the central nervous system and the hypothalamic-pituitary axis plus efferent autonomic neuronal pathways to the liver and adrenal medulla are blocked.

Less extensive blockade will not completely abolish stress-related hormonal and metabolic changes. This was shown by a prospective randomized study of patients undergoing an elective abdominal aortic aneurysm repair. These patients had only a partial reduction in serum cortisol levels ($p < .01$) and urinary catecholamines ($p < .01$) with epidural anesthesia.

Providing adequate postoperative analgesia does not necessarily equate with blocking the sympathetic response. Epidural local anesthetics block the sympathetic response, but epidural opioids incompletely block the signal. Kehlet and Holte evaluated the effects of analgesia, including intravenous PCA, NSAIDs, and epidural anesthesia on attenuating the sympathetic response to reduce morbidity. Only epidural analgesia with local anesthetics significantly reduced the magnitude of the stress response. Moller found that intravenous PCA provided effective postoperative analgesia but did not effectively alter the stress response after surgery.

Intraoperative analgesia can be provided using systemic intravenous opioids or by using epidural analgesia. It is common practice, however, to limit epidural local anesthetic administration until after cross-clamp release and reaching hemostasis because epidural local anesthetics may cause profound and prolonged hypotension at the time of cross-clamp release due to sympathetic blockade.

When an epidural is used, it is usually for postoperative analgesia. A thoracic epidural at a level corresponding to the upper dermatomal level of the incision (usually T8-T10) is placed prior to induction and systemic heparinization. This technique allows for the catheter to be left in place for several days to limit pain and significantly reduce exogenous narcotic requirements.

Specific considerations for this patient include avoiding sedation given this patient's history of chronic obstructive pulmonary disease, avoiding NSAIDs because of a higher incidence of postoperative renal complications, and careful timing and adjustments in neuraxial techniques because of perioperative anticoagulation requirements.

Further Reading

Al-Hashimi M, Thompson J. Anaesthesia for elective open abdominal aortic aneurysm repair. *Contin Educ Anaesth Crit Care Pain.* 2013;13:208–212.

Ali J, Weisel RD, Layug AB, Kripke BJ, Hechtman HB. Consequences of postoperative alterations in respiratory mechanics. *Am J Surg.* 1974;128:376–382.

Ballantyne JC, Carr DB, deFerranti S, et al. The comparative effects of postoperative analgesic therapies on pulmonary outcome: cumulative meta-analyses of randomized, controlled trials. *Anesth Analg.* 1998;86:598–612.

Beattie WS, Badner NH, Choi, P. Epidural analgesia reduces postoperative myocardial infarction: a meta-analysis. *Anesth Analg.* 2001;93:853–858.

Bunt TJ, Manczuk M, Varley K. Continuous epidural anesthesia for aortic surgery: thoughts on peer review and safety. *Surgery.* 1987;101:706–714.

Carli F, Webster J, Pearson M, et al. Protein metabolism after abdominal surgery: effects of 24-h extradural block with local anesthetic. *Br J Anaesth.* 1991;67:729–734.

Christopherson R, Beattie C, Frank SM, et al. Perioperative morbidity in patients randomized to epidural or general anesthesia for lower extremity vascular surgery. The Perioperative Ischemia Randomized Anesthesia Trial Study Group. *Anesthesiology.* 1993;79:422–434.

Cuschieri RJ, Morran CG, Howie JC, et al. Postoperative pain and pulmonary complications: comparison of three analgesic regimes. *Br J Surg.* 1985;72:495–498.

Dureuil B, Cantineau JP, Desmonts JM. Effects of upper or lower abdominal surgery on diaphragmatic function. *Br J Anaesth.* 1987;59:1230–1235.

Enquist A, Brandt MR, Fernandes A, Kehlet H. The blocking effect of epidural analgesia on the adrenocortcial and hyperglycaemic responses to surgery. *Acta Anaesthesiol Scand.* 1977;21:330–335.

Ford GT, Whitelaw WA, Rosenal TW, Cruse PJ, Guenter CA. Diaphragm function after upper abdominal surgery in humans. *Am Rev Respir Dis.* 1983;127:431–436.

George KA, Chisakuta AM, Gamble JAS, Browne GA. Thoracic epidural infusion for postoperative pain relief following abdominal aortic surgery: bupivacaine, fentanyl or a mixture of both? *Anaesthesia.* 1992;47:388–394.

Ghansah JN, Murphy JT. Complications of major aortic and lower extremity vascular surgery. *Semin Cardiothorac Vasc Anesth.* 2004;8:335–361.

Horlocker TT, Benzon HT, Brown DL, et al. Regional anesthesia in the anticoagulated patient: defining the risks (the second ASRA Consensus Conference on Neuraxial Anesthesia and Anticoagulation). *Reg Anesth Pain Med.* 2003;28:172–197.

Horlocker TT, Wedel DJ. Neuraxial block and low molecular weight heparin: balancing perioperative analgesia and thromboprophylaxis. *Reg Anesth Pain Med.* 1998;23:164–177.

Horlocker TT, Wedel DJ, Schlicting JL. Postoperative epidural analgesia and oral anticoagulant therapy. *Anesth Analg.* 1994;79:89–93.

Hosoda R, Hattori M, Shimada Y. Favorable effects of epidural analgesia on hemodynamics, oxygenation, and metabolic variables in the immediate post-anesthetic period. *Acta Anesthesiol Scand.* 1993;37:469–474.

Kalko Y, Ugurlucan M, Basaran M, et al. Epidural anaesthesia and mini-laparotomy for the treatment of abdominal aortic aneurysms in patients with severe chronic obstructive pulmonary disease. *Acta Chir Belg.* 2007;107:307–312.

Kanat F, Golcuk A, Teke T, Golcuk M. Risk factors for postoperative pulmonary complications in upper abdominal surgery. *ANZ J Surg.* 2007;77:135–141.

Kehlet H. General vs. regional anesthesia. In: Rogers MC, Tinker JH, Covino BG, et al., eds. *Principles and Practice of Anesthesiology.* St. Louis, MO: Mosby-Year Book; 1993:1218–1234.

Kehlet H. The stress response to surgery: release mechanisms and modifying effect of pain relief. *Acta Chir Scand.* 1988;550:22–28.

Kehlet H, Holte K. Effect of postoperative analgesia on surgical outcome. *Br J Anaesth.* 2001;87:62–72.

Latimer RG, Dickman M, Day WC, Gunn ML, Schmidt CD. Ventilatory patterns and pulmonary complications after upper abdominal surgery determined by preoperative and postoperative computerized spirometry and blood gas analysis. *Am J Surg.* 1971;122:622–632.

Lindholm EE. Perioperative aspects of abdominal aortic surgery: focus on choice of anesthetics. *Acta Anaesthesiol Scand.* 2016;60:411.

Lunn JK, Dannemiller FJ, Stanley TH. Cardiovascular responses to clamping of the aorta during epidural and general anesthesia. *Anesth Analg.* 1979;58:372–376.

Magnusdottir H, Kimo K, Ricksten SE, et al. High thoracic epidural anesthesia does not inhibit sympathetic nerve activity in the lower extremities. *Anesthesiology.* 1999;91:1299–1304.

Moller IW, Dinesen K, Sondergard S, et al. Effect of patient-controlled analgesia on plasma catecholamine, cortisol and glucose concentrations after cholecystectomy. *Br J Anaesth.* 1988;61:160–164.

Naito Y, Tamai S, Shingu K, et al. Responses of plasma adrenocorticotropic hormone, cortisol, and cytokines during and after upper abdominal surgery. *Anesthesiology*. 1992;77:426–431.

Pasin L, Nardelli P, Belletti A, et al. Pulmonary complications after open abdominal aortic surgery: a systematic review and meta-analysis. *J Cardiothorac Vasc Anesth*. 2017;31:562–568.

Rao TLK, El-Etr AA. Anticoagulation following placement of epidural and subarachnoid catheters: an evaluation of neurologic sequelae. *Anesthesiology*. 1981;55:618–620.

Savas JF, Litwack R, Davis K, et al. Regional anesthesia as an alternative to general anesthesia for abdominal surgery in patients with severe pulmonary impairment. *Am J Surg*. 2004;188:603–605.

Schwander D, Bachmann F. Heparin and spinal or epidural anesthesia: decision analysis. *Ann Fr Anesth Reanim*. 1991;10:284–296.

Simonneau G, Vivien A, Sartene R, et al. Diaphragm dysfunction induced by upper abdominal surgery role of postoperative pain. *Am Rev Respir Dis*. 1983;128:899–903.

Smeets HJ, Kievit J, Dulfer FT, et al. Endocrine-metabolic response to abdominal aortic surgery: a randomized trial of general anesthesia versus general plus epidural anesthesia. *World J Surg*. 1993;17:601–607.

Udelsman R. Endocrine and molecular responses to surgical stress. *Curr Probl Surg*. 1994;8:663–720.

Udelsman R, Norton FA, Jelenich SE, et al. Responses of the hypothalamic-pituitary-adrenal and renin-angiotensin and the sympathetic system during controlled surgical and anesthetic stress. *J Clin Endocrinol Metab*. 1987;64:986–994.

Vedrinne C, Vedrinne JM, Guiraud M, et al. Nitrogen-sparing effect of epidural administration of local anesthetics in colon surgery. *Anesth Analg*. 1989;69:354–359.

Wozniak MF, LaMuraglia GM, Musch G. Anesthesia for open abdominal aortic surgery. *Int Anesthesiol Clin*. 2005;43:61–78.

Wu CL, Perkins FM. Oral anticoagulant prophylaxis and epidural catheter removal. *Reg Anesth*. 1996;21:517–524.

3.2. What is fast-track management? Discuss epidural management in fast-track cases

Perioperative physicians have been researching and implementing ways to provide more efficient integrated care in many surgeries, including open abdominal aortic surgeries. Fast-track protocols often focus on ways to lessen mechanical ventilation, improve early mobilization, and prevent ileus. Strategies include no bowel preparation, less fasting, and more effective pain control. Other benefits are reductions in the systemic inflammatory response, possibly leading to a reduction in overall morbidity and mortality. Patient-controlled analgesia (PCA) is typically the most commonly cited pain management strategy used in fast-track management for open abdominal aortic procedures.

Epidural solutions of bupivacaine or ropivacaine are typically used in combination with an opioid such as sufentanil or fentanyl. However, if PCA narcotics are used in combination with epidurals for analgesia, it is prudent to avoid narcotics in the epidural, thereby reducing the chance of respiratory depression because of multiple narcotic sources.

The quantity of analgesia given at each self-administration demand is the bolus dose. It is assumed patients will demand analgesic doses until their pain has been relieved, but the demand dose size influences the patient's perception of how effective the treatment is. If the dose is too small, the patient will fail to achieve adequate analgesia. If the dose is too large, the plasma concentration will increase with repeated doses until it causes sedation and possibly respiratory depression. The optimal bolus dose is the minimum dose to produce consistently appreciable analgesia without side effects.

The time between patient demands, during which the machine will not administer a further dose despite additional patient demands, is the lockout interval. This interval is guided by the bolus dose, the pharmacokinetics and pharmacodynamics of the drug, and, particularly, the time for the drug to reach peak plasma concentrations.

Further Reading

Berti M, Casati A, Fanelli G, et al. 0.2% ropivacaine with or without fentanyl for patient-controlled epidural analgesia after major abdominal surgery: a double-blind study. *J Clin Anesth*. 2000;12:292–297.

Brustia P, Renghi A, Aronici M, et al. Fast-track in abdominal aortic surgery: experience in over 1,000 patients. *Ann Vasc Surg*. 2015;29:1151–1159.

Curatolo M, Schnider TW, Petersen-Felix S, et al. A direct search procedure to optimize combinations of epidural bupivacaine, fentanyl, and clonidine for postoperative analgesia. *Anesthesiology*. 2000;92:325–337.

Grider JS, Mullet TW, Saha SP, Harned ME, Sloan PA. A randomized, double-blind trial comparing continuous thoracic epidural bupivacaine with and without opioid in contrast to a continuous paravertebral infusion of bupivacaine for post-thoracotomy pain. *J Cardiothorac Vasc Anesth*. 2012;26:83–89.

Muehling B, Schelzig H, Steffen P, et al. A prospective randomized trial comparing traditional and fast-track patient care in elective open infrarenal aneurysm repair. *World J Surg*. 2009;33:577–585.

Muehling BM, Ortlieb L, Oberhuber A, et al. Fast track management reduces the systemic inflammatory response and organ failure following elective infrarenal aortic aneurysm repair. *Interact Cardiovasc Thorac Surg*. 2011;12:784–788.

Scott DA, Blake D, Buckland M, Etches R, et al. A comparison of epidural ropivacaine infusion alone and in combination with 1, 2, and 4 microg/mL fentanyl for seventy-two hours of postoperative analgesia after major abdominal surgery. *Anesth Analg*. 1999;88:857–864.

3.3. Compare the advantages and disadvantages of using an epidural for an open abdominal aortic bifemoral bypass

Epidurals have safely been used both intraoperatively and postoperatively to various degrees for this procedure. They provide excellent site-specific pain control. Studies report less sedation, improved respiratory mechanics, and shorter time to extubation. Epidurals may also minimize gastrointestinal complications. Additionally, they may help to modulate sympathetic outflow, thereby improving organ perfusion.

However, epidurals are an invasive procedure and require both patient consent and expertise in placement. Daily management is costlier than for PCA. Common concerns are hypotension and possible motor blockade that often requires adjustments in rates and solution composition. Epidural management poses challenges with anticoagulation, and epidurals are contraindicated in patients with coagulopathies, infections, or tumors at the site. Catheter complications result from inadvertent penetration of the dura, damage to neurovascular structures, or infection. In a series of 51,000 epidural catheters, accidental dural puncture occured in 0.16% to 1.3% of epidural catheter insertion. Subsequent postdural headaches developed in 16% to 86% of these patients. Systemic absorption of solutions can produce seizures, loss of airway protective reflexes, respiratory depression, coma, cardiac arrhythmias, hemodynamic instability, and motor or autonomic blockade (urinary retention, weakness) in 0% to 45% of patients.

Another potential problem with postoperative analgesia is opioid-induced respiratory depression. Large surveys of patients receiving morphine through epidural catheters found the incidence of respiratory depression to be less than 1%, comparable to parenteral and oral morphine. Additionally, the combination of epidural opioid and local anesthetic can reduce the amount of opioid needed. Other rare complications include abscesses and hematomas. Many potential problems can be mitigated by proper placement and the use of low-dosage solutions.

Further Reading

Albright GA. Cardiac arrest following regional anesthesia with etidocaine and bupivacaine. *Anesthesiology*. 1979;51:285–287.

Auroy Y, Narchi P, Messiah A, et al. Serious complications related to regional anesthesia. *Anesthesiology*. 1997;87:479–486.

Bardia A, Sood A, Mahmood F, et al. Combined epidural-general anesthesia vs general anesthesia alone for elective abdominal aortic aneurysm repair. *JAMA Surg*. 2016;151:1116–1123.

Bois S, Couture P, Boudreault D, et al. Epidural analgesia and intravenous patient-controlled analgesia result in similar rates of postoperative myocardial ischemia after aortic surgery. *Anesth Analg*. 1997;85:1233–1239.

Boylan JF, Katz J, Kavanagh BP, et al. Epidural bupivacaine-morphine analgesia versus patient-controlled analgesia following abdominal aortic surgery: analgesic, respiratory, and myocardial effects. *Anesthesiology*. 1998;89:585–593.

Horlocker TT. Regional anesthesia: complications of spinal and epidural anesthesia. *Anesthesiol Clin N Am*. 2000;18:461–485.

Guay J, Kopp S. Epidural pain relief versus systemic opioid-based pain relief for abdominal aortic surgery. *Cochrane Database Syst Rev.* 2016 Jan 5;1:CD005059.

Ko PJ, Hsieh HC, Liu YH, et al. Experience with early postoperative feeding after abdominal aortic surgery. *Chang Gung Med J.* 2004;27:210–216.

Manion SC, Brennan TJ. Thoracic epidural analgesia and acute pain management. *Anesthesiology.* 2011;7:181–188.

Panaretou V, Siafaka I, Theodorou D, et al. Combined general-epidural anesthesia with continuous postoperative epidural analgesia preserves sigmoid colon perfusion in elective infrarenal aortic aneurysm repair. *Saudi J Anaesth.* 2012;6:373–379.

Panaretou V, Toufektzian L, Siafaka I, et al. Postoperative pulmonary function after open abdominal aortic aneurysm repair in patients with chronic obstructive pulmonary disease: epidural versus intravenous analgesia. *Ann Vasc Surg.* 2012;26:149–155.

Ready LB, Loper KA, Nessly M, et al. Postoperative epidural morphine is safe on surgical wards. *Anesthesiology.* 1991;75:452–456.

Stride PC, Cooper GM. Dural taps revisited: a 20-year survey from Birmingham Maternity Hospital. *Anaesthesia.* 1993;48:247–255.

Tanaka K, Watanabe R, Harada T, et al. Extensive applications of epidural anesthesia and analgesia in a university hospital: incidence of complications related to technique. *Reg Anesth Pain Med.* 1993;18:34–38.

Von Hosslin T, Imboden P, Luthi A, et al. Adverse events of postoperative thoracic epidural analgesia: a retrospective analysis of 7273 cases in a tertiary care teaching hospital. *Eur J Anaesthesiol.* 2016;33:708–714.

Wallace D, Bright E, London NJ. The incidence of epidural abscess following epidural analgesia in open abdominal aortic aneurysm repair. *Ann R Coll Surg Engl.* 2010;92:31–33.

3.4. What are the advantages and disadvantages of using intravenous patient-controlled analgesia for pain control? What are the adverse effects of opioids? How can they be minimized?

The advantages of PCA include the self-delivery of medication and faster alleviation of pain because the patient can self-address pain. With PCA, the patient typically spends less time in pain and tends to use less medication than when medication is given according to a set schedule.

The disadvantages of PCA include if the PCA device is not programmed properly, it can result in the under- or overdosing of narcotics. PCA may also be inappropriate for patients with learning difficulties, those with poor manual dexterity, and those who are critically ill.

Opioids have a systemic effect by binding to opioid receptors, thereby affecting a wide number of organ systems. They should be used with caution in patients with impaired ventilation, liver failure, or increased intracranial pressure.

Opioid-related side effects include sedation, dizziness, pruritis, nausea, vomiting, constipation, urinary retention, and respiratory depression. The most common side effects of opioid use are constipation and nausea, which may be difficult to manage. Nausea and vomiting in abdominal surgery patients is very distressing, with many patients fearing it more than they do pain.

Pruritis from opioids, especially neuraxial opioids, may have a very negative effect on the postoperative recovery of patients. A small dose of a mixed opioid agonist-antagonist (e.g., 5 mg of intravenous nalbuphine or 0.3 mg of intravenous buprenorphine) administered several times per day, as needed, or a very low-dose continuous intravenous infusion of naloxone may help alleviate some of these symptoms.

Respiratory depression is the most feared complication and is most common in the opioid-naive patient. It is usually transient and antagonized by pain, but excessive sedation may contribute to increased morbidity and mortality. The initial steps are to identify and eliminate any unnecessary medication and be prepared to reverse the respiratory and/or sedative effects of excess opioids with small bolus doses of naloxone.

The strategies for managing opioid side effects vary but may also include dosage reduction/adjustment, opioid switching/rotation, altering the routes of administration, and symptomatic management of specific side effects with monitoring and dosing according to patient response. It is prudent to avoid simultaneous neuraxial and intravenous narcotics. Patients with a known history of intolerance may require preemptive treatment of the specific side effect.

Side effects may also be minimized through multimodal approaches. Multimodal analgesia uses a combination of drugs with different modes of action. In this way, it is possible to use lower doses of drugs, minimizing unwanted side effects.

For example, by using a combination of NSAIDs (in properly selected patients) and an opioid for postoperative pain, the amount of opioid required is less, and the opioid-related side effects are reduced. With trauma, metabolic changes and the activation of several biological cascade systems (cytokines, complement, arachidonic acid metabolites, nitric oxide, free oxygen radicals, etc.) occur. Applying multimodal interventions may help to lower the undesirable sequelae of the surgical injury cascade while also improving overall recovery.

Further Reading

Dahan A, Aarts L, Smith TW. Incidence, reversal, and prevention of opioid-induced respiratory depression. *Anesthesiology*. 2010;112:226–238.

Elviro-Lazo OL, White PF. The role of multimodal analgesia in pain management after ambulatory surgery. *Curr Opin Anaesthesiol*. 2010;23:697–703.

Kehlet H. Multimodal approach to control postoperative pathophysiology and rehabilitation. *Br J Anaesth*. 1997;78:606–617.

Rogers E, Mehta S, Shengelia R, et al. Four strategies for managing opioid induced side effects in older adults. *Clin Geriatr*. 2013;21: epub at www.consultant360.com/articles/four-strategies-managing-opioid-induced-side-effects-older-adults.

Sinatra RS, de Leon-Cassasola OA, Ginsburg B, et al. *Acute Pain Management*. London, UK: Cambridge University Press; 2009: 612–614.

3.5. Are there other alternative analgesic options for postoperative pain management for this procedure?

Abdominal surgical procedures result in significant acute postoperative pain; however, not all surgical patients are good candidates for general anesthesia. In selected cases, a continuous spinal epidural technique has been employed to avoid general anesthesia. This may be beneficial in a patient, such as this one, with a history of chronic pulmonary obstructive disease. Additionally, not all patients are candidates for epidurals, and many are intolerant of systemic opioids. Cases like these have prompted consideration of other pain relief techniques. Knowing more about the surgical incision assists in guiding analgesic therapy choices.

Alternative analgesic options for open aortic procedures have included intrathecal opioids and local anesthetic wound instillation. Opioids work primarily by modulation of the mu-opioid receptor, altering nociceptive stimuli in the central nervous system, spinal cord, and periphery. Local anesthetics block voltage-gated Na^+ channels, reversibly inhibiting action potential propagation, primarily in sensory fibers.

More recently, paravertebral and transverse abdominis plane blocks have been used. Regarding paravertebral blocks, Richardson et al. inserted preoperative bilateral T10 paravertebral catheters in 8 patients undergoing major abdominal vascular surgery using 25 mL of 0.5% bupivacaine divided between the 2 catheters. This provided the basis of an effective intraoperative analgesic regimen that was continued postoperatively by infusion.

With surgical trauma, metabolic changes and the activation of several biological cascade systems occurs (e.g., cytokines, complement, arachidonic acid metabolites, nitric oxide, free oxygen radicals.). Employing multimodal interventions may result in a reduction in the undesirable sequelae of surgical injury cascade with an improved recovery. As a multimodal adjuvant, acetaminophen use is justified. Acetaminophen's exact mechanism is unknown, although it is thought to interact with cyclooxygenase and nitric oxide pathways. NSAIDs inhibit prostaglandin synthesis, preventing part of the inflammatory response. Because of a relevantly higher incidence of renal insufficiency, traditional NSAIDs are not recommended for this patient population, unlike acetaminophen.

Further Reading

Blay M, Orban JC, Rami L, et al. Efficacy of low-dose intrathecal morphine for postoperative analgesia after abdominal aortic surgery: a double-blind randomized study. *Reg Anesth Pain Med*. 2006;31:127–133.

Buvanendran A, Kroin JS. Multimodal analgesia for controlling acute postoperative pain. *Curr Opin Anaesthesiol*. 2009;22:588–593.

Chaykovska L, Blohme L, Mayer D, et al. Paraincisional subcutaneous infusion of ropivacaine after open abdominal vascular surgery shows significant advantages. *Ann Vasc Surg.* 2014;28:837–844.

Flaherty J, Horn JL, Derby R. Regional anesthesia for vascular surgery. *Anesthesiol Clin.* 2014;32:639–659.

Fléron MH, Weiskopf RB, Bertrand M, et al. A comparison of intrathecal opioid and intravenous analgesia for the incidence of cardiovascular, respiratory, and renal complications after abdominal aortic surgery. *Anesth Analg.* 2003;97:2–12.

Flores JA, Nishibe T, Koyama M, et al. Combined spinal and epidural anesthesia for abdominal aortic aneurysm surgery in patients with severe chronic pulmonary obstructive disease. *Int Angiol.* 2002;21:218–221.

Kehlet H, Wilkinson RC, Fischer HB, et al. PROSPECT: evidence-based, procedure-specific postoperative pain management. *Best Pract Res Clin Anaesthesiol.* 2007;21:149–159.

Pfeiffer U, Dodson ME, Van Mourik G, et al. Wound instillation for postoperative pain relief: a comparison between bupivacaine and saline in patients undergoing aortic surgery. *Ann Vasc Surg.* 1991;5:80–84.

Richardson J, Vowden P, Sabanathan S. Bilateral paravertebral analgesia for major abdominal vascular surgery: a preliminary report. *Anaesthesia.* 1995;50:995–998.

Scholz A. Mechanisms of (local) anaesthetics on voltage-gated sodium and other ion channels. *Br J Anaesth.* 2002;89:52–61.

Shine TS, Greengrass RA, Feinglass NG. Use of continuous paravertebral analgesia to facilitate neurologic assessment and enhance recovery after thoracoabdominal aortic aneurysm repair. *Anesth Analg.* 2004;98:1640–1643.

Smith HS. Potential analgesic mechanisms of acetaminophen. *Pain Physician.* 2009;12:269–280.

White PF, Kehlet H. Improving postoperative pain management: what are the unresolved issues? *Anesthesiology.* 2010;112:220–225.

Young MJ, Gorlin AW, Modest VE, et al. Clinical implications of the transversus abdominis plane block in adults. *Anesthesiol Res Pract.* 2012;2012:731645.

Complex Spine

David A. Edwards and Christopher Sobey

15

Case Scenario

A 65-year-old man with extensive thoracolumbar osteoarthritis and neuroforaminal stenosis associated with chronic axial pain presented for a T10-iliac fusion. He currently takes extended-release oxycodone at a dose of 30 mg 3 times daily with as needed oxycodone instant release. He has a further history of hypertension, diabetes, and hypothyroidism. His remaining home medicines include metoprolol, cyclobenzaprine, metformin, and celecoxib.

1. Patient Considerations

1.1. What defines opioid tolerant? What defines opioid naive?

The US Food and Drug Administration defines an opioid-tolerant patient as one "who [is] taking at least 60 mg oral morphine equivalents/day . . . or an equianalgesic dose of another opioid for one week or longer." An opioid-naive patient is one who is exposed to little or no opioid. Because definitions have not been standardized across the literature, studies are difficult to compare when evaluating for patient risks. Recent efforts to standardize these definitions have been made so that future research can consistently report risks associated with use of opioids in the preoperative period.

Further Reading

Dowell D, Haegerich TM, Chou R. CDC Guideline for Prescribing Opioids for Chronic Pain—United States, 2016. JAMA. 2016;315(15):1624–1645.

Edwards DA, Hedrick TL, Argoff C, Gulur P, Holubar SD, Jayaram J, Gan TJ, Mythen MG, Miller TE, Shaw AD, Thacker JKM, McEvoy MD. American Society for Enhanced Recovery and Perioperative Quality Initiative Joint Consensus Statement on Perioperative Management of Patients on Preoperative Opioid Therapy. 2019. Anesth Analg. in press.

1.2. What are the perioperative risks in opioid-tolerant patients?

Outpatients on doses of more than 50 milligram morphine equivalents have a fourfold increase of all-cause mortality. Opioids are dose-dependently associated with increased perioperative risk of poor outcomes (Box 15.1). By minimizing the use of opioids through use of multimodal analgesia (MMA), including regional anesthesia, and nonmedication pain management techniques, many of these risks can be reduced.

Box 15.1 Opioid-Related Perioperative Risks

- Opioid-induced respiratory depression
- Opioid-induced hyperalgesia
- Increased risk for opioid dependence and substance use disorder
- Delayed wound healing
- Increased surgical reintervention
- Prolonged hospital stay
- Higher readmission rates
- Greater healthcare costs
- Increased all-cause morbidity
- Increased mortality
- Suffering

Further Reading

Brummett CM, Waljee JF, Goesling J, et al. New persistent opioid use after minor and major surgical procedures in US adults. JAMA Surg. 2017;152(6):e170504.

Cron DC, Englesbe MJ, Bolton CJ, et al. Preoperative opioid use is independently associated with increased costs and worse outcomes after major abdominal surgery. Ann Surg. 2017;265(4):695–701.

Dunn KM, Saunders KW, Rutter CM, et al. Opioid prescriptions for chronic pain and overdose: a cohort study. Ann Intern Med. 2010;152:85–92.

Gomes T, Mamdani MM, Dhalla IA, Paterson JM, Juurlink DN. Opioid dose and drug-related mortality in patients with nonmalignant pain. Arch Intern Med. 2011;171:686–691.

Koury K, Chaudhary S, Williams L, Jaff M, Gulur P. Opioid tolerance: a predictor of increased length of stay and higher readmission rates. Pain Physician. 2014;17(4):503.

Shanmugam VK, Couch KS, McNish S, Amdur RL. Relationship between opioid treatment and rate of healing in chronic wounds. Wound Repair Regen. 2017;25(1):120–130.

1.3. Should opioids be weaned before surgery?

Opioids are dose-dependently associated with poor surgical outcomes. Preoperative opioid dose and perioperative opioid total dose are associated with poor outcomes. So, it has been hypothesized that preoperative weaning of opioid in patients leading up to surgery will lessen the risk of poor outcomes related to opioids. Direct evidence of the benefit of preoperative opioid tapering has not been shown yet in high-quality studies, although a few preliminary and low-quality studies show a positive risk reduction. It has been recommended by a consensus of experts that opioids be minimized before surgery to the least effective dose to mitigate risk of opioid escalation.

Further Reading

Blum JM, Biel SS, Hilliard PE, Jutkiewicz EM. Preoperative ultra-rapid opiate detoxification for the treatment of post-operative surgical pain. Med Hypotheses. 2015;84(6):529–531.

Edwards DA, Hedrick TL, Argoff C, Gulur P, Holubar SD, Jayaram J, Gan TJ, Mythen MG, Miller TE, Shaw AD, Thacker JKM, McEvoy MD. American Society for Enhanced Recovery and Perioperative Quality Initiative Joint Consensus Statement on Perioperative Management of Patients on Preoperative Opioid Therapy. 2019. Anesth Analg. in press.

Hassamal S, Haglund M, Wittnebel K, Danovitch I. A preoperative interdisciplinary biopsychosocial opioid reduction program in patients on chronic opioid analgesia prior to spine surgery: a preliminary report and case series. Scand J Pain. 2016;13:27–31.

McAnally H. Rationale for and approach to preoperative opioid weaning: a preoperative optimization protocol. Perioperative Med. 2017;6:19.

Nguyen L-CL, Sing DC, Bozic KJ. Preoperative reduction of opioid use before total joint arthroplasty. J Arthroplasty. 2016;31(9 suppl):282–287.

Sadeghian S, Karimi A, Dowlatshahi S, et al. The association of opium dependence and postoperative complications following coronary artery bypass graft surgery: a propensity-matched study. J Opioid Manage. 2009;5(6):365–372.

1.4. What are strategies for pain management for opioid-tolerant patients?

Opioid-tolerant patients are at risk of suffering due to undertreatment of pain. They also may be at higher risk of opioid-related adverse events, given the higher doses of opioid needed to control their pain. By using an MMA strategy to treat pain, opioid dose escalation can be limited while maintaining excellent pain control and reducing perioperative risks.

1.4.1. Multimodal analgesia

Multimodal analgesia is the use of multiple methods, pharmacologic and nonpharmacologic, to treat pain. With use of multiple methods, lower doses of individual medications are needed for effective analgesia, limiting their individual and combined side effects. Medications useful in an MMA plan for complex spine operations are listed in Table 15.1.

Further Reading

Choi YS, Shim JK, Song JW, Kim JC, Yoo YC, Kwak YL. Combination of pregabalin and dexamethasone for postoperative pain and functional outcome in patients undergoing lumbar spinal surgery: a randomized placebo-controlled trial. Clin J Pain. 2013;29(1):9–14.

Loftus RW, Yeager MP, Clark JA, Brown JR, Abdu WA, Sengupta DK, Beach ML. Intraoperative ketamine reduces perioperative opiate consumption in opiate-dependent patients with chronic back pain undergoing back surgery. Anesthesiol. 2010;113(3):639–646.

McCarthy GC, Megalla SA, Habib AS. Impact of intravenous lidocaine infusion on postoperative analgesia and recovery from surgery: a systematic review of randomized controlled trials. Drugs. 2010;70(9):1149–1163.

Schmidt PC, Ruchelli G, Mackey SC, Carroll IR. Perioperative gabapentinoids: choice of agent, dose, timing, and effects on chronic postsurgical pain. Anesthesiol. 2013;119(5):1215–1221.

Table 15.1:
Nonopioid analgesics, antispasmodics, and adjuncts

NSAIDs	*Alpha-2 Agonists*
• Ketorolac (IV)	• Clonidine (PO, patch, IM)
• Ibuprofen (PO/IV)	• Dexmedetomidine (IV)
• Celecoxib (PO)	• Guanfacine (PO)
• Diclofenac (topical)	• Tizanidine (PO)
Neuropathic Pain Agents	*NMDA Antagonists*
• Anticonvulsants (gabapentin, pregabalin)	• Ketamine (IV, IM, PO)
• SNRIs (duloxetine, milnacipran)	• Amantadine (PO)
• TCAs (nortriptyline, amitriptyline)	• Memantine (PO)
Antispasmodics	• Dextromethorphan (PO)
• Tizanidine (PO)	• Magnesium (IV)
• Cyclobenzaprine (PO)	*Local Anesthetics*
• Baclofen (PO)	• Lidocaine (IV, IM, PN, IT, topical, patch)
• Diazepam, lorazepam	• Bupivacaine (IM, PN, IT)
Acetaminophen (PO, IV)	• Ropivacaine (IM, PN)
Dexamethasone (IV, PN)	• Chloroprocaine (IT)

Note: NSAIDs: nonsteroidal anti-inflammatory drugs; IV: intravenous; PO: oral; IM: intramuscular; PN: perineural; IT: intrathecal; SNRIs: serotonin norepinephrine reuptake inhibitors; TCAs: tricyclic antidepressants; NMDA: N-methyl-D-aspartate.

1.4.2. Regional anesthesia

Regional anesthesia can be used in complex spine surgery under the right circumstances. The 2 most effective methods are local infiltration of the surgical wound upon closure, and continuous epidural infusion. Epidural catheter placement above the incision can be done prior to surgery or by the surgeon at closure. A sterile catheter placed in the epidural space cephalad to the surgical incision is commonly tunneled and sutured in place at the skin. Continuous epidural infusion can help provide local analgesia to the proximate wound site and can be a helpful adjunct in an MMA plan. Close daily evaluation for signs of infection and weakness is imperative.

Further Reading

Gritsenko K, Khelemsky Y, Kaye AD, Vadivelu N, Urman RD. Multimodal therapy in perioperative analgesia. Best Pract Res Clin Anaesthesiol. 2014;28(1):59–79.

Kjaergaard M, Moniche S, Olsen KS. Wound infiltration with local anesthetics for postoperative pain relief in lumbar spine surgery: a systematic review. Acta Anaesthesiol Scand. 2012;56(3):282–290.

Mathiesen O, Dahl B, Thomsen BA, Kitter B, Sonne N, Dahl JB, Kehlet H. A comprehensive multimodal pain treatment reduces opioid consumption after multilevel spine surgery. Eur Spine J. 2013;22(9):2089–2096.

Wick EC, Grant MC, Wu CL. Postoperative multimodal analgesia pain management with nonopioid analgesics and techniques: a review. JAMA Surg. 2017;152(7):691–697.

2. Pain Management Considerations and Use of Regional Anesthesia

2.1. What are the types of pain?

There are 3 general types of pain: nociceptive, inflammatory, and neuropathic (Table 15.2). Nociceptive pain occurs with activation of nociceptors, specialized nerve endings that detect and transmit the many pain modalities (e.g., heat, cold, pressure, chemical), or by free nerve endings. Nociceptive pain can be somatic or visceral. Somatic nociceptive pain is

Table 15.2: Types of pain

Nociceptive	Nociceptive pain occurs when nociceptors are activated. This type of pain is protective. Nociceptors in the musculoskeletal and gastrointestinal systems sense pain associated with these tissues, resulting in somatic and visceral nociceptive pain, respectively.
Inflammatory	Inflammatory mediators in infected or injured tissue lower the threshold to neuronal signaling. In this condition, pain neurons are activated more easily.
Neuropathic	Neuropathic pain is caused by injury to neurons and can be the result of chronic disease states, such as with diabetes, or nerve injury, such as with surgery.

caused by activation of nociceptors in the musculoskeletal system. Visceral nociceptive pain occurs when receptors are activated in the viscera. During surgical damage of tissue, both somatic and visceral nociceptive pain types exist, as incision damages muscle, bone, and vasculature. As a result, movement after surgery is painful.

A second type of pain is inflammatory pain. This type also occurs with surgery as tissues are damaged in the process. With cellular release of inflammatory mediators, called the inflammatory milieu (e.g., TNF-alpha, interleukins, ATP), the threshold for nerve firing is lowered such that neuronal action potentials are more likely to occur and transmission of pain signals is increased.

Further Reading

Edwards DA, Rathmell JP, Shah BJ. Post-herniorrhaphy Pain. In: Hayek SM, Shah BJ, Desai MJ, Chelimsky TC, eds. Pain Medicine: An Interdisciplinary Case-Based Approach. New York: Oxford University Press; 2015:337–352.

2.2. What is central sensitization? What are the physiologic and cellular mechanisms that underlie central sensitization?

The centralization of pain describes a situation where peripheral pain detection has resulted, after some time, in facilitation of pain pathways in the central nervous system that includes the spinal cord and brain. One sign of pain centralization is sensitivity beyond the region of the initial pain generator. This means that neurons in the spinal cord have been sensitized to transmit pain, and as a result, a broad region of the peripheral nervous system is sensitized.

Central sensitization results from facilitation of changes in the nervous system between first-, second-, and third-order neurons. The condition may be transient, as with acute postoperative allodynia and hyperalgesia where the region around the surgical insult is painfully sensitive. It also can become permanent as with chronic painful conditions like fibromyalgia, where there is no apparent peripheral cause of pain, yet the individual feels widespread pain.

The pathophysiology underlying the development of central sensitization is incompletely understood. Under normal conditions, first-order neurons (unmyelinated C-fibers and thinly myelinated A-delta pain fibers) signal pain to the spinal cord. With repeated peripheral stimulation and/or in the setting of neuroinflammation or nerve injury, several changes occur to the neurons and synapses. Early on, enhanced responsiveness to peripheral pain signals develops at the synapses in the spinal cord. There exists increased excitatory signaling (glutamate) and reduced inhibitory signaling (GABA, 5-HT, NE). Nerve injury results in C-fiber cell death with subsequent ingrowth of deep dorsal horn A-fibers. Now activation of these A-fibers transmits pain sensation to the brain. Development of central sensitization involves changes in gene expression, sustained increases in inflammatory mediators (cytokines and chemokines), and cellular and synaptic structural changes that results in chronic facilitated signaling of pain.

Further Reading

Ji RR, Nackley A, Huh Y, et al. Neuroinflammation and central sensitization in chronic and widespread pain. Anesthesiol. 2018;129(2):343-366.
Woolf CJ. Central sensitization: implications for the diagnosis and treatment of pain. Pain. 2011;152(3 suppl):S2–S15.
Woolf CJ, Salter MW. Neuronal plasticity: increasing the gain in pain. Science. 2000;288(5472):1765–1769.

3. Postoperative Pain Management

3.1. How do NMDA antagonists work to control pain? Why are they useful in opioid-tolerant patients and patients with central sensitization?

Drugs like ketamine, amantadine, memantine, methadone, and magnesium all act at the N-methyl-D-aspartate (NMDA) receptor to block ion transmission, raise the threshold for action potential firing, and decrease the likelihood of pain signal transmission. NMDA receptors also modulate directly and indirectly the sensitivity of other receptors, such as the mu-opioid receptor. Ketamine is known to enhance the analgesic effects of opioids, possibly via this interaction between the NMDA and mu-opioid receptors. As such, caution is required when using NMDA antagonists in patients tolerant to opioids. In opioid-tolerant patients, treating pain via NMDA blockade is especially effective for this reason. Occasionally, patients with intractable central pain can find pain relief with NMDA antagonist treatment where other analgesic target treatment has failed (e.g., gabapentin on A2delta Ca2+ channels, clonidine on alpha-2 receptors; antidepressants affecting serotonergic and adrenergic receptors).

Further Reading

Nielsen RV, Fomsgaard JS, Siegel H, et al. Intraoperative ketamine reduces immediate postoperative opioid consumption after spinal fusion surgery in chronic pain patients with opioid dependency: a randomized, blinded trial. Pain. 2017;158(3):463–470.
Peltoniemi MA, Hagelberg NM, Olkkola KT, et al. Ketamine: a review of clinical pharmacokinetics and pharmacodynamics in anesthesia and pain therapy. Clin Pharmacokinet. 2016;55(9):1059–1077.
Visser E, Schug SA. The role of ketamine in pain management. Biomed Pharmacother. 2006;60(7):341–348.

3.2. How do you dose ketamine for intraoperative and postoperative pain control?

Ketamine can be dosed as a weight-based infusion or bolus dosed. A common range for pain control in adult patients under anesthesia is 5 to 10 mcg/kg/min infusion. Ketamine as a bolus is commonly given in the range of 0.2 to 0.5 mg/kg IV/IM. Lower doses should be used when in combination with other multimodal analgesia medications or in the elderly to avoid oversedation and postoperative delirium. In the postoperative phase, awake patients typically tolerate 3 to 10 mcg/kg/min ketamine infusions if up-titration is done slowly and to effect. Rapid dose escalation can lead to side effects such as hypersalivation, hallucinations, and sedation.

Further Reading

Loftus RW, Yeager MP, Clark JA, et al. Intraoperative ketamine reduces perioperative opiate consumption in opiate-dependent patients with chronic back pain undergoing back surgery. Anesthesiology. 2010;113(3):639–646.

3.3. How is methadone dosed for intraoperative and postoperative pain control?

Methadone binds to and activates several target receptors, including the mu-opioid receptor and the NMDA receptor. It has a fast onset of action, ranging from 8 to 10 minutes, when given intravenously. It also has a long duration of action. The common dose range for methadone is 5 to 20 mg IV on induction of anesthesia, depending on the duration of surgery, and 2.5 to 5 mg IV for postoperative acute pain treatment.

Further Reading

Gottschalk A, Durieux ME, Nemergut EC, Intraoperative methadone improves postoperative pain control in patients undergoing complex spine surgery. Anesth Analg. 2011;112(1):218–223.

Murphy GS, Szokol JW, Avram MJ, et al. Clinical effectiveness and safety of intraoperative methadone in patients undergoing posterior spinal fusion surgery: a randomized, double-blinded, controlled trial. Anesthesiology. 2017;126(5):822–833.

3.4. What other NMDA antagonists exist, and what is the evidence for their use in postoperative acute pain treatment?

Amantadine, memantine, and dextromethorphan are also NMDA antagonists used orally for treatment of attention deficit hyperactivity disorder, Alzheimer's disease, and cough suppression, respectively. They have also been used effectively in the treatment of acute and chronic neuropathic pain, although the supportive evidence is of moderate strength only (see Table 15.1). Magnesium is also an NMDA antagonist, and magnesium infusions have been used in the treatment of pain.

Further Reading

Bujak-Gizycka B, Kacka K, Suski M, et al. Beneficial effect of amantadine on postoperative pain reduction and consumption of morphine in patients subjected to elective spine surgery. Pain Med. 2012;13(3):459–465.

Emik U, Unal Y, Arslan M, et al. The effects of memantine on recovery, cognitive functions, and pain after propofol anesthesia. Braz J Anesthesiol. 2016;66(5):485–491.

King MR, Ladha KS, Gelineau AM, et al. Perioperative dextromethorphan as an adjunct for postoperative pain: a meta-analysis of randomized controlled trials. Anesthesiol. 2016;124(3):696–705.

Shin HJ, Kim EY, Na HS, et al. Magnesium sulphate attenuates acute postoperative pain and increased pain intensity after surgical injury in staged bilateral total knee arthroplasty: a randomized, double-blinded, placebo-controlled trial. Br J Anaesth. 2016;117(4):497–503.

3.5. Do NSAIDs prevent bone healing in spine surgery?

Early literature suggested that NSAID use in the perioperative period could result in poor outcomes such as increased bleeding, decreased bone healing, and increased nonunion of spinal fusion. However, a review of 138 subsequent studies on the topic does not support this conclusion when NSAIDs are used only in the 48 hours after surgery to treat acute postoperative inflammatory pain.

Further Reading

Sivaganesan A, Chotai S, White-Dzuro G, et al. The effect of NSAIDs on spinal fusion: a cross-disciplinary review of biochemical, animal, and human studies. Eur Spine J. 2017;26(11):2719–2728.

3.6. How can the risk of opioid-induced ventilatory impairment be managed postoperatively?

Opioid-induced ventilatory impairment (OIVI) remains a high-risk event too frequently encountered in the postoperative period. The incidence of OIVI is between 0.15% and 1.1% of postsurgical patients. Risk factors for OIVI include long-acting opioids, neuraxial anesthesia (with opioids), use of MMA (e.g., addition of gabapentin and other sedating agents), basal opioid infusions, and the number and education of the prescribers. Patient-specific risk factors for OIVI include obesity, obstructive sleep apnea, chronic use of opioids, and more, and several imperfect strategies are available to mitigate this risk (Table 15.3). Consensus conferences on this topic sponsored by the Anesthesia Patient Safety

Table 15.3:
Risk factors for postoperative opioid-induced ventilatory impairment

Patient Factors	Surgical Factors
• Obesity	• General anesthesia
• Obstructive sleep apnea	• Long-acting opioids
• Chronic opioid use	• Gabapentin
• Age	• Sedating drugs
• Renal impairment	• Multiple prescribers
• Neurologic disease	• Prescriber education
• Diabetes	

Foundation support the use of continuous electronic monitoring, including the use of continuous pulse oximetry and capnography when supplemental oxygen is used. Pulse oximetry is commonly available, so it likely to be the most helpful tool for detecting OIVI despite its limitations. Nursing evaluation for somnolence and sedation at regular intervals is especially important in the first 4 hours after discharge from the postanesthesia care unit when most OIVI events occur (50% of OIVI events occur within 12 hours after surgery, and 75% within 24 hours). A combination of risk stratification (heightened alert for the most at-risk patients) and continuous monitoring for patients on postoperative opioids is recommended.

Further Reading

Cavalcante AN, Sprung J, Schroeder DR, et al. Multimodal analgesic therapy with gabapentin and its association with postoperative respiratory depression. Anesth Analg. 2017;125:141–146.

Chidambaran V, Olbrecht V, Hossain M, et al. Risk predictors of opioid-induced critical respiratory events in children: naloxone use as a quality measure of opioid safety. Pain Med. 2014;15:2139–2149.

Dahan A, Aarts L, Smith TW. Incidence, reversal, and prevention of opioid-induced respiratory depression. Anesthesiology. 2010;112:226–238.

Gupta K, Prasad A, Nagappa M, et al. Risk factors for opioid-induced respiratory depression and failure to rescue: a review. Curr Opin Anaesthesiol. 2018;31:110–119.

Jungquist CR, Correll DJ, Fleisher LA, et al. Avoiding adverse events secondary to opioid-induced respiratory depression: implications for nurse executives and patient safety. J Nurs Adm. 2016;46:87–94.

Maddox RR, Williams CK. Clinical experience with capnography monitoring for PCA patients. APSF Newsletter. 2012;26:47–50.

Stoelting RK, Overdyk FJ for the Anesthesia Patient Safety Foundation. Conclusions and Recommendations from the June 8, 2011, Conference on Electronic Monitoring Strategies (Essential Electronic Monitoring Strategies to Detect Clinically Significant Drug-Induced Respiratory Depression in the Postoperative period). www.apsf.org/initiatives.php?id=10. Accessed Jul 14, 2018.

Sun Z, Sessler DI, Dalton JE, et al. Postoperative hypoxemia is common and persistent: a prospective blinded observational study. Anesth Analg. 2015;121:709–715.

Taenzer AH, Pyke JB, McGrath SP, et al. Impact of pulse oximetry surveillance on rescue events and intensive care unit transfers: a before-and-after concurrence study. Anesthesiology. 2010;112:282–287.

Taylor S, Kirton OC, Staff I, et al. Postoperative day one: a high-risk period for respiratory events. Am J Surg. 2005;190:752–756.

Craniotomy

Roxana Grasu and Sally Raty

16

Case Scenario

A 45-year-old woman presents for resection of a newly diagnosed right temporal mass. She presented to her family doctor with complaints of "tension-like" headaches for the past month. Brain MRI at that time revealed the right temporal mass. Her history is remarkable for fibromyalgia, chronic migraines, depression, and anxiety. She takes fluoxetine and clonazepam daily.

1. Patient Considerations

1.1. Postcraniotomy headache

1.1.1. How are acute and persistent PCH defined?

Postcraniotomy headache (PCH), as a significant complication after neurosurgery, first received attention in the literature in the 1980s, being described as significant headache after surgery for acoustic neuroma. The International Headache Society recognized craniotomy as a cause of headache in its 2004 headache classification. In the current 2013 International Classification of Headache Disorders (ICDH-3), the "acute headache attributed to craniotomy" is a headache of less than 3 months' duration caused by surgical craniotomy, performed for nontraumatic head pathology, and which develops within 7 days after craniotomy. Exclusion of other etiologies of headache following a craniotomy, such as cervicogenic headache, as a result of positioning during surgery, headache from cerebrospinal fluid (CSF) leak,

Box 16.1 Classification of Headache Attributed to Craniotomy

I. **Acute**—headache of less than 3 months' duration caused by surgical craniotomy
   Diagnostic criteria:
   A. Any headache fulfilling criteria C and D
   B. Surgical craniotomy (not following traumatic head injury) has been performed
   C. Headache is reported to have developed within 7 days after one of the following:
      1. Craniotomy
      2. Regaining of consciousness following the craniotomy
      3. Discontinuation of medication(s) that impairs ability to sense or report pain
   D. Either of the following:
      1. Headache has resolved within 3 months after the craniotomy
      2. Headache has not yet resolved, but 3 months have not yet passed since the craniotomy
   E. Not better accounted for by another ICHD-3 diagnosis

II. **Persistent**—headache of greater than 3 months' duration caused by surgical craniotomy
   Diagnostic criteria:
   A. Any headache fulfilling criteria C and D
   B. Surgical craniotomy (not following traumatic head injury) has been performed
   C. Headache is reported to have developed within 7 days after one of the following:
      1. Craniotomy
      2. Regaining of consciousness following the craniotomy
      3. Discontinuation of medication(s) that impairs ability to sense or report pain
   D. Headache persists for >3 months after the craniotomy
   E. Not better accounted for by another ICHD-3 diagnosis

ICHD: International Classification of Headache Disorders.

Adapted from Headache Classification Committee of the International Headache Society (IHS) The International Classification of Headache Disorders, 3rd edition. *Cephalalgia*. 2018;38(1):1-211.

infections, hydrocephalus, and intracranial hemorrhage, is necessary prior to assigning the diagnosis of acute PCH. PCH lasting for more than 3 months after craniotomy is classified as "persistent headache attributed to craniotomy" (Box 16.1). PCH represents an important group of secondary headaches, and its management often constitutes a challenge for neurosurgeons, anesthesiologists, neurologists, and headache specialists.

Further Reading

Headache Classification Committee of the International Headache Society (IHS) The International Classification of Headache Disorders, 3rd edition. *Cephalalgia*. 2018;38(1):1–211.

Rocha-Filho PA. Post-craniotomy headache: a clinical view with a focus on the persistent form. *Headache*. 2015;55:733–738.

Silverstein H, Norrell H, Smouha E, Jones R. Retrolabyrinthine or retrosigmoid vestibular neurectomy: indications. *American Journal of Otology*. 1987;8:414–418.

1.1.2. What is the incidence of acute and persistent PCH?

Pain following craniotomy is more common than previously thought. Up to 80% of craniotomy patients experience moderate to severe pain in the immediate postoperative period, and up to 30% develop persistent headache. Compared with supratentorial craniotomy, infratentorial approaches including posterior fossa and skull base procedures are associated with a higher incidence of persistent PCH.

Clinical trials measuring analgesic use after craniotomy provide an indirect measurement of PCH pain, and data suggest that 50% to 90% of patients require pain relief medication in the immediate postoperative period.

A scarce few prospective cohort studies have evaluated the incidence of PCH. Moderate to severe pain is defined as ≥4 on a 0–10 scale and is commonly experienced by patients during the first 48 hours after craniotomy. According to Gottschalk et al., 69% of patients experience moderate pain on the first postoperative day, and 48% have moderate pain on the second postoperative day. Mordhorst et al. found that 87% of patients undergoing elective craniotomy experienced pain during the first 24 hours.

The estimated incidence of postsurgical chronic pain ranges from 10% to 50% following nonneurosurgic procedures, and a review of the literature suggests a similar or higher incidence of persistent or chronic PCH. The reported incidence of persistent headache after acoustic neuroma resection is 33% to 44% and after supratentorial craniotomy is 11.9% to 29.3%. Batoz et al. found an incidence of 56% of chronic PCH, possibly because of their broader definition of chronic pain. The prevalence of persistent PCH declines consistently with time.

Further Reading

Batoz H, Verdonck O, Pellerin C, Roux G, Maurette P. The analgesic properties of scalp infiltrations with ropivacaine after intracranial tumor resection. *Anesth Analg.* 2009;109:240–244.

Biswas BK, Bithal PK. Preincision 0.25% bupivacaine scalp infiltration and postcraniotomy pain: a randomized double-blind, placebo-controlled study. *J Neurosurg Anesthesiol.* 2003;15:234–239.

Flexman AM, Ng JL, Gelb AW. Acute and chronic pain following craniotomy. *Curr Opin Anesthesiol.* 2010;23:551–557.

Gee JR, Ishaq Y, Vijayan N. Postcraniotomy headache. *Headache.* 2003;43:276–278.

Gerlach K, Uhlig T, Huppe M, et al. Remifentanil-propofol vs sufentanil-propofol anaesthesia for supratentorial craniotomy: a randomized trial. *Eur J Anaesthesiol.* 2003;20:813–820.

Gottschalk A, Berkow LC, Stevens RD, et al. Prospective evaluation of pain and analgesic use following major elective intracranial surgery. *J Neurosurg.* 2007;106:210–216.

Guy J, Hindman BJ, Baker KZ, et al. Comparison of remifentanil and fentanyl in patients undergoing craniotomy for supratentorial space-occupying lesions. *Anesthesiology.* 1997;86:514–524.

Kaur A, Selwa L, Fromes G, Ross DA. Persistent headache after supratentorial craniotomy. *Neurosurgery.* 2000;47:633–636.

Kehlet H, Jensen TS, Woolf CJ. Persistent postsurgical pain: risk factors and prevention. *Lancet.* 2006;367:1618–1625.

Mordhorst C, Latz B, Kerz T, Wisser G, et al. Prospective assessment of postoperative pain after craniotomy. *J Neurosurg Anesthesiol.* 2010;22:202–206.

Rimaaja T, Haanpaa M, Blomstedt G, Farkilla M. Headache after acoustic neuroma surgery. *Cephalalgia.* 2007;27:1128–1135.

Rocha-Filho PA, Gherpeli JL, de Siqueira JT, Rabello GD. Postcraniotomy headache: characteristics, behavior and effect on quality of life in patients operated for treatment of supratentorial intracranial aneurysms. *Cephalalgia.* 2008;28:41–48.

Schaller B, Baumann A. Headache after removal of vestibular schwannoma via the retrosigmoid approach: a long term follow-up study. *Otolaryngol Head Neck Surg.* 2003;128:387–395.

1.1.3. What are the characteristics and severity of PCH?

Superficial, sharp, aching incisional pain is the most common manifestation, often associated with pressing or pounding, tension-type headache and sometimes throbbing, migraine-type headache. As many as 80% of postcraniotomy patients experience moderate to severe pain in the first 2 days after surgery, and despite gradual, significant improvement over time, up to one-third of patients may go on to experience persistent headache.

The majority of PCHs are incisional and unilateral (55%–79%). Approximately 35% to 55% of patients have new bilateral postoperative headaches. PCH contralateral to the surgical side is most common after acoustic neuroma surgery.

Patients commonly describe PCH as "pressing," "pounding," "throbbing," or "pulsating." PCH often presents as short-lasting attacks and can be triggered or worsened by emotional and physical stress, position, or coughing. PCH can have "migraine-like" features, including severe pain and a throbbing quality accompanied by photophobia, nausea, and vomiting. In addition to the nociceptive pain, postcraniotomy neuropathic pain has been described in 25% of patients. Two-thirds of patients who have acute PCH rate the pain as moderate or severe, and a majority of them report pain onset within 48 hours postoperatively.

In general, the incidence of severe persistent headache is highest after acoustic neuroma surgery; however, Kaur et al. studied persistent PCH after supratentorial craniotomy and found that 4% of patients had medically uncontrolled headaches, and 3.2% continued to require prescription pain medications for headaches 1 year postoperatively. The prevalence, frequency and intensity of PCH significantly decrease over time.

Further Reading

Batoz H, Verdonck O, Pellerin C, Roux G, Maurette P. The analgesic properties of scalp infiltrations with ropivacaine after intracranial tumor resection. *Anesth Analg*. 2009;109:240–244.

De Beneditis G, Lorenzetti A, Migliore M, Spagnoli D, Tiberio F, Vilani RM. Postoperative pain in neurosurgery: a pilot study in brain surgery. *Neurosurgery*. 1996;38:466–469, discussion 469–470.

De Gray LC, Matta BF. Acute and chronic pain following craniotomy: a review. *Anaesthesia*. 2005;60:693–704.

Flexman AM, Ng JL, Gelb AW. Acute and chronic pain following craniotomy. *Curr Opin Anesthesiol*. 2010;23:551–557.

Gee JR, Ishaq Y, Vijayan N. Postcraniotomy headache. *Headache*. 2003;43:276–278.

Kaur A, Selwa L, Fromes G, Ross DA. Persistent headache after supratentorial craniotomy. *Neurosurgery*. 2000;47:633–636.

Molnar I, Simon E, Nemes R, Fulesdi B, Molnar C. Postcraniotomy headache. *J Anaesth*. 2014;28:102–111.

Rimaaja T, Haanpaa M, Blomstedt G, Farkilla M. Headache after acoustic neuroma surgery. *Cephalalgia*. 2007;27:1128–1135.

Rocha-Filho PA. Post-craniotomy headache: a clinical view with a focus on the persistent form. *Headache*. 2015;55:733–738.

Rocha-Filho PA, Gherpeli JL, de Siqueira JT, Rabello GD. Postcraniotomy headache: characteristics, behavior and effect on quality of life in patients operated for treatment of supratentorial intracranial aneurysms. *Cephalalgia*. 2008;28:41–48.

Schaller B, Baumann A. Headache after removal of vestibular schwanoma via the retrosigmoid approach: a long term follow-up study. *Otolaryngol Head Neck Surg*. 2003;128:387–395.

Schankin CJ, Gall C, Straube A. Headache syndromes after acoustic neuroma surgery and their implications for quality of life. Cephalalgia. 2009;29:760–771.

Thibault M, Girard F, Moumdjian R, Chouinard P, Boudreault D, Ruel M. Craniotomy site influences postoperative pain following neurosurgical procedures: a retrospective study. *Can J Anaesth*. 2007;54:544–548.

1.1.4. Describe risk factors thought to contribute in general to the development of significant acute and chronic postsurgical pain

Both patient-specific and surgery-specific risk factors can contribute to development of significant acute and chronic postsurgical pain. Risk factors for the development of chronic postsurgical pain can be subdivided into preoperative, intraoperative, and postoperative factors (Box 16.2). Several studies suggest that there could be a genetic disposition to increased pain susceptibility; however, no specific genetic marker for development of chronic pain after surgery has been identified yet. Preoperative risk factors include female sex and younger age. Females have an increased incidence of most chronic pain syndromes and also have an increased risk of developing persistent postsurgical pain. Younger patients seem to carry an increased risk of developing persistent postsurgical pain; some studies found a reduction in odds of developing postsurgical pain per each 1-year increase in age. Mechanisms explaining the increased incidence of chronic pain in younger patients are unknown but may relate to reduction in peripheral nociceptive function with increased age. Preoperative pain is consistently found to be a predictor for persistent postsurgical pain. Psychosocial factors including depression, psychological vulnerability (e.g., catastrophizing), anxiety, and stress are predictors for persistent postsurgical

Box 16.2 Risk Factors for Chronic Postsurgical Pain

I. Preoperative

1. Pain, moderate to severe, lasting more than 1 month
2. Repeat surgery
3. Female sex
4. Younger age (adults)
5. Preoperative anxiety, depression
6. Psychological vulnerability (e.g., stress, catastrophizing)
7. Genetic predisposition
8. Inefficient diffuse noxious inhibitory control (DNIC)
9. Workers' compensation (late return to work)

II. Intraoperative

1. Surgical approach with risk of nerve damage
2. Avoidance of nitrous oxide anesthesia

III. Postoperative

1. Pain (acute, moderate to severe)
2. Radiation therapy to area
3. Neurotoxic chemotherapy
4. Depression
5. Anxiety
6. Psychological vulnerability

Sources: Adapted from Schug SA, Palmer GM, Scott DA, Halliwell R, Trinca J; APM:SE Working Group of the Australian and New Zealand College of Anaesthetists and Faculty of Pain Medicine, *Acute Pain Management: Scientific Evidence, 4th edition*, p. 19, Table 1.3, ANZCA & FPM, Melbourne. 2015.

pain. Hypervigilance, thought to be one of the psychosocial factors contributing to fibromyalgia, may also play a role in persistent postsurgical pain. The most significant postoperative predictive factor for persistent postsurgical pain appears to be the severity of acute postoperative pain.

Further Reading

De Kock M. Expanding our horizons: transition of acute postoperative pain to persistent pain and establishment of chronic postsurgical pain services. *Anesthesiology*. 2009;111:461–463.

Diatchenko L, Slade GD, Nackley AG, et al. Genetic basis for individual variations in pain perception and the development of a chronic pain condition. *Hum Mol Genetic*. 2005;14:135–143.

Hinrichs-Rocker A, Schulz K, Jarvinen I, Lefering R, Simanski C, Neugebauer EA. Psychosocial predictors and correlates for chronic post-surgical pain (CPSP): a systematic review. *Eur J Pain*. 2009;13:719–730.

Kehlet H, Jensen TS, Woolf CJ. Persistent postsurgical pain: risk factors and prevention. *Lancet*. 2006;367:1618–1625.

Macrae WA. Chronic post-surgical pain 10 years on. *Br J Anaesth*. 2008;101(1):77–86.

Schug SA, Palmer GM, Scott DA, Halliwell R, Trinca J; APM:SE Working Group of the Australian and New Zealand College of Anaesthetists and Faculty of Pain Medicine, *Acute Pain Management: Scientific Evidence, 4th edition*, ANZCA & FPM, Melbourne. 2015.

Schug SA, Pogatzki-Zahn EM. Chronic pain after surgery or injury. *PainClin Updates*. 2011;9:1–5.

1.1.5. What specific patient factors are currently associated with the development of chronic PCH?

According to the neurosurgical literature, several of the patient factors identified as risk factors in general for chronic postsurgical pain, such as female sex, younger age, presence of preoperative depression and anxiety, correlate with the incidence, frequency, and severity of PCH.

In one study, female sex, anxiety ,and depression were strongly associated with headache frequency after supratentorial craniotomy. Other studies found that younger women had worse outcomes in regard to incidence and severity of PCH. One retrospective study of headache after acoustic neuroma with a retrosigmoid approach found that female sex, previous headache, and tumor size were independent predictors of chronic PCH. The same study found that postoperative depression was significantly more common in patients with chronic PCH. Although chronic pain and depression are clearly related, further investigation is needed.

Further Reading

De Beneditis G, Lorenzetti A, Migliore M, Spagnoli D, Tiberio F, Vilani RM. Postoperative pain in neurosurgery: a pilot study in brain surgery. *Neurosurgery*. 1996;38:466–469, discussion 469–470.

Flexman AM, Ng JL, Gelb AW. Acute and chronic pain following craniotomy. *Curr Opin Anesthesiol.* 2010;23:551–557.

Gottschalk A, Berkow LC, Stevens RD, et al. Prospective evaluation of pain and analgesic use following major elective intracranial surgery. *J Neurosurg*. 2007;106:210–216.

Rimaaja T, Haanpaa M, Blomstedt G, Farkilla M. Headache after acoustic neuroma surgery. *Cephalalgia*. 2007;27:1128–1135.

Rocha-Filho PA, Gherpeli JL, de Siqueira JT, Rabello GD. Postcraniotomy headache: characteristics, behavior and effect on quality of life in patients operated for treatment of supratentorial intracranial aneurysms. *Cephalalgia*. 2008;28:41–48.

1.1.6. What is the significance of preexistent headache in a patient scheduled for craniotomy?

PCH is more frequent in patients with a history of preexistent headache. Nevertheless, the preoperative headache attributed to the brain tumor, which frequently resembles primary headaches, such as migraine- or tension-type, is also more common in patients with preexisting headache history. Therefore, a patient with history of migraine and new onset of tumor-related tension-type headache may be at higher risk for developing significant acute and chronic PCH.

Many patients with PCH describe pain in the surgical area. A significant number also describe a primary headache pattern similar to a tension-type or migraine-type headache. Patients with a preexisting headache pattern can have a substantial change in the headache pattern after craniotomy.

Further Reading

Flexman AM, Ng JL, Gelb AW. Acute and chronic pain following craniotomy. Curr Opin Anesthesiol. 2010;23:551-557.

Nelson S, Taylor LP. Headaches in brain tumor patients: primary or secondary? *Headache*. 2014;54:776–785.

Rocha-Filho PA. Post-craniotomy headache: a clinical view with a focus on the persistent form. *Headache*. 2015;55:733–738.

Schankin CJ, Straube A. Secondary headaches: secondary or still primary? *J Headache Pain*. 2012;13:263–270.

1.1.7. Should anxiety and mood disorders be investigated and treated before the surgery?

In general, depression and anxiety are more prevalent among patients with PCH. The prevalence of depression and anxiety after craniotomy is greater than before craniotomy. Severe depression and anxiety are significantly correlated not only with higher frequency and severity of acute PCH but also with a greater risk of developing chronic PCH. Although there are no clinical trials to date evaluating whether depression and anxiety treatment diminishes the incidence of PCH, every attempt should be made to diagnose and treat these conditions throughout the perioperative period.

Further Reading

Flexman AM, Ng JL, Gelb AW. Acute and chronic pain following craniotomy. *Curr Opin Anesthesiol.* 2010;23:551–557.

Rimaaja T, Haanpaa M, Blomstedt G, Farkilla M. Headache after acoustic neuroma surgery. *Cephalalgia.* 2007;27:1128–1135.

Rocha-Filho PA. Post-craniotomy headache: a clinical view with a focus on the persistent form. *Headache.* 2015;55:733–738.

Rocha-Filho PA, Gherpeli JL, de Siqueira JT, Rabello GD. Postcraniotomy headache: characteristics, behavior and effect on quality of life in patients operated for treatment of supratentorial intracranial aneurysms. *Cephalalgia.* 2008;28:41–48.

1.1.8. What is the significance of preexistent fibromyalgia and migraine in a patient scheduled for craniotomy?

The preoperative presence of both fibromyalgia and migraine greatly increases the risk of developing significant acute and chronic PCH. Optimal perioperative management of these conditions is recommended for the prevention and treatment of significant and persistent PCH.

Fibromyalgia, an idiopathic, chronic pain condition, frequently coexists with other chronic pain conditions like tension-type headache or migraine. A recent large epidemiologic study evidenced a 55.8% prevalence of migraine among fibromyalgia patients, while other studies showed the prevalence of fibromyalgia in migraine patients to be more than 30%.

Fibromyalgia and chronic migraine frequently co-occur, suggesting common pathophysiologic mechanisms like central sensitization and decreased descending inhibition leading to enhanced pain perception. Comorbidity between fibromyalgia and migraine results in heightened somatic hyperalgesia compared with the presence of only one condition. Chronic migraine enhances both hyperalgesia and spontaneous fibromyalgia pain. Effective migraine prophylaxis results in a significant improvement of fibromyalgia symptoms.

Comorbidities of anxiety, depression, and somatization disorder are frequently associated with fibromyalgia and are independently known to increase the risk of acute and chronic pain after surgery.

Further Reading

Giamberardino MA, Affaitati G, Martelletti P. Impact of migraine on fibromyalgia symptoms. *J Headache Pain.* 2016;17:281–289.

Pogatzki-Zahn EM Englbrecht JS, Schug SA. Acute pain management in patients with fibromyalgia and other diffuse chronic pain syndromes. *Curr Opin Anesthesiol.* 2009;22:627–633.

Vji B, Whipple MO, Tepper SJ, Mohabbat AB, Stillman M, Vincent A. Frequency of migraine headaches in patients with fibromyalgia. *Headache.* 2015;55:860–865.

1.1.9. Discuss the short- and long-term repercussions of acute and chronic PCH for patients

In the immediate postoperative period, a lack of effective analgesia can lead to distress, agitation, confusion, hypertension, shivering, and vomiting and result in raised intracranial pressure and bleeding. Poorly controlled acute postoperative pain prolongs recovery and hospitalization and exposes the patient at high risk for developing chronic pain.

In the long term, there are great repercussions from chronic PCH on patients' quality of life. There is a direct correlation between the frequency and severity of chronic PCH and negative impact on the individual's social functioning. Headaches can be incapacitating and are greatly associated with the failure to return to the preoperative activity level. Individuals with PCH have more problems with work and other daily activities than those without headache. Among the patients with PCH, 29% to 60% report that the headaches interfere with activities of daily living, including recreational (25%), work (19%–38%), and social activities (8%). In 15% of cases, PCH has a negative impact on the mood, and in 22% the pain is incapacitating.

Further Reading

Betchen SA, Walsh J, Post KD. Self-assessed quality of life after acoustic neuroma surgery. *J Neurosurg*. 2003;99:818–823.

Flexman AM, Ng JL, Gelb AW. Acute and chronic pain following craniotomy. *Curr Opin Anesthesiol*. 2010;23:551–557.

Rocha-Filho PA. Post-craniotomy headache: a clinical view with a focus on the persistent form. *Headache*. 2015;55:733–738.

Rocha-Filho PA, Gherpeli JL, de Siqueira JT, Rabello GD. Postcraniotomy headache: characteristics, behavior and effect on quality of life in patients operated for treatment of supratentorial intracranial aneurysms. *Cephalalgia*. 2008;28:41–48.

Schankin CJ, Gall C, Straube A. Headache syndromes after acoustic neuroma surgery and their implications for quality of life. *Cephalalgia*. 2009;29:760–771.

2. Pain Considerations

2.1. Pathophysiology of PCH

2.1.1. Describe current pain mechanisms associated with headache development following craniotomy

Most patients with PCH describe the pain as predominantly superficial and incisional, suggesting a somatic rather than a visceral origin. The pain is thought to arise mainly from the pericranial muscles, and soft tissue rather than from the brain tissue itself, which is poorly innervated.

Possible pathophysiologic mechanisms of acute PCH involve injury to cutaneous nerves that supply sensation to the scalp and underlying tissues, and to perivascular nerves that supply sensation to the dura mater. Sensory innervation of the scalp and dura involves a rich plexus arising primarily from the trigeminal nerve (its ganglion and the 3 principal divisions and their branches), the upper 3 cervical nerves, and minor branches from the facial, vagus, and glossopharyngeal nerves. The type of injury has been described as mechanical and chemical irritation of the scalp, muscles, periosteum, and dura mater. Occasionally CSF leakage and reduced intracranial pressure (ICP) have also been observed. CSF leak is not uncommon following skull base surgery. Worsening of headache symptoms with upright positioning can be indicative of CSF leak. Dural tension, aseptic meningitis, and adherence of cervical muscles to the dura can also contribute to acute PCH development. The mass of the muscle involved during surgery is also crucial; suboccipital and subtemporal routes are associated with the highest incidence of pain, possibly related to surgical stress in major muscle tissues (i.e., the temporalis, splenium capitis, and cervicis muscles).

The development of chronic PCH is probably related to central sensitization, an increased ability to sense nociceptive signals that can be triggered by extensive and acute pain stimuli. Persistent tension headache and neck muscle spasm likely result from surgical positioning of the head and neck during craniotomy.

Further Reading

De Beneditis G, Lorenzetti A, Migliore M, Spagnoli D, Tiberio F, Vilani RM. Postoperative pain in neurosurgery: a pilot study in brain surgery. *Neurosurgery*. 1996;38:466–469, discussion 469–470.

Dirks J, Moiniche S, Hilsted KL, Dahl JB. Mechanisms of postoperative pain: clinical indications for a contribution of central neuronal sensitization. *Anesthesiology*. 2002;97(6):1591–1596.

Gottschalk A, Yaster M. The perioperative management of pain from intracranial surgery. *Neurocrit Care*. 2009;10:387–402.

Kaur A, Selwa L, Fromes G, Ross DA. Persistent headache after supratentorial craniotomy. *Neurosurgery*. 2000;47:633–636.

Rimaaja T, Haanpaa M, Blomstedt G, Farkilla M. Headache after acoustic neuroma surgery. *Cephalalgia*. 2007;27:1128–1135.

Rocha-Filho PA, Gherpeli JL, de Siqueira JT, Rabello GD. Postcraniotomy headache: characteristics, behavior and effect on quality of life in patients operated for treatment of supratentorial intracranial aneurysms. *Cephalalgia*. 2008;28:41–48.

Ryzenman JM, Pensak ML, Tew JM Jr. Headache: a quality of life analysis in a cohort of 1,657 patients undergoing acoustic neuroma surgery; results from the acoustic neuroma association. *Laryngoscope*. 2005;115(4):703–711.

Teo MK, Eljamel MS. Role of craniotomy repair in reducing postoperative headaches after a retrosigmoid approach. *Neurosurgery*. 2010;67(5):1286–1291.

2.1.2. What surgical risk factors have been identified to contribute to the development of PCH?

The surgical site, approach, and nature of the procedure also have considerable influence on the incidence and severity of acute postoperative pain. Infratentorial (posterior fossa and skull base) procedures are associated with more severe pain at rest and with movement than are supratentorial procedures. A study comparing supra- and infratentorial routes found that average pain intensity as recorded on a 10-point scale 24 hours postoperatively was 4.5 ± 2.7 versus 6.3 ± 2.6, with a total opioid consumption of 6.6 ± 12.6 mg versus 26.9 ± 88.9 mg, respectively. Similar differences were noticed with a 1-year follow-up time: the prevalence of chronic PCH after supratentorial surgeries was 11.9%, notably lower than the 60% and 70% experienced after translabyrinthine and retrosigmoid approaches, respectively. The relationship between pain intensity and the location of craniotomy could be explained by the difference in muscle mass underlying the surgical incision; this also explains the higher pain scores after suboccipital and subtemporal interventions.

Further Reading

De Beneditis G, Lorenzetti A, Migliore M, Spagnoli D, Tiberio F, Vilani RM. Postoperative pain in neurosurgery: a pilot study in brain surgery. *Neurosurgery*. 1996;38:466–469, discussion 469–470.

Gottschalk A, Berkow LC, Stevens RD, et al. Prospective evaluation of pain and analgesic use following major elective intracranial surgery. *J Neurosurg*. 2007;106:210–216.

Ryzenman JM, Pensak ML, Tew JM Jr. Headache: a quality of life analysis in a cohort of 1,657 patients undergoing acoustic neuroma surgery; results from the acoustic neuroma association. *Laryngoscope*. 2005;115(4):703–711.

Thibault M, Girard F, Moumdjian R, Chouinard P, Boudreault D, Ruel M. Craniotomy site influences postoperative pain following neurosurgical procedures: a retrospective study. *Can J Anaesth*. 2007;54:544–548.

2.1.3. How can surgical technique influence the development and severity of PCH?

Surgeons have concluded that bone flap replacement (craniotomy) not only serves cosmetic purposes but also can reduce the incidence of PCH. In posterior fossa surgery, reduced pain has been demonstrated with craniotomy compared with craniectomy, and with cranioplasty after craniectomy. Schaller and coworkers found a reduction from 94% to 27% in chronic PCH frequency when the bone flap was replaced at the end of surgery. Patients who underwent craniotomy had a lower rate of headache at discharge (19%) and at 1 year postoperatively (1%) than patients with craniectomy, who had rates of 43% and 10%, respectively. The lower rate of CSF leakage in craniotomy patients (6%) compared with craniectomy patients (20%) could be one explanation for the lower rate of PCH at discharge and 1 year later. Cranioplasty at the conclusion of surgery with insertion of methyl methacrylate between the cervical muscles and dura can also decrease the occurrence of PCH. When an abdominal adipose graft was applied, chronic pain and its severity were reduced compared with standard neurosurgical wound closure techniques (11.9 vs. 30.3%). A retrospective analysis demonstrated a decreased incidence of postoperative pain in patients having a duraplasty (0%) compared with patients having direct dural closure (100%). Duraplasty decreases the tension on the dura when compared with direct dural closure.

The translabyrinthine approach to resection of acoustic neuromas has been associated with less chronic PCH than the retrosigmoid or suboccipital approach. The amount of muscle damage from resection of the temporalis and posterior cervical muscles may also impact the severity of postoperative pain. The surgical approach is crucial; therefore, to minimize complications, the possibly less invasive method should be chosen.

Further Reading

Gottschalk A, Berkow LC, Stevens RD, et al. Prospective evaluation of pain and analgesic use following major elective intracranial surgery. *J Neurosurg*. 2007;106:210–216.

Gottschalk A, Yaster M. The perioperative management of pain from intracranial surgery. *Neurocrit Care*. 2009;10:387–402.

Harner SG, Beatty CW, Ebersold MJ. Impact of cranioplasty on headache after acoustic neuroma removal. *Neurosurgery*. 1995;36(6):1097–1099.

Koperer H, Deinsberger W, Jodicke A, Boker DK. Postoperative headache after the lateral suboccipital approach: craniotomy versus craniectomy. *Minim Invasive Neurosurg*. 1999;42:175–178.

Porter RG Sr, Leonetti JP, Ksiazek J, Anderson D. Association between adipose graft usage and postoperative headache after retrosigmoid craniotomy. *Otol Neurotol*. 2009;30(5):635–639.

Ruckenstein MJ, Harris JP, Cueva RA, et al. Pain subsequent to resection of acoustic neuromas via suboccipital and translabyrinthine approaches. *Am J Otol*. 1996;17:620–624.

Ryzenman JM, Pensak ML, Tew JM Jr. Headache: a quality of life analysis in a cohort of 1,657 patients undergoing acoustic neuroma surgery; results from the acoustic neuroma association. *Laryngoscope*. 2005;115(4):703–711.

Schaller B, Baumann A. Headache after removal of vestibular schwanoma via the retrosigmoid approach: a long term follow-up study. *Otolaryngol Head Neck Surg*. 2003;128:387–395.

Schessel DA, Nedzelski JM, Rowed D, Feghali JG. Pain after surgery for acoustic neuroma. *Otolaryngol Head Neck Surg*. 1992;107:424–429.

Talke PO, Gelb AW. Postcraniotomy pain remains a real headache! *Eur J Anaesthesiol*. 2005;22:325–327.

Thibault M, Girard F, Moumdjian R, Chouinard P, Boudreault D, Ruel M. Craniotomy site influences postoperative pain following neurosurgical procedures: a retrospective study. *Can J Anaesth*. 2007;54:544–548.

2.2. Local and regional anesthesia

2.2.1. Does local anesthesia have a role in preventing PCH?

Local anesthetics are routinely used for both intraoperative scalp infiltration of wound margins and scalp blockade. Preincisional scalp nerve block or wound infiltration with local anesthetic decreases intraoperative analgesic requirements and may reduce pain in the early postoperative period. A preemptive analgesic mechanism has been suggested to be involved in local anesthetic's effect on postcraniotomy pain. Therefore, the opioid-sparing effect of scalp wound infiltration or scalp nerve blocks makes these techniques useful intra- and postoperative adjuncts to opiate analgesia. However, the majority of studies suggest that their postoperative analgesic effects are brief and clinically inferior to those of opioids. Law-Koune et al. noted a significant but transient reduction in morphine consumption, without any change in pain scores, during the first 2 postoperative hours in patients who received local anesthetic wound infiltration at skin closure; however, the effect did not extend beyond this time.

Additionally, it has been theorized that local anesthetic wound infiltration may prevent inflammation, sensitization, and development of neuropathic pain and chronic PCH. Batoz et al. have prospectively examined the effect of local anesthetic infiltration of the surgical wound at the end of the surgery on the incidence of chronic PCH; although the authors failed to show a significant reduction in opioid consumption in the immediate postoperative period, they reported an impressive reduction in persistent pain (56% vs. 8%) and neuropathic pain (25% vs. 4%) 2 months after surgery.

Further Reading

Batoz H, Verdonck O, Pellerin C, Roux G, Maurette P. The analgesic properties of scalp infiltrations with ropivacaine after intracranial tumor resection. *Anesth Analg*. 2009;109:240–244.

De Gray LC, Matta BF. Acute and chronic pain following craniotomy: a review. *Anaesthesia*. 2005;60:693–704.

Dunn LK, Naik BI, Nemergut EC, Durieux ME. Post-craniotomy pain management: beyond opioids. *Curr Neurol Neurosci Rep*. 2016;93:1–10.

Flexman AM, Ng JL, Gelb AW. Acute and chronic pain following craniotomy. *Curr Opin Anesthesiol*. 2010;23:551–557.

Gottschalk A, Berkow LC, Stevens RD, et al. Prospective evaluation of pain and analgesic use following major elective intracranial surgery. *J Neurosurg*. 2007;106:210–216.

Haldar R, Kaushal A, Gupta D, Srivastava S, Singh PK. Pain following craniotomy: reassessment of the available options. *Biomed Res Int.* 2015;1:1–10.

Law-Koune JD, Szekely B, Fermanian C, Peuch C, Liu N, Fischler M. Scalp infiltration with bupivacaine plus epinephrine or plain ropivacaine reduces postoperative pain after supratentorial craniotomy. *J Neurosurg Anesthesiol.* 2005;17(3):139–143.

Kehlet H, Jensen TS, Woolf CJ. Persistent postsurgical pain: risk factors and prevention. *Lancet.* 2006;367:1618–1625.

Vadivelu N, Kai AM, Tran D, Kodumudi G, Legler A, Ayrian E. Options for perioperative pain management in neurosurgery. *J Pain Res.* 2016;9:37–47.

2.2.2. What is a scalp block, and what is its role in management of PCH?

A scalp block refers to selective infiltration of local anesthetics to the nerves that supply sensation to the scalp. The addition of a scalp block to a general anesthetic for craniotomy surgery has the advantages of blunting the hemodynamic response to the placement of Mayfield head pins and skin incision, and providing early postoperative analgesia without the need for opioids. Preventing severe early postoperative pain may have a role in decreasing risk for development of persistent pain. A scalp block includes targeted bilateral injection of the 7 nerves that provide innervation to the scalp: the supraorbital, supratrochlear, zygomaticotemporal, and auriculotemporal nerves, which are branches of the trigeminal nerve, along with greater auricular, lesser, and greater occipital nerves, which are branches of second- and third-cervical spinal nerves. Ropivacaine 0.5% or 0.75% and bupivacaine 0.25% to 0.5% are common local anesthetic choices for a scalp block, and epinephrine 1:200,000 is a frequent additive. Complications of scalp blocks are rare; however, unintentional intravascular injection can result in local anesthetic toxicity, including seizures, cardiac dysrhythmias, or cardiac arrest. Through possible preemptive mechanisms, scalp block can decrease PCH, and its effect lasts longer than would be predicted based on the pharmacokinetics of the local anesthetics used. Use of a scalp block can reduce pain scores in the early postoperative period compared with placebo and provides similar pain relief when compared with intravenous fentanyl or morphine. Thus, scalp block can be useful as an adjuvant nonopioid analgesic.

Several small observational studies support the use of a scalp block for patients undergoing craniotomy. Nguyen et al. performed a prospective double-blind, randomized study in 30 patients receiving a block with 0.75% ropivacaine or saline. Pain was assessed starting at 4 and up to 48 hours postoperatively. The average pain score in the ropivacaine group was significantly lower when compared with the saline group for up to 24 hours, and the analgesic effect seemed to persist for at least 48 hours postoperatively. Ayoub et al. found that scalp block provided transitional analgesia equivalent to that conferred by morphine 0.1 mg/kg intravenously, administered after dural closure, with similar side effects. In a systematic review of 138 studies of scalp blocks for postcraniotomy analgesia and meta-analysis of 7 randomized controlled trials of 320 patients (scalp blocks were performed before skin incision in 3 studies and after wound closure in 4 studies), Guilfoyle et al. found that scalp blocks are useful for postoperative analgesia, particularly in the early postoperative period when craniotomy pain is most severe; however, the opioid-sparing effect was limited.

Further Reading

Ayoub C, Girard F, Boudreault D, Chouinard P, Ruel M, Moumdjian R. A comparison between scalp nerve block and morphine for transitional analgesia after remifentanil-based anesthesia in neurosurgery. *Anesth Analg.* 2006;103(5):1237–1240.

Dunn LK, Naik BI, Nemergut EC, Durieux ME. Post-craniotomy pain management: beyond opioids. *Curr Neurol Neurosci Rep.* 2016;93:1–10.

Girard F, Quentin C, Charbonneau S, Ayoub C, Boudreault D, Chouinard P, Ruel M, Moumdjian R. Superficial cervical plexus block for transitional analgesia in infratentorial and occipital craniotomy: a randomized trial. *Can J Anaesth.* 2010;57(12):1065–1070.

Guilfoyle MR, Helmy A, Duane D, Hutchinson PJ. Regional scalp block for postcraniotomy analgesia: a systematic review and meta-analysis. *Anesth Analg.* 2013;116:1093–1102.

Haldar R, Kaushal A, Gupta D, Srivastava S, Singh PK. Pain following craniotomy: reassessment of the available options. *Biomed Res Int.* 2015;1:1–10.

Lee EJ, Lee MY, Shyr MH, Cheng JT, Toung TJ, Mirski MA, Chen TY. Adjuvant bupivacaine scalp block facilitates stabilization of hemodynamics in patients undergoing craniotomy with general anesthesia: a preliminary report. *J Clin Anesth.* 2006;18(7):490–494.

Nguyen A, Girard F, Boudreault D, et al. Scalp nerve blocks decrease the severity of pain after craniotomy. *Anesth Analg.* 2001;93:1272–1276.

Osborn, I, Sebeo, J. "Scalp block" during craniotomy: a classic technique revisited. *J Neurosurg Anesth.* 2010;22(3):187–194.

Vadivelu N, Kai AM, Tran D, Kodumudi G, Legler A, Ayrian E. Options for perioperative pain management in neurosurgery. *J Pain Res.* 2016;9:37–47.

3. Perioperative Pain Management

3.1. Opioid analgesia

3.1.1. Which opioids are commonly used for intraoperative anesthesia management for elective craniotomy?

Anesthesia management during elective craniotomy requires the use of short-acting and ultra-short-acting opioids to provide effective intraoperative analgesia without increasing ICP, maintain cerebral perfusion pressure (CPP), and facilitate rapid emergence and early neurologic assessment postoperatively. The choice of intraoperative opioid analgesics can have a significant impact on the time course and severity of postoperative pain. The commonly used intraoperative opioids are remifentanil, fentanyl, and sufentanil.

Patients who receive remifentanil, an ultra-short-acting opioid, for intraoperative analgesia request additional analgesics earlier and in greater amounts in the postoperative period compared with patients who receive fentanyl or sufentanil as the primary intraoperative opioid. The increase in postoperative analgesic requirements following intraoperative remifentanil use is likely due to the rapid degradation of remifentanil to inactive metabolites, withdrawal-induced hyperalgesia, and acute opioid tolerance. The clinical significance of this is debatable, given the rapid extinction of the phenomenon a few hours after cessation of remifentanil.

Reference

Flexman AM, Ng JL, Gelb AW. Acute and chronic pain following craniotomy. *Curr Opin Anesthesiol.* 2010;23:551–557.

3.1.2. What are the pharmacologic characteristics that make remifentanil an opioid of choice during elective craniotomy?

Remifentanil hydrochloride is a μ-opioid receptor agonist with unique pharmacokinetic properties. Remifentanil has a rapid onset of action (half-time for equilibration between blood and the effect compartment = 1.3 minutes) and a short context-sensitive half-life (i.e., the time required for the drug's plasma level to decrease by 50% after cessation of an infusion = 3.2 minutes). The latter property is attributable to hydrolytic metabolism of remifentanil by nonspecific tissue and plasma esterases. The primary metabolite of remifentanil has little biologic activity. Therefore, rapid onset makes remifentanil a prudent choice for anesthesia induction and maintenance, and its rapid offset facilitates the examination of neurologic function soon after emergence.

The pharmacodynamic properties of remifentanil, including analgesia, sedation, respiratory depression, and effects on hemodynamics, ICP, and CPP, are dose dependent and similar to those of fentanyl, alfentanil, or sufentanil.

Further Reading

Glass PSA, Hardman D, Kamyama Y, et al. Preliminary pharmacokinetics and pharmacodynamics of an ultra-short acting opioid: remifentanil (G187084B). *Anesth Analg.* 1993;77:1031–1040.

Guy J, Hindman BJ, Baker KZ, et al. Comparison of remifentanil and fentanyl in patients undergoing craniotomy for supratentorial space-occupying lesions. *Anesthesiology.* 1997;86:514–524.

Kapila A, Glass PSA, Jacobs JR, et al. Measured context-sensitive half-times of remifentanil and alfentanil. *Anesthesiology*. 1995;83:968–975.

Kim SH, Stoicea N, Soghomonyan S, Bergese SD. Remifentanil-acute opioid tolerance and opioid induced hyperalgesia: a systematic review. *Am J Ther*. 2015;22:e62–e74.

Warner DS, Hindman BJ, Todd MM, et al. Intracranial pressure and hemodynamic effects of remifentanil versus alfentanil in patients undergoing supratentorial craniotomy. *Anesth Analg*. 1996;83:348–353.

Westmoreland GL, Hoke JF, Sebel PS, Hug CC, Muir KT. Pharmacokinetics of remifentanil (G187084B) and its major metabolite (G190291) in patients undergoing elective inpatient surgery. *Anesthesiology*. 1993;79:893–903.

3.1.3. What are the advantages and disadvantages of using remifentanil for craniotomy?

Compared with other short-acting opioids, remifentanil is preferred in neuroanesthesia because it allows for a more predictable emergence and cognitive recovery when early assessment of postoperative neurologic function is imperative. Because of its unique pharmacokinetic profile, remifentanil produces intense analgesia effects that are highly titratable and dissipate rapidly, enabling a predictable wake-up even after prolonged infusion. These favorable pharmacokinetic properties are minimally altered by extremes of age, renal function, and hepatic function. Compared with fentanyl and alfentanil, remifentanil supplementation of general anesthesia may improve intraoperative hemodynamic control, with better control of hypertensive and tachycardic responses to noxious stimuli.

The cerebrovascular effects of remifentanil are minimal, dose dependent, and at low-dose infusion comparable to other short-acting opioids, with no effect on ICP and minimal decrease of CPP.

As a bolus-infusion regimen, it can be used reliably for analgesia and sedation in all phases of anesthesia. During intraoperative management, remifentanil is commonly administered as a 1-μg/kg bolus followed by an infusion of 0.5 to 1 μg/kg/min for induction and 0.05 to 2.0 μg/kg/min for maintenance of anesthesia.

During awake craniotomy, the unique ease of titration of remifentanil provides effective analgesia and sedation with minimal respiratory depression and allows for sufficient patient responsiveness during speech or motor mapping.

Like other opioids, remifentanil has little effect on somatosensory evoked potentials (SSEPs) and motor evoked potentials (MEPs). Total intravenous anesthesia (TIVA) techniques combining propofol and remifentanil infusions provide some of the best conditions for monitoring SSEPs and MEPs.

Respiratory depression following discontinuation of remifentanil is reliably brief, and residual opioid effect after return of adequate respiratory drive is unlikely. Therefore, respiratory adverse events in the recovery unit may be minimized after intraoperative use of remifentanil compared with other opioids.

Remifentanil shares a side effect profile that is similar to other opioids and includes pruritus and postoperative nausea and vomiting). However, the incidence of intraoperative hypotension, bradycardia, and chest wall muscle rigidity is greater with remifentanil than with other opioids and can become prominent especially when remifentanil is used at higher doses. Remifentanil has higher overall costs compared with other opioids.

Finally, when remifentanil is used for intraoperative analgesia, it results in greater and earlier requests for postoperative analgesia compared with fentanyl and sufentanil. This has been attributed to rapid metabolism of remifentanil to inactive metabolites, opioid-induced hyperalgesia (OIH), and acute opioid tolerance (AOT). Despite some evidence in the literature, the development of AOT and OIH by remifentanil administration remains controversial.

Further Reading

Beers R, Camporesi E. Remifentanil update: clinical science and utility. *CNS Drugs*. 2004;18:1085–1104.

Dijan MC, Blanchet B, Pesce F, et al. Comparison of the time to extubation after use of remifentanil or sufentanil in combination with propofol as anesthesia in adults undergoing nonemergency intracranial surgery: a prospective, randomized, double-blind trial. *Clin Ther*. 2006;28:560–568.

Engelhard K, Werner C, Mollenberg O, et al. Effects of remifentanil/propofol in comparison with isoflurane on dynamic cerebrovascular autoregulation in humans. *Acta Anaesthesiol Scand*. 2001;45:971–976.

Gelb AW, Salevsky F, Chung F, et al. Remifentanil with morphine transitional analgesia shortens neurological recovery compared to fentanyl for supratentorial craniotomy. *Can J Anaesth*. 2003;50:946–952.

Girard F, Quentin C, Charbonneau S, Ayoub C, Boudreault D, Chouinard P, Ruel M, Moumdjian R. Superficial cervical plexus block for transitional analgesia in infratentorial and occipital craniotomy: a randomized trial. *Can J Anaesth (J Can Anesth)*. 2010;57(12):1065–1070.

Guy J, Bradley JH, Baker KZ, et al. Comparison of remifentanil and fentanyl in patients undergoing craniotomy for supratentorial space-occupying lesions. *Anesthesiology*. 1997;86:514–524.

Hans P, Bonhomme V, Bill KM, et al. Target-controlled infusion of propofol and remifentanil combined with bispectral index monitoring for awake craniotomy. *Anaesthesia*. 2000;55:255–259.

Mackey JJ, Parker SD, Nass CM, et al. Effectiveness of remifentanil versus traditional fentanyl-based anesthetic in high-risk outpatient surgery. *J Clin Anesth*. 2000;12:427–432.

Ozkose Z, Cok OY, Tuncer B, et al. Comparison of hemodynamics, recovery profile, and early postoperative pain control and costs of remifentanil versus alfentanil-based total intravenous anesthesia (TIVA). *J Clin Anesth*. 2002;14:161–168.

van der Zwan T, Baerts WD, Perez RS, de Lange JJ. Postoperative condition after the use of remifentanil with a small dose of piritramide compared with fentanyl-based protocol in patients undergoing craniotomy. *Eur J Anaesthesiol*. 2005;22:438–441.

3.1.4. What are the current opioids used for postoperative analgesia after craniotomy?

Traditionally, opioids were avoided for postcraniotomy analgesia because their common side effects of sedation, nausea, vomiting, and miosis could mask signs of an acute intracranial event and prevent adequate neurologic examination. Opioid-induced respiratory depression has the potential to decrease minute ventilation, leading to hypercapnia, an increase in cerebral blood flow and ICP, and promotion of cerebral edema. Studies investigating major side effects from postcraniotomy opioid use largely dispelled this concern. In fact, severe pain postoperatively can lead to increased patient distress, sympathetic stimulation, arterial hypertension, and risk for intracranial bleeding.

The most common opioids used for postoperative analgesia after craniotomy are morphine and its derivatives (e.g., hydromorphone, hydrocodone, oxycodone, oxymorphone, codeine) and tramadol. Opioids are often used in combination with nonopioid analgesics (e.g., acetaminophen).

Morphine is a 10-fold more potent opiate than codeine and serves as the gold standard for moderate and severe pain management. Morphine provides superior analgesia to both tramadol and codeine in neurosurgical population, without increasing sedation, vomiting, or hypoventilation. Codeine, although widely used because of its limited sedative and respiratory-depressing effects, provides suboptimal pain control. The analgesic effect of codeine is dependent on demethylation to morphine in the liver, a process under polymorphic inheritance. Almost 10% of population are slow mobilizers and another 10% are fast metabolizers, which makes codeine ineffective in this subgroup.

Tramadol is a synthetic analog of codeine with limited μ-opioid receptor affinity and an inhibitor of serotonin and norepinephrine reuptake. Some centers avoid the use of tramadol, citing the potential risk of seizures and the high incidence of vomiting as unacceptable side effects. However, one study that included patients undergoing craniotomy for epilepsy found that the addition of tramadol to oxycodone/acetaminophen (Percocet) analgesia provided better pain control after craniotomy than Percocet alone. Rahimi et al. pointed out the drug has a potentially beneficial effect as a supplemental pain medication after craniotomy.

Further Reading

Cascorbi I. Pharmacogenetics of cytochrome p4502D6: genetic background and clinical implication. *Eur J Clin Invest*. 2003;33:17–22.

Goldsack C, Sculplak SM, Smith M. A double-blind comparison of codeine and morphine for postoperative analgesia following intracranial surgery. *Anaesthesia*. 1996;51:1029–1032.

Gottschalk A, Berkow LC, Stevens RD, et al. Prospective evaluation of pain and analgesic use following major elective intracranial surgery. *J Neurosurg*. 2007;106:210–216.

Gottschalk A, Yaster M. The perioperative management of pain from intracranial surgery. *Neurocrit Care*. 2009;10:387–402.

Molnar I, Simon E, Nemes R, Fulesdi B, Molnar C. Postcraniotomy headache. *J Anaesth*. 2014;28:102–111.

Rahimi SY, Alleyne CH, Vernier E, Witcher MR, Vender JR. Postoperative pain management with tramadol after craniotomy: evaluation and cost analysis. *J Neurosurg*. 2010;112:268–272.

Sudheer PS, Logan SW, Terblanche C, Ateleanu B, Hall JE. Comparison of the analgesic efficacy and respiratory effects of morphine, tramadol and codeine after craniotomy. *Anaesthesia*. 2007;62:555–560.

3.1.5. What are the differences between patient-controlled analgesia (PCA) and pro re nata (PRN), or as needed, analgesia when treating PCH?

The patient-controlled analgesia (PCA) administration route is secure, effective, and without additional adverse events when compared with other conventional analgesic therapies. PCA is widely used to reduce postoperative pain after general surgery and is a well-tolerated and effective method of pain control after craniotomy in alert patients. PCA after craniotomy appears to be a more effective analgesic technique than intermittent PRN administration of opioids. After supratentorial craniotomy, fentanyl PCA is more effective than PRN fentanyl.

Further Reading

Flexman AM, Ng JL, Gelb AW. Acute and chronic pain following craniotomy. *Curr Opin Anesthesiol*. 2010;23:551–557.

Jellish WS, Leonetti JP, Sawicki K, et al. Morphine/odansetron PCA for postoperative pain, nausea, and vomiting after skull base surgery. *Otolaryngol Head Neck Surg*. 2006;135:175–181.

Molnar I, Simon E, Nemes R, Fulesdi B, Molnar C. Postcraniotomy headache. *J Anaesth*. 2014;28:102–111.

Morad AH, Winters BD, Yaster M, et al. Efficacy of intravenous patient-controlled analgesia after supratentorial intracranial surgery: a prospective randomized controlled trial. Clinical article. *J Neurosurg*. 2009;111:343–350.

3.1.6. What are acute opioid tolerance and opioid-induced hyperalgesia?

Common concerns regarding the use of opioids in the perioperative setting are side effects like physical dependence and addiction. More recently, acute tolerance and hyperalgesia with opioid therapy, even when administered within a clinically accepted dose range, have become a concern because hyperalgesia might be a risk factor for the development of chronic pain after surgery.

AOT is defined as a requirement for increased doses of an opioid in order to achieve the original degree of analgesic effect. AOT is typically observed after patients have been taking opioids for an extended period. Dose escalation is typically useful, and the pain is limited to the original site. OIH is defined as increased sensitivity to noxious stimuli as a result of opioid use. Although controlled preclinical experiments defined OIH in animals as a decrease in pain threshold from baseline after chronic administration of opioids, researchers of OIH in human trials have not agreed on a definition. It is a paradoxical phenomenon in which escalating doses of opioids lead to an increased perception of pain. Increased pain may be limited to the original area or may become widespread. Opioids provide analgesic and antihyperalgesic effects initially but are subsequently associated with hyperalgesia, which may place the patient at risk for the development of chronic pain after surgery. The use of opioids seems to be a double-edged sword: patients receiving opioids to control their pain paradoxically become more sensitive to pain as a direct result of opioid therapy.

Further Reading

Angst MS, Clarc JD. Opioid-induced hyperalgesia: a qualitative systematic review. *Anesthesiology*. 2006;104:570–587.

Chu LF, Angst MS, Clark JD. Opioid-induced hyperalgesia in humans: molecular mechanisms and clinical considerations. *Clin J Pain*. 2008;24:479–496.

Hayhurst CJ, Durieux ME. Differential opioid tolerance and opioid-induced hyperalgesia: a clinical reality. *Anesthesiology*. 2016;124:483–488.

Fishbain DA, Cole B, Lewis JF, et al. Do opioids induce hyperalgesia in humans? An evidence-based structured review. *Pain Med*. 2009;10:829–839.

Kim SH, Stoicea N, Soghomonyan S, Bergese SD. Remifentanil-acute opioid tolerance and opioid induced hyperalgesia: a systematic review. *Am J Ther*. 2015;22:e62–e74.

Malik OS, Kaye AD, Urman RD. Perioperative hyperalgesia and associated clinical factors. *Curr Pain Headache Rep*. 2017;21:4. (online).

Martinez V, Fletcher D. Prevention of opioid-induced hyperalgesia in surgical patients: does it really matter? *Br J Anaesth*. 2012;109:302–304.

3.1.7. How can OIH be diagnosed and measured?

The difference between AOT and OIH is conceptually easy to understand, but the two are clinically difficult to distinguish. The development of either OIH or AOT will lead to increased pain and consequently to escalating doses of opioids. Treating AOT by increasing the opioid dose will result in better pain control. However, in OIH, increasing the opioid dose worsens the pain. Changing from one opioid to another, decreasing the opioid dose, or eliminating the specific opioid being used improves pain control in OIH.

In practice, clinicians should suspect OIH when a patient reports an increased level of pain despite increasing opioids or when an opioid's effect seems to wane in the absence of disease progression, particularly in the context of unexplained pain or the development of allodynia (pain caused by nonnoxious stimulus) unassociated with the original pain.

Remifentanil, with its unique pharmacokinetic profile, is the opioid most extensively studied in both animal and human OIH research. While some studies suggest a common hyperalgesic propensity for all opioids, randomized controlled trials suggest that in postsurgical patients, only remifentanil induces measurable OIH.

The circumstances under which OIH may occur are not yet entirely understood but may include high opioid doses, long-term treatment, or abrupt changes in concentrations inducing withdrawal. Thermal (heat or cold), mechanical, or transdermal electrical stimulation is used in quantitative sensory testing to objectively measure hyperalgesia.

Further Reading

Fletcher D, Martinez V. Opioid-induced hyperalgesia in patients after surgery: a systematic review and a meta-analysis. *Br J Anaesth*. 2014;112:991–1004.

Kim SH, Stoicea N, Soghomonyan S, Bergese SD. Remifentanil-acute opioid tolerance and opioid induced hyperalgesia: a systematic review. *Am J Ther*. 2015;22:e62–e74.

Lee M, Silverman S, Hansen H, Patel V, Manchikanti L. A comprehensive review of opioid-induced hyperalgesia. *Pain Physician*. 2011;14:145–161.

3.1.8. What cellular mechanisms contribute to AOT and OIH?

The underlying mechanisms of AOT and OIH are still unclear. AOT is likely to involve multiple mechanisms, such as decoupling from transduction and antianalgesia systems, and alterations of the N-methyl-D-aspartate (NMDA) receptor and its intracellular second messenger systems (central desensitization). OIH also may be explained by multiple mechanisms, including activation of central NMDA nociceptive systems (central sensitization), extensive spinal internalization and inactivation of μ-opioid receptors, up-regulation of the cyclic adenosine monophosphate pathway, and spinal dynorphin release. There also may be a genetic component associated with these processes. Thus, development of AOT and OIH may involve similar mechanisms.

Among the potential mechanisms, NMDA pain-facilitator mechanism, mediated through activation of the central glutaminergic system, seems to play a key role. Experimental studies performed in animals and humans have shown that NMDA receptor antagonists analogous to ketamine inhibit central sensitization and prevent OIH and may be useful adjuncts to morphine to control postoperative pain after opioid-based anesthesia. Human studies investigating NMDA receptor antagonists and the development of hyperalgesia differ in their findings. Several studies suggest that remifentanil-induced hyperalgesia was prevented by small-dose ketamine, while others found that NMDA antagonists had no significant effect in prevention.

Further Reading

Angst MS, Koppert W, Pahl I, et al. Short-term infusion of the mu-opioid agonist remifentanil in humans causes hyperalgesia during withdrawal. *Pain*. 2003;106:49–57.

Guignard B, Coste C, Costes H, et al. Supplementing desflurane-remifentanil anesthesia with small-dose ketamine reduces perioperative opioid analgesic requirements. *Anesth Analg*. 2002;95:103–108.

Joly V, Richebe P, Guignard B, et al. Remifentanil-induced postoperative hyperalgesia and its prevention with small-dose ketamine. *Anesthesiology*. 2005;103:147–155.

Koppert W, Sittl R, Scheuber K, et al. Differential modulation of remifentanil-induced analgesia and postinfusion hyperalgesia by S-ketamine and clonidine in humans. *Anesthesiology*. 2003;99:152–159.

Luginbuhl M, Gerber A, Schnider TW, et al. Modulation of remifentanil-induced analgesia, hyperalgesia, and tolerance by small dose ketamine in humans. *Anesth Analg*. 2003;96:726–732.

3.1.9. Can remifentanil induce AOT and OIH?

Although unable to clearly differentiate between AOT and OIH, the current experimental and clinical data generally support the development of AOT and/or OIH in specific settings, such as remifentanil exposure in human volunteer and postsurgical pain cohorts, when remifentanil was infused at ≥0.1 μg/kg/min either alone or with inhalation anesthetics.

Experimental studies performed in animals and human volunteers showed that AOT developed a couple of hours after the initiation of remifentanil administration through controlled infusion. The speed at which the tolerance develops varies based on the pharmacokinetics of the opioid: the shorter-acting the opioid, the faster the development of tolerance. The hyperalgesia in healthy volunteers was tested after remifentanil infusion was stopped for some time, and not during the infusion. Therefore, it is difficult to ascertain whether the researchers studied OIH, opioid withdrawal, or AOT.

A small number of clinical studies looked at AOT and OIH in the setting of acute perioperative opioid exposure. Although a few studies looked at fentanyl and sufentanil, the majority studied remifentanil-induced hyperalgesia. A recent systematic review and meta-analysis of randomized, controlled studies revealed that the administration of high doses of remifentanil to patients during surgery was associated with a clinically small but statistically significant increase in their perception of pain at rest during the first 24 hours, and moderately increased morphine use, with no difference in morphine-related side effects like nausea, vomiting, or drowsiness. The pain intensity at rest was greatest at 1 hour after surgery and then gradually decreased over 24 hours. Available data also suggested that in patients after surgery, compared with other opioids like fentanyl and sufentanil, only remifentanil induces measurable OIH.

Further Reading

Fletcher D, Martinez V. Opioid-induced hyperalgesia in patients after surgery: a systematic review and a meta-analysis. *Br J Anaesth*. 2014;112:991–1004.

Kim SH, Stoicea N, Soghomonyan S, Bergese SD. Remifentanil-acute opioid tolerance and opioid induced hyperalgesia: a systematic review. *Am J Ther*. 2015;22:e62–e74.

Malik OS, Kaye AD, Urman RD. Perioperative hyperalgesia and associated clinical factors. *Curr Pain Headache Rep*. 2017;21:4. (online).

3.1.10. Is OIH in the surgical setting clinically significant enough to warrant efforts at prevention or treatment?

Modern-day perioperative pain control continues to be unsatisfactory. Nearly half of all surgical patients have moderate to severe pain postoperatively, and 24% experience inadequate pain relief. Patient surveys indicate that chronic pain after surgery is more common than previously appreciated. More than 50% of patients have chronic pain after thoracotomy, mastectomy, and limb amputation. chronic PCH occurs in up to 50% of patients undergoing posterior fossa surgeries and up to 30% of patients undergoing supratentorial surgeries.

The development of hyperalgesia and subsequent treatment with escalating doses of opioids in the acute postoperative period can increase the opioid-related side effects on respiratory, gastrointestinal, and urologic function. It can also lead to impaired early mobilization, prolonged hospital stay, and decreased overall patient satisfaction. Furthermore, hyperalgesia in the postoperative period is now considered a potential risk factor for the development of chronic pain.

A mounting body of evidence supports the existence of perioperative hyperalgesia. Key sources of perioperative hyperalgesia include nociceptive-induced pain with surgical trauma, OIH, and inadequate control of pain in the pre-operative setting. Research also hints that inhaled anesthetics may also play a role in the development of perioperative hyperalgesia.

A recent systematic review and meta-analysis of randomized controlled trials aimed at quantifying OIH in patients after surgery confirms that high intraoperative doses of remifentanil (e.g., infusion ≥0.1 μg/kg/min) results in hyperalgesia in patients after surgery. The available data were insufficient for conclusions to be drawn for fentanyl and sufentanil. However, the clinical impact of remifentanil-induced hyperalgesia in the immediate postoperative period appeared to be limited to a slight increase in pain intensity at rest, greatest 1 hour after surgery and gradually decreasing over 24 hours, with a moderate increase in morphine use after surgery without any impact on the incidence of opioid-related side effects.

Various pharmacologic approaches have been tested to prevent remifentanil-induced hyperalgesia in patients after surgery, including perioperative ketamine, magnesium, propofol, and nitrous oxide. Although the evidence is not particularly robust, it has been suggested that remifentanil be administered intraoperatively at the lowest possible dose and associated with propofol anesthesia. However, another systematic review of remifentanil-induced hyperalgesia could not find any strong, consistent evidence to support the need to reduce the dose of remifentanil or apply preventive modulations.

In general, for the management of true OIH, it has been suggested to taper opioids; switch to a long-acting opioid, such as hydromorphone or methadone; consider rotating long-acting opioids; or use low doses of complete opioid receptor antagonists such as naloxone;, or partial opioid agonist buprenorphine. Other drugs may have a role in modulation of OIH, such as NMDA receptor antagonists (ketamine, morphine, dextromethorphan), cyclooxygenase-2 (COX-2) inhibitors, and α2 receptor agonists (clonidine, dexmedetomidine).

Further Reading

Fletcher D, Martinez V. Opioid-induced hyperalgesia in patients after surgery: a systematic review and a meta-analysis. *Br J Anaesth.* 2014;112:991–1004.

Kim SH, Stoicea N, Soghomonyan S, Bergese SD. Remifentanil-acute opioid tolerance and opioid induced hyperalgesia: a systematic review. *Am J Ther.* 2015;22:e62–e74.

Malik OS, Kaye AD, Urman RD. Perioperative hyperalgesia and associated clinical factors. *Curr Pain Headache Rep.* 2017;21:4. (online).

3.2. Nonopioid analgesia

3.2.1. Which nonopioid analgesics are currently used for perioperative pain control of craniotomy patients?

Local anesthetics and acetaminophen are the most frequently used nonopioid analgesics for the management of postcraniotomy pain. However, they provide only limited analgesic benefit, and often additional agents are required for supplemental or transitional analgesia. Nonsteroidal anti-inflammatory drugs (NSAIDs) may have opioid-sparing effects. Concerns about platelet inhibition from the inhibition of cyclooxygenase-1 (COX-1) and cardiovascular thrombotic events from inhibition of COX-2 make the use of NSAIDs less common in the neurosurgical population. Dexmedetomidine, gabapentin, and ketamine show potential benefit for intra- and postoperative analgesia in initial studies, but larger randomized prospective trials are needed to assess their role as part of the multimodal strategy to optimize pain control after craniotomy.

Further Reading

Dunn LK, Naik BI, Nemergut EC, Durieux ME. Post-craniotomy pain management: beyond opioids. *Curr Neurol Neurosci Rep.* 2016;93:1–10.

Haldar R, Kaushal A, Gupta D, Srivastava S, Singh PK. Pain following craniotomy: reassessment of the available options. *Biomed Res Int.* 2015;1:1–10.

Vadivelu N, Kai AM, Tran D, Kodumudi G, Legler A, Ayrian E. Options for perioperative pain management in neurosurgery. *J Pain Res.* 2016;9:37–47.

3.2.2. What are the limitations of NSAID use in the perioperative management of craniotomy?

Although NSAIDs are effective for treating headaches in general, their use in neurosurgery is controversial. The anti-inflammatory and analgesic effects of NSAIDs are mediated through inhibition of COX-2, while inhibition of COX-1 causes platelet dysfunction and may increase risk for bleeding. Several commonly used NSAIDs (e.g., diclofenac, ibuprofen, and naproxen) inhibit both COX-1 and COX-2. A limited number of studies, primarily from Europe, have investigated the use of these nonselective NSAIDs for postcraniotomy pain. NSAIDs, including ketoprofen and diclofenac, are effective for rescue analgesia and may have even greater benefit when administered preemptively. A one-time preoperative dose of diclofenac was effective for pain control and reduced opioid requirements without increasing the risk of bleeding. Despite the efficacy of NSAIDs for pain control, many neurosurgical practices in the United States avoid NSAIDs in the immediate perioperative period due to concerns of bleeding, renal function impairment, and alterations of cerebral blood flow. In the immediate postoperative setting, craniotomy patients can be relatively hypovolemic, making renal blood flow "prostaglandin dependent," and administration of a nonspecific NSAID can interfere with renal blood flow in this scenario. Indomethacin decreases cerebral blood flow by cerebral vasoconstriction.

Selective COX-2 inhibitors, a subset of NSAIDs, such as celecoxib and parecoxib, can provide analgesia without increasing bleeding risk. The initial enthusiasm for COX-2 inhibitors was replaced by caution when studies demonstrated an increased risk for cardiovascular thrombotic events with the use of COX-2 inhibitors. Parecoxib remains available for use in Europe. One study demonstrated a small benefit, while another found no benefit to the addition of parecoxib to scalp block and morphine PCA for postcraniotomy analgesia. Therefore, the evidence does not support routine use of this medication.

Further Reading

Chang CY, Challa CK, Shah J, Eloy JD. Gabapentin in acute postoperative pain management. *Biomed Res Int.* 2014;2014:631756.

Dunn LK, Naik BI, Nemergut EC, Durieux ME. Post-craniotomy pain management: beyond opioids. *Curr Neurol Neurosci Rep.* 2016;93:1–10.

Haldar R, Kaushal A, Gupta D, Srivastava S, Singh PK. Pain following craniotomy: reassessment of the available options. *Biomed Res Int.* 2015;1:1–10.

Jones SJ, Cormack J, Murphy MA, Scott DA. Parecoxib for analgesia after craniotomy. *Br J Anaesth.* 2009;102:76–79.

Malik OS, Kaye AD, Urman RD. Perioperative hyperalgesia and associated clinical factors. *Curr Pain Headache Rep.* 2017;21:4. (online).

Molnar C, Simon E, Kazup A, Gal J, Molnar L, Novak L, et al. A single preoperative dose of diclofenac reduces the intensity of acute postcraniotomy headache and decreases analgesic requirements over five postoperative days in adults: a single center, randomized, blinded trial. *J Neurol Sci*. 2015;353:70–73.

Tanskanen P, Kytta J, Randell T. Patient-controlled analgesia with oxycodone in the treatment of postcraniotomy pain. *Acta Anaesthesiol Scand*. 1999;43:42–45.

Williams DL, Pemberton E, Leslie K. Effect of intravenous parecoxib on post-craniotomy pain. *Br J Anaesth*. 2011;107:398–403.

Yadav G, Choupoo S, Das SK, Das SK, Behera SS, Khuba S, et al. Evaluating the role of flupirtine for postcraniotomy pain and compare it with diclofenac sodium: a prospective, randomized, double blind, placebo-controlled study. *J Neurosurg Anesthesiol*. 2014;26:32–36.

3.2.3. What is the role of acetaminophen in treatment of PCH?

Acetaminophen (N-acetyl-p-aminophenol) is a centrally acting cyclooxygenase inhibitor used alone and in combination with opioids for postcraniotomy analgesia. Acetaminophen is nonsedating, does not cause respiratory depression, and is devoid of the negative side effects associated with NSAIDs. However, the opioid-sparing effect of acetaminophen is limited. Although frequently prescribed, acetaminophen is not sufficient as a sole analgesic for postcraniotomy pain. Pain, opioid consumption, and opioid side effects are reduced when acetaminophen is coadministered with PCA opioids. Acetaminophen is metabolized extensively in the liver, and overdosing may cause hepatotoxicity.

Further Reading

Dunn LK, Naik BI, Nemergut EC, Durieux ME. Post-craniotomy pain management: beyond opioids. *Curr Neurol Neurosci Rep*. 2016;93:1–10.

Haldar R, Kaushal A, Gupta D, Srivastava S, Singh PK. Pain following craniotomy: reassessment of the available options. *Biomed Res Int*. 2015;1:1–10.

Vadivelu N, Kai AM, Tran D, Kodumudi G, Legler A, Ayrian E. Options for perioperative pain management in neurosurgery. *J Pain Res*. 2016;9:37–47.

3.2.4. What are emerging novel nonopioid analgesics for prevention and treatment of PCH?

Novel analgesic adjuncts like anticonvulsants (gabapentin and pregabalin), NMDA receptor antagonists (ketamine), and α2 adrenoreceptor agonists (dexmedetomidine) have emerged recently and provide potential benefit for postoperative analgesia in initial studies, but larger randomized prospective trials are needed to confirm their role as part of a balanced, multimodal approach to managing postcraniotomy pain.

Further Reading

Dunn LK, Naik BI, Nemergut EC, Durieux ME. Post-craniotomy pain management: beyond opioids. *Curr Neurol Neurosci Rep*. 2016;93:1–10.

3.2.5. What is the role of anticonvulsants in the perioperative management of PCH?

Gabapentin is an anticonvulsant with a chemical structure similar to gamma-aminobutyric acid and is related to, though less potent than, pregabalin. Gabapentin binds to presynaptic voltage-gated calcium channels and inhibits neurotransmitter release and excitatory neurotransmission in dorsal horn neurons. Both gabapentin and pregabalin are commonly used to treat neuropathic, postoperative pain following spine surgery, and both decrease opioid requirements. However, there are few studies on the acute benefit of gabapentinoids with intracranial procedures. Preoperative gabapentin reduced pain scores, lowered opioid consumption, and decreased the incidence of nausea and vomiting, but it is associated with increased sedation and time to tracheal extubation.

Further Reading

Chang CY, Challa CK, Shah J, Eloy JD. Gabapentin in acute postoperative pain management. *Biomed Res Int*. 2014;2014:631756.

Dunn LK, Naik BI, Nemergut EC, Durieux ME. Post-craniotomy pain management: beyond opioids. *Curr Neurol Neurosci Rep*. 2016;93:1–10.

Haldar R, Kaushal A, Gupta D, Srivastava S, Singh PK. Pain following craniotomy: reassessment of the available options. *Biomed Res Int*. 2015;1:1–10.

Türe H, Sayin M, Karlikaya G, Bingol CA, Aykac B, Türe U. The analgesic effect of gabapentin as a prophylactic anticonvulsant drug on postcraniotomy pain: a prospective randomized study. *Anesth Analg*. 2009;109:1625–1631.

Vadivelu N, Kai AM, Tran D, Kodumudi G, Legler A, Ayrian E. Options for perioperative pain management in neurosurgery. *J Pain Res*. 2016;9:37–47.

3.2.6. Can NMDA receptor antagonists be used to treat PCH?

NMDA receptors are ligand gated ion channels that allow passage of calcium, sodium, and potassium into the cell. They are involved in pain modulation at the level of spinal cord and central sensitization of nociceptors. NMDA receptor antagonists lack intrinsic analgesic properties. Their analgesic effects are mediated through inhibition of central sensitization. Methadone and ketamine are commonly used for management of chronic pain. Methadone, a multimodal analgesic, can act as both an NMDA receptor antagonist and an opioid. Methadone can provide long-lasting analgesia and may decrease opioid tolerance and opioid-induced hyperalgesia. A previous review demonstrated that NMDA receptor antagonists like dextromethorphan and ketamine can be effective not only for preventive analgesia but also for acute postoperative pain when administered with NSAIDs and opioids perioperatively. Ketamine can serve an important role in reducing opioid tolerance and opioid-induced hyperalgesia, and it demonstrates opioid-sparing properties in a variety of nonneurosurgical and major spine procedures. Historically, ketamine administration was avoided during intracranial surgery due to ketamine's perceived effects on increasing cerebral blood flow and intracranial pressure.[10] However, the subanesthetic effects of low-dose intraoperative ketamine on postoperative sedation, mental status, and pain have not been investigated.

Further Reading

Dunn LK, Naik BI, Nemergut EC, Durieux ME. Post-craniotomy pain management: beyond opioids. *Curr Neurol Neurosci Rep*. 2016;93:1–10.

Flexman AM, Ng JL, Gelb AW. Acute and chronic pain following craniotomy. *Curr Opin Anesthesiol*. 2010;23:551–557.

Haldar R, Kaushal A, Gupta D, Srivastava S, Singh PK. Pain following craniotomy: reassessment of the available options. *Biomed Res Int*. 2015;1:1–10.

Loftus RW, Yeager MP, Clark JA, Brown JR, Abdu WA, Sengupta DK, et al. Intraoperative ketamine reduces perioperative opiate consumption in opiate-dependent patients with chronic back pain undergoing back surgery. *Anesthesiol*. 2010;113(3):639–646.

McCartney CJL, Sinha A, Katz J. A qualitative systematic review of the role of N-methyl-D-aspartate receptor antagonists in preventive analgesia. *Anesth Analg*. 2004;98(5):1385–1400.

Vadivelu N, Kai AM, Tran D, Kodumudi G, Legler A, Ayrian E. Options for perioperative pain management in neurosurgery. *J Pain Res*. 2016;9:37–47.

3.2.7. Can α2 adrenoreceptor agonists have a role in prevention and treatment of PCH?

Dexmedetomidine is a potent central and peripheral presynaptic α2 adrenoreceptor antagonist that provides sedation without respiratory depression. Dexmedetomidine reduces opioid consumption, has both nonopioid analgesic properties and preemptive analgesic activity, and mitigates opioid-induced hyperalgesia. Intraoperative infusion of dexmedetomidine does not appear to significantly delay emergence or extubation times in patients undergoing craniotomy.

Further Reading

Dunn LK, Naik BI, Nemergut EC, Durieux ME. Post-craniotomy pain management: beyond opioids. *Curr Neurol Neurosci Rep.* 2016;93:1–10.

Haldar R, Kaushal A, Gupta D, Srivastava S, Singh PK. Pain following craniotomy: reassessment of the available options. *Biomed Res Int.* 2015;1:1–10.

Peng K, Jin XH, Liu SL, Ji FH. Effect of intraoperative dexmedetomidine on post-craniotomy pain. *Clin Ther.* 2015;37:1114–1121.

Rajan S, Hutcherson MT, Sessler DI, Kurz A, Yang D, Ghobrial M, et al. The effects of dexmedetomidine and remifentanil on hemodynamic stability and analgesic requirement after craniotomy: a randomized controlled trial. *J Neurosurg Anesthesiol.* 2016 Oct;28(4):282–290.

Song J, Ji Q, Sun Q, Gao T, Liu K, Li L. The opioid-sparing effect of intraoperative dexmedetomidine infusion after craniotomy. *J Neurosurg Anesthesiol.* 2016;28:14–20

Vadivelu N, Kai AM, Tran D, Kodumudi G, Legler A, Ayrian E. Options for perioperative pain management in neurosurgery. *J Pain Res.* 2016;9:37–47.

Zhao LH, Shi ZH, Chen GQ, Yin NN, Chen H, Yuan Y, et al. Use of dexmedetomidine for prophylactic analgesia and sedation in patients with delayed extubation after craniotomy: a randomized controlled trial. *J Neurosurg Anesthesiol.* 2017 Apr;29(2):132–139.

3.2.8. Do steroids have any role in treatment of PCH?

Most patients undergoing craniotomy are administered high-dose dexamethasone before, during, and after their procedure, to reduce both inflammation and vasogenic cerebral edema. Dexamethasone has a central antiemetic effect and plays a significant role in the prevention of postoperative nausea and vomiting. Dexamethasone serves as an analgesic through its modulation of peripheral nociceptors and anti-inflammatory effect. A systematic review of the impact of a single intravenous dose of dexamethasone on postoperative pain has shown a small but statistically significant analgesic benefit. Corticosteroids may relieve headache postoperatively by decreasing chemical meningitis triggered by the formation of bone dust during surgery.

Further Reading

Apfel CC, Korttila K, Abdalla M, et al; IMPACT Investigators. A factorial trial of six interventions for the prevention of postoperative nausea and vomiting. *N Engl J Med.* 2004;350:2441–2451.

Rhen T, Cidlowski JA. Antiinflammatory action of glucocorticoids—new mechanisms for old drugs. *N Engl J Med.* 2005;353:1711–1723.

Waldron NH, Jones CA, Gan TJ, Allen TK, Habib AS. Impact of perioperative dexamethasone on postoperative analgesia and side-effects: systematic review and meta-analysis. *Br J Anaesth.* 2013;1:191–200.

3.2.9. Can serotonin 5-HT receptor agonists be used as adjuncts to opioid treatment of PCH?

Serotonin 5-HT receptor agonists may be a useful alternative treatment for postcraniotomy headache manifesting as migraine type. According to Venkatraghavan et al., the postoperative subcutaneous administration of sumatriptan (a 5-HT_1 agonist) after cranial microvascular decompression surgery improved the quality of recovery and reduced headache assessed 24 hours after surgery. The mechanism remains unknown but could be related to reduction in headache, mood modulation, or both, mediated by a serotonin effect. In another study, sumatriptan has been found useful in patients with persistent headache following acoustic neuroma excision. More well-designed, high-quality studies are needed to assess the role of serotonin 5-HT receptor agonists for treatment of PCH.

Further Reading

Levo H, Pyykko I, Blomsted G. Postoperative headache after surgery for vestibular schwannoma. *Ann Otol Rhinol Laryngol.* 2000;109:853–858.

Venkatraghavan L, Li L, Bailey T, Manninen PH, Tymianski M. Sumatriptan improves postoperative quality of recovery and reduces postcraniotomy headache after cranial nerve decompression. *Br J Anaesth.* 2016;117:73–79.

3.3. Nonpharmacologic therapy and multimodal analgesia

3.3.1. What other nonpharmacologic therapies for chronic PCH are available?

There is little evidence within the existing literature to guide clinical decision-making once first- and second-line pharmacologic agents have been trialed. Nonpharmacologic therapies including transcutaneous electrical nerve stimulation (TENS), electro-acupuncture, cryotherapy, radiofrequency and cryoablation, botulinum neurotoxin injections, and physiotherapy have been tried with variable success. Electrical acupuncture may be clinically effective as an adjunct to intraoperative anesthesia and postoperative analgesia for craniotomy. Botulinum neurotoxin has been used successfully to treat primary headache syndromes. In a case series peri-incisional botulinum neurotoxin type A appears to be a potentially valuable tool in the management of chronic PCH after traumatic brain injury.

Further Reading

An LX, Chen X, Ren XJ, Wu HF. Electro-acupuncture decreases postoperative pain and improves recovery in patients undergoing supratentorial craniotomy. *Am J Chin Med.* 2014;42:1099–1109.

Haldar R, Kaushal A, Gupta D, Srivastava S, Singh PK. Pain following craniotomy: reassessment of the available options. *Biomed Res Int.* 2015;1:1–10.

Liu X, Li S, Wang B, An L, Ren X, Wu H. Intraoperative and postoperative anesthetic and analgesic effect of multipoint transcutaneous electrical acupuncture stimulation combined with sufentanil anaesthesia in patients undergoing supratentorial craniotomy. *Acupunct Med.* 2015;33:270–276.

MacKenzie HM, Teasell R, Miller TA, Sequeira K. Peri-incisional botulinum toxin for chronic postcraniotomy headache after traumatic brain injury: a case series. *PM&R.* 2015;7:785–788.

3.3.2. What is the importance of multimodal analgesia?

Failure to adequately manage postoperative pain can increase postoperative complications, length of stay, and health expenses. Therefore, pain management following craniotomy is a balancing act of achieving adequate analgesia while avoiding sedation, respiratory depression, hypercapnia, nausea, vomiting, and hypertension. Current evidence suggests that a balanced, multimodal approach to treatment of PCH is often required to optimize pain control while limiting undesirable side effects.

Preoperatively, it is important to diagnose, adequately treat, and optimize primary and secondary headaches, as well as any other preexisting chronic pain conditions. In addition, anxiety and mood disorders should be investigated and treated.

Intraoperatively, total intravenous or combined inhalational-intravenous anesthesia technique, including a balanced opioid-based technique, low-dose NMDA antagonists, α2 adrenergic agonists, and a combination of local infiltration and scalp block, can be utilized.

Postoperatively, opioids (morphine, codeine, and analogs), tramadol, acetaminophen, nonsteroidal anti-inflammatories, and COX-2 inhibitors are considered first-line agents for the management of PCH. Additional pain relief may be provided by using a variety of adjuncts, including tricyclic antidepressants, anticonvulsants, and muscle relaxants; for migraine-type headache, 5-HT_1 receptor agonists and caffeine may be helpful. When persistent headache is not alleviated by first- and second-line agents, other nonpharmacologic therapy, such as TENS, electro-acupuncture, cryotherapy, radiofrequency and cryoablation, botulinum neurotoxin injections, and physiotherapy, can be considered. The surgical scar should always be palpated, and if the patient's pain is reproduced, infiltration of the scar using local anesthetic can be useful.

Future areas of study should focus on elucidating patient- and surgery-related risk factors for severe pain, improving methods for assessing pain, discovering the effect of intraoperative anesthetic management on postoperative pain, and exploring the role of adequate analgesic management on long-term functional outcomes after craniotomy surgery.

Further Reading

Dunn LK, Naik BI, Nemergut EC, Durieux ME. Post-craniotomy pain management: beyond opioids. *Curr Neurol Neurosci Rep.* 2016;93:1–10.

Haldar R, Kaushal A, Gupta D, Srivastava S, Singh PK. Pain following craniotomy: reassessment of the available options. *Biomed Res Int.* 2015;1:1–10.

Rocha-Filho PA. Post-craniotomy headache: a clinical view with a focus on the persistent form. *Headache.* 2015;55:733–738.

Vadivelu N, Kai AM, Tran D, Kodumudi G, Legler A, Ayrian E. Options for perioperative pain management in neurosurgery. *J Pain Res.* 2016;9:37–47.

3.3.3. Considering the available evidence, what recommendations can be made for the perioperative management and prevention of PCH in this patient?

This patient has several risk factors for the development of both acute and chronic PCH: fibromyalgia, chronic migraines, and a history of both depression and anxiety. Preoperative assessment and treatment of the preexisting and modifiable risk factors are critical. If the patient has peritumoral edema with or without intracranial hypertension, preoperative treatment with a corticosteroid can decrease intracranial edema and inflammation and may also have a role in reducing the pre- and postcraniotomy pain. Although preoperative anticonvulsants like gabapentin have shown some mild effect on decreasing PCH and opioid consumption when used as part of multimodal pain management, these drugs can cause delayed emergence and cloud postoperative neurologic assessment. If this patient takes gabapentin routinely, the drug can be continued in the perioperative period, but it should not be started as a new medication prior to surgery.

Intraoperatively, a preemptive approach with the goal of reducing the postoperative pharmacologic burden is prudent. A combination of prepinning scalp block and a pre- or postprocedure surgical wound infiltration with local anesthetic can be used, taking care to stay within the total maximum allowable dose for local anesthetics. As a part of TIVA or a combined inhalational-intravenous anesthesia regimen, propofol and a balanced opioid (fentanyl and remifentanil) technique can be utilized. Additionally, low-dose dexmedetomidine intravenous infusion can be administered and stopped 30 to 60 minutes before the end of the procedure. Patients undergoing craniotomy for tumor commonly receive scheduled high-dose dexamethasone perioperatively to reduce surgical cerebral edema and inflammation; if continued for a few days postoperatively, this should have a beneficial effect on PCH. Supplemental scheduled intravenous acetaminophen can also be started intraoperatively. The use of an intraoperative remifentanil infusion, especially high-dose (≥0.1 μ/kg/min), may place the patient at risk for postoperative OIH. The use of a bispectral index monitor in conjunction with standard anesthesia monitors may allow for a more tailored titration of anesthetic depth and a decrease of opioid dose to a minimum necessary as part of the multimodal analgesic regimen.

Morphine or hydromorphone PCA and scheduled intravenous acetaminophen can be the first-line drugs for immediate postoperative pain relief. Pain should be carefully assessed using objective and validated methods, and opioids should be carefully titrated to avoid serious side effects. When the pain subsides, and the patient is alert and can tolerate oral intake, she can be transitioned to oral analgesics. NSAIDs are commonly avoided after craniotomy for tumor due to their antiplatelet properties and the concern for bleeding. Second-line agents, including tricyclic antidepressants, anticonvulsants, and muscle relaxants, as well as other additional agents like 5-HT receptor agonists, should be considered in any patient with preexistent migraine, depression, and/or anxiety.

17

Polytrauma

Cynthia H. Shields and Lisa Bleckner

Case Scenario

A 25-year-old man suffered a head-on motor vehicle collision. His injuries included a left below-the-knee complex fracture with tissue loss, right radial head and midhumerus fracture, and right pulmonary contusion. Following initial stabilization and fixation of his fractures, he was transferred to the intensive care unit, intubated, and sedated. On postoperative day 2, the patient was extubated and is now complaining of severe pain. The pain service has been consulted to help with his management.

1. Trauma History and Physical Exam

1.1. What are the essential elements of an acute pain history in the trauma patient?

A history of the cause and mechanism of injury can provide valuable insight into the patient's prior and current pain management needs. Knowing the patient's previous level of function will inform the clinician on the likely psychological as well as physical impact of the current trauma. Obtain a comprehensive summary of injuries with a focus on renal, hepatic, pulmonary, neurologic, and musculoskeletal systems. Perform a primary pain evaluation that includes documentation of the primary source(s) and location of pain, the quality of the pain (i.e., sharp, shooting, aching, throbbing, squeezing) to determine the pain type (nociceptive somatic or visceral, neuropathic, inflammatory), the severity of the pain (most commonly assessed using the Numeric Rating Scale [NRS], the Visual Analogue Scale [VAS], or preferentially a validated multidimensional scale such as the Defense and Veterans Pain Rating Scale [DVPRS] or Quality of Recover scales such as the QoR-9 that give a more complete assessment of the impact of pain), and the duration of pain (i.e., constant, episodic).

Useful medical history that can impact pain management includes a patient's psychosocial comorbidities such as depression, anxiety, substance use disorder, or post-traumatic stress disorder (PTSD). Coping strategies, family support, beliefs, and expectations are all qualifiers that may impact the patient's pain trajectory.

Review current medications with attention to possible drug-drug interactions and side effects. Side effects that are of concern include excessive sedation, delirium, opioid-induced bowel dysfunction, anticholinergic syndrome, serotonin syndrome, and QT prolongation.

Further Reading

Hinrichs-Rocker A, Schultz K, Jarvinenn I, Lefering R, Simanski C, Neugebauer EA. Psychosocial predictors and correlates for chronic post-surgical pain (CPSP): a systematic review. *Eur J Pain*. 2009;13(7):719–730.

Myles PS, Hunt JO, Nightingale CE, et al: Development and psychometric testing of a quality of recovery score after general anesthesia and surgery in adults. *Anesth Analg*. 1999;88:83–90.

Polomano RC, Galloway KT, Kent ML, et al. Psychometric Testing of the Defense and Veterans Pain Rating Scale (DVPRS): a new pain scale for military population. *Pain Med*. 2016;17(8):1505–1519.

1.2. What are the essential elements of an acute pain examination in the trauma patient?

Complete a focused physical exam with attention on the musculoskeletal and neurologic exam. It can be extremely helpful to examine the patient in the trauma bay or operating room to get a picture of the full extent of the injuries and to assess what approaches for pain control may be appropriate. This includes identifying the intravenous (IV) access to determine route of analgesic administration, and location of pain and injuries to know if regional anesthesia can be used. Obtain a baseline electrocardiogram for evaluation of the QT interval, since multiple pain management medications can prolong the QT interval and may put the patient at risk for dysrhythmia.

1.2.1. Multidisciplinary coordination

Because of the complex nature of polytrauma, multiple teams are likely to be involved in the patient's care. Having coordinated discussions with the multidisciplinary team is extremely helpful in integrating pain management into the overall team effort. These discussions should include future surgical plans, current coagulation status and surgical plans for future anticoagulation, physical therapy and occupational therapy goals, and discharge planning goals. Early discussion of discharge planning goals can help focus and direct management. For example, it is helpful to know if the patient will be going to a rehabilitation facility and, if so, which pain modalities are allowed at that institution.

1.2.2. Patient and family discussion

Finally, after completing an appropriate history and physical examination and a discussion with the multidisciplinary team, it will be necessary to sit down and have a long conversation with the patient and his or her family regarding reasonable goals for pain management and to provide reassurance that the pain management team will continue to work with them during the recovery process.

Further Reading

Ip HY, Abrishami A, Peng PW, Wong J, Chung F. Predictors of postoperative pain and analgesic consumption: a qualitative systematic review. *Anesthesiology*. 2009;111(3):657–677.

Yap YG, Camm AJ. Drug induced QT prolongation and torsades de pointes. *Heart*. 2003;89:1363–1372.

2. Multimodal Analgesia

2.1. What are the goals for multimodal pain management?

The goals of a multimodal analgesia (MMA) plan are to decrease the subjective sensation of pain, improve objective function, and decrease the risk of individual medication side effects. Multimodal analgesia should be considered a "balanced" plan, whereby, according to Buvanendran et al., "a combination of different analgesics possessing separate mechanisms and sites of actions act in synergy to improve analgesia and lower the adverse effects of a single agent." The members of the American Society of Anesthesiologists Task Force on Acute Pain Management "strongly agree that whenever possible" the use of MMA as part of the perioperative pain management plan should be instituted.

In trauma patients specifically, a goal is to diminish the amount of opioids needed throughout the perioperative period, which in turn will reduce the adverse effects of opioids in the postoperative period. Studies have demonstrated a 20% to 50% reduction in opioid use in patients receiving combinations of nonsteroidal anti-inflammatory drugs (NSAIDs), cyclooxygenase inhibitors, acetaminophen, ketamine, gabapentin, pregabalin, and regional anesthesia.

Further Reading

Buvanendran A, Kroin JS. Multimodal analgesia for controlling acute postoperative pain. *Curr Opin Anaesthesiol.* 2009;22(5):588–593.

Kehlet H. Postoperative opioid sparing to hasten recovery: what are the issues? *Anesthesiology.* 2005;102(6):1083–1084.

Ashburn MA, Caplan RA, Carr DB, et al. Practice guidelines for acute pain management in the perioperative setting: an updated report by the American Society of Anesthesiologists Task Force on Acute Pain Management. *Anesthesiology.* 2012;116(2):248–273.

White P. The changing role of non-opioid analgesic techniques in the management of postoperative pain. *Anesth Analg.* 2005;101:S5–S22.

2.2. What should be the initial approach for multimodal pain management in this patient?

The initial approach for implementing a multimodal pain management plan begins with an assessment of the type and severity of pain that the patient is experiencing. Because trauma patients are likely to have nociceptive, inflammatory, and neuropathic pain, the analgesic plan should reflect treatment of these pain types. Nonopioids should be used on a schedule to avoid the need for high-dose opioids. For mild pain, nonopioids may be sufficient. For moderate to severe pain, opioids are indicated. The additive and synergistic effects of combination multimodal treatment can reduce the side effects of high doses of any one drug alone and reduce the overall amount of opioid needed.

Further Reading

Botting RM. Inhibitors of cyclooxygenase. *J Physiol Pharmacol.* 2006;57:113–124.

Kehlet H. Multimodal approach to control postoperative pathophysiology and rehabilitation. *Br J Anaesthes.* 1997;78:606–617.

Young A, Buvanendran A. Recent advances in multimodal analgesia. *Anesthesiology Clinics.* 2012;30(1):91–100.

2.2.1. IV opioids

Patient-controlled analgesia (PCA) devices are the delivery method of choice for systemic IV opioids in conscious patients able to manage self-delivery. PCA provides better analgesic efficacy and improved patient satisfaction compared with nurse-delivered medicine. In general, there is little evidence that warrants the use of one opioid versus another in PCA. However, on a patient-by-patient basis, certain opioids may be better tolerated than others, with fewer adverse side effects. Common starting demand doses used within our institution are hydromorphone 0.2 to 0.4 mg every 10 minutes, morphine 1 to 2 mg every 10 minutes, or fentanyl 10 mcg every 10 minutes. Caution should be taken if incorporating a basal rate due to oversedation. In fact, most studies have been unable to demonstrate any benefit from addition of a basal rate in combination with the demand dose. In our practice, a basal rate is rarely prescribed.

Further Reading

Grass JA. Patient-controlled analgesia. *Anesth Analg.* 2005;101(5S):S44–S61.

Woodhouse A, Ward ME, Mather LE. Intra-subject variability in post-operative patient-controlled analgesia (PCA): is the patient equally satisfied with morphine, pethidine and fentanyl? *Pain.* 1999;80(3):545–553.

2.2.2. Oral opioids

In addition to the PCA, if the patient can take and absorb oral medications, the oral route is preferred. Along with an MMA plan, the lowest opioid dose for the shortest duration to treat moderate to severe pain is preferred. Typical adult starting doses are oxycodone 5 to 10 mg or morphine 5 to 15 mg every 4 hours as needed (PRN). Cautious titration to effect is warranted in the trauma patient with depressed sensorium, in the elderly patient, or in combination with MMA so overdose does not occur.

Mechanism of action: Opioids bind to mu, delta, and kappa receptors, thereby affecting the modulation of pain within the central and peripheral nervous systems. Analgesia is the result of blunted nociceptor excitability, diminished release of inflammatory neuropeptides, and a decrease in action potential proliferation.

Further Reading

DePriest AZ, Puet BL, Holt AC. Metabolism and disposition of prescription opioids: a review. *Forensic Sci Rev.* 2015;27:143–145.

2.2.3. Acetaminophen

This class of drug possesses both antipyretic properties and some mild analgesic anti-inflammatory properties. When given in combination with PCA opioids, there is a reduction of opioid consumption, but there is no decrease in opioid-related adverse effects. The patient should receive a scheduled dose of oral or IV acetaminophen, 1 g every 6 hours as the maximum dose (4 g/d), adjusting downward for altered hepatic function, when combined with medications that decrease hepatic metabolism, or when other medications with acetaminophen are used.

Mechanism of action: Acetaminophen is a centrally acting cyclooxygenase inhibitor and a weak peripheral cyclooxygenase inhibitor, but its complete mechanism of action to treat pain remains unclear.

Further Reading

Graham GG, Davies MJ, Day RO, Mohamudally A, Scott KF. The modern pharmacology of paracetamol: therapeutic actions, mechanism of action, metabolism, toxicity and recent pharmacological findings. *Inflammopharmacol.* 2013;21(3):201–232.

2.2.4. NSAIDs

Nonsteroidal anti-inflammatory medications demonstrate a wide range of analgesic, anti-inflammatory, and antipyretic properties. Nonselective NSAIDs play a key role in MMA. Scheduled ibuprofen or ketorolac is an effective component of the MMA plan that targets the inflammatory component of pain. Renal function must be assessed prior to using NSAIDs in patients with reduced renal function and in elderly patients.

Mechanism of action: NSAIDs inhibit prostaglandin synthesis in peripheral and central tissues. There is a synergistic enhancement of analgesia when NSAIDs are used in combination with acetaminophen.

Further Reading

Maund E, McDaid C, Rice S, Wright K, Jenkins B, Woolacott N. Paracetamol and selective and non-selective non-steroidal anti-inflammatory drugs for the reduction in morphine-related side-effects after major surgery: a systematic review. *Br J Anaesthes.* 2011;106(3):292–297.

2.2.5. Gabapentinoids

Both gabapentin and pregabalin have been shown to significantly reduce neuropathic pain. As part of an MMA plan, trauma patients may benefit from use of either gabapentin or pregabalin for treatment of neuropathic pain due to nerve injury or from surgical intervention. The main side effect of these medications is sedation. Starting low and titrating up to effect over several days is warranted. In middle-aged individuals, gabapentin 300 mg 3 times a day (TID) is a usual starting dose, and it is escalated in 300-mg increments (per dose) every 3 to 5 days to a maximum dose of 1200 mg 3 times a day. Alternatively, pregabalin can be utilized at a starting dose of 25 mg up to TID dosing and escalated to a dose of 150 mg for each dose. Given the propensity to contribute to daytime sedation, alternatively it can be given at bedtime only to improve sleep. Reduced doses are required in elderly patients and in patients with limited renal function.

Mechanism of action: Gabapentinoids bind to A2delta subunit of voltage-sensitive presynaptic Ca^{++} channels to reduce the release of neurotransmitters (specifically glutamate, norepinephrine, substance P) from presynaptic nerve terminals that influence pain.

Further Reading

Baron R. Mechanisms of disease: neuropathic pain—a clinical perspective. *Nat Clin Pract Neurol.* 2006;2(2):95–106.

Baron R, Binder A, Wasner G. Neuropathic pain: diagnosis, pathophysiological mechanisms, and treatment. *Lancet Neurol.* 2010;9(8):807–819. doi:10.1016/S1474-4422(10)70143-5

Gordh TE, Stubhaug A, Jensen TS, et al. Gabapentin in traumatic nerve injury pain: a randomized, double-blind, placebo-controlled, cross-over, multi-center study. *Pain.* 2008;138(2):255–266.

2.2.6. Ketamine

Ketamine is an important piece of the MMA plan specifically for patients with VAS scores >7/10, as they have been shown to receive the strongest benefit. Initial dosing of ketamine begins at ~2.5 mcg/kg/min (~10 mg/h in a 70-kg patient) and can be increased to a common dose of 5 mcg/kg/min. Higher doses, 5 to 15 mcg/kg/min (up to 60 mg/h), may be tolerated, but side effects, such as hallucinations, are more frequent. The maximum dose of ketamine is usually determined by the patient's discomfort with the medication. Neuropsychiatric effects such as feelings of anxiousness, often accompanied by visual disturbances and/or nightmares, indicate the upper dosing limit has been reached and ketamine should be decreased.

Mechanism of action: Ketamine is a noncompetitive antagonist of the NMDA receptor at subanesthetic doses.

Further Reading

Laskowski K, Stirling A, McKay WP, Lim HJ. Revue méthodique de l'utilisation de la kétamine intraveineuse pour l'analgésie postopératoire. *Can J Anesth/J Can Anesth.* 2011;58(10):911–923.

3. Regional Anesthesia

3.1. How do you determine if the primary pain source is suitable for regional anesthesia?

The main benefit of regional anesthesia in a trauma patient is the delivery of a site-specific high-quality analgesic that has very few systemic side effects. Multiple factors must be considered when determining the suitability of regional anesthesia in a trauma patient. Dr. Andre Boezaart teaches that regional anesthesia must only be used in the right patient, at the right time, and for the right indication. Thus, the right trauma patient is the willing patient (self-consenting or consented by the health care surrogate) who has severe pain or who may experience severe pain from surgery. The right patient must be able to cooperate and tolerate regional anesthesia and must be able to be positioned so that the procedure can be safely performed. The benefits of pain control in this method must be balanced against the risk of performing the block and/or use of a catheter infusion. Performing regional anesthesia at the right time is important as well. In anticoagulated patients, regional anesthesia may be contraindicated until the anticoagulant is metabolized according to the guidelines from the American Society of Regional Anesthesia and Pain Medicine. The indication for regional anesthesia is pain control, so the procedure must be deemed useful to alleviate pain for an adequate time period.

If a patient is deemed an adequate candidate for regional anesthesia, the next determination is administration of a single-injection nerve block versus a continuous peripheral nerve block (CPNB). Benefits of a CPNB in a trauma patient include a continuous infusion of local anesthetic targeting the desired peripheral nerve(s), the ability to administer boluses of local anesthetic (by patient or provider) if pain spikes occur, and the ability to bolus the catheter with a surgical dose of local anesthetic for frequent operating room visits.

Be mindful that chronic pain is a significant risk for patients who experience acute injury. Up to 77% of patients suffer from this malady, which is defined as pain lasting longer than 3 months from the initial injury. Because the greatest risk factor for transitioning from acute to chronic pain is the intensity of the acute pain at the time of injury, much care must be taken to minimize the acute pain as early and effectively as possible.

Further Reading

Gadsden J, Warlick A. Regional anesthesia for the trauma patient: improving patient outcomes. *Local Reg Anesth.* 2015 12;8:45–11.

Horlocker TT, Wedel DJ, Rowlingson JC, et al. Executive summary: regional anesthesia in the patient receiving antithrombotic or thrombolytic therapy. *Reg Anesthes Pain Med.* 2010;35(1):102–105.

3.2. The orthopedic surgical staff has now decided that the patient's left lower extremity is not salvageable, and the patient is scheduled for a left below-knee amputation in 2 days. What are the regional anesthesia options for this patient?

Adequate analgesia for a below-knee amputation requires coverage of the common peroneal (L4-S2), tibial (L4-S2), and saphenous nerves (L2-L4). This can be achieved with either an epidural or a peripheral nerve block (lumbar plexus in combination with a sciatic nerve block, or femoral/saphenous block in combination with sciatic nerve block).

Epidural analgesia is efficacious in treating postamputation pain, particularly in the postoperative period. Benefits include superior analgesia at rest and with movement as compared with opioids alone, as well as reduction of the neuroendocrine stress response. Additives such as clonidine and fentanyl to the local anesthetic have been shown to further enhance the analgesic properties of epidurals. Potential pitfalls of epidural analgesia include hypotension, infection, urinary retention (patients may require a urinary catheter for the duration of in situ epidural, depending on the level of the infusion), and bilateral lower extremity motor blockade, which has the potential to limit physical therapy.

The use of prolonged regional analgesia via a peripheral nerve catheter(s) is likely beneficial in amputation patients. Peripheral nerve catheters may provide a broader scope of function than epidural catheters as they are able to target upper as well as lower extremity pain. In addition, these catheters can remain in situ for prolonged periods and have more flexible guidelines in the setting of anticoagulation.

Further Reading

Bernard JM, Ottmar K, Bonnet F. Comparison of intravenous and epidural clonidine for postoperative patient-controlled analgesia. *Anesth Analg.* 1995;81:706–712.

Curatolo M, Sveticic G. Drug combinations in pain treatment: a review of the published evidence and a method for finding the optimal combination. *Best Pract Res Clin Anaesthesiol.* 2002;16(4):507–519.

Kent ML, Hsia H-LJ, Van de Ven TJ, et al. Perioperative pain management strategies for amputation: a topical review. *Pain Med.* 2017;18(3):504–519.

Ong BY, Arneja A, Ong EW. Effects of anesthesia on pain after lower-limb amputation. *Journal of J Clin Anesthes.* 2006;18(8):600–604.

Pöpping DM, Elia N, Van Aken HK, et al. Impact of epidural analgesia on mortality and morbidity after surgery. *Ann Surg.* 2014;259(6):1056–1067.

Velickovic I, Yan J, Grass J. Modifying the neuroendocrine stress response. *Semin Anesth Perioperat Med Pain.* 2002;21(1):16–25.

Wu CL, Cohen DR, Richman JM. Efficacy of postoperative patient-controlled and continuous infusion epidural analgesia versus intravenous patient-controlled analgesia with opioids: a meta-analysis. *Anesthesiology.* 2005;103(5):1079–1088.

3.3. Sciatic and femoral peripheral nerve block catheters had been placed. What type of local anesthesia and what concentration and rate should be used?

Because severe postoperative surgical pain is a risk factor for persistent postoperative pain and possibly for phantom limb pain, a high initial concentration of local anesthetic is one strategy for optimizing initial pain control through fast onset and dense blockade. The primary innervation below the knee is sciatic, with a relatively small contribution from the saphenous. For the first 48 hours after amputation, we recommend a sciatic catheter infusion concentration of 0.25% bupivacaine with an initial rate of 8 mL/h with a bolus of 4 mL every 30 minutes. For the femoral catheter, ropivacaine 0.2% continuous rate of 6 mL/hour with no bolus is used to limit risk for local anesthetic toxicity. After 48 hours the sciatic infusion should be changed to either 0.2% ropivacaine or 0.125% bupivacaine. Systemic local anesthetic toxicity from continuous infusions is rare; however, vigilance for the signs and symptoms of systemic local anesthetic toxicity as well as continued evaluation of the efficacy and benefits of peripheral nerve catheters are required.

Further Reading

Bleckner L, Solla C, Fileta BB, Howard R, Morales CE, Buckenmaier CC. Serum free ropivacaine concentrations among patients receiving continuous peripheral nerve block catheters. *Anesth Analg.* 2014;118:225–229.

3.4. What regional anesthesia adjuncts would be appropriate?

Although there is limited evidence to support the addition of clonidine to peripheral nerve blocks, in some studies it has been shown to improve epidural analgesia and reduce opioid requirements without increasing side effects. A typical epidural dose would be 1 to 2 mcg of clonidine per milliliter of epidural local anesthetic solution.

Further Reading

Chan CW, Chong YK. Alpha-2 agonists in acute pain management. *Expert Opin Pharmacother.* 2010;11(17): 2849–2868.

Farmery AD, Wilson-MacDonald J. The analgesic effect of epidural clonidine after spinal surgery: a randomized placebo-controlled trial. *Anesth Analg.* 2009;108(2):631–634.

4. Phantom Limb Pain

4.1. Who is at risk for phantom limb pain?

Patients with high levels of preoperative limb pain are more likely to have more severe postoperative phantom limb pain (PLP). Preoperative opioid use and preoperative anxiety are both associated with increased postoperative PLP. The severity of PLP in the immediate postoperative period is a good predictor of the severity of chronic PLP.

Further Reading

Hanley MA, Jensen MP, Smith DG, et al. Preamputation pain and acute pain predict chronic pain after lower extremity amputation. *J Pain.* 2007;8(2):102–109.

Kent ML, Hsia HJ, Van de Ven TJ, et al. Perioperative pain management strategies for amputation: a topical review. *Pain Med.* 2017;18(3):504–519.

Raichle KA, Osborne TL, Jensen MP, et al. Preoperative state anxiety, acute postoperative pain, and analgesic use in persons undergoing lower limb amputation. *Clin J Pain*. 2015;31(8):699–706.

Roullet S, Nouette-Gaulain K, Biais M, et al. Preoperative opioid consumption increases morphine requirement after leg amputation. *Can J Anesth*. 2009;56(12):908–913.

4.2. What are the incidence and onset time of PLP?

Approximately one-third of amputation patients will experience the onset of PLP within the acute postoperative phase. The incidence of PLP is estimated to be between 51% and 85% of amputation patients.

Further Reading

Kent ML, Hsia HJ, Van de Ven TJ, et al. Perioperative pain management strategies for amputation: a topical Review. *Pain Med*. 2017;18(3):504–519.

4.3. What strategies can be used for the prevention of PLP?

Although there are no well-documented methods to prevent or even treat PLP, recent articles suggest strategies that may help minimize PLP. Because severe and poorly controlled pain immediately postoperatively is associated with a higher prevalence of persistent postoperative pain, using all available strategies to optimize immediate postoperative pain control is a reasonable approach.

Further Reading

Batoz H, Semjen F, Bordes-Demolis M, et al. Chronic postsurgical pain in children: prevalence and risk factors. *Br J Anaesth*. 2016;117:489–496.

Hanley MA, Jensen MP, Smith DG, et al. Preamputation pain and acute pain predict chronic pain after lower extremity amputation. *J Pain*. 2007;8(2):102–109.

4.3.1. Surgical strategies

Use of evidence-based surgical techniques for limb amputation is critical both for neuroma avoidance and for functional recovery and may have some impact on phantom limb pain.

Further Reading

Kent ML, Hsia HJ, Van de Ven TJ, et al. Perioperative pain management strategies for amputation: a topical review. *Pain Med*. 2017;18(3):504–519.

Smith DG, Skinner HB. Amputations. In: Skinner HB, McMahon PJ. eds. *Current Diagnosis and Treatment in Orthopedics*. 5th ed. New York, NY: McGraw-Hill; 2014:568–594.

4.3.2. Acute pain service strategies

Amputation patients may benefit from the involvement of specialized acute pain services that can provide the optimal plan for use of MMA. Because acute pain services are highly variable, the current data are only suggestive of the benefits such a service offers. Suggested benefits include better pain control, decreased incidence of adverse events, decreased post-operative morbidity and mortality, decreased persistent postsurgical pain, and decreased costs.

Acute pain services can provide regional anesthesia. While perioperative epidural analgesia has not been shown to prevent PLP, it has been shown to reduce the incidence of severe PLP. Peripheral nerve catheters do effectively manage acute postamputation pain; however, there is only limited evidence showing efficacy in reducing the incidence of severe PLP. Prolonged infusions of local anesthetic by peripheral nerve catheters hold some promise in reducing PLP, but more studies are needed to effectively evaluate the efficacy of this technique.

Further Reading

Borghi B, D'Addabbo M, Borghi R. Can neural blocks prevent phantom limb pain? *Pain Manag.* 2014;4(4):261–266.

Schug SA, Palmer GM, Scott DA, Halliwell R, Trinca J. *Acute Pain Management: Scientific Evidence* [online]. 4th ed. Melbourne: Australian and New Zealand College of Anaesthetists; 2015:61, 125, 261, 264, 284.

4.3.3. Pharmacologic strategies

4.3.3.1. Gabapentinoids

Gabapentin has been shown to have opioid-sparing and analgesic effects perioperatively. However, no studies have looked at acute pain outcomes immediately postamputation. One study by Buvanderan et al. demonstrated that a 2-week course of pregabalin started on the day of surgery diminished neuropathic pain symptoms 6 months postoperatively. One approach is to extrapolate the results of these studies to the acute pain management of the amputation patient.

4.3.3.2. Ketamine

Ketamine is an effective analgesic with a good safety profile, and it may be opioid sparing in the perioperative period. However, there is no evidence that ketamine reduces or prevents PLP.

4.3.3.3. Tricyclic antidepressants and specific serotonin reuptake inhibitors

Tricyclic antidepressants (TCAs) and specific serotonin reuptake inhibitors (SSRIs) have not been shown to be effective in acute pain management, although they can be helpful in chronic pain management. Amitriptyline and duloxetine have the most evidence supporting their use in the treatment of neuropathic pain. It may be reasonable to extrapolate the data from chronic neuropathic pain management and consider starting amputation patients on one of these medications, which should be initiated at a low dose.

Further Reading

Bell RF, Dahl JB, Moore RA. Perioperative ketamine for acute postoperative pain. *Cochrane Database Syst Rev.* 2006;(1):CD004603.

Buvanendran A, Kroin JS, Valle Della CJ, et al. Perioperation oral pregabalin reduces chronic pain after total knee arthroplasty: a prospective randomized controlled trial. *Anesth Analg.* 2010;110(1);199–207.

Hayes C, Armstrong-Brown A, Burstal R. Perioperative intravenous ketamine infusion for the prevention of persistent post amputation pain: A randomized, controlled trial. *Anaesth Intensive Care.* 2004; 32(3):330–338.

Kim K, Mishina M, Kokubo R, et al. Ketamine for acute neuropathic pain in patients with spinal cord injury. *J Clin Neurosci.* 2013;20(6):804–807.

Laskowski K, Stirling A, McKay WP, Lim HJ. A systematic review of intravenous ketamine for postoperative analgesia. *Can J Anaesth.* 2011;58:911–923.

McCormik Z, Chang-Chien G, Marshall B, Huang M, Harden RN. Phantom limb pain: a systematic neuroanatomical-based review of pharmacologic treatment. *Pain Med.* 2014;15(2):292–305.

4.3.4. Nonpharmacologic strategies

4.3.4.1. Preoperative counseling

Combined sensory and procedural information given preoperatively can reduce postoperative pain. In our practice we use a robust peer-counseling program, where amputees come and speak to patients prior to their amputation and discuss their recovery experience. Expectation management can have a significant impact on a patient's experience and perception of control.

4.3.4.2. Stress and arousal reduction

Stress and arousal reduction includes relaxation techniques, guided imagery, and hypnosis. Common examples of relaxation techniques include deep breathing and sequential muscle relaxation. Relaxation has moderate evidence to show improvement in psychological well-being, but it does not decrease analgesic use. Guided imagery, however, improves psychological well-being and decreases analgesic use. In adults, hypnosis has only mild evidence to support an improvement in psychological well-being; in children, however, there is moderately strong evidence to support its use in reducing periprocedural pain.

4.3.4.3. Distraction

Distraction is another behavioral technique used to manage pain. Examples of this strategy include listening to music, watching television, squeezing a ball, or otherwise directing attention elsewhere. There is strong evidence supporting the effectiveness of distraction to reduce self-reported pain across all age groups. In our practice, video gaming has been used as an effective form of distraction for amputees.

4.3.4.4. Acupuncture

Acupuncture decreases postoperative pain and opioid use and reduces opioid-related side effects.

4.3.4.5. Mirror therapy

Several studies have shown mirror therapy to be an effective modality in treating PLP. Mirror therapy theoretically provides cortical reorganization that helps reduce maladaptive changes caused by neuromodulation following amputation.

Further Reading

Barbin J, Setha V, Casillas JM, Paysant J, Perennou D. The effects of mirror therapy on pain and motor control of phantom limb in amputees: a systematic review. *Ann Phys Rehabil Med.* 2016;59(4):270–275.

Kohl A, Winfried R, Glombiewski JA. Acceptance, cognitive restructuring, and distraction as coping strategies for acute pain. *J Pain.* 2013;14(3):305–315.

Nelson EA, Dowsey MM, Knowles SR. et al. Systematic review of the efficacy of pre-surgical mind-body based therapies on postoperative outcome measures. *Complement Ther Med.* 2013;21(6):697–711.

Stineman MG, Kwong PL, Kurichi JE, et al. The effectiveness of inpatient rehabilitation in the acute postoperative phase of care after transtibial or transfemoral amputation: study of an integrated health care delivery system. *Arch Phys Med Rehabil.* 2008;89(10):1863–1872.

Suls J, Wan CK. Effects of sensory and procedural information on coping with stressful medical procedures and pain: a meta-analysis. *J Consult Clin Psychol.* 1989;57(3):372–379.

Sun Y, Gan TJ, Dubose JW, et al. Acupuncture and related techniques for postoperative pain: a systematic review of randomized controlled trials. *Br J Anaesth.* 2008;101(2):151–160.

Tome-Pires C, Miro J. Hypnosis for the management of chronic and cancer procedure–related pain in children. *Int J Clin Exp Hypn.* 2012;60(4):432–457.

Uman LS, Birniew KA, Noel M, et al. Psychological interventions for needle-related procedural pain and distress in children and adolescents. *Cochrane Database Syst Rev.* 2013;10:CDOO5179.

4.3.4.6. Recommendations for the prevention of PLP

Despite the lack of strong evidence for the effectiveness of any therapy to prevent the development of PLP, we recommend using a comprehensive multimodal pain management strategy supervised by an acute pain service. The strategy should include use of regional analgesia (epidural analgesia if appropriate or proximal continuous peripheral nerve blockade), IV and oral analgesics designed to limit adverse drug effects, and nonpharmacologic modalities.

Further Reading

Karinkolas M, Aretha D, Tsolakis I, et al. Optimized perioperative analgesia reduces chronic phantom limb pain intensity, prevalence and frequency: a prospective randomized clinical trial. *Anesthesiology.* 2011;114 (5):1144–1154.

Gehling M, Tryba M. Prophylaxis of phantom pain: is regional analgesia ineffective? *Schmerz.* 2003;17(1):11–19.

Borghi B, D'Addabbo M, White PF, et al. The use of prolonged peripheral neural blockade after lower extremity amputation: the effect on symptoms associated with phantom limb syndrome. *Anesth Analg.* 2010;111(5):1308–1315.

5. Compartment Syndrome

5.1. Which trauma patients are at risk of compartment syndrome? What is the incidence of compartment syndrome?

Acute compartment syndrome (ACS) is one of the most serious complications of extremity trauma and is most likely to occur in male patients under the age of 35 years after fractures to the tibia or forearm. The incidence of the lower extremity compartment syndrome in trauma patients ranges from 1.5% to 29% for closed tibial fractures and from 1.2% to –10.2% in open tibial fractures. Following trauma to the extremity, swelling of the osteofascial compartment leads to an increased pressure within the compartment. This pressure increase will eventually cause a collapse of capillary vessels, resulting in cellular hypoxia and increased vascular permeability, further worsening the intracompartmental pressure. Once arteriolar compression occurs, muscle and nerve ischemia ensue, with resultant muscle infarction and nerve damage if immediate treatment is not delivered. The mortality rate of ACS is 11% to 15%; amputation rates are 11% to 21%.

Further Reading

Choi JJ, Lin E, Gadsden J. Regional anesthesia for trauma outside the operating theatre. *Curr Opin Anaesthesiol.* 2013;26(4):495–500.

Tiwari A, Haq I, Myint F. Acute compartment syndromes. *Br J Surg.* 2002;89:397–412.

5.2. Is regional anesthesia acceptable in a patient at risk for compartment syndrome?

Peripheral nerve catheters in trauma patients have the potential to mask the signs and symptoms of ACS, particularly in the lower extremity. For this reason, if a CPNB is placed in a patient who is at risk for compartment syndrome, there must be very open lines of communication between the anesthesia provider and the surgeon. Any escalation in narcotic requirements or sudden worsening of pain should immediately be brought to the surgeon's attention.

Further Reading

Heemskerk J, Kitslaar P. Acute compartment syndrome of the lower leg: retrospective study on prevalence, technique, and outcome of fasciotomies. *World J Surg.* 2003;27(6):744–747.

6. Transitioning Care and Weaning Medications

6.1. This patient is now 8 days postamputation and is highly resistant to weaning off IV ketamine. Inability to wean off of IV ketamine precludes his transfer to a rehabilitation facility. How should you manage this issue?

It is not unusual for patients to feel anxious at the thought of ketamine or other pain medications being terminated. A slow wean, with focus on functional restoration and next steps, is often beneficial to the psychological well-being of the patient. In our practice, ketamine is typically decreased by 10 mg/d until it is off.

Methadone is an opioid analgesic that also possesses NMDA receptor antagonism (similar to ketamine) and therefore may be useful in the treatment of pain. Although methadone is not used as a first-line analgesic at our institution, we often will switch the patient's prescribed opioid to methadone if ketamine is a strong component of the analgesic regimen. Initial starting dose is methadone 5 mg PO TID with a slow titration in 5-mg increments every 3 days. Caution must be used when prescribing methadone in the acute pain setting because it takes several days to reach steady state. Moreover, continuation into the outpatient setting or rehabilitation setting may be precluded by provider unwillingness to prescribe. Because methadone can potentially lead to QT prolongation, a baseline EKG should be obtained to document the pretreatment QT value and then repeated 3 days later, with each adjustment of dose. Be aware that there are several other classes of medications that can prolong the QT interval that may be prescribed while the patient is in the hospital.

Further Reading

Krantz MJ, Martin J, Stimmel B. QTc interval screening in methadone treatment. *AnnIntern Med.* 2009;150:387–395.

Morley JS, Bridson J, Nash TP, Miles JB, White S, Makin MK. Low-dose methadone has an analgesic effect in neuropathic pain: a double-blind randomized controlled crossover trial. *Palliat Med.* 2003;17(7):576–587.

Yap YG, Camm AJ. Drug induced QT prolongation and torsades de pointes. *Heart.* 2003;89:1363–1372.

6.2. Nothing is working with this patient. He seems grossly oversedated and still is complaining of severe pain and is not making any progress with functional goals. How do you approach this?

First, repeat your trauma-focused history and physical and obtain relevant imaging specifically looking for new or progressive pathology. Potential etiologies of worsening pain include compartment syndrome, wound hematoma, wound infection, sepsis, abscess, decubiti, and failure of orthopedic hardware. Also evaluate for previously unrecognized sources of pain. Treat any newly identified pathology.

If no new or worsening pathology is identified, consider other factors that may be impacting the patient's pain perception. Are there psychosocial factors involved that can be mitigated? If no treatable causes are identified, 2 options are available.

6.2.1. Care escalation

Escalate the level of monitoring and transfer the patient to the intensive care unit, where more aggressive pain management strategies are possible. In this setting, options to consider can include dexmedetomidine and higher dose (>60 mg/h) ketamine infusions. Dexmedetomidine has been shown to decrease postoperative pain intensity and opioid consumption; however, it may cause arterial hypotension and bradycardia. One should not escalate care and initiate these therapies without specific goals. One goal might be to decrease opioid or other sedative use, to transiently gauge the degree of analgesia a patient may require for control of pain, and then to reformulate a plan for de-escalation and recovery. Frequent reassessment of therapy efficacy is required. Decisions on whether to continue or discontinue therapy should be based on goal achievement.

6.2.2. Care de-escalation

Explain to the patient and his or her family or caregivers that the current therapies are not working and are exposing the patient to risk without the benefit hoped for. Identify the risks, such as oversedation, that are interfering with the functional goals. Begin a systematic weaning protocol for opioids and sedatives with functional goals in place. A common strategy for opioid weaning for inpatients and in the postoperative acute and subacute phase is to decrease the opioid daily dose by 10% per day.

Further Reading

Blaudszun G, Lysakowski C, Elia N, et al. Effect of perioperative systemic alpha2 agonists on postoperative morphine consumption and pain intensity: systematic review and meta-analysis of randomized controlled trials. *Anesthesiology.* 2012;116(6):1312–1322.

Chaparro LE, Smith SA, Moore RA, et al. Pharmacotherapy for the prevention of chronic pain after surgery in adults. *Cochrane Database Syst Rev.* 2013;7:CD008307.

Suttner J, White Lovett A, Vernachio K. Best practices in tapering methods in patients undergoing opioid therapy. *Adv Pharmacol Pharm.* 2013;1(2):42–57.

6.3. Is there a role for benzodiazepines in trauma pain management?

It is unlikely that benzodiazepines improve analgesia; in fact, they may antagonize opioid-induced analgesia. Concurrent use of both benzodiazepines and opioids increases the risk of opioid-related death. However, benzodiazepines may be of benefit in treating anxiety or muscle spasm. If benzodiazepines are initiated for the treatment of muscle spasm, they should be used at the lowest possible dose and weaned off as soon as possible. If they are being used to treat anxiety, they should not be started except at the recommendation of a psychiatrist. The patient should then be transitioned as quickly as possible to other antianxiety medications, which pose a lower risk.

Further Reading

Dowell D, Haegerich TM, Chou R. Guideline for prescribing opioids for chronic pain: -United States, 2016. *JAMA.* 2016;315(15):1624–1645.

Jones CM, McAninch JK. Emergency department visits and overdose deaths from combined use of opioids and benzodiazepines. *Am J Prev Med.* 2015;49:493–501.

Reddy S, Patt RB. The benzodiazepines as adjuvant analgesics. *J Pain Symptom Manage.* 1994;9:510–514.

6.4. Are long-acting opioids helpful in the trauma population, and do the risks outweigh the benefits?

There are risks and benefits to initiating extended-release, long-acting (ER/LA) opioids. Polytrauma patients typically have moderate to severe pain with multiple pain generators, and their pain is likely to persist for months if not years. More than 50% of trauma patients rate their pain as severe 2 years after injury. Trauma patients are frequently receiving around-the-clock immediate-release (IR) opioids; however, missed doses may cause plasma concentrations to fall, leading to inadequate analgesia. ER/LA opioids may prevent troughs and lead to improved pain control, but analgesia and long-term safety compared with IR opioids have not been shown. Notably, ER/LA formulations may be more difficult to taper. Discontinuation of IV pain medications is an important clinical milestone for trauma patients because it allows them to participate more easily in physical and occupational therapy. ER/LA opioids can facilitate the transition from IV to oral opioids. The Food and Drug Indication indication for ER/LA opioids is "pain severe enough to require a daily round-the-clock, long-term opioid treatment and for which alternative options are inadequate." Many polytrauma patients meet these criteria.

However, there are many risks involved with the use of ER/LA opioids. There are currently no randomized controlled trial looking at the efficacy of using ER/LA opioids in trauma patients. Guidelines from the Centers for Disease Control and Prevention have highlighted the risks associated with ER/LA opioids, including their increase abuse potential given the large dose of opioid in each unit. The risk of opioid abuse is increased in patients with a history of substance abuse disorder, in younger patients, in those with depression, and in patients using psychotropic medications. Compared with the general population, trauma patients have a higher rate of substance abuse. Immediate-release opioids in combination with ER/LA opioids increase the risk for opioid overdose compared with IR medications alone. Patients receiving ER/LA opioids have a higher daily opioid use compared with those receiving IR opioids alone. The risk of death from overdose increases as dosage increases. Certain ER/LA opioids pose an even higher risk. Methadone is involved in one-third of opioid-related deaths but accounts for less than 2% of opioids prescribed for pain management. Fentanyl patches may also pose an additional risk because the dosing is unfamiliar both for clinicians and for patients.

6.4.1. Recommendations

ER/LA opioids may be useful, but they also pose a significant risk, perhaps more so in polytrauma patients. The initiation of ER/LA opioids should facilitate the rapid discontinuation of IV opioids, a decrease in the amount of IR oral opioid use, and subsequent patient improvement in attaining functional goals (e.g., participation in physical and occupational therapy). If those goals are not being met, a re-evaluation and discontinuation of these medications may be indicated. If ER/LA opioids facilitate meeting these goals, opioid risk mitigation strategies must be put in place during the transition from inpatient to outpatient care. These strategies should include transition to an outpatient prescriber who will initiate an opioid contract, continue random urine drug screening, and facilitate an opioid-weaning plan. Clinicians should use their regional Prescription Drug Monitoring Program to monitor for patterns of substance abuse and doctor-shopping. Rescue naloxone should be prescribed to reduce the risk of overdose death in the community. Trauma patients on prolonged opioid therapy should receive care from a clinician who is comfortable with and experienced in managing opioid-weaning and risk mitigation strategies.

Further Reading

Demetriades D, Gkiokas G, Velmahos GC, Brown C, Murray J, Noguchi T. Alcohol and illicit drugs in traumatic deaths: prevalence and association with type and severity of injuries. *J Am Coll Surg*. 2004;199:687–692.

Dowell D, Haegerich TM, Chou R. CDC guideline for prescribing opioids for chronic pain--United States, 2016. *JAMA*. 2016;315(15):1624–1645.

Kaske S, Lefering R, Bouillion F, et al. Pain assessment of severely injured patients 2 years after trauma. *Schmerz*. 2016;3:273–278.

Paulozzi L, Mack KA, Jones CM. Vital signs: risk for overdose from methadone used for pain relief: United States, 1999–2010. *MMWR Morb Mortal Wkly Rep*. 2012;61:493–497.

Ramchand R, Marshall GN, Schell TL, et al. Alcohol abuse and illegal drug use among Los Angeles County trauma patients: prevalence and evaluation of single item screener. *J Trauma*. 2009;66:1461–1467.

Sunshine A, Olson NZ, Colon A, et al. Analgesic efficacy of controlled-release oxycodone in post-operative pain. *J Clin Pharmacol*. 1996;36:595–603.

Walley AY, Xuan Z, Hackman HH, et al. Opioid overdose rates and implementation of overdose education and nasal naloxone distribution in Massachusetts: interrupted time series analysis. *BMJ*. 2013;346:f174.

7. Clinical Pearls

Not all of these clinical pearls have medical literature to support them; however, the core group of anesthesiologists in the national capital region, who have been responsible for the acute pain management of military polytrauma patients since 2001, agree that these pearls represent valid clinical truths.

- Pain trajectory in severe trauma rapidly escalates over the first week to 2 weeks and then waxes and wanes during the acute surgical phase.
- Items that improve the overall pain trajectory:
  - patient optimism and anticipation of complete recovery
  - decrease in surgical tempo
  - ability to participate in rehabilitation
  - ability to get adequate sleep
  - appropriate peer counseling
  - good level of preinjury resilience and coping strategies
  - adequate family support
- Items that worsen overall pain trajectory:
  - patient with difficulty coping preinjury
  - overinvolved family or no family support, dysfunctional family
  - low preinjury level of resilience
  - post-traumatic stress disorder
  - depression
  - high level of anxiety in either the patient or the family
- Trauma patients can develop significant opioid tolerance, and continued opioid dose increase may not improve pain control but will increase the risks.
- Trauma patients are likely to have setbacks, leading to patient and family frustration and often increased difficulty with pain management.
- Trauma patients and families may get frustrated because often the multiple services need to be involved and communication may seem uncoordinated. Team meetings that involve the patient and family can be helpful.
- Some patients will express a desire to control their pain management and may be very persistent in their pursuit of all pain management options.
- Some patients may initially be resistant to integrative therapies (meditation, hypnosis, relaxation, breathing, acupuncture, mirror therapy); however, gentle encouragement to participate in the combination of all pain treatment options will often result in improved pain control and satisfied patients.
- The onset of neuropathic pain frequently occurs at the 10- to 14-day mark.
- Patients with sciatic nerve injuries are likely to have difficult-to-manage neuropathic pain.
- Epidural clonidine and opioids combined with local anesthesia can be extremely helpful in patients with difficult-to-manage pain.
- Failed limb salvage patients experience complex and difficult-to-treat pain after amputation.
- Calcaneal injury causes pain that is difficult to treat. In fact, calcaneal surgery is noted to be the most painful orthopedic procedure.

Further Reading

Ephraim PL, Wegener ST, MacKenzie EJ, Dillingham TR, Pezzin LE. Phantom pain, residual limb pain, and back pain in amputees: results of a national survey. *Arch Phys Med Rehabil.* 2005;86(10):1910–1919.

Gerbershagen HJ, Aduckathil S, van Wijck AJ, Peelen LM, Kalkman CJ, Meissener W. Pain intensity on the first day after surgery: a prospective cohort study comparing 179 surgical procedures. *Anesthesiology.* 2013;118(4):934–944.

Schug SA, Palmer GM, Scott DA, Halliwell R, Trinca J. *Acute Pain Management: Scientific Evidence* [online]. 4th ed. Melbourne: Australian and New Zealand College of Anaesthetists; 2015:298..

Topuz K, Kutlay M, Simşek H, Atabey C, Demircan M, Senol Güney M. Early surgical treatment protocol for sciatic nerve injury due to injection: a retrospective study. *J Neurosurg.* 2011;25(4):509–515.

18

Complex Regional Pain Syndrome

Steven R. Hanling, Ian M. Fowler, and C. Ryan Phillips

Case Scenario

A 37-year-old woman who is admitted as an inpatient has progressively debilitating complex regional pain syndrome (CRPS) type I (previously known as reflex sympathetic dystrophy [RSD]) of the right foot, which developed after an ankle fracture requiring 6 weeks of casting. Though the patient previously was very active, the CRPS has progressed to the point where she is nonambulatory and wheelchair-bound due to severe pain in both lower extremities, with the right side worse than the left. Orthopedic Surgery has requested an acute pain evaluation. Other medical history includes obesity (secondary to inability to perform any physical activity) and major depressive disorder.

1. Differential Diagnoses

1.1. What differential diagnoses must be considered in a patient with presumed complex regional pain syndrome?

The differential diagnoses for complex regional pain syndrome (CRPS) are multiple as the condition is one of exclusion per the Budapest criteria. Any condition that causes peripheral pain, whether it is neurogenic, vasogenic, autoimmune, or other, must be acknowledged and either investigated or removed from the list of differential diagnoses by history, physical exam, laboratory, and/or imaging studies. Table 18.1 provides a selection of potential conditions that may need to be addressed prior to making the diagnosis of CRPS.

Further Reading

Raja SN, Grabow TS. Complex regional pain syndrome I (reflex sympathetic dystrophy). *Anesthesiology*. 2002;96(5):1254–1260.

1.2. How is the diagnosis of CRPS made?

A thorough history and a complete physical exam, including neurologic and vascular exams, should be performed on the patient in whom CRPS is suspected, to assist in ruling out these other potential causes and to document the current condition. Table 18.2 presents an extensive list of tests that may be of assistance in excluding or decreasing the likelihood of one of the other diseases in the differential.

1.3. How well do the objective tests work in attempts to diagnose CRPS?

The positive and negative predictive values for MRI in CRPS are 100% and 45%, respectively; MRI is performed to look for muscle and soft tissue edema, muscle atrophy, and soft tissue enhancement, all of which may be late findings, making this test very sensitive but not very specific. A triple-phase bone scan has a sensitivity of 60% as bone involvement is highly variable. Electrodiagnostic nerve studies are beneficial to evaluate for a mono- or polyneuropathy, which may be present in CRPS. A duplex ultrasound is useful for evaluating for a deep vein thrombosis. Additionally, while the use of a sympathetic block serves both a diagnostic and a therapeutic purpose, there are cases of CRPS that are not sympathetically maintained or for which sympathetic blocks stop providing therapeutic benefit after several sequential blocks.

Table 18.1: CRPS differential diagnoses

Neurogenic	Vasogenic	Other
Painful diabetic neuropathy	Thoracic outlet syndrome	Cellulitis
Small-fiber peripheral neuropathies	Raynaud's disease	Erythromelalgia
Entrapment neuropathies (e.g., cubital tunnel syndrome, carpal tunnel syndrome)	Acrocyanosis	
	Deep vein thrombosis	
	Vascular insufficiency	
Discogenic disease	Lymphedema	

Table 18.2:
Studies and tests to assist in making the diagnosis of CRPS

History	Complete physical exam
Neurologic exam	Vascular exam
MRI	Triple-phase bone scan
Nerve conduction velocity and electromyogram	Duplex ultrasound
Quantitative sensory testing	Autonomic function testing
Temperature measurement	Sympathetic blockade

Use of the Budapest criteria is an efficient and cost-effective method of diagnosing CRPS as the current criteria have a sensitivity of 0.99 and a specificity of 0.68.

Further Reading

Birklein F, O'Neill D, Schlereth T. Complex regional pain syndrome: an optimistic perspective. *Neurology*. 2015;84(1):89–96.

Bruehl S. Complex regional pain syndrome. *BMJ*. 2015;351:h2730.

Harden RN, Bruehl S, Perez RS, Birklein F, Marinus J, Maihofner C, Lubenow T, Buvanendran A, Mackey S, Graciosa J, Mogilevski M, Ramsden C, Chont M,Vatine JJ.Validation of proposed diagnostic criteria (the "Budapest criteria") for complex regional pain syndrome. *Pain*. 2010;150(2):268–274.

1.4. What are the typical signs and symptoms seen in a patient with CRPS?

The Budapest criteria as shown in Table 18.3 include the typical signs and symptoms as well as the requirements for the diagnosis.

Sensory: Pain is exacerbated with movement, temperature changes, contact, and stress. Allodynia and hyperalgesia are frequently present as well, along with a baseline burning pain. Sensory deficits are present in a glove- or stocking-type pattern, and there are often proprioceptive disturbances, causing the affected limb to feel foreign or oversized.

Motor: Patients may develop tremors, irregular myoclonus, decreased range of motion, and fixed dystonia-like postures. The chronic stage may result in fibrotic contractures, further loss of range of motion, and central motor symptoms.

Autonomic: CRPS frequently results in edema and hyperhidrosis of the affected limb, along with change in skin color and temperature. The inflammatory component of CRPS may induce a red color change, while long-term

Table 18.3:
Budapest criteria for CRPS

Continuing pain is disproportionate to the inciting event
No other diagnosis better explaining signs and symptoms
1 sign in 2 or more categories and 1 symptom in 3 or more categories

Category	Signs/Symptoms
Sensory	Hyperalgesia, hyperesthesia, allodynia
Vasomotor	Temperature, skin color asymmetry Skin color changes
Sudomotor/edema	Edema, sweating changes, or asymmetry
Motor/trophic	Decreased range of motion Motor dysfunction (weakness, tremor, dystonia) Trophic changes (hair, nail, skin)

autonomic dysfunction may cause the limb to appear blue. The mottled appearance may present early in the course of CRPS.

Trophic: The trophic changes of CRPS are a result of connective tissue effects and include increased hair growth, increased or decreased nail growth, and skin atrophy.

Further Reading

Birklein F, O'Neill D, Schlereth T. Complex regional pain syndrome: an optimistic perspective. *Neurology*. 2015;84(1:89–96.

1.5. What factors predispose patients to developing CRPS?

CRPS affects women more commonly than men in a 3:1 to 4:1 ratio, and it is most common in those aged 50 to 70 years. The incidence of CRPS I and II has been reported to be 5.46 and 0.82 per 100,000 person-years, respectively. Within the past decade (2012), the International Association for the Study of Pain adopted the more specific Budapest criteria, which has halved the rates of CRPS.

CRPS is found most commonly following a fracture (40% of all cases), with as many as 3% to 7% of people with a distal radial fracture developing CRPS. Other traumatic injuries (sprains, contusions, and crushes) may be responsible for an additional 20% of cases. Distal extremity surgeries are associated with CRPS, with up to 8.3% of patients undergoing carpal tunnel release developing it in one large prospective study.

Patients with more physically demanding jobs in the service industry have also been seen to develop CRPS at almost double the rate of others.

Further Reading

Allen G, Galer BS, Schwartz L. Epidemiology of complex regional pain syndrome: a retrospective chart review of 134 patients. *Pain*. 1999;80(3):539–544.

Birklein F, O'Neill D, Schlereth T. Complex regional pain syndrome: an optimistic perspective. *Neurology*. 2015;84(1):89–96.

Bruehl S. Complex regional pain syndrome. *BMJ*. 2015;351:h2730.

1.6. Are there genetic factors involved in the predisposition to develop CRPS?

Genetics may play a role in the development of CRPS, but determining hereditary data is still difficult due to the changing diagnostic criteria over the past 20 years. However, there have been some links to human leukocyte antigen DR13, DR15, and DQ1. Migraineurs also have a marked association with the development of CRPS, as 63% of those with CRPS meet criteria for migraine while only 30% of the general population will meet those criteria. Of those with migraine and CRPS, 82% had headaches prior to onset of CRPS symptoms.

Further Reading

Birklein F, O'Neill D, Schlereth T. Complex regional pain syndrome: an optimistic perspective. *Neurology*. 2015;84(1):89–96.

Peterlin BL, Rosso AL, Nair SA, Young WB, Schwartzman RJ. Migraine may be a risk factor for the development of complex regional pain syndrome. *Cephalalgia*. 2010 Feb;30(2):214–223.

1.7. What is the typical CRPS personality?

It is important to note that there is no "CRPS personality" and that "anxiety, depression, and personality are not predictors for the development of CRPS." Some researchers have postulated that traumatic life events like abuse and violence are more frequent in those who develop CRPS than in those with limb pain that does not develop into CRPS.

Further Reading

Birklein F, O'Neill D, Schlereth T. Complex regional pain syndrome: an optimistic perspective. *Neurology*. 2015;84(1):89–96.

2. Noninterventional Pharmacologic Modalities for Maximizing Analgesia

2.1. Are opioids a good option for management of CRPS?

Opioids typically provide at least 50% pain relief with a number needed to treat (NNT) between 3.3 and 4.7 in reviews of multiple studies of patients with neuropathic pain conditions. In a study of morphine efficacy in patients with spinal cord stimulator for CRPS, the devices were turned off, and the patients were randomized to sustained-release morphine 90 mg or placebo. Only 1 patient in the morphine group had adequate pain control without turning the device back on prior to the completion of the study at 8 days. Therefore, while opioids may be beneficial in an acute setting to gain some control during a pain flare, they are not an ideal long-term treatment option due to the risks of tolerance, dependence, addiction, and respiratory depression, among others. For patients demonstrating improved clinical outcomes while on long-term opioids, it is recommended to follow CDC guidelines to improve patient and societal safety.

Further Reading

Finnerup NB, Attal N, Haroutounian S, McNicol E, Baron R, Dworkin RH, Gilron I, Haanpaa M, Hansson P, Jensen TS, Kamerman PR, Lund K, Moore A, Raja SN, Rice ASC, Rowbotham M, Sena E, Siddall P, Smith BH, Wallace M. Pharmacotherapy for neuropathic pain in adults: a systematic review and meta-analysis. *Lancet Neurol*. 2015;14(2):162–173.

Harke H, Gretenkort P, Ladleif HU, Rahman S, Harke O. The response of neuropathic pain and pain in complex regional pain syndrome I to carbamazepine and sustained-release morphine in patients pretreated with spinal cord stimulation: a double-blinded randomized study. *Anesth Analg*. 2001;92(2):488–495.

Sindrup SH, Jensen TS. Efficacy of pharmacological treatments of neuropathic pain: an update and effect related to mechanism of drug action. *Pain*. 1999;83(3):389–400.

2.2. What is a good first-line medication therapy for a CRPS flare?

Glucocorticoids are an appropriate first-line medication, especially if the duration of symptoms is less than 6 to 9 months. A few studies have shown high degrees of efficacy using a variety of steroids and dosing regimens. Prednisolone 100 mg daily and 25% reduction every 4 days is one dosing strategy that is in use.

Further Reading

Birklein F, O'Neill D, Schlereth T. Complex regional pain syndrome: an optimistic perspective. *Neurology*. 2015;84(1):89–96.

Perez RS, Zollinger PE, Dijkstra PU, Thomassen-Hilgersom IL, Zuurmond WW, Rosenbrand KC, Geertzen JH. Evidence based guidelines for complex regional pain syndrome type 1. *BMC Neurology*. 2010;10(1):20.

2.3. What other medications can be used for a CRPS flare?

Anticonvulsants like gabapentin, pregabalin, and even topiramate are used in multiple neuropathic pain conditions. Gabapentin has been shown to reduce sensory deficit in the affected limb of CRPS, but pain relief is mild. Pregabalin has not been studied in CRPS, but a review of gabapentin and pregabalin in other neuropathic pain conditions revealed an NNT of 7.2 and 7.7, respectively.

Antidepressants can be extremely helpful for the patient with CRPS because of their potential direct pain-relieving effect and their benefits for the concomitant mood disorders that may develop over time. As has been seen with other neuropathic pain conditions, the selective serotonin and norepinephrine reuptake inhibitors (SNRIs) *duloxetine, venlafaxine, desvenlafaxine*, and *citalopram* can be very effective with an NNT of 6.4. Tricyclic antidepressants (TCAs)—*amitriptyline, nortriptyline, imipramine, desipramine*, and *doxepin*—can have cardiovascular and antihistamine effects but as a class have an NNT of 3.6 for neuropathic conditions. The selective serotonin reuptake inhibitors (SSRIs) are less efficacious in neuropathic conditions than the other classes of antidepressants.

Further Reading

Finnerup NB, Attal N, Haroutounian S, McNicol E, Baron R, Dworkin RH, Gilron I, Haanpaa M, Hansson P, Jensen TS, Kamerman PR, Lund K, Moore A, Raja SN, Rice ASC, Rowbotham M, Sena E, Siddall P, Smith BH, Wallace M. Pharmacotherapy for neuropathic pain in adults: a systematic review and meta-analysis. *Lancet Neurol.* 2015;14(2):162–173.

Van de Vusse AC, Stomp-van den Berg SG, Kessels AH, Weber WE. Randomised controlled trial of gabapentin in complex regional pain syndrome type 1 [ISRCTN84121379]. *BMC Neurol.* 2004;4(1):13.

2.4. Are there intravenous agents that can be used in a perioperative setting to reduce the pain of CRPS?

The *N-methyl-D-aspartic acid (NMDA) receptor antagonist* ketamine used as a subanesthetic infusion either in the inpatient setting or as outpatient intermittent infusions can provide excellent pain relief in many patients. Ketamine has been shown to provide long-lasting pain relief along with an increase in quality of life and participation in activities over a range of doses from outpatient infusions every 3 to 4 weeks at 0.5 mg/kg over 30 to 45 minutes to inpatient, intubated 5-day treatment courses of up to 7 mg/kg/h. However, it is important to recognize that infusions greater than 0.5 mg/kg/h do not substantially change pain in our experience but do have increased side effects and potential for other adverse events associated with higher doses, intensive care unit admission, and intubation.

Bisphosphonates are another intravenous (IV) option with increasing evidence (5 randomized controlled trials) for their use in CRPS, and they may be more efficacious in the acute phase due to their inhibition of osteoclast activity. Each of the studies used a different drug (alendronate, clodronate, pamidronate, and neridronate) and varied between oral and IV route of administration. Additionally, there is evidence that bisphosphonate treatment is more efficacious in early disease, in patients with fracture as their predisposing event, and in the "warm" subtype. A recent study by Varenna and colleagues showed no significant difference between clodronate 300 mg IV every day for 10 consecutive days, pamidronate 60 mg IV every third day for 4 times, and neridronate 100 mg IV every third day for 4 times.

Intravenous immunoglobulin is a novel therapy for CRPS and is currently being studied as a treatment option after showing efficacy at levels comparable with other treatments when trialed without strict protocol for number of infusions or spacing.

Further Reading

Birklein F, O'Neill D, Schlereth T. Complex regional pain syndrome: an optimistic perspective. *Neurology*. 2015;84(1):89–96.

Goebel A, Shenker N, Padfield N, Shoukrey K, McCabe C, Serpell M, Sanders M, Murphy C, Ejibe A, Milligan H, Kelly J, Ambler G. Low-dose intravenous immunoglobulin treatment for complex regional pain syndrome (LIPS): study protocol for a randomized controlled trial. *Trials*. 2014;15(1):404.

Kiefer RT, Rohr P, Ploppa A, Dieterich HJ, Grothusen J, Koffler S, Altemeyer KH, Unertl K, Schwartzman RJ. Efficacy of ketamine in anesthetic dosage for the treatment of refractory complex regional pain syndrome: an open-label phase II study. *Pain Med.* 2008;9(8):1173–1201.

Patil S, Anitescu M. Efficacy of outpatient ketamine infusions in refractory chronic pain syndromes: a 5-year retrospective analysis. *Pain Med.* 2012;13(2):263–269.

Varenna M, Manara M, Rovelli F, Zucchi F, Sinigaglia L. Predictors of responsiveness to bisphosphonate treatment in patients with complex regional pain syndrome type I: a retrospective chart analysis. *Pain Med.* 2017;18(6):1131–1138.

3. Interventional Pain Techniques

3.1. What interventional procedures can be helpful in the management of CRPS?

Interventional procedures used in the management of CRPS include sympathetic nerve blocks (e.g., stellate ganglion, lumbar sympathetic), neuraxial blocks (e.g., epidural or subarachnoid), somatic nerve blocks (e.g., brachial plexus), neurodestructive techniques of the sympathetic nerves (e.g., chemical, radiofrequency, surgical), and implantable devices (e.g., neuromodulation, intrathecal drug delivery systems).

3.2. Are sympathetic blocks useful in CRPS?

Somatosensory dysfunction in CRPS has been described in the literature, and sympathetic nerve blocks are performed to temporarily disrupt sympathetic transmission. Stellate ganglion blocks (for upper extremity CRPS) and lumbar sympathetic blocks (for lower extremity CRPS) are often administered using a mixture of long-acting local anesthetic and short-acting local anesthetic or long-acting local anesthetic alone in close intervals in conjunction with physical and occupational therapy (e.g., weekly) to facilitate pain reduction and improved function. Although these blocks are not recommended for routine use in the treatment of CRPS, there are limited treatment options in treatment-refractory CRPS, and these blocks should be considered a reasonable option and administered in close proximity to functional therapies. Functional progress of patients should be followed closely after these blocks are performed to ensure the blocks' efficacy and usefulness.

Further Reading

Bruehl S. Complex regional pain syndrome. *BMJ*. 2015;351:h2730.

Dworkin RH, O'Connor AB, Kent J, Mackey SC, Raja SN, Stacey BR, Levy RM, Backonja M, Baron R, Harke H, Loeser JD, Treede RD, Turk DC, Wells CD, International Association for the Study of Pain Neuropathic Pain Special Interest Group. Interventional management of neuropathic pain: NeuPSIG recommendations. *Pain*. 2013;154(11):2249–2261.

Harden RN, Bruehl S, Perez RS, Birklein F, Marinus J, Maihofner C, Lubenow T, Buvanendran A, Mackey S, Graciosa J, Mogilevski M, Ramsden C, Chont M, Vatine JJ. Validation of proposed diagnostic criteria (the "Budapest criteria") for complex regional pain syndrome. *Pain*. 2010;150(2):268–274.

Perez RS, Zollinger PE, Dijkstra PU, Thomassen-Hilgersom IL, Zuurmond WW, Rosenbrand KC, Geertzen JH. Evidence based guidelines for complex regional pain syndrome type 1. *BMC Neurology*. 2010;10(1):20.

Raja SN, Grabow TS. Complex regional pain syndrome I (reflex sympathetic dystrophy). *Anesthesiology*. 2002;96(5):1254–1260.

Van Eijs F, Stanton-Hicks M, Van Zundert J, Faber CG, Lubenow TR, Mekhail N, van Kleef M, Huygen F. Evidence-based interventional pain medicine according to clinical diagnosis. 16. Complex regional pain syndrome. *Pain Pract*. 2010;11(1):70–87.

3.3. Can epidural injections or infusions be part of the treatment of CRPS?

The use of lumbar epidural infusions (for lower extremity CRPS) of local anesthetic, clonidine, and/or opioids to facilitate pain relief and functional improvement through interruption of transmission of the somatosensory and sympathetic nervous systems has been described in the literature through randomized controlled trials. Unilateral cervical epidural infusions (for upper extremity CRPS) of local anesthetic and clonidine have also been described through retrospective review. Epidural infusions have several advantages: (1) variation of volume, dose, and concentration of local anesthetic to achieve the desired effect; (2) allowance for the use of multiple pharmacologic agents of different mechanisms of action; (3) effective titration and control of pain during functional therapies; and (4) patient-controlled administration options. Risks of continuous infusions into the epidural space include (1) infection, including epidural abscess, especially for long-term use; (2) hematoma formation, especially in the setting of coagulopathies; and (3) motor weakness with use of local anesthetics. Harden et al. suggest using epidural infusion techniques as an option in patients who have failed intermittent sympathetic blockade, described previously.

Further Reading

Harden RN, Bruehl S, Perez RS, Birklein F, Marinus J, Maihofner C, Lubenow T, Buvanendran A, Mackey S, Graciosa J, Mogilevski M, Ramsden C, Chont M, Vatine JJ. Validation of proposed diagnostic criteria (the "Budapest criteria") for complex regional pain syndrome. *Pain*. 2010;150(2):268–274.

Van Eijs F, Stanton-Hicks M, Van Zundert J, Faber CG, Lubenow TR, Mekhail N, van Kleef M, Huygen F. Evidence-based interventional pain medicine according to clinical diagnosis. 16. Complex regional pain syndrome. *Pain Pract*. 2010;11(1):70–87.

3.4. Do peripheral nerve blocks have a role in the treatment of CRPS?

Somatic nerve blocks, similar to neuraxial infusions, exert their effects through blockade of both the sympathetic and somatosensory nervous systems; however, these types of blocks are performed peripherally at the level of a specific plexus or nerve. Several case reports describe the use of a continuous catheter–based infusion of local anesthetic around the brachial plexus through an axillary approach using a low concentration of bupivacaine (ranging from 0.05% to 0.125%) up to a period of 3 weeks' duration resulting in improved function in physical therapy for many of the patients. Nerve blocks to other nerves are certainly possible, but there is limited description of such techniques in the literature.

Further Reading

Harden RN, Bruehl S, Perez RS, Birklein F, Marinus J, Maihofner C, Lubenow T, Buvanendran A, Mackey S, Graciosa J, Mogilevski M, Ramsden C, Chont M, Vatine JJ. Validation of proposed diagnostic criteria (the "Budapest criteria") for complex regional pain syndrome. *Pain*. 2010;150(2):268–274.

Van Eijs F, Stanton-Hicks M, Van Zundert J, Faber CG, Lubenow TR, Mekhail N, van Kleef M, Huygen F. Evidence-based interventional pain medicine according to clinical diagnosis. 16. Complex regional pain syndrome. *Pain Pract*. 2010;11(1):70–87.

3.5. If the sympathetic block is successful, should destruction of the sympathetic ganglia be performed for long-term pain relief?

Destruction of sympathetic ganglia using chemical means, radiofrequency, and surgery has been well described in the literature and evolved as a potential method to induce a sympathectomy of longer duration than local anesthetics, but only in the form of case reports. Unfortunately, the results of these case reports are mixed; these techniques carry a substantial risk of postneurodestructive complications, including deafferentation pain and recurrence of symptoms, so their use in treatment of CRPS has fallen out of favor.

Further Reading

Dworkin RH, O'Connor AB, Kent J, Mackey SC, Raja SN, Stacey BR, Levy RM, Backonja M, Baron R, Harke H, Loeser JD, Treede RD, Turk DC, Wells CD, International Association for the Study of Pain Neuropathic Pain Special Interest Group. Interventional management of neuropathic pain: NeuPSIG recommendations. *Pain*. 2013;154(11):2249–2261.

Harden RN, Bruehl S, Perez RS, Birklein F, Marinus J, Maihofner C, Lubenow T, Buvanendran A, Mackey S, Graciosa J, Mogilevski M, Ramsden C, Chont M, Vatine JJ. Validation of proposed diagnostic criteria (the "Budapest criteria") for complex regional pain syndrome. *Pain*. 2010;150(2):268–274.

3.6. When is neuromodulation appropriate for the treatment of CRPS?

Neuromodulation, including spinal cord and peripheral nerve stimulation, has shown efficacy in treating CRPS of the upper and lower extremities. Dworkin et al. state there is moderate-quality evidence for the use of spinal cord stimulation as a treatment for CRPS and suggest using this technique for patients who do not respond to noninvasive or less invasive treatments or for patients in which nerve blocks are not appropriate.

Further Reading

Dworkin RH, O'Connor AB, Kent J, Mackey SC, Raja SN, Stacey BR, Levy RM, Backonja M, Baron R, Harke H, Loeser JD, Treede RD, Turk DC, Wells CD, International Association for the Study of Pain Neuropathic Pain Special Interest Group. Interventional management of neuropathic pain: NeuPSIG recommendations. *Pain.* 2013;154(11):2249–2261.

Harden RN, Bruehl S, Perez RS, Birklein F, Marinus J, Maihofner C, Lubenow T, Buvanendran A, Mackey S, Graciosa J, Mogilevski M, Ramsden C, Chont M, Vatine JJ. Validation of proposed diagnostic criteria (the "Budapest criteria") for complex regional pain syndrome. *Pain.* 2010;150(2):268–274.

Van Eijs F, Stanton-Hicks M, Van Zundert J, Faber CG, Lubenow TR, Mekhail N, van Kleef M, Huygen F. Evidence-based interventional pain medicine according to clinical diagnosis. 16. Complex regional pain syndrome. *Pain Pract.* 2010;11(1):70–87.

Sickle Cell Pain Crisis

Vikram Bansal, Deva Sharma, and Uma Shastri

19

Case Scenario

A 22-year-old African American woman is seen in consultation in the emergency department for acute right quadriceps pain. The patient has a known history of homozygous SS sickle cell disease and is known to the emergency department staff for having recurrent acute vaso-occlusive pain episodes, for which extremely large doses of opioids have been administered. Other pertinent medical history includes mild asthma and avascular necrosis of the hips.

1. Pathophysiology and Epidemiology

1.1. What is the pathophysiology of sickle cell disease?

Sickle cell disease results from a single-point mutation of glutamic acid replaced with valine in the beta globin gene. A hemoglobin molecule is composed of 2 alpha and 2 beta subunits. An individual with sickle cell disease has normal alpha subunits and altered beta subunits. If 1 beta subunit is normal and 1 is mutated (heterozygote), that individual has sickle cell trait. Most patients with sickle cell trait are asymptomatic, but they have an increased lifetime risk for select complications, including but not limited to splenic rupture at high altitudes, venous thromboembolism, renal papillary necrosis, traumatic hyphema, hyposthenuria, exercise-induced heat stroke, and rhabdomyolysis.

Through a complex interplay of adhesive events among blood cells, structurally altered erythrocytes can obstruct the vasculature, producing episodes of acute pain, hemolytic anemia, organ injury, and early mortality.

Patients with sickle cell disease experience a wide spectrum of clinical sequelae as a result of chronic inflammation, hemolysis, and vaso-occlusion, including but not limited to acute and chronic lung injury, recurrent infections secondary to autosplenectomy, leg ulcerations, chronic kidney disease, pulmonary hypertension, cholelithiasis, seizures, cerebral infarcts and vasculopathy, proliferative retinopathy, venous thromboembolic events, priapism, and avascular necrosis.

Further Reading

Beet EA. The genetics of the sickle-cell trait in a Bantu tribe. Ann Eugen. 1949;14:279–284.

Bucknor MD, Goo JS, Coppolino ML. The risk of potential thromboembolic, renal and cardiac complications of sickle cell trait. Hemoglobin. 2014;38:28–32.

Ingram VM. A specific chemical difference between the globins of normal human and sickle-cell anaemia haemoglobin. Nature. 1956;178:792–794.

Kato GJ, Steinberg MH, Gladwin MT. Intravascular hemolysis and the pathophysiology of sickle cell disease. J Clin Invest. 2017;127:750–760.

Manwani D, Frenette PS. Vaso-occlusion in sickle cell disease: pathophysiology and novel targeted therapies. Hematology Am Soc Hematol Educ Program. 2013;2013:362–369.

Pauling L, Itano HA, et al. Sickle cell anemia, a molecular disease. Science. 1949;109:443.

1.2. What is the epidemiology of sickle cell disease and acute pain episodes?

Sickle cell anemia (SCA), the most severe phenotype of sickle cell disease (HbSS and HbS β^0 thalassemia), represents one of the most common monogenic blood disorders worldwide, with an estimated 300,000 new cases each year. Epidemiologic data indicate that 5.2% of patients with sickle cell disease have 3 to 10 episodes of severe pain every year. The frequency, severity, location, and duration of an acute vaso-occlusive pain episode can vary significantly among affected individuals, and many are able to identify specific triggers for their acute pain, including but not limited to changes in climate, strenuous physical activity, dehydration, and acute infection.

Further Reading

Steinberg MH. Management of sickle cell disease. N Engl J Med. 1999;340:1021–1030.

Therrell BL Jr., Lloyd-Puryear MA, Eckman JR, et al. Newborn screening for sickle cell diseases in the United States: a review of data spanning 2 decades. Semin Perinatol. 2015;39:238–251.

Weatherall DJ. The inherited diseases of hemoglobin are an emerging global health burden. Blood. 2010;115:4331–4336.

1.3. What is the pathophysiology of acute sickle cell pain episodes?

Acute vaso-occlusive pain episodes, also referred to as sickle cell crises, are initiated and sustained by adhesive interactions among sickled erythrocytes, endothelial cells, and plasma constituents. Erythrocyte injury leads to intra- and extravascular hemolysis, ischemia/reperfusion injury, and inflammation. Acute pain is often caused by ischemic tissue injury due to vaso-occlusion within the vasculature, resulting in decreased blood flow to end-organ tissues, endothelial injury, and release of inflammatory mediators. Acute vaso-occlusive pain episodes can last for days to weeks, depending on their severity. Pain commonly involves the back, legs, arms, knees, chest, or abdomen. The pain generally affects 2 or more sites, and bone pain tends to be bilateral and symmetric. If an individual has recurrent acute pain episodes, they often involve similar anatomic distributions and patterns as previously experienced. Acute vaso-occlusive pain episodes are described in 4 phases. The first is a prodromal phase consisting of paresthesia and aches, usually presenting 24 hours before the second infarctive phase, which lasts 2 to 3 days. The third phase is he postinfarctive inflammatory phase, which is followed by a fourth, recovery phase.

Further Reading

Ballas SK. The sickle cell painful crisis in adults: phases and objective signs. Hemoglobin. 1995;19:323–333.

Kato GJ, Steinberg MH, Gladwin MT. Intravascular hemolysis and the pathophysiology of sickle cell disease. J Clin Invest. 2017;127:750–760.

Steinberg MH. Management of sickle cell disease. N Engl J Med. 1999;340:1021–1030.

1.4. What are the predisposing factors of acute vaso-occlusive pain episodes?

The major risk factors for acute vaso-occlusive pain episodes include intrinsic and extrinsic stimuli that predispose deoxygenated erythrocytes to sickle and adhere to other blood cells. The major risk factors include, but are not limited to, hypoxia, acidosis, hypothermia, hypovolemia, severe anemia, infections, high altitudes, stress, pregnancy, and alcohol.

Further Reading

Steinberg MH. Management of sickle cell disease. N Engl J Med. 1999;340:1021–1030.

2. Evaluation and Treatment

2.1. How should anesthesiologists evaluate patients with sickle cell disease and acute pain?

When a patient presents to the hospital with acute vaso-occlusive pain, a physician must act quickly and promptly to address the patient's symptoms. A complete history and physical examination constitute the first step in diagnosis. Specifically, ask about the patient's previous vaso-occlusive pain symptoms and determine whether the current symptoms are similar. Information such as location, duration, severity, and intensity are vital to a diagnosis. In addition, look for potential factors that may have precipitated acute pain as stated in the previous question, including infection, acidosis, stress, hypovolemia, and dehydration. Physical examination should specifically focus on any signs of infection or dehydration. As part of standard care, a complete blood count with differential, reticulocyte indices, and comprehensive metabolic panel should be ordered. If any shortness of breath, fever, or new oxygen requirement is found on examination, a chest radiograph should be ordered to rule out acute chest syndrome, in addition to blood and urine cultures. No single laboratory test is diagnostic of an acute vaso-occlusive pain episode, although many patients have elevation of their baseline leukocytes, which promote vascular inflammation and vessel damage when activated. A decline in baseline platelet counts may also be observed in individuals with uncomplicated acute pain episodes. Absence of hemolysis or a stable hemoglobin level does not preclude a patient from having an acute pain episode.

Treatment of acute vaso-occlusive pain episodes can be extremely challenging and often requires a multidisciplinary team, including but not limited to acute pain specialists, internists, and hematologists. Pain scales, such as the Visual Analogue Scale, verbal pain scales, and body drawings can help determine the location and severity of pain. In addition, pain scales help the physician to determine if other disease-specific etiologies of acute pain warrant further evaluation, such as acute hepatic sequestration, avascular necrosis, and cholelithiasis. Many patients followed at comprehensive sickle cell disease centers will have formal pain action plans for acute vaso-occlusive pain episodes. Significant deviation from those plans may result in undertreatment of the patient's pain due to concerns about addiction, opiate abuse, and dependence, as well as respiratory depression.

Further Reading

Shanley LA, Ebeling M, Titus MO. Changes in platelet count as a predictive tool in sickle cell acute vaso-occlusive crises: a pediatric study. Clin Pediatr (Phila). 2011;50:657–661.

Steinberg MH. Management of sickle cell disease. N Engl J Med. 1999;340:1021–1030.

Wun T. The role of inflammation and leukocytes in the pathogenesis of sickle cell disease: haemoglobinopathy. Hematology. 2001;5:403–412.

Yale SH, Nagib N, Guthrie T. Approach to the vaso-occlusive crisis in adults with sickle cell disease. Am Fam Physician. 2000;61:1349–1356, 1363–1364.

2.2. What are some noninterventional pharmacologic methods to treat acute vaso-occlusive pain episodes?

Maintaining adequate volume status is critical for preventing worsening of acute pain, as dehydration precipitates further sickling of erythrocytes. However, excessive hydration can lead to pulmonary edema, and respiratory status should be closely monitored during this period. Hydroxyurea is a key component for the chronic treatment of patients with sickle cell disease who experience frequent acute vaso-occlusive pain episodes. Hydroxyurea increases the production of fetal hemoglobin, also referred to as hemoglobin F, which lacks the beta subunit responsible for abnormal erythrocyte morphology in sickle cell disease. Patients on hydroxyurea are followed closely during initiation to monitor for thrombocytopenia. In patients with significant toxicities prohibiting hydroxyurea use, such as leg ulcers, which develop due to impaired wound healing, chronic outpatient blood transfusion therapy is an alternative disease-modifying therapy, which can be used to reduce the frequency of acute pain episodes until leg ulcers have adequately healed. Chronic blood transfusion therapy can also be used to reduce acute vaso-occlusive pain episodes in pregnant women, in whom hydroxyurea is generally avoided due to concerns about teratogenicity in animal models.

Other nonpharmacologic treatment options include heat or warm compresses. Cold compresses can worsen symptoms by increasing sickling and should be avoided. Oxygen therapy is not indicated unless there is hypoxia, due to the concern that the routine use of oxygen can suppress erythrocyte production, depress reticulocytosis, or induce rebound pain after oxygen discontinuation. Additional nonpharmacologic treatments that should be considered on an individualized basis include psychosocial support via cognitive-behavior modification, relaxation and breathing exercises, and hypnosis.

Transfusion of packed red blood cells should not be used for the treatment of acute vaso-occlusive pain but should be reserved for individuals with symptomatic anemia and other acute disease–related complications such as stroke, acute chest syndrome, and multiorgan failure. The severity of these complications may be attenuated by blood transfusions, which increase oxygen carrying capacity, decrease bone marrow production of erythrocytes containing hemoglobin S, and improve rheological properties of blood. In patients with serum hemoglobin levels greater than 10.0 g/dL, simple blood transfusions can increase blood viscosity and exacerbate acute vaso-occlusive pain.

Deep venous thrombosis prophylaxis should always be promptly initiated in patients with sickle cell disease who are admitted for acute vaso-occlusive pain episodes. Compared with the general population, patients with sickle cell disease have a significantly higher risk of deep venous thrombosis than do age- and race-matched controls, and an acute pulmonary embolism in an individual with sickle cell disease can precipitate acute chest syndrome and rapid respiratory compromise.

Incentive spirometry should also be incorporated into the routine management of individuals with sickle cell disease who are admitted to the hospital, as a cost-effective measure to prevent V/Q mismatching, acute respiratory failure, and development of acute chest syndrome.

Further Reading

Bader U, Banyai M, Boni R, et al. Leg ulcers in patients with myeloproliferative disorders: disease- or treatment-related? Dermatology. 2000;200:45–48.

Bellet PS, Kalinyak KA, Shukla R, et al. Incentive spirometry to prevent acute pulmonary complications in sickle cell diseases. N Engl J Med. 1995;333:699–703.

Embury SH, Garcia JF, Mohandas N, et al. Effects of oxygen inhalation on endogenous erythropoietin kinetics, erythropoiesis, and properties of blood cells in sickle-cell anemia. N Engl J Med. 1984;311:291–295.

Goldberg MA, Brugnara C, Dover GJ, et al. Treatment of sickle cell anemia with hydroxyurea and erythropoietin. N Engl J Med. 1990;323:366–372.

Josephson CD, Su LL, Hillyer KL, et al. Transfusion in the patient with sickle cell disease: a critical review of the literature and transfusion guidelines. Transfus Med Rev. 2007;21:118–133.

Naik RP, Streiff MB, Lanzkron S. Sickle cell disease and venous thromboembolism: what the anticoagulation expert needs to know. J Thromb Thrombolysis. 2013;35:352–358.

Ohene-Frempong K, Weiner SJ, Sleeper LA, et al. Cerebrovascular accidents in sickle cell disease: rates and risk factors. Blood. 1998;91:288–294.

Okusanya BO, Oladapo OT. Prophylactic versus selective blood transfusion for sickle cell disease in pregnancy. Cochrane Database Syst Rev. 2013:CD010378.

Quirolo K. How do I transfuse patients with sickle cell disease? Transfusion. 2010;50:1881–1886.

Rodgers GP, Dover GJ, Noguchi CT, et al. Hematologic responses of patients with sickle cell disease to treatment with hydroxyurea. N Engl J Med. 1990;322:1037–1045.

Sirieix ME, Debure C, Baudot N, et al. Leg ulcers and hydroxyurea: forty-one cases. Arch Dermatol. 1999;135:818–820.

Stein PD, Beemath A, Meyers FA, et al. Deep venous thrombosis and pulmonary embolism in hospitalized patients with sickle cell disease. Am J Med. 2006;119:897 e7–e11.

2.3. What are the noninterventional pharmacologic treatments for management of analgesia during an acute sickle cell pain crisis?

Opioids are the primary treatment modality for an acute vaso-occlusive pain episode. Opioid treatment should be started as rapidly as possible once the patient arrives in the emergency department. Several outcomes are improved with early initiation of opioid therapy, including decreased length of hospital stay and decreased amount of total opioid consumption. Patient-controlled analgesia (PCA) is a mode of opioid delivery that has been shown to have the best outcomes when compared with oral or intravenous nurse-administered opioids or a continuous infusion alone. PCA dosing is based on the patient, the severity of symptoms, and whether or not the patient is opioid naive. If a patient is on chronic opioid therapy, this should be added in the form of a background infusion on the PCA or continuation of is or her long-acting opioid. Similarly, these strategies can be considered in the subset of patients whose pain can be refractory to standard opioid therapy, even when utilized as part of a multimodal pain management strategy. Although opioids are the mainstay of treatment for an acute vaso-occlusive pain episode, it is important to consider the addition of various adjuncts so that a multimodal pain management strategy is employed.

Further Reading

Mathias MD, McCavit TL. Timing of opioid administration as a quality indicator for pain crises in sickle cell disease. Pediatrics. 2015;135:475–482.

van Beers EJ, van Tuijn CF, Nieuwkerk PT, et al. Patient-controlled analgesia versus continuous infusion of morphine during vaso-occlusive crisis in sickle cell disease, a randomized controlled trial. Am J Hematol. 2007;82:955–960.

2.4. What are some multimodal adjuncts that can be added to treat acute vaso-occlusive pain episodes?

Acetaminophen has been shown to be beneficial during an acute vaso-occlusive pain episode when used in combination with opioids. The role for nonsteroidal inflammatory drugs (NSAIDs) is less clear, while first-line therapy with intravenous fluids and intravenous ketorolac was shown to effectively resolve acute vaso-occlusive pain episodes in an observational study of 50 children presenting to the emergency department. Another study of 29 children with sickle cell disease who were randomized to either intravenous ketorolac or placebo in a double-blinded fashion did not show a reduction in total dose of morphine received or reduction in pain severity (scored by the 10-cm linear Visual Analogue Scale) between the 2 groups. Although NSAIDs may be associated with a number of advantages over narcotic medications, including potent anti-inflammatory effects, as well as lack of addictive potential, respiratory depression, and central nervous system effects, irreversible renal failure has been reported in association with their use in sickle cell disease. Further, acute kidney injury is a poor prognostic marker in hospitalized patients with sickle cell disease who are transferred to the intensive care unit; it can be precipitated by a number of factors, including volume depletion, rhabdomyolysis, and infections, in addition to the use of NSAIDs. In patients with sickle cell disease, creatinine levels are an inaccurate marker of glomerular filtration rate because of the relatively high tubular secretion of creatinine; acute subclinical tubular injury may still occur in individuals with normal serum creatinine levels. In summary, there are no standardized guidelines for the use of NSAIDs in individuals with sickle cell disease and acute vaso-occlusive pain episodes. While intravenous ketorolac may be effective for acute pain management as an adjunct to other therapies, it should be used with caution and for a limited time to prevent development of acute kidney injury.

In addition to NSAIDs, steroids should also be used with caution for the treatment of acute vaso-occlusive pain episodes. Activation of inflammatory pathways has been implicated in the pathogenesis of acute vaso-occlusive pain, promoting activation of the vascular endothelium and increased cellular adhesion, suggesting the utility of steroids in the treatment of acute vaso-occlusive pain. However, retrospective data have raised concern about the association between steroid use and rebound pain and stroke in individuals with sickle cell disease. In a randomized, single-institution study of 2 doses of intravenous methylprednisolone versus placebo in 74 children and teenagers presenting with acute vaso-occlusive pain, a shorter duration of analgesic therapy was reported in the methylprednisolone group. While the underlying mechanism of rebound pain associated with steroids is not entirely clear, this is felt to be related to rebound inflammation and embolization of bone marrow fat. Based on data from limited single-institution studies, the recommendations for steroid use for the treatment of acute vaso-occlusive pain in sickle cell disease is grade 2B. If steroids are used for the treatment of acute vaso-occlusive pain, the associated risks of rebound pain should be discussed with the patient beforehand.

Further Reading

Alleyne GA. The kidney in sickle cell anemia. Kidney Int. 1975;7:371–379.

Allon M. Renal abnormalities in sickle cell disease. Arch Intern Med. 1990;150:501–504.

Ataga KI, Orringer EP. Renal abnormalities in sickle cell disease. Am J Hematol. 2000;63:205–211.

Audard V, Moutereau S, Vandemelebrouck G, et al. First evidence of subclinical renal tubular injury during sickle-cell crisis. Orphanet J Rare Dis. 2014;9:67.

Ballas SK. Corticosteroids and sickle cell disease. J Natl Med Assoc. 2009;101:283.

Beiter JL Jr., Simon HK, Chambliss CR, et al. Intravenous ketorolac in the emergency department management of sickle cell pain and predictors of its effectiveness. Arch Pediatr Adolesc Med. 2001;155:496–500.

Buckalew VM Jr., Someren A. Renal manifestations of sickle cell disease. Arch Intern Med. 1974;133:660–669.

Cecchini J, Lionnet F, Djibre M, et al. Outcomes of adult patients with sickle cell disease admitted to the ICU: a case series. Crit Care Med. 2014;42:1629–1639.

Darbari DS, Fasano RS, Minniti CP, et al. Severe vaso-occlusive episodes associated with use of systemic corticosteroids in patients with sickle cell disease. J Natl Med Assoc. 2008;100:948–951.

de Jong PE, Statius van Eps LW. Sickle cell nephropathy: new insights into its pathophysiology. Kidney Int. 1985;27:711–717.

Griffin TC, McIntire D, Buchanan GR. High-dose intravenous methylprednisolone therapy for pain in children and adolescents with sickle cell disease. N Engl J Med. 1994;330:733–737.

Guyatt GH, Oxman AD, Vist GE, et al. GRADE: an emerging consensus on rating quality of evidence and strength of recommendations. BMJ. 2008;336:924–926.

Hardwick WE Jr., Givens TG, Monroe KW, et al. Effect of ketorolac in pediatric sickle cell vaso-occlusive pain crisis. Pediatr Emerg Care. 1999;15:179–182.

Hebbel RP, Vercellotti G, Nath KA. A systems biology consideration of the vasculopathy of sickle cell anemia: the need for multi-modality chemo-prophylaxsis. Cardiovasc Hematol Disord Drug Targets. 2009;9:271–292.

Simckes AM, Chen SS, Osorio AV, et al. Ketorolac-induced irreversible renal failure in sickle cell disease: a case report. Pediatr Nephrol. 1999;13:63–67.

Strouse JJ, Hulbert ML, DeBaun MR, et al. Primary hemorrhagic stroke in children with sickle cell disease is associated with recent transfusion and use of corticosteroids. Pediatrics. 2006;118:1916–1924.

Strouse JJ, Takemoto CM, Keefer JR, et al. Corticosteroids and increased risk of readmission after acute chest syndrome in children with sickle cell disease. Pediatr Blood Cancer. 2008;50:1006–1012.

Vandy Black L, Smith WR. Evidence-based mini-review: are systemic corticosteroids an effective treatment for acute pain in sickle cell disease? Hematology Am Soc Hematol Educ Program. 2010;2010:416–417.

2.5. Can meperidine be used in the management of acute vaso-occlusive pain episodes?

Meperidine should be avoided in the treatment of acute vaso-occlusive pain episodes because the metabolite normeperidine can potentially accumulate and cause anxiety, tremors, myoclonus, and generalized seizures. This is more likely to occur in patients with sickle cell disease because of both continued repeat doses and the possibility of impaired renal function. Sedation and reduction in both systolic and diastolic blood pressures has also been reported in individuals with sickle cell disease receiving meperidine for the treatment of acute vaso-occlusive pain.

Further Reading

Ballas SK. Meperidine for acute sickle cell pain in the emergency department: revisited controversy. Ann Emerg Med. 2008;51:217.

Uzun B, Kekec Z, Gurkan E. Efficacy of tramadol vs meperidine in vasoocclusive sickle cell crisis. Am J Emerg Med. 2010;28:445–449.

2.6. Can methadone be used in the management of acute vaso-occlusive pain episodes?

Recent studies have shown that the addition of methadone to a standard multimodal opioid pain management strategy produces more pain relief. Thus, methadone can be added for improved pain management, although a plan for weaning should be in place prior to discharge and repeated electrocardiograms should be used to monitor for QT prolongation during initiation.

Further Reading

Horst J, Frei-Jones M, Deych E, et al. Pharmacokinetics and analgesic effects of methadone in children and adults with sickle cell disease. Pediatr Blood Cancer. 2016;63:2123–2130.

2.7. What are other medications that can be employed in the management of an acute sickle cell pain crisis?

Gabapentin can be considered as part of a multimodal pain strategy, particularly in patients with a neuropathic component of pain, although this is not a common presentation of acute vaso-occlusive pain in most patients. Ketamine infusions have also been used successfully in cases of acute vaso-occlusive pain episodes that are refractory to opioids.

Other investigational therapies that have been studied in the management of acute vaso-occlusive episodes include tinzaparin, a low-molecular-weight heparin, which was shown to reduce the number of days with severe pain, as well as overall duration of pain and hospitalization in a randomized, placebo-controlled trial of 253 patients. Purified poloxamer 188 has also been shown to decrease the severity of acute vaso-occlusive pain episodes in a randomized, placebo-controlled trial of 255 patients with sickle cell disease, presumably by increasing tissue oxygenation, although the benefit was relatively small. L-arginine therapy, a required substrate for nitric oxide synthesis, may also potentially improve acute vaso-occlusive pain by restoring nitric oxide levels according to results of a randomized, placebo-controlled trial of 38 children with sickle cell disease, in which L-arginine reduced narcotic use by more than than 50%.

Further Reading

Brandow AM, Farley RA, Panepinto JA. Neuropathic pain in patients with sickle cell disease. Pediatr Blood Cancer. 2014;61:512–517.

Morris CR, Kuypers FA, Lavrisha L, et al. A randomized, placebo-controlled trial of arginine therapy for the treatment of children with sickle cell disease hospitalized with vaso-occlusive pain episodes. Haematologica. 2013;98:1375–1382.

Orringer EP, Casella JF, Ataga KI, et al. Purified poloxamer 188 for treatment of acute vaso-occlusive crisis of sickle cell disease: A randomized controlled trial. JAMA. 2001;286:2099–2106.

Qari MH, Aljaouni SK, Alardawi MS, et al. Reduction of painful vaso-occlusive crisis of sickle cell anaemia by tinzaparin in a double-blind randomized trial. Thromb Haemost. 2007;98:392–396.

Uprety D, Baber A, Foy M. Ketamine infusion for sickle cell pain crisis refractory to opioids: a case report and review of literature. Ann Hematol. 2014;93:769–771.

2.8. Hydroxyurea is used to decrease the frequency of vaso-occlusive. Can it also be used in the treatment of acute events?

Although hydroxyurea is not beneficial for the treatment of an acute vaso-occlusive pain episode, it is indicated for patients who have experienced at least 3 or more acute vaso-occlusive pain episodes in a given year; it also has been demonstrated to decrease the frequency of acute pain episodes when used at maximal tolerated dose.

Further Reading

Goldberg MA, Brugnara C, Dover GJ, Schapira L, Charache S, Bunn HF. Treatment of sickle cell anemia with hydroxyurea and erythropoietin. N Engl J Med. 1990;323:366–372.

2.9. Is there a role for peripheral nerve blockade in the management of acute vaso-occlusive pain episodes?

Peripheral nerve blockade (PNB), with either a single injection or a continuous catheter technique, has also been shown to be a successful addition to noninterventional pharmacologic therapy for the treatment of refractory pain. Peripheral nerve blockade should be considered early in the treatment plan as part of the standard algorithm. Peripheral nerve blockade can target the pain associated with acute vaso-occlusion through mechanisms that can complement the pharmacologic management. A PNB can improve regional blood flow and counteract the vasoconstrictive pain that is associated with nitric oxide depletion. In addition, peripheral nerve blockade could be effective in a subset of patients with sickle cell disease who have a component of neuropathic pain. PNB has been shown to be effective in treating neuropathic pain. The use of a PNB will also allow a reduction in the amount of opioids used, and thus a decrease in opioid related side effects.

Further Reading

Forero M, Adhikary SD, Lopez H, et al. The erector spinae plane block: a novel analgesic technique in thoracic neuropathic pain. Reg Anesth Pain Med. 2016;41:621–627.

Giabicani M, Compere V, Fourdrinier V, et al. Is sickle cell disease a possible risk factor for peripheral neuropathy after popliteal sciatic nerve block? Br J Anaesth. 2013;111:508–510.

Li J, Karmakar MK, Li X, et al. Regional hemodynamic changes after an axillary brachial plexus block: a pulsed-wave Doppler ultrasound study. Reg Anesth Pain Med. 2012;37:111–118.

Morris CR, Kuypers FA, Lavrisha L, et al. A randomized, placebo-controlled trial of arginine therapy for the treatment of children with sickle cell disease hospitalized with vaso-occlusive pain episodes. Haematologica. 2013;98:1375–1382.

2.10. Are there additional risks to placing peripheral nerve blocks in patients with sickle cell disease?

Although peripheral nervous system involvement is rare in individuals with sickle cell disease, Okuyucu and colleagues showed that subclinical peripheral nerve involvement might be seen in a subset of patients (19.6%; 10 out of 51). However, the frequency of acute vaso-occlusive pain episodes was not significantly correlated with peripheral neuropathy. There has been one published case report of a peripheral neuropathy after a PNB in a patient with sickle cell disease.

Further Reading

Giabicani M, Compere V, Fourdrinier V, Dureuil B. Is sickle cell disease a possible risk factor for peripheral neuropathy after popliteal sciatic nerve block? Br J Anaesth. 2013;111:508–510.

Okuyucu EE, Turhanoglu A, Duman T, et al. Peripheral nervous system involvement in patients with sickle cell disease. Eur J Neurol. 2009;16:814–818.

2.11. How soon should a patient be discharged after an acute vaso-occlusive pain episode?

It is imperative to ensure adequate pain control during the discharge period. This decreases the likelihood of a recurrent acute vaso-occlusive pain episode resulting in readmission. Prior to discharge, the patient must first be transitioned from PCA to oral opioids. The patient can be safely discharged home after being monitored for approximately 24 to 48 hours and when it is deemed that his or her pain is adequately controlled with only oral opioids and adjuncts. The World Health Organization pain ladder can help guide selection of the discharge pain regimen, although therapies should be individualized, with careful review of the patient's medical comorbidities. Opioids should be prescribed in an amount to last only until the 1- to 2-week follow-up visit.

In addition to opioids, patients should be advised to use acetaminophen. Gabapentin can also be considered if a neuropathic component of pain is present. Studies are conflicting on whether NSAIDs should be used in patients with sickle cell disease due to the propensity for renal papillary necrosis and end-stage renal disease. Patients should be advised against taking NSAIDs on a scheduled basis and should use them only as needed if they do not have any prohibiting medical comorbidities, such as chronic kidney disease or concurrent use of therapeutic anticoagulation therapy.

Patients should continue hydroxyurea on discharge for the prevention of recurrent acute vaso-occlusive pain episodes and should be advised to ensure adequate hydration, rest, and avoidance of extreme temperatures. Many patients with sickle cell disease experience chronic pain in addition to periodic episodes of acute pain. These patients may also require chronic opioid therapy.

Further Reading

Baddam S, Aban I, Hilliard L, et al. Acute kidney injury during a pediatric sickle cell vaso-occlusive pain crisis. Pediatr Nephrol. 2017. Aug;32(8):1451–1456

Brookoff D, Polomano R. Treating sickle cell pain like cancer pain. Ann Intern Med. 1992;116:364–368.

Correia CR, Soares AT, Azurara L, Palare MJ. Use of gabapentin in the treatment of chronic pain in an adolescent with sickle cell disease. BMJ Case Rep. 2017 Apr 21;2017.

Okorji LM, Muntz DS, Liem RI. Opioid prescription practices at discharge and 30-day returns in children with sickle cell disease and pain. Pediatr Blood Cancer. 2017;64.

Quarmyne MO, Dong W, Theodore R, et al. Hydroxyurea effectiveness in children and adolescents with sickle cell anemia: a large retrospective, population-based cohort. Am J Hematol. 2017;92:77–81.

Smith WR, Penberthy LT, Bovbjerg VE, et al. Daily assessment of pain in adults with sickle cell disease. Ann Intern Med. 2008;148:94–101.

Steinberg MH. Management of sickle cell disease. N Engl J Med. 1999;340:1021–1030.

Hip Fracture

Franchesca Arias, Catherine C. Price, and Jeffrey C. Gadsden

20

Case Scenario

An 83-year-old woman presents to the emergency room with severe left hip pain after tripping over a rug while walking to the bathroom. She has no other injuries related to the fall and did not lose consciousness. Her medical history includes hypertension, osteoporosis, and a remote history of a transient ischemic attack, and she is a 40-pack-a-year smoker. Her family state that she has most of her mental faculties, but that in recent years she has become more forgetful at times. Her only medications are amlodipine and aspirin. On examination, her left leg is shortened and externally rotated, and she is loudly complaining of severe pain. Vital signs are blood pressure 189/101, heart rate 97 bpm, respiratory rate 24/min, and SpO_2 of 96% on 2 liters oxygen by nasal cannula. Her lab work reveals a hemoglobin of 11 g/dL, with normal electrolytes and coagulation studies.

1. Preoperative Care

1.1. What is the epidemiology of hip fracture?

Hip fracture is a significant public health problem, affecting 2.2 million people annually worldwide. In the United States, there are approximately 300,000 hospital visits for hip fracture every year. Risk factors for hip fracture broadly fall into two categories: those that decrease bone mineral density (e.g., female sex, older age, genetic predisposition, low body frame size, and poor diet) and those that increase risk for falls. The elderly usually suffer a hip fracture after minor trauma, such as a fall from standing. The lifetime risk of hip fracture in females is 1 in 7, compared with 1 in 15 for males.

While the mechanism of injury is often minor, the consequences are substantial: 1-month mortality in elderly hip fracture patients approaches 10% and is over 35% at 1 year. Of independent community dwellers who present to the hospital with hip fracture, 11% remain bedridden for the rest of their life, 16% remain in long-term care facilities, and approximately 80% require a walking aid 12 months postfracture. Early mortality is largely the result of complications due to immobility such as pneumonia and thromboembolic events. Nonoperative hip fracture patients have a fourfold increase in mortality over those who undergo surgery. For this reason, early operative fixation is the rule, with more than 98% of hip fractures in the United States undergoing some type of surgical procedure.

Further Reading

Bhandari M, Swiontkowski M. Management of Acute Hip Fracture. *N Engl J Med.* 2017;377:2054–2062.

Nurmi I, Narinen A, Lüthje P, Tanninen S. Functional outcome and survival after hip fracture in elderly: a prospective study of 106 consecutive patients. *J Orthop Traumatol.* 2004;5:7–14.

Sanford AM, Morley JE, McKee A. Orthogeriatrics and hip fractures. *J Nutr Health Aging.* 2018;22:457–462.

Simunovic N, Devereaux PJ, Sprague S, Guyatt GH, Schemitsch E, Debeer J, Bhandari M. Effect of early surgery after hip fracture on mortality and complications: systematic review and meta-analysis. *CMAJ.* 2010;182:1609–1616.

Veronese N, Maggi S. Epidemiology and social costs of hip fracture. *Injury* 2018; [epub ahead of print]

1.2. What are some common approaches to preoperative analgesia in the patient with hip fracture?

Pain from a fractured hip has been shown to contribute to an increase in postoperative complications, prolonged bed rest, delayed ambulation, truncated or missed physical therapy sessions, and impaired long-term functional recovery. Despite the fact that many patients presenting with hip fracture report moderate to severe pain, a significant number of these patients receive little or no analgesic intervention in the prehospital setting or in the emergency department. Age appears to be a driving factor: regardless of the presenting complaint, emergency room patients over the age of 75 years are 19% less likely to receive any analgesic compared with their younger cohorts. Factors that contribute to this "oligoanalgesia" include fear of sedation or other opioid-related side effects in this elderly population, preexisting confusion/dementia, poorly performed pain assessments, language barriers, and the wish to avoid confounding a diagnosis.

Effective analgesic options in this population include the use of nonopioids such as acetaminophen and nonsteroidal anti-inflammatory medications; regional anesthetic techniques such as fascia iliaca block, femoral nerve block, and obturator nerve block; and intravenous opioids. Despite the attendant risk for delirium in this population, opioids remain the mainstay of treatment both in the prehospital setting and in the emergency department. Opioids may provide good relief from static pain, but they are less effective at combating pain during movement (dynamic pain), which is critical during the recovery period when the patient is undergoing physical therapy and rehabilitation. Moreover, because there is no well-established method to stabilize the fractured hip, even simple movements such as shifting position in bed, using a bedpan, or reaching for call buttons may lead to excruciating pain in this population.

Further Reading

Gadsden J, Warlick A. Regional anesthesia for the trauma patient: improving patient outcomes. *Local Reg Anesth.* 2015;8:45–55.

Guay J, Parker MJ, Griffiths R, Kopp SL. Peripheral nerve blocks for hip fractures: Cochrane Review. *Anesth Analg.* 2018;126:1695–1704.

Morrison RS, Magaziner J, McLaughlin MA, Orosz G, Silberzweig SB, Koval KJ, Siu AL. The impact of post-operative pain on outcomes following hip fracture. *Pain.* 2004;103:303–311.

Platts-Mills TF, Esserman DA, Brown L, Bortsov AV, Sloane PD, McLean SA. Older US emergency department patients are less likely to receive pain medication than younger patients: results from a national survey. *Ann Emerg Med.* 2012;60:199–206.

1.3. How do pain intensity and pain management influence the risk of perioperative delirium?

Elderly patients presenting with hip fracture are at high risk for delirium during their hospital admission, with an overall incidence of up to 53%, a rate substantially higher than for other age-matched elective surgeries. Additional factors that increase the likelihood of delirium include male sex, preexisting dementia, low body-mass index, a higher number of medical comorbidities, a higher number of prescription medications, and an American Society of Anesthesiologists physical status score of 4 or greater. Delirium is a serious adverse event and is associated with greater morbidity and mortality, longer hospital length of stay, and institutionalization. This often creates a dilemma for the physician: pain itself is known to provoke delirium, while treating the pain with opioids may also increase that risk. This highlights the value of nonopioid and locoregional therapies in this population. Notwithstanding, it appears that of these two competing priorities, untreated pain is by far the more potent exacerbating factor, and opioids should not be withheld if other options have been exhausted or are not indicated or available. In the absence of preexisting dementia, hip fracture patients with untreated pain are 9 times more likely to develop perioperative delirium than those whose pain is well controlled. Meperidine is more likely than other opioids to provoke delirium in this population.

Further Reading

Bruce AJ, Ritchie CW, Blizard R, Lai R, Raven P. The incidence of delirium associated with orthopedic surgery: a meta-analytic review. *Int Psychogeriatr.* 2007;19:197–214.

Gottschalk A, Hubbs J, Vikani AR, Gottschalk LB, Sieber FE. The impact of incident postoperative delirium on survival of elderly patients after surgery for hip fracture repair. *Anesth Analg.* 2015;121:1336–1343.

Lee HB, Mears SC, Rosenberg PB, Leoutsakos JS, Gottschalk A, Sieber FE. Predisposing factors for postoperative delirium after hip fracture repair in individuals with and without dementia. *J Am Geriatr Soc.* 2011;59:2306–2313.

Morrison RS, Magaziner J, McLaughlin MA, Orosz G, Silberzweig SB, Koval KJ, Siu AL. The impact of post-operative pain on outcomes following hip fracture. *Pain* 2004;103:303–311.

Sieber FE, Mears S, Lee H, Gottschalk A. Postoperative opioid consumption and its relationship to cognitive function in older adults with hip fracture. *J Am Geriatr Soc.* 2011;59:2256–2262.

Table 20.1:
Innervation of the hip joint and relevant surrounding structures

Nerve Branch	Area Innervated
Lumbar plexus	
Femoral nerve	Anterolateral femoral neck, head, and shaft; joint capsule; acetabulum and labrum
Obturator nerve	Medial femoral neck, head, and shaft; joint capsule; acetabulum and labrum
Accessory obturator nerve	Medial femoral neck, head, and shaft; joint capsule
Lateral femoral cutaneous nerve	Skin overlying greater trochanter and lateral thigh
Sacral plexus	
Sciatic nerve	Posterior femoral neck, head, and shaft; joint capsule; acetabulum and labrum
Nerve to quadratus femoris	Posterior femoral neck, head, and shaft; joint capsule; acetabulum and labrum
Superior gluteal nerve	Posterior femoral neck, head, and shaft; joint capsule; acetabulum and labrum
Other	
Subcostal nerve (T12)	Skin of the proximal lateral thigh between greater trochanter and iliac crest

1.4. What is the innervation of the hip joint?

The hip joint is primarily innervated by elements from both the lumbar and sacral plexuses (Table 20.1).

The bone and periosteum of the proximal femur and acetabulum, as well as the joint capsule, are richly innervated by branches originating from the femoral, obturator, accessory obturator, and sciatic nerves, as well as nerve to quadratus femoris and the superior gluteal nerve. The skin overlying the hip on the lateral thigh is primarily innervated by the lateral femoral cutaneous nerve and the subcostal nerve. Pain from hip fracture principally originates from the periosteal surfaces and disrupted joint capsule, as well as muscular spasm or hematoma. While not part of the hip joint, the area of skin supplied by the lateral femoral cutaneous nerve is often a source of pain for hip fracture patients due to hematoma/ swelling that develops over the site of impact from the fall.

Further Reading

Birnbaum K, Prescher A, Hepler S, Heller KD. Sensory innervation of the hip joint: an anatomical study. *Surg Radiol Anat.* 1997:19:371–375.

Nielsen TD, Moriggl B, Søballe K, Kolsen-Petersen JA, Børglum J, Bendtsen TF. A cadaveric study of ultrasound-guided subpectineal injectate spread around the obturator nerve and its hip articular branches. *Reg Anesth Pain Med.* 2017;42:357–361.

1.5. How effective are nerve blocks at reducing pain in the hip fracture patient?

Nerve blocks are an attractive analgesic modality in the treatment of hip fracture pain as they can provide high-quality targeted analgesia while sparing any side-effects of systemic medications such as respiratory depression, hypoxia, or delirium. Survey studies done of emergency departments suggest the number of centers offering nerve blocks for hip fracture patients appears to be increasing in the last 2 decades.

While small, single-center trials show a variety of effects, analyses of pooled data show that nerve blocks are an effective intervention in this population. A 2018 Cochrane Review of 31 trials (1760 participants) demonstrated that when compared with systemic analgesia, patients receiving nerve blocks following admission for hip fracture had a standard mean reduction in pain level with movement at 30 minutes of −3.4 on a scale of 0 to 10. There also appeared to be a reduction in pneumonia (10.9% vs. 26.9%), shorter time to mobilization, lower costs for the analgesic regimen, decreased opioid consumption, and an increase in reported patient satisfaction. The reviewers did not find any difference with respect to acute confusional state, myocardial ischemia, or mortality. The studies were somewhat heterogeneous and included a variety of nerve blocks and their combinations, varied techniques (e.g., landmark, nerve stimulator guided, ultrasound guided), blocks of varying durations, and different block settings (e.g., in the emergency department vs. preoperative vs. postoperative). Another meta-analysis of 21 trials (1422 participants) used a multiple treatment comparison methodology of common peripheral nerve blocks for hip fracture patients to determine what the most effective blocks were for particular outcomes. This analysis revealed that for acute pain intensity, the combination of obturator nerve block and lateral femoral cutaneous nerve block was the most effective; for delirium, fascia iliaca block was the block of choice, with a greater than 70% reduction.

This provides a rationale for the choice of peripheral nerve blocks that are commonly employed. Many centers routinely employ either single-injection or continuous femoral nerve blocks for hip fracture analgesia. This has been shown to be superior to systemic analgesics at reducing pain intensity (rest and dynamic) and opioid consumption both preoperatively and postoperatively. The fascia iliaca block has emerged as a block of choice for many clinicians in emergency medicine and anesthesiology, since it aims to block both the femoral nerve and the lateral femoral cutaneous nerve. Depending on the approach taken, the obturator nerve may be blocked as well following fascia iliaca blockade.

Further Reading

Abou-Setta AM, Beaupre LA, Rashiq S, et al. Comparative effectiveness of pain management interventions for hip fracture: a systematic review. *Ann Intern Med.* 2011;155:234–245.

Guay J, Parker MJ, Griffiths R, Kopp SL. Peripheral nerve blocks for hip fractures: a Cochrane Review. *Anesth Analg.* 2018;126:1695–1704.

Holdgate A, Shepherd SA, Huckson S. Patterns of analgesia for fractured neck of femur in Australian emergency departments. *Emerg Med Austr.* 2010;22:3–8.

Rashid A, Beswick E, Galitzine S, Fitton L. Regional analgesia in the emergency department for hip fractures: survey of current UK practice and its impact on services in a teaching hospital. *Emerg Med J.* 2014;31:909–913.

Rashiq S, Vendermeer B, Abou-Setta AM, Beaupre LA, Jones A, Dryden DM. Efficacy of supplemental peripheral nerve blockade for hip fracture surgery: multiple treatment comparison. *Can J Anesth.* 2013;60:230–243.

Ritcey B, Pageau P, Woo MY, Perry JJ. Regional nerve blocks for hip and femoral neck fractures in the emergency department: a systematic review. *CJEM.* 2016;18:37–47.

1.6. What is the role of epidural analgesia for hip fracture patients?

Randomized studies of epidural analgesia versus parenteral opioids for hip fracture patients demonstrate statistically significant lower pain scores with few side effects out to 72 hours. Early epidural analgesia may also reduce adverse cardiac events compared with systemic therapies. However, epidural analgesia is not utilized routinely for hip fracture care for a number of reasons. Many elderly patients presenting with hip fracture are on anticoagulant or antiplatelet medications that preclude neuraxial intervention. In addition, these patients are increasingly benefiting from femoral or fascia iliaca blockade in the emergency department or shortly after admission. Since emergency medicine physicians are less likely to feel comfortable placing and managing an epidural block, and the availability of an anesthesiologist is not always predictable, peripheral nerve blocks have become the first-line locoregional intervention in many centers. While the operative case may be carried out using neuraxial anesthesia, epidural analgesia is likely to impair mobilization postoperatively. There is increasing evidence that early ambulation leads to better functional outcome and independence after hip fracture repair, and the desire to get patients out of bed and walking on the day of surgery or the day after tends to preclude the use of epidural analgesia.

Further Reading

Foss NB, Kristensen MT, Kristensen BB, Jensen PS, Kehlet H. Effect of postoperative epidural analgesia on rehabilitation and pain after hip fracture surgery. *Anesthesiology.* 2005;102:1197–204.

Matot I, Oppenheim-Eden A, Ratrot R, Baranova J, Davidson E, Eylon S, Peyser A, Liebergall M. Preoperative cardiac events in elderly patients with hip fracture randomized to epidural or conventional analgesia. *Anesthesiology.* 2003;98:156–163.

Morri M, Forni C, Marchioni M, Bonetti E, Marseglia F, Cotti A. Which factors are independent predictors of early recovery of mobility in the older adults' population after hip fracture? A cohort prognostic study. *Arch Orthop Trauma Surg*. 2018;138:35–41.

Scheinin H, Virtanen T, Kentala E, Uotila P, Laitio T, Hartiala J, Heikkila H, Sriola-Heinonen K, Pullisaar O, Yli-Mayry S, Jalonen J. Epidural infusion of bupivacaine and fentanyl reduces perioperative myocardial ischaemia in elderly patients with hip fracture: a randomized controlled trial. *Acta Anaesthesiol Scand*. 2000;44:1061–1070.

1.7. What are the goals of the fascia iliaca block? How is this block performed?

Fascia iliaca block is an anterior approach to the lumbar plexus. The block was first described as a landmark technique at the junction of the lateral one-third and medial two-thirds of a line drawn over the inguinal crease. The concept was to advance a needle through the fascia lata and fascia iliaca of the proximal anterior thigh, and with a large (i.e., 40 mL or greater) volume of local anesthetic, generate a broad spread underneath the fascia iliaca and thereby achieve blockade of the femoral, lateral femoral cutaneous, and obturator nerves with one injection. Proximal spread was encouraged by applying pressure on the thigh distal to the needle. While this technique was reasonably effective at blocking the femoral and lateral femoral cutaneous nerves, clinical and radiographic studies have demonstrated that obturator nerve block happens infrequently, if at all. It may be that when the injectate is deposited distal to the inguinal ligament, there is simply not enough hydraulic force to overcome the "pinch point" created by the ligament and the iliacus muscle.

The suprainguinal fascia iliaca technique was first described in 2011 by Hebbard and colleagues. This technique is performed using an ultrasound transducer placed in a parasagittal orientation over the inguinal ligament between the femoral artery and anterior superior iliac spine and translated cephalad until the iliacus muscle is observed deep to the transversus abdominis and internal oblique muscles (Figure 20.1). Starting from the caudal aspect of the transducer, the needle is advanced in plane underneath the inguinal ligament until the tip is observed underneath the fascia of iliacus within the pelvis (Figure 20.2). At this point, a large volume (typically 30–40 mL) of dilute local anesthetic is then administered, and success is associated with the "peeling away" of the fascia from the overlying muscle and observation of longitudinal spread of the local anesthetic. Unlike the infrainguinal approaches, the suprainguinal approach appears to more reliably block all 3 elements. Desmet and colleagues demonstrated that when using 40 mL of ropivacaine for hip arthroplasty, a sensory block was achieved in 93%, 95%, and 76% of cases for the femoral, lateral femoral cutaneous, and obturator nerves, respectively.

Despite the potential advantages of the ultrasound-guided, suprainguinal fascia iliaca technique, both techniques have been shown to be effective at reducing pain intensity and reducing opioids for hip fracture patients. The landmark technique is simple to learn and perform and does not require additional equipment or expertise, making it an attractive

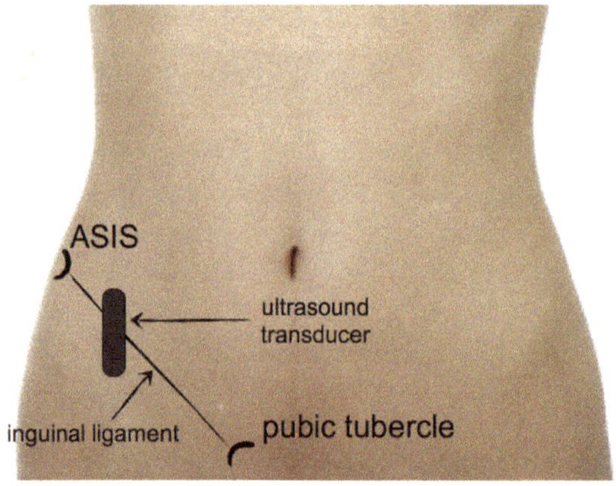

Figure 20.1 Ultrasound transducer position for the suprainguinal fascia iliaca block. ASIS = anterior superior iliac spine.

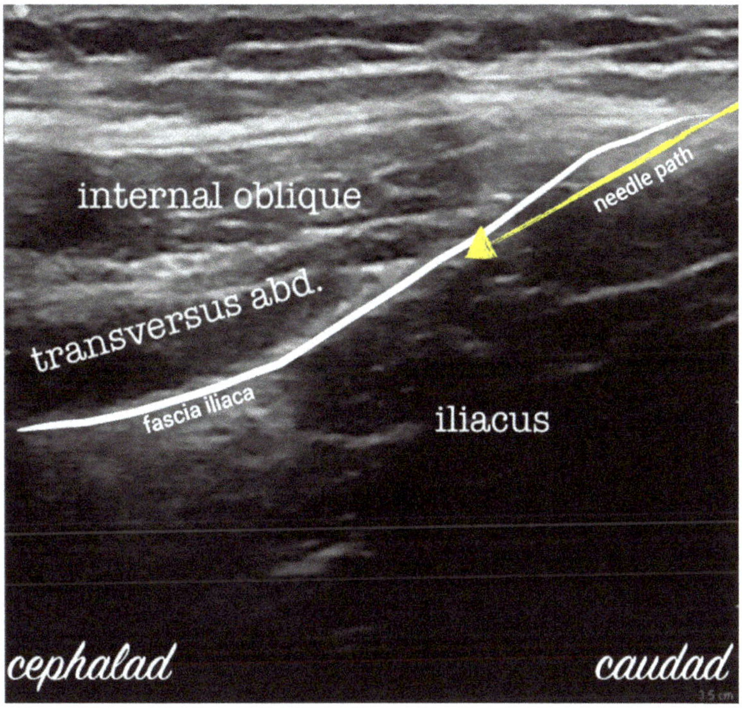

Figure 20.2 Suprainguinal fascia iliaca ultrasound image. Once an image of the iliacus, internal oblique, and transversus abdominis muscles is obtained, a needle is inserted in plane from caudad to cephalad until the tip is immediately below the fascia iliaca.

option to those clinicians who lack training on ultrasound-guided nerve blocks. In some health systems, prehospital personnel (nurses or paramedics) have been trained to routinely perform fascia iliaca block in order to establish rapid analgesia and avoid systemic medications.

Continuous fascia iliaca block is also reasonably simple to perform and has the advantage of prolonged duration of analgesia compared with single-injection blocks. This is particularly important for hip fracture patients, who may wait up to 24 to 48 hours (or longer) while medical comorbidities have been optimized prior to surgical repair.

Further Reading

Chesters A, Atkinson P. Fascia iliaca block for pain relief from proximal femoral fracture in the emergency department: a review of the literature. *Emerg Med J.* 2014;31:e84–e87.

Desmet M, Vermeylen K, Van Herreweghe I, Carlier L, Soetens F, Lambrecht S, Croes K, Pottel H, Van de Velde M. A longitudinal supra-inguinal fascia iliaca compartment block reduces morphine consumption after total hip arthroplasty. *Reg Anesth Pain Med.* 2017;42:327–333.

Hebbard P, Ivanusic J, Sha S. Ultrasound-guided supra-inguinal fascia iliaca block: a cadaveric evaluation of a novel approach. *Anaesthesia.* 2011;66:300–305.

Nie H, Yang YX, Wang Y, Liu Y, Zhao B, Luan B. Effects of continuous fascia iliaca compartment blocks for postoperative analgesia in patients with hip fracture. *Pain Res Manag.* 2015;20:210–212.

Swenson JD, Davis JJ, Stream JO, Crim JR, Burks RT, Greis PE. Local anesthetic injection deep to the fascia iliaca at the level of the inguinal ligament: the pattern of distribution and effects on the obturator nerve. *J Clin Anesth.* 2015;27:652–657.

Vaughan B, Manley M, Stewart D, Iyer V. Distal injection site may explain lack of analgesia from fascia iliaca block for total hip. *Reg Anesth Pain Med.* 2013;38:556–557.

1.8. What is the incidence of major neurocognitive disorder or dementia in patients presenting with hip fracture?

Major neurocognitive disorder (NCD), also known as dementia, is a common neurodegenerative condition that interferes with daily functioning and is most common in older adults. According to the diagnostic criteria, major NCD is an acquired neurologic syndrome characterized by a decline in one or multiple cognitive domains that is reported by an individual patient, or a knowledgeable informant, and established via formal clinical assessment (i.e., impaired scores in at least 1 domain on neuropsychological assessment). Cognitive deficits must limit functional independence and are not secondary to other psychiatric disorders (e.g., major depressive disorder, schizophrenia, or delirium). Prevalence of major NCD ranges from 2% to 3% in adults >65 years and occurs in up to 47% of adults >85 years. Like the term *dementia, major NCD* is an umbrella term, and the nature, extent, and course of the cognitive and functional symptoms are used to denote the hypothesized pathology. For example, major NCD due to Alzheimer's disease presents with primary amnestic features. In contrast, major NCD due to Parkinson's disease presents with primary executive dysfunction that emerges in the context of a well-established history of Parkinson's disease. Prevalence of major NCDs varies by disease type. In the United States, Alzheimer's disease, vascular disease, and Parkinson's disease are among the most prevalent.

The incidence of hip fractures is high in the elderly. The incidence is highest in cognitively compromised individuals, and older adults with preexisting major NCDs are 3 times more likely than their counterparts without major NCDs to sustain a hip fracture. Few studies have compared the incidence of hip fracture across the different major NCDs (e.g., Alzheimer's disease vs. vascular disease). Compared with healthy controls, up to 85% of older adults with Parkinson's disease experience a hip fracture, and older adults with Alzheimer's disease are twice as likely as their cognitively intact counterparts to experience a hip fracture.

Further Reading

American Psychiatric Association. *Diagnostic and Statistical Manual of Mental Disorders*. 5th ed. Washington, DC: American Psychiatric Association; 2013.

Freter S, Koller K. Hip fractures and Alzheimer's disease. *Canadian Review of Alzheimer's Disease and Other Dementias.* 2008;11(1):15–20.

Friedman SM, Menzies IB, Bukata SV, Mendelson DA, Kates SL. Dementia and hip fractures: development of a pathogenic framework for understanding and studying risk. *Geriatr Orthop Surg Rehabil.* 2010;1(2):52–62.

Mak J, Cameron I, March L. Evidence-based guidelines for the management of hip fractures in older persons: an update. *Med J Aust.* 2010;192(1):37–41.

Yiannopoulou KG, Papageorgiou SG, Anastasiou IP, Ganetsos TK, Karydakis KD. Prevalence of Parkinsonism in older patients with hip fracture. *Hip Int.* 2011;21(3):351–355.

1.9. How do we grade the severity of a major neurocognitive disorder?

Functional status is essential to diagnosing a major NCD and establishing disease severity. According to the *Diagnostic and Statistical Manual of Mental Disorders* (*DSM-5*), the significant cognitive decrements present in a major NCD must result in functional limitations. Thus, the role of cognition in human life is emphasized at the time of rendering the diagnosis. Similarly, level of functional independence forms the basis for establishing disease severity. That is, the severity of a major NCD, regardless of disease type, is determined by the degree of functional impairment associated with the condition. "Mild" captures functional limitations in instrumental activities of daily living; "moderate" denotes further decline and functional limitations that extend to basic activities of daily living. Finally, a severe major NCD reflects a state of complete dependence on others for all activities of daily living.

Establishing functional status can be challenging, particularly in older adults who may prefer to opt out of specific activities without ever experiencing any difficulties completing them. Ideally, a comprehensive clinical interview, which includes careful history taking, caregiver reports, and observation, combined with the integration of other cultural and medical factors, would help in this process. Alternatively, many psychometrically sound scales are available to help assess functional status. The Clinical Dementia Rating scale (CDR) is a 30-minute semistructured interview administered by the clinician. Similarly, the Dementia Severity Rating Scale (DSRS) is a 5-minute scale administered by trained staff. The CDR and the DSRS require the presence of an informant who is somewhat familiar with the patient.

Further Reading

American Psychiatric Association. *Diagnostic and Statistical Manual of Mental Disorders* 5th ed. Washington, DC: American Psychiatric Association; 2013.

Moelter ST, Glenn MA, Xie SX, et al. The Dementia Severity Rating Scale predicts Clinical Dementia Rating Sum of Boxes scores. *Alzheimer Dis Assoc Disord.* 2015;29(2):158.

O'Bryant SE, Waring SC, Cullum CM, et al. Staging dementia using Clinical Dementia Rating Scale Sum of Boxes scores: A Texas Alzheimer's research consortium study. *Arch Neurol.* 2008;65(8):1091–1095.

1.10. How does dementia influence the assessment and treatment of pain?

Self-report of pain is the gold-standard method of pain assessment, and the presence of a major NCD, particularly a severe major NCD, represents a barrier to pain assessment. Hallmark symptoms of major NCDs, such as memory loss, executive dysfunction, and impairment in language, can interfere with accurate self-reporting. Moreover, symptoms often endorsed by patients with chronic pain such as psychomotor slowing, distractibility, and rigidity are also present in neurodegenerative processes. In light of the limitations in assessment, pain in adults with major NCDs is often poorly assessed, and traditional instruments used to examine a patient's pain experience may not be appropriate in this group. According to the American Geriatrics Society, accurate assessment of pain in cognitively compromised older adults will incorporate results from a validated observational pain scale that ought to be interpreted in the context of the cultural and maturational factors that influence pain experience in this group.

Pain is present in approximately one-third of community-dwelling older adults and up to 80% of institutionalized older adults. Pain in older adults is associated with physical inactivity, social isolation, increased psychiatric distress, and disruptions in sleep. In the context of hip fracture, evidence indicates that postoperative pain experience is an independent predictor for functional outcomes 2 months after surgery. Therefore, appropriate assessment and management of pain in older adults with major NCD is of paramount importance.

Further Reading

Cavalieri TA. Pain management in the elderly. *J Am Osteopath Assoc.* 2002;102:481–485.

Corbett A, Husebo BS, Achterberg WP, Aarsland D, Erdal A, Flo E. The importance of pain management in older people with dementia. *Br Med Bull.* 2014;111(1). 139–148.

Feldt KS, Oh HL. Pain and hip fracture outcomes for older adults. *Orthop Nurs.* 2000;19(6):35.

Hadjistavropoulos T, Herr K, Prkachin KM, et al. Pain assessment in elderly adults with dementia. *Lancet Neurol.* 2014;13(12):1216–1227.

Herr K. Pain assessment in cognitively impaired older adults: new strategies and careful observation help pinpoint unspoken pain. *AJN The American Journal of Nursing.* 2002;102(12):65–67.

Zwakhalen SM, Hamers JP, Abu-Saad HH, Berger MP. Pain in elderly people with severe dementia: a systematic review of behavioural pain assessment tools. *BMC Geriatr.* 2006;6(1):3.

1.11. What is the incidence of postoperative delirium, and why is this a concern?

Delirium is an acute neurocognitive disorder characterized by alteration in consciousness, behavior, and attention. Advancing age is a significant risk factor for delirium, and approximately 14% to 56% of all hospitalized adults >65 years develop delirium. Delirium can interfere with postoperative recovery and has been associated with prolonged hospitalization, hospital readmission, future institutionalization, and increased mortality.

The incidence of delirium is higher in more medically compromised patients and occurs up to 87% of the time in older adults admitted to the intensive care unit. After hip fracture repair, delirium occurs in 35% to 65% of patients and may interfere with functional recovery. To date, delirium rates are similar between patients who received general anesthesia and those who received neuraxial anesthesia for operative fixation. As such, early detection and prompt treatment are instrumental to care planning and may promote improved postoperative outcomes.

Further Reading

Fong TG, Tulebaev SR, Inouye SK. Delirium in elderly adults: diagnosis, prevention, and treatment. *Nat Rev Neurol.* 2009;5(4):210–220.

Marcantonio ER, Flacker JM, Wright RJ, Resnick NM. Reducing delirium after hip fracture: a randomized trial. *J Am Geriatr Soc.* 2001;49(5):516–522.

Marcantonio ER, Flacker JM, Michaels M, Resnick NM. Delirium is independently associated with poor functional recovery after hip fracture. *J Age Related Disord.* 2001;13(2):9–15.

O'Donnell CM, McLoughlin L, Patterson CC, Clarke M, McCourt KC, McBrien ME, McAuley DF, Shields MO. Perioperative outcomes in the context of mode of anaesthesia for patients undergoing hip fracture surgery: systematic review and meta-analysis. *Br J Anaesth.* 2018 Jan;120(1):37–50. Epub 2017 Nov 24.

Oh ES, Fong TG, Hshieh TT, Inouye SK. Delirium in older persons: advances in diagnosis and treatment. *JAMA.* 2017;318(12):1161–1174.

Pisani MA, McNicoll L, Inouye SK. Cognitive impairment in the intensive care unit. *Clin. Chest Med.* 2003;24(1):727–737.

Witlox J, Eurelings LS, de Jonghe JF, et al. Delirium in elderly patients and the risk of post discharge mortality, institutionalization, and dementia: a meta-analysis. *JAMA.* 2010; 304(4):443–451.

2. Regional and Anesthetic Variables

2.1. What are the different approaches to surgical management of hip fracture, and what are the implications for pain burden?

There are two broad categories of surgical repair for hip fracture. Internal fixation is the technique of choice for nondisplaced femoral neck fractures and intertrochanteric fractures. This can be done by the percutaneous placement of several small, cancellous screws that hold the neck and head of the femur in place. Alternatively, a single, large screw with a side plate (often called a dynamic or sliding screw) can be used. In some cases of intertrochanteric fractures, an intramedullary nail is indicated to stabilize the femur. For displaced femoral neck fractures, arthroplasty is generally indicated to improve function and reduce chronic postoperative pain. This can be done either as a total hip arthroplasty, where both femoral and acetabular components are inserted, or as a hemiarthroplasty, where just the femoral component is replaced.

The degree of postoperative pain following hip fracture repair is variable and is related to a number of factors such as degree of preoperative pain, the duration of preoperative pain, emotional state, extent of repair, and degree of mobilization postoperatively. Percutaneous fixation (or "pinning") is associated with the least amount of surgical trespass. As a result, the pain intensity following these procedures is often mild to moderate. The skin exposure and periosteal disruption associated with a dynamic hip screw are greater than with a percutaneous pinning, and so the expected degree of pain intensity will generally be higher. At the other end of the spectrum, arthroplasty involves the greatest degree of soft tissue and bony trauma and is associated with a higher intensity of pain for a longer duration compared with internal fixation techniques.

Further Reading

Bhandari M, Swiontkowski M. Management of Acute Hip Fracture. *N Engl J Med.* 2017;377:2054–2062.

Kang H, Ha YC, Kim JY, Woo YC, Lee JS, Jang EC. Effectiveness of multimodal pain management after bipolar hemiarthroplasty for hip fracture: a randomized controlled study. *J Bone Joint Surg Am.* 2013;20:291–296.

2.2. Does the use of general versus neuraxial anesthesia affect outcomes in patients undergoing repair of hip fracture?

The debate about the optimal intraoperative technique for hip fracture repair has not been completely resolved. This is largely due to conflicting trials, especially small, single-institution studies. For this reason, larger database-driven studies may provide better answers to this question. Neuman and colleagues reported that in their analysis of more than 18,000 hip fracture patients, neuraxial anesthesia was associated with a significantly lower adjusted odds of death and respiratory complications in patients with intertrochanteric fractures but not femoral neck fractures. Contradicting that message was an analysis of more than 55,000 patients in a UK data set by White and colleagues that showed no difference in 5- or 30-day mortality. However, secondary analyses of factors associated with death in that group demonstrated that hypotension was strongly associated with mortality, and that both general anesthesia and larger doses of spinal bupivacaine were implicated in causing decreased blood pressure. These data suggest that hip fracture patients do have improved outcomes when neuraxial anesthesia is used, but only if the dose of spinal local anesthetic is judicious and hypotension (>20% decrease in preoperative blood pressure) is avoided. It is likely that many clinicians inadvertently use substantially more local anesthetic than is needed for spinal anesthesia, especially for a percutaneous fixation, a procedure that often requires only 15 to 30 minutes to complete. One recent dose-finding study demonstrated that the minimum effective dose of isobaric 0.5% bupivacaine to provide successful spinal anesthesia for hip fracture repair was 0.43 mL (or 2.15 mg).

Further Reading

Neuman MD, Silber JH, Elkassabany NM, Ludwig JM, Fleisher LA. Comparative effectiveness of regional versus general anesthesia for hip fracture surgery in adults. *Anesthesiology*. 2012;117:72–92.

Szucs S, Rauf J, Iohom G, Shorten GD. Determination of the minimum initial intrathecal dose of isobaric 0.5% bupivacaine for the surgical repair of a proximal femoral fracture. *Eur J Anaesthesiol*. 2015;32:759–763.

White SM, Moppett IK, Griffiths R. Outcome by mode of anaesthesia for hip fracture surgery: an observational audit of 65,535 patients in a national dataset. *Anaesthesia*. 2014;69:224–230.

White SM, Moppett IK, Griffiths R, Johansen A, Wakeman R, Boulton C, Plant F, Williams A, Pappenheim K, Majeed A, Currie CT, Grocott MPW. Secondary analysis of outcomes after 11,085 hip fracture operations from the prospective UK Anaesthesia Sprint Audit of Practice (ASAP-2). *Anaesthesia*. 2016;17:506–514.

Wood RJ, White SM. Anaesthesia for 1131 patients undergoing proximal femoral fracture repair: a retrospective, observational study of effects on blood pressure, fluid administration and perioperative anemia. *Anaesthesia*. 2011;66:1017–1022.

2.3. Can hip fracture repair be carried out using peripheral nerve blocks alone?

While a carefully performed spinal anesthetic may be the technique of choice, this is not always an option. Most hip fracture patients are operated on urgently, and with the increasing number of anticoagulant and antiplatelet medications that many elderly patients are prescribed, neuraxial anesthesia is frequently contraindicated. Other factors such as patient refusal or difficulty accessing the spinal space due to spinal deformity may also preclude neuraxial anesthesia.

At the same time, comorbidities such as cardiac, pulmonary, and neurologic disease often make general anesthesia an undesirable option. It is possible for hip fracture surgery to be performed with peripheral nerve blocks alone. Important factors to consider are the type of procedure (e.g., a minimally invasive percutaneous pinning versus a total arthroplasty), the anticoagulation status (lumbar plexus block is generally contraindicated in anticoagulated patients), and patient and surgical factors such as tolerance of possible movement of the operative (and contralateral) limb during surgery.

Because the hip and overlying skin are innervated by a variety of nerves from two different plexuses (see Table 20.1), careful consideration of the surgical approach is warranted. Combined lumbar and sacral plexus blocks may be the ideal option, as this provides complete analgesia to the lower limb. However, these deep blocks are relatively contraindicated in anticoagulated patients, and in these circumstances a careful weighing of the risks and benefits is necessary. Additionally, these plexus blocks require a large combined volume of local anesthetic, which increases the risk of local anesthetic systemic toxicity. Because many elderly hip fracture patients are small in stature, the margin for safety with local anesthetic dosing is frequently slim. Alternatives include separate femoral, lateral femoral cutaneous, obturator, and sciatic nerve blocks; however, with multiple-block techniques such as these, the level of complexity increases and the chance of complete success may be decreased.

Further Reading

de Visme V. Peripheral blocks of the lower limb for repair of fractured neck of femur. *Br J Anaesth.* 1998;81:483–484.

Mullanu C, Gaillat F, Scemama F, Thiabault S, Lavand'homme P, Auffray JP. Acute toxicity of local anesthetic ropivacaine and mepivacaine during a combined lumbar plexus and sciatic block for hip surgery. *Acta Anaesthesiol Belg.* 2002;53:221–223.

3. Postoperative Care

3.1. What regional analgesic options are indicated for hip fracture patients following surgical repair?

If a preoperative catheter (fascia iliaca or femoral nerve catheter) can be left in place throughout the operative procedure without impacting on the surgical field, this may provide some value through the first day or more of the postoperative period. Many patient, especially those with nondisplaced fractures undergoing percutaneous fixation, state that the bulk of the pain they experienced preoperatively disappeared with the fixation, and they can transition to oral multimodal medications. Especially for the more robust surgical approaches, maintaining a regional analgesic catheter can decrease pain intensity and opioid requirements.

Some modification of the infusion and concentration regimens may be required if the patient is expected to ambulate while the catheter is in situ. A decreased concentration (e.g., ropivacaine 0.1% rather than 0.2%) may continue to provide sufficient analgesia without any motor block that would impair rehab efforts.

Beneficial effect can also be achieved with daily, repeated single-injection blocks. Mouzopoulos et al. randomized hip fracture patients to receive fascia iliaca blocks with bupivacaine or sham blocks daily from admission to discharge. Delirium rates and duration of delirium were significantly reduced in the experimental group.

Further Reading

Abou-Setta AM, Beaupre LA, Rashiq S, et al. Comparative effectiveness of pain management interventions for hip fracture: a systematic review. *Ann Intern Med.* 2011;155:234–245.

Arsoy D, Huddleston JI, Amanatullah DF, Giori NJ, Maloney WJ, Goodman SB. Femoral nerve catheters improve home disposition and pain in hip fracture patients treated with total hip arthroplasty. *J Arthoplasty.* 2017;32:3434–3437.

Mouzopoulos G, Vasiliadis G, Lasanioanos N, Nikolaras, Morakis E, Kaminaris M. Fascia iliaca block prophylaxis for hip fracture patients at risk for delirium: a randomized placebo-controlled study. *J Orthopaed Traumatol.* 2009;10:127–133.

3.2. What other multimodal options are indicated for these patients in the postoperative period?

All patients should receive a standardized, scheduled regimen of multimodal analgesia in the postoperative period until the pain has resolved. The provision of scheduled (rather than "as-needed") nonopioids establishes a foundation of analgesia on which additional rescue analgesia can occur. Scheduled analgesic regimens are also more effective than demand-based analgesic regimens, provide better patient satisfaction, and reduce the risk of undertreatment. Moreover, many hip fracture patients are cognitively impaired and are less likely to request pain medication on an "as-needed" basis.

The most common nonopioid multimodal agents initiated postoperatively are acetaminophen and NSAIDs/COX-2 selective inhibitors. Acetaminophen has an excellent safety profile and, if dosed at approximately 1000 mg q6h, is effective at managing both rest and dynamic pain. No dosing adjustment is needed based on age. NSAIDs are also an excellent complementary therapy and likewise should be dosed every 6 to 8 hours. Care must be taken in those patients with gastric ulcer disease, and the selective COX-2 inhibitors are often used in place of nonselective agents in these cases. Patients with renal impairment should be prescribed NSAIDs with care, as these medications can worsen renal function. Gabapentinoids have been shown to be effective in reducing pain intensity and opioid consumption in elective total joint arthroplasty, but their beneficial effect is less clear with hip fracture patients. In addition, the sedative effect can sometimes impair mobilization. However, these are also generally free from serious adverse effects and may be considered in cases where there is an element of neuropathic pain or high pain intensity requiring larger doses of opioid medications.

Opioids should be prescribed if needed, but not on a scheduled basis. The use of scheduled sustained-release oxycodone or morphine is associated with an increase in delirium in elderly hip fracture patients, as well as other common opioid-related adverse effects such as nausea, vomiting, constipation, ileus, urinary retention, and respiratory depression. However, pain itself is a strongly provocative factor for delirium, and opioids should not be withheld if a patient is receiving the scheduled, foundational nonopioid regimen in addition to locoregional analgesia and is still in discomfort.

Further Reading

Chin RP, Ho CH, Cheung LP. Scheduled analgesic regimen improves rehabilitation after hip fracture surgery. *Clin Orthop Relat Res.* 2013;471:249–260.

Cowan R, Lim JH, Ong T, Kumar A, Sahota O. The challenges of anaesthesia and pain relief in hip fracture care. *Drugs Aging.* 2017;34:1–11.

Fabi DW. Multimodal analgesia in the hip fracture patient. *J Orthop Trauma.* 2016;30 (suppl 1):S6–S11.

Inguinal Hernia Repair in a Neonate

Andrew D. Franklin and J. Matthew Kynes

21

Case Scenario

A 14-week-old child presents for operative repair of bilateral inguinal hernias. The infant was born at 27 weeks postconceptual age (PCA) and spent 11 weeks in the neonatal intensive care unit (NICU) after birth. The child had an episode of acute groin pain requiring manual reduction of the hernia in the emergency room last week, and the surgeon considers it is urgent to proceed with repair of the hernias to prevent bowel incarceration. Examination of the child shows a small for stated age infant who is otherwise vigorous and well appearing.

1. Patient Factors: The Premature Infant

1.1. What are the major immediate pulmonary considerations for children born prior to adequate production of pulmonary surfactant?

Pulmonary surfactant is a phospholipoprotein that decreases surface tension of alveoli. Type II pneumocytes begin to produce surfactant between 23 and 24 weeks postconceptional age (PCA). Production may be inadequate until 36 weeks PCA, and children born without adequate surfactant experience reduced lung compliance, reduced lung volumes, ventilation-perfusion mismatch, and increased shunting leading to hypoxemia. All of these conditions may be exacerbated under general anesthesia, putting these children at increased risk for intraoperative and postoperative respiratory failure. Preterm infants are often managed initially with continuous positive airway pressure (CPAP) and supplemental oxygen, but they may require tracheal intubation, mechanical ventilation, or even extracorporeal membrane oxygenation (ECMO) in severe cases. For children who are mechanically ventilated, frequent opening and collapse of alveoli without adequate end expiratory pressure can lead to worsening pulmonary status due to mechanical lung injury. Recommendations for ventilatory management of premature infants include providing low tidal volumes (4–6 mL/kg), increased respiratory rates, minimal fraction of inspired oxygen ($FiO_{2)}$, sufficient positive end expiratory pressure (PEEP) to prevent alveolar collapse, and permissive hypercapnia.

Surfactant therapy was introduced clinically in 1980, and its use has increased survival and decreased long-term pulmonary complications of prematurity. Prophylactic surfactant replacement is occasionally provided to infants born at less than 26 weeks PCA at high risk of respiratory distress syndrome (RDS), but more commonly it is administered as rescue therapy after failure of CPAP ventilation. Multiple surfactant preparations are commercially available, with natural sources outperforming synthetic versions in most studies. In most settings surfactant administration requires intubation and brief mechanical ventilation, but increasingly efforts are being made to transition neonates to CPAP as quickly as possible following surfactant administration. In addition to its use for RDS, investigations into other neonatal conditions, including meconium aspiration, congenital pneumonia, pulmonary hypoplasia, pulmonary hemorrhage, and with ECMO cannulation, are underway and may expand its role in neonatal management.

Further Reading

Coté CJ, Lerman H, Anderson BJ, eds. Coté and Lerman's A Practice of Anesthesia for Infants and Children. 5th ed. Philadelphia, PA: Elsevier; 2013:733.

Sweet D, Speer CP. "Surfactant replacement: resent and future." In: Bancalari E ed., The Newborn Lung: Neonatology Questions and Controversies. 2nd ed. Philadelphia, PA: Elsevier; 2012:283–299.

1.2. Differentiate bronchopulmonary dysplasia from transient tachypnea of the newborn and respiratory distress syndrome

Transient tachypnea of the newborn (TTN) refers to a self-limited respiratory process presenting with increased respiratory rate after birth and typically lasting 2 to 5 days. TTN may be related to decreased lung compliance from delayed lung fluid resorption and is associated with prematurity, maternal sedation, maternal asthma, and delivery by cesarean section. Respiratory distress syndrome is a pulmonary developmental disorder that is associated with preterm birth and increases in incidence and severity with prematurity, occurring in 50% of infants born between 26 and 28 weeks PCA and 20% to 30% of infants born at 30 to 31 weeks PCA. It presents at birth with increased respiratory effort and hypoxia that may resolve quickly or progress to requiring surfactant therapy, CPAP, and/or prolonged ventilatory support. Bronchopulmonary dysplasia (BPD) is a clinical diagnosis that refers to infants born at less than 32 weeks PCA whose lung disease becomes chronic, requiring supplemental oxygen treatment for at least 28 days by 36 weeks postmenstrual age or time of discharge home. In addition to prematurity and surfactant deficiency, factors that are associated with BPD include barotrauma, oxygen toxicity, inflammation, infection, nutritional status, and genetic predisposition.

Further Reading

MacDonald MG, Seshia MMK, Mullett MD, eds. Avery's Neonatology: Pathophysiology and Management of the Newborn. 7th ed. Philadelphia, PA: Lippincott Williams & Wilkins; 2015:560.

Ehrenkranz RA, Walsh MC, Vohr BR, et al. Validation of the National Institutes of Health consensus definition of bronchopulmonary dysplasia. Pediatrics. 2005;116:1353–1360.

1.3. Discuss the ontogeny of pain in the developing fetus

Neurologic development of the fetus begins with early stages of brain and spinal cord formation at 3 weeks gestation followed by neural crest cell migration and neural proliferation. Spinal cord formation is complete by the beginning of the second trimester, with maximal neuronal development occurring between 8 and 18 weeks PCA. Sensory receptors begin development at 7 weeks gestation and are present throughout the skin and mucosa by 20 weeks PCA with active synaptogenesis occurring in this period. Stimulation in animals and humans in this stage produces withdrawal reflexes, hormonal stress responses (catecholamines, steroid hormones, glucagon, growth hormone), and autonomic arousal consistent with pain response at later stages of development. However, the ability to perceive painful stimuli by nociceptive pathways requires transmission of pain sensation to the cortex. The first projections from the thalamus to the cortex appear at 12 to 16 weeks gestation and do not undergo complete dendritic arborization and thalamocortical synaptogenesis until 23 weeks. Peripheral nerves undergo full maturation into the spinal cord from 23 to 25 weeks gestation, creating an intact circuit from peripheral sensation to spinothalamic transmission and cortical activation by around 26 weeks. Indeed, cortical pain response as measured by increased blood flow by near-infrared spectroscopy after heelstick has been found in neonates at 25 weeks gestation. Although the neuroanatomic system for pain perception is in place by this stage of fetal development, considerable debate and limited information exist regarding the timing of the development of a subjective and conscious pain experience in the neonate.

Further Reading

Coté CJ, Lerman H, Anderson BJ, eds. Coté and Lerman's A Practice of Anesthesia for Infants and Children. 5th ed. Philadelphia, PA: Elsevier; 2013:771.

Derbyshire SWG. Can fetuses feel pain? BMJ. 2006;332(7546):909–912.

Slater R, et al. Cortical pain responses in human infants. J Neurosci. 2006;26(14):3663–3666.

1.4. At what gestational age is it appropriate to provide analgesia to the premature neonate for painful procedures?

Critically ill preterm neonates may experience hundreds of painful procedures during their hospitalization, and specific analgesic measures are used in less than 50% of these procedures. Assessment of pain in neonates is challenging, but multimodal tools incorporating facial expressions, physiologic measurements, and behavior (crying and consolability) have been developed (e.g., Neonatal Facial Coding System, Premature Infant Pain Profile, Neonatal Pain and Sedation Scale). Premature neonates display a lower threshold for responses to noxious stimuli compared with older infants as well as evidence of central sensitization with repeated stimuli. Given the hormonal stress response and autonomic arousal that accompany noxious stimuli as early as 20 weeks PCA and evidence that peripheral stimuli trigger cortical responses by 26 weeks PCA, efforts to reduce or relieve pain perception for neonates at any viable age are warranted. This is particularly true for neonates undergoing moderate to severely painful procedures such as circumcision, chest drain insertion and removal, and nonemergent intubations. Short-term consequences of inadequate analgesia include physiologic instability, apnea, hypoxia, and increased cortisol secretion. Central pain sensitization from noxious stimuli occurs quickly in neonates due to immaturity of descending neuroinhibitory feedback systems, which causes increased excitability of nociceptive neurons in the dorsal horn of the spinal cord and exaggerated stress responses with subsequent stimuli. In animal models there is evidence that painful stimulation at certain stages of development can produce permanent changes in basal and stress-induced hormone responses, which can last into adulthood through a process of physiologic programming. Analgesic strategies may include nonpharmacologic methods of pain control, including facilitated tucking (a soothing technique where an infant's arms and legs are held in a flexed position), non-nutritive sucking, breastfeeding, or skin-to-skin care. Pharmacologic management of neonatal pain includes oral sucrose solutions, which can provide 4 to 5 minutes of reduction in pain scores during a mild to moderately painful procedure. Fentanyl and morphine are the most common medications used for analgesia in neonates, although infusions may carry risks for neurodevelopmental alteration and other adverse effects that outweigh benefits of pain control when used for prolonged sedation during mechanical ventilation. Topical anesthetic agents may also be used to reduce pain response to procedures in neonates.

Further Reading

AAP Committee on Fetus and Newborn and Section on Anesthesiology and Pain Medicine. Prevention and management of procedural pain in the neonate: an update. Pediatrics. 2016. 137(2):e20154271.

Coté CJ, Lerman H, Anderson BJ, eds. Coté and Lerman's A Practice of Anesthesia for Infants and Children. 5th ed. Philadelphia, PA: Elsevier; 2013:909.

1.5. What is neonatal abstinence syndrome, and how does opioid withdrawal present in neonates?

In neonates who have been treated with opioids for more than 7 to 10 days, physiologic tolerance develops, and increasing doses are required to provide equivalent analgesia or sedation. Rapid opioid weaning may induce withdrawal symptoms in infants, characterized by metabolic and respiratory manifestations (fever, diaphoresis, tachypnea), gastrointestinal manifestations (vomiting, loose stools, weight loss, poor feeding), and neurologic manifestations (tremors, sleep disturbance, seizures). Gradual opioid de-escalation may be facilitated by methadone, which has a longer half-life and shorter duration of weaning than morphine. Clonidine may be added for control of centrally mediated sympathetic symptoms of withdrawal. Neonatal abstinence syndrome (NAS) results when opioid-related complications occur from prenatal maternal opioid ingestion. The incidence of NAS increased fivefold from 2000 to 2012. Symptoms of opioid withdrawal usually occur within the first 24 to 48 hours after birth and do not fully resolve until 8 to 16 weeks of age. Up to 80% of infants with NAS require pharmacologic therapy, with an average hospitalization of 17 days. Standardized protocols for long-term opioid weaning often include nonpharmacologic measures (swaddling, soothing, feeding), frequent scoring for withdrawal symptoms, and gradual dose reduction. Withdrawal Assessment Tool-1 (WAT-1), a symptom assessment scale, has been validated in pediatric patients requiring opioid withdrawal in both intensive care and general ward settings. Neonates presenting for surgery with NAS or opioid tolerance will require careful titration of analgesics to attain adequate pain control in the perioperative period, and regional anesthesia options should be considered.

Further Reading

Franck LS, Scoppettuolo LA, Wypij D, Curley MA. Validity and generalizability of the Withdrawal Assessment Tool-1 (WAT-1) for monitoring iatrogenic withdrawal syndrome in pediatric patients. Pain. 2012 Jan;153(1):142–148.

MacDonald MG, Seshia MMK, Mullett MD, eds. Avery's Neonatology: Pathophysiology and Management of the Newborn. 7th ed. Philadelphia, PA: Lippincott Williams & Wilkins; 2015:1577.

McQueen K, Murphy-Oikonen J. Neonatal abstinence syndrome. N Engl J Med. 2016;375:2468–2479.

1.6. What are the unique aspects of opioid therapy and toxicity for neonates?

Opioids are commonly employed for painful procedures and sedation in neonates as they promote hemodynamic stability and have limited effect on myocardial function. Opioid analgesics also preserve hypoxic pulmonary vasoconstriction and control of pulmonary vascular hypertension with painful stimuli. Due to immature hepatic clearance systems, elimination half-lives for several opioids may be up to 4 times longer in neonates than in older children. Morphine clearance is particularly impaired in preterm infants. These pharmacodynamic differences, combined with a less developed blood-brain barrier and altered ventilatory response to hypoxemia and hypercapnia compared with older children, contribute to an increased risk of respiratory depression in neonates when opioids are administered. Neonates can develop rapid tolerance to opioids as demonstrated by decreased cardiovascular and sedative effect or dependence with withdrawal symptoms after therapeutic opioid administration for as little as 5 days. In the long term, there are some indications that increased morphine exposure in neonates may lead to worse neurodevelopmental outcomes, including impaired short-term memory, social problems, decreased cerebellar volume, and internalizing behavior later in childhood.

Further Reading

Borenstein-Levin L, et al. Narcotics and sedative use in preterm neonates. J Pediatr. 2017;180:92–98.

MacDonald MG, Seshia MMK, Mullett MD, eds. Avery's Neonatology: Pathophysiology and Management of the Newborn. 7th ed. Philadelphia, PA: Lippincott Williams & Wilkins; 2015:1561.

1.7. What are the unique aspects of local anesthetic therapy and toxicity for neonates?

The risk of local anesthetic (LA) toxicity in neonates is elevated for several reasons. Neonates have a reduced concentration of alpha-1-acid glycoprotein (AAG) compared with older children and adults, starting around one-third of adult levels at birth and normalizing around 1 year of age. AAG, red blood cells, and albumin all play a role in binding local anesthetics, and overall serum free fraction levels of LAs are higher in neonates than in adults. In addition, amide LA metabolism by the liver is reduced in neonates due to immature development of the cytochrome P450 system. Neonates under 1 month of age have a bupivacaine clearance rate that is one-third that of adults, and bupivacaine accumulation to toxic doses after 48 hours of infusion has been found even at recommended doses of <0.2 mg/kg/h. Ropivacaine has an improved safety profile compared with bupivacaine but also displays age-dependent clearance. Because of these risks, bolus and infusion doses of LA should be reduced in neonates by at least 30% to avoid accumulation and excessive serum concentration leading to systemic toxicity. Ester local anesthetics, like 2-chloroprocaine, are rapidly metabolized by plasma cholinesterases even in premature neonates and may be considered as an alternative to amide local anesthetics.

When local anesthetic systemic toxicity (LAST) does occur, preverbal neonates are unable to express early signs and symptoms of altered mental status and neural disturbance and are therefore more likely to present with arrhythmia, respiratory arrest, or seizures. Due to the enhanced sodium channel blocking effect of local anesthetics on nerves discharging at increased frequency, cardiac sensitivity to local anesthetic toxicity is also elevated in neonates given their higher resting heart rate. As in adults, neonates exhibiting neurologic and cardiovascular manifestations of LAST should receive supportive care and lipid emulsion administration as quickly as possible. Though lipid emulsion has a wide margin of safety when used to reverse LAST, recommendations and guidelines regarding lipid emulsion therapy in neonates have not been published.

Further Reading

Gregory GA, Andropoulos DB, eds. Gregory's Pediatric Anesthesia. 5th ed. Chicester, West Sussex: Wiley-Blackwell; 2012: 419.

Mazoit JX, Dalens BJ. Pharmacokinetics of local anesthetics in infants and children. Clin Pharmacokinet. 2004;42(1):17–32.

Veneziano G, Tobias JD. Chloroprocaine for epidural anesthesia in infants and children. Paediatr Anaesth. 2017 [epub ahead of print].

1.8. Discuss the long-term manifestations of inadequately treated pain in the neonate

Animal data demonstrate that undertreated pain in the neonatal stage can lead to altered nociception at older ages with synaptic modulation of sensory pathways. In humans, clinical studies have shown that neonates who experience painful stimuli may have increased pain sensitivity at older ages, presumably related to increased excitability of dorsal horn nociceptive neurons to noxious and nonnoxious stimuli. In one study, infants circumcised with little or no analgesia displayed increased pain behavior during later immunizations compared with uncircumcised patients or those who received adequate analgesia for their circumcision. In other studies, low birth weight infants who were exposed to painful stimuli as neonates displayed differences in pain perception, with increased pain intensity at age 8 to 10 years compared with those who were not. In addition to pain perception, development and behavior may be affected by inadequately treated neonatal pain. Regardless of illness severity, poor cognition and motor function are associated with a greater number of painful neonatal procedures for very preterm infants. In addition, preterm infants who experience more painful stimuli in the neonatal period display less cortical thickness at age 7 as compared with preterm infants who did not. Given these findings, several pediatric societies have issued guidelines regarding pain control in this population.

Further Reading

AAP Committee on Fetus and Newborn and Section on Anesthesiology and Pain Medicine. Prevention and management of procedural pain in the neonate: an update. Pediatrics. 2016;137(2):e20154271.

Borenstein-Levin L, et al. Narcotics and sedative use in preterm neonates. J Pediatr. 2017;180:92–98.

Gregory GA, Andropoulos DB, eds. Gregory's Pediatric Anesthesia. 5th ed. Chicester, West Sussex: Wiley-Blackwell; 2012:846.

2. Preoperative Evaluation and Preparation

2.1. What are the unique implications of ambulatory surgery for ex-premature infants?

There are several aspects the anesthesiologist must take into consideration before confirming that an ex-premature infant is appropriate for ambulatory surgery. The risk of postoperative apnea must be weighed against the benefits of ambulatory surgery in this population. Children who were born prematurely commonly experience periods of obstructive, central, and mixed apneas postoperatively. Most postoperative apneic episodes are typically managed well in the hospital with vigilant nursing, apnea monitoring, and gentle stimulation with occasional need for brief bag-mask ventilation. However, these episodes may lead to an acute life-threatening event if the child is discharged home. The risk of having postoperative apneic events is directly related to the child's PCA, history of prior apneic events, and anemia. The risk of postoperative apnea falls to less than 1% (95% statistical confidence) when the ex-premature child reaches 56 weeks; therefore, many centers employ policies that permit ambulatory surgery for children between 56 and 60 weeks PCA. Infants younger than this age should be admitted for overnight observation and apnea monitoring. However, this suggestion is for infants without significant cardiopulmonary manifestations, anemia, or congenital syndromes. Children with additional co-morbid conditions may warrant overnight apnea monitoring even if they are older than 60 weeks PCA. The appropriate timing and postsurgical disposition of such children should be discussed between the surgeon and anesthesiologist in the preoperative planning phase.

2.2. What specific information would you need regarding the child's neonatal intensive care unit course?

Infants born preterm typically spend their first few days to first few months in the neonatal intensive care unit (NICU) based on the degree of prematurity and the associated sequelae as well as manifestations of superimposed congenital disorders. The anesthesiologist's review of the NICU course should include each organ system, with particular emphasis placed on the cardiac and pulmonary systems. Periods of endotracheal intubation in the NICU and presence of anatomic abnormalities such as laryngomalacia, tracheomalacia, and subglottic stenosis may affect airway management and increase risk of postoperative stridor. Bronchopulmonary dysplasia is a complex entity of the premature child that is caused by extended periods on mechanical ventilation and oxygen free radical injury and may lead to the need for postoperative oxygen supplementation or CPAP, which would preclude discharge home. Pulmonary hypertension may result from a patent ductus arteriosus or severe pulmonary disease.

2.3. What are the regional anesthetic options for this patient? Which technique is superior?

For inguinal hernia repairs, the regional anesthetic options include neuraxial blockade or peripheral blockade. Neuraxial options include single-injection subarachnoid (spinal) or caudal blockade and, less commonly, lumbar epidural single injection or lumbar epidural catheters advanced from the caudal epidural space. Paravertebral, transverse abdominal plane (TAP), and ilioinguinal/iliohypogastric nerve blocks are options for peripheral blockade.

Caudal or spinal blocks provide similar surgical conditions; however, caudal blocks may be technically easier to place and have higher success rates. Though paravertebral nerve blocks are feasible for inguinal hernia surgery and may possibly reduce risk of nausea or urinary retention, these blocks may be more difficult to perform and require significantly more time to place. Ilioinguinal/iliohypogastric nerve blocks provide more effective analgesia than TAP blocks but have not clearly shown superiority over caudal blocks and carry the disadvantage of needing 2 injections if bilateral surgery is planned. However, the ilioinguinal/iliohypogastric nerve block technique is easily facilitated with ultrasound guidance, and less local anesthetic may be used as compared with a caudal block. Lack of clear superiority of one regional anesthetic technique over another suggests that level of comfort with the various techniques and availability of appropriate equipment should be the major considerations when choosing a regional anesthetic technique for pediatric inguinal hernia surgery.

Further Reading

Hoelzle M, Weiss M, Dillier C, Gerber A. Comparison of awake spinal with awake caudal anesthesia in preterm and ex-preterm infants for herniotomy. Paediatr Anaesth. 2010 Jul;20(7):620–624.

Law LS, Tan M, Bai Y, Miller TE, Li YJ, Gan TJ. Paravertebral block for inguinal herniorrhaphy: a systematic review and meta-analysis of randomized controlled trials. Anesth Analg. 2015 Aug;121(2):556–569.

Shanthanna H, Singh B, Guyatt G. A systematic review and meta-analysis of caudal block as compared to noncaudal regional techniques for inguinal surgeries in children. Biomed Res Int. 2014;2014:890626.

2.4. Describe the medical evidence surrounding the use of regional anesthesia to mitigate postoperative apnea for infants undergoing inguinal hernia surgery

A few studies have specifically studied the impact of regional anesthesia on postoperative apnea in infants undergoing inguinal hernia surgery. If general anesthesia is considered directly related to the development of postoperative apnea in this population, regional anesthesia may theoretically mitigate these risks. Two major studies have studied this topic, the General Anesthesia Compared to Spinal (GAS) study and the Cochrane Review.

The GAS study was a multinational randomized trial that enrolled more 700 children undergoing inguinal hernia surgery at less than 60 weeks postmenstrual age (PMA). Half of the enrolled patients were born preterm, defined as less than 37 weeks PMA. Both term and preterm infants were randomized to receive either a regional anesthetic (spinal, spinal with caudal, spinal with ilioinguinal nerve block, or caudal) or a general anesthetic (GA) with sevoflurane. Infants in the regional anesthetic (RA) arm received no sedatives, hypnotics, or opioids at any point in the perioperative period. The results of this study showed no statistically significant difference in postoperative apnea between the regional anesthetic and general anesthetic groups in the first 12 postoperative hours after inguinal hernia surgery, with both groups exhibiting an apnea risk of 3% to 4%. The researchers split the groups into early apnea (0–30 minutes after surgery) and late apnea (30 minutes to 12 hours). Late apnea was equal in both RA and GA groups (2%), but there was a statistically significant reduction in early apnea in the RA group (1%) compared with the GA group (3%). However, the clinical significance of reduction in early apnea is questionable as infants are typically highly monitored in the postanesthesia care unit during the first 30 minutes or more after surgery.

Like the GAS study, the goal of the Cochrane Review was to determine whether pure regional anesthesia techniques led to less postoperative apnea than GA for infants undergoing inguinal hernia surgery. Unlike the GAS study, the Cochrane Review evaluated only preterm children (born at less than 37 weeks gestational age). This meta-analysis, though perhaps inadequately powered, did suggest that regional anesthesia without additional sedative agents may reduce the incidence of postoperative apnea by up to 47% in former preterm children undergoing inguinal hernia surgery in early infancy.

These contradictory studies fail to provide a definitive answer on the debate. Well-aligned perioperative teams that have been well educated on the benefits and challenges of a pure regional anesthetic technique in the operating room may perhaps confer mild reductions in postoperative apnea to preterm infants undergoing inguinal hernia surgery, but the clinical impact of this apnea reduction on the overall outcome of the child has not been well elucidated.

Further Reading

Davidson AJ, Morton NS, Arnup SJ, de Graaff JC, Disma N, Withington DE, Frawley G, Hunt RW, Hardy P, Khotcholava M, von Ungern Sternberg BS, Wilton N, Tuo P, Salvo I, Ormond G, Stargatt R, Locatelli BG, McCann ME; General Anesthesia Compared to Spinal Anesthesia (GAS) Consortium. Apnea after awake regional and general anesthesia in infants: the General Anesthesia Compared to Spinal Anesthesia Study—comparing apnea and neurodevelopmental outcomes, a randomized controlled trial. Anesthesiology. 2015 Jul;123(1):38–54.

Jones LJ, Craven PD, Lakkundi A, Foster JP, Badawi N. Regional (spinal, epidural, caudal) versus general anaesthesia in preterm infants undergoing inguinal herniorrhaphy in early infancy. Cochrane Database Syst Rev. 2015 Jun 9;6:CD003669.

3. Intraoperative Management

3.1. During the preoperative interview, the anesthesiologist discusses placing a caudal block after induction of anesthesia. The child's mother refuses to provide consent for the regional anesthetic technique, reporting that placement of an epidural catheter for her during labor was a very unpleasant experience. How might the anesthesiologist approach this?

Hesitation to provide informed consent to regional anesthesia by the parent/guardian is typically a result of misinformation about the procedure or a history of an adverse event in either the parent/guardian or other family member. The majority of these misunderstandings are easily cleared up by effective preoperative discussion with the anesthesiologist. In addition, in light of ongoing research focused on the possible long-terms effects of anesthetics in children under 3 years of age, a discussion of regional anesthesia replacing the need for general anesthesia is appropriate in this scenario. The anesthesiologist should focus on the safety of the regional anesthetic technique, explain the reasons for performing the procedure, and explain the experience he or she has had with the technique. Multiple reports provided by the Pediatric Regional Anesthesia Network (PRAN) underscore the overall safety of multiple regional anesthesia techniques, and these data may be discussed with parents during the preoperative interview. The PRAN has reported a complication risk of 1.9% for caudal blocks, after reviewing more than 18,000 patients within the PRAN database who received caudal anesthesia. Risk of complication from a caudal block is inversely related to the child's age, and the most common reported complications were failure to achieve adequate blockade and aspiration of blood during placement. Importantly, no temporary or permanent neurologic sequelae were noted in the large group of studied patients. Most parents/guardians are sympathetic to the notion that regional anesthetics may assist with opioid reduction, earlier extubation, and fewer opioid-related side effects. Requirement for written informed consent for pediatric regional anesthesia varies across hospital systems and associated pediatric pain services. Written consent for anesthesia is occasionally obtained outside of implied anesthesia consent with the surgical consent; local policies should be followed regarding regional anesthetic techniques.

Further Reading

Andropoulos DB, Greene MF. Anesthesia and developing brains: implications of the FDA warning. N Engl J Med. 2017 Mar 9;376(10):905–907.

Lönnqvist PA, Morton NS, Ross AK. Consent issues and pediatric regional anesthesia. Paediatr Anaesth. 2009 Oct;19(10):958–960.

Suresh S, Long J, Birmingham PK, De Oliveira GS Jr. Are caudal blocks for pain control safe in children? An analysis of 18,650 caudal blocks from the Pediatric Regional Anesthesia Network (PRAN) database. Anesth Analg. 2015 Jan;120(1):151–156.

3.2. What are the absolute and relative contraindications for pediatric regional anesthesia?

The primary absolute contraindication for pediatric regional anesthesia is parental refusal of the technique. Obtaining assent should be considered, and risks/benefits should be discussed with the older adolescent during the preoperative interview as well. Other contraindications are similar to contraindications for regional anesthesia in adults, with few unique aspects in children. Overlying skin infection at the site, underlying coagulopathy, and anatomic abnormalities such as lumbosacral myelomeningocele are absolute contraindications. Indwelling continuous catheters should be avoided in the presence of significant systemic infection. Relative contraindications vary significantly, and the benefit of the procedure should be weighed carefully around the potential risk for each unique patient situation. These include progressive neurologic disease, risk of compartment syndrome, and volume depletion prior to neuraxial blocks. Caudal blocks in children with ventriculoperitoneal (VP) shunts are commonly performed, but strict adherence to sterile technique is indicated to reduce risk of shunt infection, and temporary increases in intracranial pressure due to the large volume (0.5–1 mL/kg) typically injected into the epidural space during this procedure must be taken into consideration. Routine administration of antibiotic prophylaxis prior to caudal blocks in children with VP shunts is a controversial topic, with limited medical evidence to either support or refute this practice.

Further Reading

Ecoffey C. Safety in pediatric regional anesthesia. Paediatr Anaesth. 2012 Jan;22(1):25–30.

Platis CM, Kachko L, Livni G, Efrat R, Katz J. Caudal anesthesia in children with shunt devices. Paediatr Anaesth. 2006 Nov;16(11):1198–1199.

Veyckemans F, Scholtes JL. Caudal block and ventricular shunt devices: beware of the consequences of increasing epidural pressure! Paediatr Anaesth. 2007 Jul;17(7):707–709.

3.3. If regional anesthesia if not possible, what perioperative analgesic strategy would you employ?

If regional anesthesia cannot be employed due to inability to obtain parental informed consent or due to the presence of a contraindication, an opioid-sparing perioperative analgesic regimen should be employed. These regimens reduce opioid-related side effects, particularly respiratory depression, giving the neonate the best chance of early extubation and reducing the risk of postoperative reintubation. Local anesthetic infiltration during surgical closure of the incision by the surgeon is an effective way to provide a short period of analgesia to the child and reduce overall need for postoperative opioids. Indeed, a few studies have shown equivalency of local field block to caudal block for unilateral pediatric inguinal hernia repair, and field blocks certainly require less expertise to place, utilize less total local anesthetic, and have less impact on operating room time. Oral acetaminophen (20 mg/kg load) may be given preoperatively to children, often along with oral benzodiazepine premedication if planned, or administered rectally (40 mg/kg load) after induction of anesthesia. Though the medical evidence regarding the efficacy of enteral acetaminophen is mixed, the bulk of evidence suggests that acetaminophen may play a small role in opioid reduction, particularly if paired with a nonsteroidal anti-inflammatory drug (NSAID). Intravenous (IV) acetaminophen has gained popularity due to ease of use in the perioperative period and lack of first-pass metabolism, but routine use has been tempered by the relatively high cost of the agent currently, and superiority over enteral preparations has not been established. However, if addition of IV acetaminophen leads to fewer opioid-related side effects and earlier discharge from the hospital, aggregate costs may actually be reduced. NSAIDs consistently show greater efficacy than acetaminophen in providing postoperative analgesia, with ketorolac being the most commonly prescribed IV NSAID in the perioperative period. There is considerable controversy regarding ketorolac's role in both renal dysfunction and postoperative bleeding in infants, with inconclusive data in the medical literature. Conservative management consists of restricting the use of ketorolac to children greater than 1 year of age provided there are no coagulation or renal abnormalities.

Further Reading

Baird R, Guilbault MP, Tessier R, Ansermino JM. A systematic review and meta-analysis of caudal blockade versus alternative analgesic strategies for pediatric inguinal hernia repair. J Pediatr Surg. 2013 May;48(5):1077–1085.

Hong JY, Won Han S, Kim WO, Kil HK. Fentanyl sparing effects of combined ketorolac and acetaminophen for outpatient inguinal hernia repair in children. J Urol. 2010 Apr;183(4):1551–1555.

3.4. You plan to perform a caudal block to provide analgesia, but a sacral dimple is noted when the child is turned to the lateral position. Do you proceed with a caudal block?

Sacral dimples noticed during placement of a caudal injection in an infant may point toward a diagnosis of an occult spinal dysraphism. Though the majority of dimples in otherwise healthy children without an associated syndrome do not extend into the spinal canal, tethered spinal cord lesions are occasionally associated with midline soft tissue defects. If a caudal block is planned, the anesthesiologist should include an examination of the sacrococcygeal area preoperatively to evaluate for overlying skin infection or presence of midline spine lesions such as hairy patches, pits, soft tissue masses (subcutaneous lipomas), hemangiomas, drainage, or skin tags. A single midline dimple less than 5 mm in diameter, less than 2.5 cm from the anus without the above additional cutaneous findings is considered a simple sacral dimple. If a lesion is noted on preoperative examination or during placement of the caudal, the anesthesiologist should consult the medical record to see if a spinal ultrasound has been performed. In a study of nearly 4000 children with simple sacral dimples undergoing sonographic evaluation, 3.4% were found to have an abnormal finding, and only 0.13% were found to have a tethered cord requiring neurosurgical intervention. If an ultrasound has not been performed, the anesthesiologist, neonatologist, and surgeon may discuss the risks and benefits of placing the caudal block. The conservative choice is to avoid the caudal block if no spinal ultrasound has been performed, particularly if significant skin stigmata are noticed.

Further Reading

Gibson PJ, Britton J, Hall DM, Hill CR. Lumbosacral skin markers and identification of occult spinal dysraphism in neonates. Acta Paediatr. 1995 Feb;84(2):208–209.

Kucera JN, Coley I, O'Hara S, Kosnik EJ, Coley BD. The simple sacral dimple: diagnostic yield of ultrasound in neonates. Pediatr Radiol. 2015 Feb;45(2):211–216.

3.5. Discuss the unique aspects of placing a spinal block in an awake child with the goal of reducing or avoiding sedatives

Though the long-term manifestations of general anesthesia on the developing brain remain unclear and it is unclear if regional anesthesia can mitigate or eliminate these risks, there is concern about the routine use of general anesthesia in young children, and some anesthesiologists advocate for a pure regional anesthetic technique in this population. Placing a regional block on an awake infant and then providing no sedatives during the operation may come as a culture shock to many surgeons, nurses, and scrub technicians who are accustomed to general anesthetics for most surgical procedures in children. The anesthesiologist must take into account the viewpoints of various stakeholders on the perioperative team before planning an awake, pure regional technique in infants. Optimally, this concept is planned well in advance with the surgeon, nursing leadership, and other members of the perioperative team.

Infants may require a higher weight-based dose of local anesthetic than adults to achieve adequate spinal blockade but are more prone to the development of local anesthetic toxicity. The larger dosage requirement is due to larger relative volumes of cerebrospinal fluid (CSF) (4 mL/kg in infants versus 2 mL/kg in adults) and faster redistribution away from the spinal cord due to proportionally greater blood flow to vessel-rich tissue beds. Spinal blocks in infants are typically performed at the L4-L5 or L5-S1 interspace, and the anesthesiologist must remember that the spinal cord terminates at L3 in this population. A standard 25-gauge Quincke or Whitacre needle is adequate, taking care to not place the larger introducer needle (if used) through the dura. Some anesthesiologists prefer to apply eutectic preparations of lidocaine and prilocaine to the site of spinal puncture 30 minutes prior to the procedure to avoid the need for subcutaneous infiltration. There are reports of placing the IV line in the lower extremity of the infant after placement of the spinal block to avoid painful venous cannulation. Placing the blood pressure cuff on the lower extremity after spinal placement can further reduce the child's discomfort during the procedure.

The benefits of a spinal block over general anesthesia are likely minimal if sedatives such as midazolam, nitrous oxide, or ketamine are used to produce a sedate child after the spinal block. Bundling the child, providing a pacifier, placing sucrose water periodically to the mouth, avoiding loud noises in the operating room, and reassuring the surgeon when the child makes minor movements of his or her upper extremities during the procedure are important facets of providing awake spinal blockade to an infant.

Further Reading

Lederhaas G. Spinal anaesthesia in paediatrics. Best Pract Res Clin Anaesthesiol. 2003 Sep;17(3):365–376.

Tobias JD. Spinal anaesthesia in infants and children. Paediatr Anaesth. 2000;10(1):5–16.

3.6. What are the local anesthetic options for a caudal block or a spinal block?

For single caudal epidural injections, a volume of 1 mL/kg of local anesthetic volume is sufficient to consistently attain a T10 blockade with a maximum volume of 20 mL. It is prudent to use the least amount of local anesthetic required to appropriately provide analgesia over the surgical incisions. If surgery is confined to only the penile or anal areas (sacral dermatomes), less local anesthetic volume is required (0.5–0.75 mL/kg provides blockade to L1), which significantly reduces the risk of local anesthetic toxicity. Ropivacaine 0.2%, bupivacaine 0.25%, or bupivacaine 0.125% are common agents and concentrations used for single-injection caudal blockade and will provide analgesia for about 4 to 6 hours. Chloroprocaine is a short-acting ester local anesthetic that has gained popularity due to its extremely short plasma half-life and negligible risk of local anesthetic toxicity. Given that a 20 mg/kg bolus dose of chloroprocaine confers only 1 hour of blockade, a continuous infusion of chloroprocaine is necessary to maintain intraoperative analgesia for prolonged surgical procedures or to provide postoperative analgesia for any reasonable length of time.

For spinal blocks, hyperbaric tetracaine 0.5% (0.4–0.6 mg/kg), hyperbaric bupivacaine 0.75% (0.3–0.6 mg/kg), or isobaric bupivacaine 0.5% (0.3–0.6 mg/kg) consistently provides 60 to 80 minutes of surgical anesthesia, with the addition of epinephrine (20–50 mcg) providing another 20 minutes. Surgical blockade with a spinal is typically limited to 90 minutes, and so the operative team must be prepared to prep, drape, and proceed with surgery in rapid fashion after spinal placement. It is advisable to have the surgeon present, scrubbed, and ready to operate, with the anesthesiologist reminding the surgeon of the time constraint, particularly if surgical trainees are present for the procedure.

Further Reading

Jöhr M. Practical pediatric regional anesthesia. Curr Opin Anaesthesiol. 2013 Jun;26(3):327–332.

Lederhaas G. Spinal anaesthesia in paediatrics. Best Pract Res Clin Anaesthesiol. 2003 Sep;17(3):365–376.

Tobias JD. Spinal anaesthesia in infants and children. Paediatr Anaesth. 2000;10(1):5–16.

Veneziano G, Iliev P, Tripi J, Martin D, Aldrink J, Bhalla T, Tobias J. Continuous chloroprocaine infusion for thoracic and caudal epidurals as a postoperative analgesia modality in neonates, infants, and children. Paediatr Anaesth. 2016 Jan;26(1):84–91.

3.7. Discuss the utility of using epinephrine in pediatric regional blocks, particularly caudal blocks

Negative aspiration of blood during placement of regional anesthetic blocks does not reliably eliminate the possibility of intravascular uptake. Test doses of local anesthetic are still frequently given in both adult and pediatric patients.

Epinephrine within "test doses" can potentially cause tachycardia, hypertension, or T-wave changes on the electrocardiogram, alarming the anesthesiologist of the possibility of intravascular injection. An appropriate test dose method should involve injecting 0.1 mL/kg of local anesthetic solution containing 1:200,000 epinephrine and monitoring for heart rate, blood pressure, or electrocardiogram changes for 60 to 90 seconds. A 10-20-25 rule may be followed, with a positive test dose signifying intravascular injection increasing the heart rate by 10 beats per minute, increasing the systolic blood pressure by 20 mmHg, and/or altering the T-wave morphology by 25%. Electrocardiogram changes, specifically T-wave or ST segment changes, tend to be the most sensitive markers of intravascular injection. Caudal blocks are inherently high-risk blocks given the relatively large volumes needed to provide adequate analgesia, the common use in infants/neonates, and the relative vascularity of the sacral epidural space.

In addition to serving as an early warning sign for intravascular uptake, epinephrine is often thought to promote vasoconstriction, thereby slowing the redistribution of local anesthetic and prolonging blockade. This effect is likely minimal in the infant and becomes even more diminished in older children.

Further Reading

Tobias JD. Caudal epidural block: a review of test dosing and recognition of systemic injection in children. Anesth Analg. 2001 Nov;93(5):1156–1161.

3.8. What are appropriate opioid adjuncts that may be placed for caudal or spinal blocks? What are the associated implications for ambulatory anesthesia?

The most commonly utilized opioid adjuncts used in single-shot caudal blocks or spinal blocks are fentanyl, hydromorphone, and morphine.

Fentanyl is a lipophilic opioid that is a common adjuvant added to local anesthetic for single-shot caudal blocks. Two studies have noted that fentanyl 1 mcg/kg added to either ropivacaine 0.2% or bupivacaine 0.25% for caudal blocks resulted in no prolonged duration of blockade, reduction in time to first postoperative analgesic, or postoperative pain scores. One study comparing caudal fentanyl to caudal clonidine added to 0.25% bupivacaine noted a marginal increase in length of blockade, but also a significant increase in the incidence of postoperative vomiting. Fentanyl administered via single injection in the caudal space likely has similar efficacy as fentanyl injected intravascularly given its lipophilicity and rapid plasma uptake.

Vetter et al. performed a double-blind, randomized study without a nonadjuvant control arm that compared caudal clonidine, hydromorphone, and morphine in children undergoing ureteral reimplantation. Hydromorphone (10 mcg/kg) and morphine (50 mcg/kg) adjuvants in 0.2% ropivacaine provided longer periods to first postoperative morphine dose, but this effect did not reach statistical significance. Importantly, opioid adjuvants were associated with significantly greater administration of diphenhydramine for pruritus and ondansetron for nausea compared with clonidine. The anesthesiologist must exercise caution when administering hydrophilic epidural opioids, particularly to ambulatory patients, as even small doses may result in delayed respiratory depression. Somnolence, apneic episodes, upper airway obstruction, or hypoxemia may require escalation in care if the patient remains in the hospital but may result in an acute life-threatening event if the child is discharged home.

Further Reading

Karl HW, Tyler DC, Krane EJ. Respiratory depression after low-dose caudal morphine. Can J Anaesth. 1996 Oct;43(10):1065–1067.

Kawaraguchi Y, Otomo T, Ota C, Uchida N, Taniguchi A, Inoue S. A prospective, double-blind, randomized trial of caudal block using ropivacaine 0.2% with or without fentanyl 1 microg kg-1 in children. Br J Anaesth. 2006 Dec;97(6):858–861.

Vetter TR, Carvallo D, Johnson JL, Mazurek MS, Presson RG Jr. A comparison of single-dose caudal clonidine, morphine, or hydromorphone combined with ropivacaine in pediatric patients undergoing ureteral reimplantation. Anesth Analg. 2007 Jun;104(6):1356–1363.

3.9. Discuss the dosing and medical evidence for neuraxial clonidine in caudal blocks

Besides opioids, a variety of other additives have been utilized in caudal blocks, such as neostigmine, ketamine, and midazolam. Many of these agents cause additional problems, are ineffective in improving duration of block, or may be neurotoxic. Of all the additives historically used in single-injection caudal blocks, clonidine (1–2 mcg/kg) has emerged as the most useful and most popular additive in clinical use today. The clonidine dose of 2 mcg/kg may provide a slightly longer duration of blockade over the 1-mcg/kg dose, but there are insufficient data regarding the incidence of side effects when children are administered the higher dosage. In a meta-analysis of 20 randomized trials, addition of clonidine to local anesthetics in a single-injection caudal block was found to increase the duration of action of the block by 4 hours, corresponding to reduced need for rescue analgesics in the postoperative period. Slightly prolonged motor block is the most significant negative effect of caudal clonidine. Hypotension, bradycardia, and sedation were all mild. A few case reports of postoperative apnea in premature children administered caudal clonidine exist. Though this is a valid concern, current evidence only suggests an association, and determination of causality has not been established. The incidence and severity of apnea and respiratory depression are inversely related to the age of the child. Preterm and term neonates are perhaps more sensitive to the sedative effects of clonidine due to immature respiratory control centers in the central nervous system.

Further Reading

Ansermino M, Basu R, Vandebeek C, Montgomery C. Nonopioid additives to local anaesthetics for caudal blockade in children: a systematic review. Paediatr Anaesth. 2003 Sep;13(7):561–573.

Schnabel A, Poepping DM, Pogatzki-Zahn EM, Zahn PK. Efficacy and safety of clonidine as additive for caudal regional anesthesia: a quantitative systematic review of randomized controlled trials. Paediatr Anaesth. 2011 Dec;21(12):1219–1230.

3.10. Discuss the role of ultrasound in caudal blocks

Some anesthesiologists advocate for the routine use of ultrasonography in the placement of single-injection caudal blocks not only to view the passage of the needle but also to view the flow of the solution as it is injected into the caudal epidural space. A linear high-frequency ultrasound probe that has a small footprint will allow for good visualization of important structures, as well as provide adequate room to maneuver the caudal needle. The probe is held in a transverse orientation, and the sacral cornua, sacrococcygeal ligament, and sacral hiatus are typically visualized well given the shallow depth of the structures. There is no clear evidence that ultrasound-guided blocks provide superior metrics to standard, landmark-based techniques, but the ultrasound method likely takes longer to complete. In the hands of an experienced anesthesiologist, ultrasound guidance may be useful when a caudal block is desired in a child in whom surface landmarks are not readily apparent or the landmark technique has been challenging.

Further Reading

Erbüyün K, Açıkgöz B, Ok G, Yılmaz Ö, Temeltaş G, Tekin İ, Tok D. The role of ultrasound guidance in pediatric caudal block. Saudi Med J. 2016 Feb;37(2):147–150.

Tsui B, Suresh S. Ultrasound imaging for regional anesthesia in infants, children, and adolescents: a review of current literature and its application in the practice of extremity and trunk blocks. Anesthesiology. 2010 Feb;112(2):473–492.

3.11. What are the nonneuraxial regional anesthesia techniques that may be utilized to provide analgesia for children undergoing inguinal hernia repair?

If neuraxial techniques are not possible, unilateral or bilateral ilioinguinal/iliohypogastric (II/IH) nerve blocks are the most appropriate regional anesthetic techniques. Caudal blocks provide superior analgesia compared with II/IHnerve blocks, as quantified by need for rescue analgesia, but they carry the potential side effects of motor block and urinary retention. II/IH nerve blocks also take longer to perform, particularly if bilateral hernia surgery is planned. One study involved the placement of a caudal block at the start of surgery followed by II/IH nerve blocks at the end of surgery. This technique provided improved analgesia over II/IH nerve blocks alone. The safety and feasibility of this 2-block technique has been questioned due to concerns about local anesthetic toxicity and time constraints in the operating room.

Further Reading

Jagannathan N, Sohn L, Sawardekar A, Ambrosy A, Hagerty J, Chin A, Barsness K, Suresh S. Unilateral groin surgery in children: will the addition of an ultrasound-guided ilioinguinal nerve block enhance the duration of analgesia of a single-shot caudal block? Paediatr Anaesth. 2009 Sep;19(9):892–898.

Shanthanna H, Singh B, Guyatt G. A systematic review and meta-analysis of caudal block as compared to noncaudal regional techniques for inguinal surgeries in children. Biomed Res Int. 2014;2014:890626.

3.12. Describe the warning signs of local anesthetic toxicity during or following a regional anesthetic technique in children

The vast majority of children are heavily sedated or under general anesthesia when regional anesthetic procedures are performed, and so early detection of local anesthetic toxicity is challenging. In addition, preverbal or nonverbal children may not have the ability to articulate such symptoms as tinnitus, palpitations, or dizziness. Unfortunately, seizures or arrhythmias may be the first signs an anesthesiologist may observe during impending life-threatening local anesthetic toxicity. If epinephrine-containing solutions are used, an increase in heart rate, increases in blood pressure, or abnormalities in the electrocardiogram may be seen during or after injection of the local anesthetic solution. T-wave abnormalities may be the most sensitive and specific marker for toxicity, and so the anesthesiologist must place electrocardiogram leads on the child prior to injection and monitor carefully during the injection phase.

Further Reading

Lönnqvist PA. Toxicity of local anesthetic drugs: a pediatric perspective. Paediatr Anaesth. 2012 Jan;22(1):39–43.

3.13. Discuss the management of local anesthetic toxicity in an infant who just received a caudal block

Local anesthetic systemic toxicity must always be considered in a patient who develops any level of physiologic derangement after injection of local anesthetic, particularly with the large volumes normally injected for regional anesthetic techniques. Bupivacaine is by far the most common amide local anesthetic implicated in pediatric LAST, though reports of lidocaine and ropivacaine toxicity exist. Dysrhythmias are nearly ubiquitous in reports of amide LAST in children, with seizures, hypotension, and tachycardia also reported. As with any other catastrophic event, the anesthesiologist must immediately focus on the basic tenets set forth by Advanced Cardiac Life Support protocols, notably restoring circulation through effective chest compressions for nonperfusing rhythms, providing appropriate emergency medications like epinephrine, and ensuring adequate oxygen/ventilation. Lipid emulsions, classically used as a component of parenteral nutrition, have repeatedly shown efficacy in the treatment of acute drug toxicities. In addition to the treatment of amide local anesthetic toxicity, lipid emulsions have also been used to successfully treat amitriptyline, lamotrigine, quetiapine, olanzapine, and diltiazem toxicities. The prevailing theory regarding the mechanism of action of lipid emulsions in LAST is the "lipid sink" theory in that the lipid emulsion provides a medium by which free fraction of lipid soluble local anesthetic may reside, instead of binding to extraneural sodium channels. Other proposed theories suggest that lipid emulsions have a role in the modulation of calcium metabolism and also provide a lipid energy source for cardiac myocytes. The dosage of a 20% lipid emulsion solution in the event of local anesthetic toxicity is 1.5 mL/kg by bolus. Two bolus doses may be provided, and if a perfusing rhythm returns, an infusion of 0.25 mL/kg/min may be started. For extreme cases of local anesthetic toxicity refractory to all other therapies, ECMO may be required.

Further Reading

Presley JD, Chyka PA. Intravenous lipid emulsion to reverse acute drug toxicity in pediatric patients. Ann Pharmacother. 2013 May;47(5):735–743.

4. Postoperative Management

4.1. What is the role of caffeine therapy in the perioperative management of premature infants?

Caffeine increases central CO_2 sensitivity and reduces the incidence of apneic episodes for premature neonates, which can occur more frequently following surgery and anesthesia. When used for apnea of prematurity, caffeine may reduce apneic events by 50% to 90% and decreases the need for positive pressure ventilation. A systematic review of randomized trials comparing prophylactic caffeine treatment to placebo found a 58% absolute risk reduction in apnea with bradycardia for infants treated with caffeine without any adverse effects. Typical reported doses for caffeine are 5 to 10 mg/kg IV prior to surgery. Caffeine therapy may be particularly useful for those infants with increased risk factors for apnea, including prior history of apnea or younger gestational age, or those who are at risk for pulmonary complications, such as infants with chronic lung disease. Of note, the clearance of caffeine is very slow in the neonatal period, and a single dose may last 72 hours or more.

Further Reading

Gregory GA, Andropoulos DB, eds. Gregory's Pediatric Anesthesia. 5th ed. Chicester, West Sussex: Wiley-Blackwell; 2012:493.

Henderson-Smart DJ, Steer P. Prophylactic caffeine to prevent postoperative apnea following general anesthesia in preterm infants. Cochrane Database Syst Rev. 2001;4:CD000048.

MacDonald MG, Seshia MMK, Mullett MD, eds. Avery's Neonatology: Pathophysiology and Management of the Newborn. 7th ed. Philadelphia, PA: Lippincott Williams & Wilkins; 2015:542.

4.2. The child develops urinary retention postoperatively after a caudal block with bupivacaine and morphine. Discuss your management strategy

The rate of serious complications after caudal blockade is very small. A PRAN analysis of 18,650 caudal blocks revealed a complication rate of 1.9%, with the most commonly reported complications being block failure, blood aspiration, and intravascular injection, with no reports of temporary or permanent sequelae. The rate of urinary retention, however, is increased with neuraxial administration of opioids and may occur in up to 27% of patients receiving neuraxial morphine. Urinary retention should be suspected in children who have received adequate fluid resuscitation and have not voided; have unexplained tachycardia, discomfort, or suprapubic fullness; and have risk factors for urinary retention such as caudal blockade or opioid administration. If the patient has signs and symptoms suggestive of urinary retention, urinary catheterization should be performed. Prolonged oliguria should prompt consultation with the urology or nephrology service, depending on the suspected etiology.

Further Reading

Gregory GA, Andropoulos DB, eds. Gregory's Pediatric Anesthesia. 5th ed. Chicester, West Sussex: Wiley-Blackwell; 2012:378.

Suresh S, et al. Are caudal blocks for pain control safe in children? An analysis of 18,650 caudal blocks from the Pediatric Regional Anesthesia (PRAN) database. Anesth Analg. 2015;120(1):151–156.

4.3. The child is unable to move his legs in the postoperative period but otherwise appears comfortable and stable. The surgeon performed bilateral ilioinguinal nerve blocks for the procedure. What is your management strategy?

II/IH nerve blocks are used for postoperative pain control most commonly after inguinal hernia repair or orchidopexy. Injection is performed blindly 2 to 3 cm medial to the anterior superior iliac spine between the internal oblique muscle and the external oblique aponeurosis. After intermittent aspiration and injection of 0.3 mL/kg local anesthetic in cephalad, medial, and caudad directions, the iliohypogastric nerve is commonly blocked in the subcutaneous tissue during needle withdrawal. Complications are rare, but injection into the femoral artery or around the femoral nerve is possible and occurs in up to 9% of children, which could produce lower extremity weakness. However, the use of ultrasound has been described and may decrease the incidence of such complications. In this instance, a neurologic exam would reveal sensory deficit in the femoral nerve distribution and quadriceps weakness. Observation is acceptable with follow-up for resolution of nerve blockade at the expected interval.

Further Reading

Coté CJ, Lerman H, Anderson BJ, eds. Coté and Lerman's A Practice of Anesthesia for Infants and Children. 5th ed. Philadelphia, PA: Elsevier; 2013, 859.

Lipp AK, Woodcock J, Hensman B, Wilkinson K. Leg weakness is a complication of ilio-inguinal nerve block in children. Br J Anaesth. 2004;92(2):273–274.

Willschke H, Marhofer P, Bösenberg A, Johnston S, Wanzel O, Cox SG, Sitzwohl C, Kapral S. Ultrasonography for ilioinguinal/iliohypogastric nerve blocks in children. Br J Anaesth. 2005 Aug;95(2):226–230.

4.4. A spinal block was placed for the procedure, but the procedure was difficult and required multiple attempts by multiple providers. The child is discharged home after an uneventful surgical procedure but returns to the emergency department the next day due to extreme irritability and feeding intolerance. What is your management strategy?

Complications of spinal blockade may include total spinal blockade, infection, bleeding, nerve injury, and postdural puncture headache. High levels of subarachnoid injection, which may occur with excessive or rapid dosing or change in position, can cause loss of respiratory effort and respiratory failure but are usually hemodynamically stable. Nerve injury after spinal injection in children is a theoretical possibility but has not been described. Postdural puncture headache also appears to be rare, although incidence as high as 5% has been reported. The low incidence may be due to reduced CSF pressure or increased rate of CSF production in young children. When postdural puncture headache occurs in young children, it may be difficult to diagnose but typically presents 1 to 3 days following the procedure, with irritability that correlates with position, vomiting, or feeding intolerance. Presentation is generally mild and managed conservatively with acetaminophen, fluid therapy, and rest. If symptoms do not resolve within 24 to 48 hours, epidural blood patch may be considered, with recommended doses of 0.2 to 0.3 mL/kg autologous blood injected into the epidural space.

Further Reading

Coté CJ, Lerman H, Anderson BJ, eds. Coté and Lerman's A Practice of Anesthesia for Infants and Children. 5th ed. Philadelphia, PA: Elsevier; 2013:847.

Ylönen P, Kokki H. Management of postdural puncture headache with epidural blood patch in children. Paediatr Anaesth. 2002;12:526–529.

4.5. What is an appropriate enteral analgesic regimen for the child to receive after discharge home?

Recommendations for management of pain after discharge must take into account the age, comorbidities, and development of the child, as well as the type of surgery performed. For procedures with mild postoperative pain, such as inguinal hernia repair, scheduled or as-needed acetaminophen is the most common medication prescribed and is without significant gastric, renal, or hematologic side effects. Despite its safety, acetaminophen may have a narrow therapeutic index in certain children, and maximum daily dosages based on weight and age must be closely followed (75 mg/kg for children, 60 mg/kg for term infants, and 45 mg/kg for preterm infants). NSAIDs have been shown to be safe in children older than 6 months and are often prescribed in an alternating fashion with acetaminophen for mild postoperative pain. Patients who have received a regional anesthetic, such as a caudal, may not require enteral analgesics following block resolution. For moderate and severe postoperative pain, as may occur in open abdominal or orthopedic procedures, opioids are commonly required for adequate pain control. Of note, reports of death and other morbidity in young children treated with codeine for postoperative pain have severely limited its use as an analgesic. Adverse effects from codeine are related to genetic variability in metabolism to morphine and active metabolites by the CYP2D6 system, and in ultra-rapid metabolizers plasma morphine may increase to toxic levels, causing respiratory depression. If an enteral opioid analgesic must be prescribed after pediatric inguinal hernia repair, the most appropriate opioid is likely oxycodone liquid suspension 0.1 to 0.15 mg/kg every 6 hours as needed. Hydrocodone is typically formulated with acetaminophen and is less appropriate, as children may inadvertently be given additional doses of acetaminophen along with the hydrocodone/acetaminophen combination, increasing the risk of acetaminophen toxicity.

Further Reading

Coté CJ, Lerman H, Anderson BJ, eds. Coté and Lerman's A Practice of Anesthesia for Infants and Children. 5th ed. Philadelphia, PA: Elsevier; 2013:919.

Gregory GA, Andropoulos DB, eds. Gregory's Pediatric Anesthesia. 5th ed. Chicester, West Sussex: Wiley-Blackwell; 2012:845.

Tobias JD, Green TP, Coté CJ. Codeine: time to say "no." Pediatrics. 2016;138(4).

22

Pediatrics: Major Abdominal Surgery

Michale Sofer and Francis Wickham Kraemer III

Case Scenario

A 7-year-old boy presents for exploratory laparotomy for the excision of a Wilms' tumor. The patient is otherwise healthy and does not take any medications at home.

1. Patient Factors

1.1. What are the different ways to assess pain in a pediatric patient? How do you choose which method to use?

Pain, as well as response to treatment, should be assessed regularly and documented, typically alongside the patient's vitals. There are several reliable, valid, and clinically sensitive assessment tools available to assess pediatric pain in neonates through adolescents. The scales utilized to monitor pain can be categorized as being self-assessment, behavioral or observational, or physiologic, with some scales encompassing components of more than one category. Multiple studies have shown the commonly used scales to be reliable and valid for the assessment of pediatric pain. However, the scores from different scales do not correlate, and ideally a chosen scale should be used consistently for a patient, without scales being interchanged.

Pain is subjective, complex, and multifactorial, affected in part by physiologic, developmental, situational, behavioral, and psychological factors. It can be difficult to assess and is often inadequately assessed and treated in the pediatric population. Although no "gold standard" is defined, self-assessment is typically favored. However, in the pediatric population, patients commonly cannot self-assess their pain due to young age, cognitive impairment, difficulty with oration or motor skills, severe emotional distress, or language barrier. Caretaker observation of patient behavior can be used to complement the self-assessment and can be used as an alternative measure when self-assessment is not available. Self-report typically is achievable after 4 years of age. In an attempt to minimize provider bias and increase reliability, several scales have been introduced for observational pain assessment.

1.2. What are commonly used pediatric pain assessment scales?

1.2.1. N-PASS

The Neonatal Pain, Agitation and Sedation Scale (N-PASS) is an observational pain assessment scale designed for infants less than 1 year old. The patient is scored in each of the 5 categories (−2 to 2) to receive a cumulative pain score (0 to 10) and sedation score (0 to −10).

1.2.2. FLACC

The Face, Legs, Activity, Cry, Consolability (FLACC) scale is a behavioral pain assessment initially designed for younger patients who are nonverbal, preverbal, or unable to self-report their own pain (Table 22.1). The scale is structured into 5 categories. A care provider gives the patient a score of 0 to 2 in each category, to receive a cumulative score of 0 to 10.

1.2.3. Revised-FLACC

The revised-FLACC scale is a modification of the FLACC scale and is the more commonly used scale today (Table 22.2). It is utilized for pediatric patients who are unable to report their pain score due to age, difficulty with oration or motor

Table 22.1:
A pain scale for preverbal and nonverbal infants (FLACC scale)

Score			
Category	**0**	**1**	**2**
Face	No particular expression or smile	Occasional grimace or frown, withdrawn, disinterested	Frequent to constant quivering chin, clenched jaw
Legs	Normal position or relaxed	Uneasy, restless, tense	Kicking or legs drawn up
Activity	Lying quietly, normal position, moves easily	Squirming, shifting back and forth, tense	Arched, rigid, or jerking
Cry	No cry (awake or asleep)	Moans or whimpers, occasional complaint	Crying steadily, screams or sobs
Consolability	Content, relaxed	Reassured by occasional touching, hugging, or being talked to; distractible	Difficult to console or comfort

Reproduced with permission of Merkel SI et al. The FLACC: a behavioral scale for scoring postoperative pain in young children. *Pediatr Nurs*. 1997;23:392.

skills, or developmental disabilities. Similarly to FLACC, the patient is scored in each of the 5 categories, for a cumulative score of 0 to 10. Revised-FLACC was generated in response to a study revealing Legs and Activity to be the less sensitive and reliable assessment categories, especially in patients with cognitive impairment. As such, r-FLACC was modified to include several additional behavioral descriptors, including verbal outbursts, tremors, increased spasticity, jerking movements, and respiratory pattern changes (such as breath holding or grunting).

Table 22.2:
Revised FLACC Scale

Categories	0	1	2
Face	No particular expression or smile	Occasional grimace or frown, withdrawn, disinterested, **sad, appears worried**	Frequent to constant quivering chin, clenched jaw, **distressed looking face, expression of fright/panic**
Legs	Normal position or relaxed, **usual tone and motion to limbs**	Uneasy, restless, tense, **occasional tremors**	Kicking, or legs drawn up, **marked increase in spasticity, constant tremors, jerking**
Activity	Lying quietly, normal position, moves easily, **regular, rhythmic respirations**	Squirming, shifting back and forth, tense, **tense/guarded movements, mildly agitated, shallow/splinting respirations, intermittent sighs**	Arched, rigid or jerking, **severe agitation, head banging, shivering, breath holding, gasping, severe splinting**
Cry	No cry (awake or asleep)	Moans or whimpers; occasional complaint, **occasional verbal outbursts, constant grunting**	Crying steadily, screams or sobs, frequent complaints, **repeated outbursts, constant grunting**
Consolability	Content, relaxed	Reassured by occasional touching, hugging, or being talked to, distractible	Difficult to console or comfort, **pushing caregiver away, resisting care or comfort measures**

Reproduced with permission of Malviya S., The revised FLACC observational pain tool: improved reliability and validity for pain assessment in children with cognitive impairment. *Paediatr Anaesth*. 2006;16(3):258–265.

1.2.4. Numeric rating scale

The numeric rating scale is probably the most widely known self-assessment scale of pain intensity. It is best utilized for patients older than 7 years who are able to report their pain and correlate their level of pain to a number from 0 to 10, with 0 being "no pain" and 10 being the "worst pain."

1.2.5. FACES

The FACES pain scale is best used for children older than 3 years who are able to discuss and self-assess their pain but may not be able to translate their pain into an abstract number. As displayed in the pictorial scale, the leftmost "happy face" depicts no pain, and the scale progresses from left to right to a "crying face" depicting the worst pain.

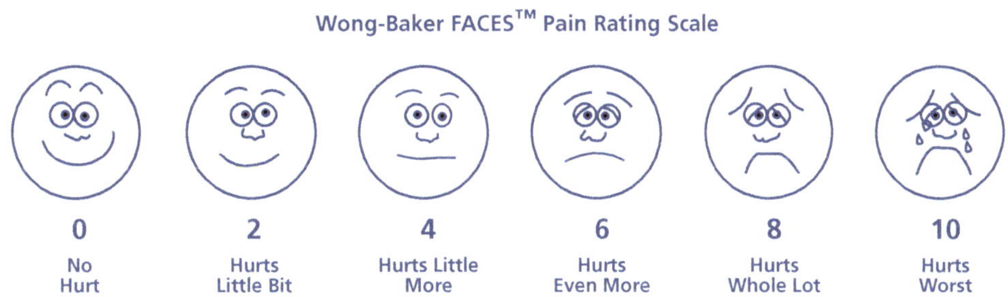

Further Reading

American Academy of Pediatrics. Committee on Psychosocial Aspects of Child and Family Health; Task Force on Pain in Infants, Children, and Adolescents. Assessment and management of acute pain in infants, children, and adolescents. *Pediatrics.* 2001;108:793–797.

Astuto M, Ingelmo PM. *Perioperative Medicine in Pediatric Anesthesia.* Anesthesia, Intensive Care and Pain in Neonates and Children. Cham: Springer International Publishing; 2016.

Chambers CT, Hardial J, Craig KD, et al. Faces scales for the measurement of postoperative pain intensity in children following minor surgery. *Clin J Pain.* 2005;21:277–285.

Lerman J, Coté CJ, Steward DJ. "Postoperative care and pain management." In: Lerman J, Coté CJ, Steward DJ. *Manual of Pediatric Anesthesia.* New York: Springer; 2016:211–225.

Malviya S, Voepel-Lewis T, Burke C, et al. The revised FLACC observational pain tool: improved reliability and validity for pain assessment in children with cognitive impairment. *Paediatr Anaesth.* 2006;16(3):258–265.

Merkel SI, Voepel-Lewis T, Shayevitz JR, et al. The FLACC: a behavioral scale for scoring postoperative pain in young children. *Pediatr Nurs.* 1997;23:293–297.

2. Surgical/Regional Anesthetic Considerations

2.1. Interventional analgesia

2.1.1. Which regional or neuraxial modalities should be considered? What are the risks and benefits of these interventions?

Current evidence supports the infusion of local anesthetics to the surgical site, continuous peripheral nerve blocks, and neuraxial anesthesia for postoperative pain control. All have been shown to decrease postoperative opioid requirements, often while improving functional recovery.

Current evidence recommends that epidural anesthesia be considered for all major abdominal, retroperitoneal, pelvic, and thoracic surgeries, and additionally may be considered for major orthopedic surgeries of the lower extremities. Epidural infusions may be utilized intraoperatively, typically as an adjunct to general anesthesia, but are most beneficial for postoperative pain control from major surgeries expected to result in protracted or severe pain. The infusion of a local anesthetic into the epidural space, with or without adjuvants such as opioids or clonidine, has been found to reliably decrease opioid requirements in the acute postoperative period.

Spinal anesthesia and combination spinal-epidural anesthesia are less commonly administered in the pediatric population, as compared with adults and obstetric anesthesia. Spinal anesthesia, which may be considered as a sole analgesic and anesthetic in newborns, may be considered for procedures that require quick onset and short duration. One common indication for spinal anesthesia in the pediatric population is its use for preterm infants at less than 60 weeks gestation who are undergoing short surgical procedures such as an inguinal hernia repair. In these patients, the utilization of spinal anesthesia eliminates the need for general anesthesia (except as a backup), eliminates the need for intraoperative opioids, and decreases (although does not eliminate) the risk of postoperative apnea.

2.1.2. What are the benefits of neuraxial anesthesia? Risks?

Regional and neuraxial anesthesia are associated with improved pain control and, importantly, with decreased perioperative opioid requirements and, consequently, decreased opioid-related side effects. These include decreased nausea and vomiting and decreased respiratory suppression, with fewer adverse respiratory events, and earlier extubation in patients who remain intubated postoperatively. Continuous epidural infusions postoperatively are also associated with an earlier return of gastrointestinal function, as compared with systemic opioid analgesia.

Prior to performing a neuraxial procedure, it is important to review for any contraindications, which include patient/parent refusal, infection at the procedural site or sepsis, coagulopathy, hypovolemia or shock, severe malformations of the spine or spinal cord, intraspinal tumors or lesions, elevated intracranial pressure with risk for herniation, and tethered cord syndrome.

Risks of neuraxial procedures in the pediatric setting are rare, but include epidural hematoma; epidural abscess or infection; lower extremity weakness; urinary retention; intravenous injection (with additional risk of local anesthetic toxicity); inadvertent subarachnoid injection (when placing an epidural); postdural puncture headache; sustained neurologic deficit or nerve injury; failed block; and inadvertent high epidural, subdural, or subarachnoid block. Hypotension is also possible but is a rare side effect in children less than 8 years old, as long as the patient does not become hypovolemic.

In a recent review of the Pediatric Regional Anesthesia Network (PRAN), Taenzer et al. reported an overall complication rate of 1.2%. A total of 27,214 neuraxial blocks were performed (94% of which were placed under general anesthesia), with the following complication rates reported:

Bleeding/hematoma: None observed
Death: Zero
Infection: 4 cases (.01%)
Unintended dural puncture: 2 cases (.007%)
Local anesthetic systemic toxicity: .01%

- 2 seizure
- 1 hypotension
- 2 cardiac arrest

Pressure sore: None observed
Compartment syndrome: None observed
Postneurologic symptoms: .013% short duration, .002% long duration

When considering variables to mitigate risk, the following should be considered:

- Presence of a dedicated acute pain service to follow/monitor patients, establish care pathways, and ensure quality improvement by tracking analgesic results

- Maintenance of strict sterile technique
- Consider caudal technique in neonates or younger infants
- Recognize increased risk of adverse drug events in neonates and younger infants

2.1.3. Which dermatomes should be blocked for this procedure? How about for a pancreatectomy? Inguinal hernia?

When performing neuraxial anesthesia for intraoperative or postoperative pain control, it is important to review the location of the surgical incision and place the spinal or epidural at the level appropriate to cover the necessary dermatomes. Making this assessment is aided with commonly used dermatomal landmarks. Anteriorly, T4 is at the level of the nipples, T10 is at the level of the umbilicus, and T12-L1 is the level of the pubis. Posteriorly, T7 is the lower edge of the wing of the scapula, and L4 is at the level of Tuffier's line, the line joining the posterior superior iliac crests (note: Tuffier's line crosses L5-S1 in patients less than 1 year old).

For a full exploratory laparotomy, optimal neuraxial coverage would include the full incision (xiphoid to pubis) from T4 to T12. Other typical incisions can be determined using the same landmarks. Neuraxial anesthesia for an open appendectomy should cover T10 to T12, open pancreatectomy should cover T6 to T8, and an open inguinal hernia repair should cover T11 to L1.

2.1.4. Which peripheral/truncal nerve blocks could be considered?

In addition to neuraxial anesthesia, peripheral regional anesthetic techniques that appropriately cover the abdominal wall and necessary dermatomes may be considered. For a variety of abdominal surgeries, options include transversus abdominis plane (TAP) block, bilateral paravertebral blocks, rectus sheath block, and quadratus lumborum block. Both TAP blocks and paravertebral blocks have been shown to be effective at reducing postoperative pain and decreasing opioid requirements in pediatric and adult patients undergoing abdominal surgeries. However, in a recent systematic review, single-injection truncal blockade in a mixed pediatric surgical cohort reported opioid reduction only in the first 6 to 8 hours following surgery, with a clinically insignificant change in pain scores. Thus, for invasive surgical interventions where prolonged nociception is expected, continuous neuraxial or truncal techniques should be considered.

Further Reading

Bernards C, Hostetter L. Epidural and spinal anesthesia. In: Barash ed. *Clinical Anesthesia*. Philadelphia, PA: Lippincott; 2013: 905–934.

Chakraborty A, Goswami J, Patro V. Ultrasound-guided continuous quadratus lumborum block for postoperative analgesia in a pediatric patient. *A Case Rep*. 2015 Feb 1; 4(3):34–36.

Hamill JK, Rahiri JL, Liley A, Hill AG. Rectus sheath and transversus abdominis plane blocks in children: a systematic review and meta-analysis of randomized trials. *Ped Anesth*. 2016;26;363–371.

Lerman J, Coté CJ, Steward DJ. Regional analgesia techniques. In: Lerman J, Coté CJ, Steward DJ. *Manual of Pediatric Anesthesia*. New York: Springer; 2016:141–166.

Maitra S, Baidya DK, Pawar DK, Arora MK, Khanna P. Epidural anesthesia and analgesia in the neonate: a review of current evidences. *J Anesth*. 2014;28:768–779.

Dadure C, Sola C, Dalens B, Capdevila X. Regional anesthesia in children. In: Miller, ed. *Anesthesia*. 7th ed. Philadelphia, PA: Elsevier/Saunders; 2010:2519–2557.

Rowney DA, Doyle E. Epidural and subarachnoid blockade in children. *Anaesthesia*. 1998;53:980–1001.

Suresh S, Schaldenbrand K, Wallis B, De Oliveira GSJ. Regional anaesthesia to improve pain outcomes in paediatric surgical patients: a qualitative systematic review of randomized controlled trials. *Br J Anaesth*. 2014;113(3):375–390.

2.2. Relationship of spinal anatomy in infants and children versus adults

2.2.1. Is spinal anatomy the same in the pediatric patient as in an adult? How?

There are notable differences in spinal anatomy in pediatric patients, as compared with an adult, which contribute to procedural decisions and drug dosing. The spinal cord in an infant (less than 1 year old) may extend as far as L3 but it reaches the adult level of L1/2 by 1 year of age. The dural sac extends to S3/4 in a neonate, as compared with the adult level of S1 also reached by 1 year of age. The more caudally ending dural sac makes it more likely to have an inadvertent dural puncture during placement of caudal blocks. In addition, the shape of the spinal column changes with growth and development. The neonatal vertebral column is kyphotic due to the flexed intrauterine posture, but as infants gain head control by 3 to 4 months of age, they develop anterior convexity of the cervical spine. By 12 to 18 months, with ambulation and further development, the spine displays a lumbar lordosis.

2.2.2. Is there a way to predict the intervertebral depth of the epidural space?

Although there is no absolute equation for predicting depth from skin to epidural space, there are some suggestions for estimation. When performing neuraxial anesthetic procedures, it is important to keep in mind that this estimate may not be accurate, as it is impacted by the weight of the child and amount of subcutaneous fat, as well as the angle of needle entry (perpendicular will be a shorter pathway than 30 degrees, etc.). The depth of the subarachnoid space is approximately 10 mm at birth and 16 mm at 3 years in the lumbar region. In children between 6 months and 10 years old, who weigh more than 10 kg, the distance from skin to lumbar epidural space in millimeters is approximately equal to the child's weight in kilograms. Use of an ultrasound probe allows for a more accurate estimate of the distance from skin to the ligamentum flavum.

2.2.3. How do these anatomic differences along with differences in cerebrospinal fluid volume affect spinal drug in pediatric patients as compared with adults?

The volume of cerebrospinal fluid (CSF) varies considerably with age. In neonates, CSF volume is greater than 10 mL/kg. Infants weighing less than 15 kg have approximately 4 mL/kg of CSF volume, which decreases to 3 mL/kg in children. In adolescence, the CSF volume is 2 mL/kg, half that of an infant. In addition, the distribution of CSF changes with aging. At birth, 50% of CSF is contained within the spine, while in adolescents and adults this amount is 25%. These variations result in differences in the pharmacodynamic and pharmacokinetic properties of intrathecally administered local anesthetic drugs. As such, the larger CSF volume (and resultant drug dilution) may account in part for the higher local anesthetic dose requirements and shorter duration of action of spinal anesthesia in pediatric patients as compared with adults.

Further Reading

Dalens B. Regional anesthetic techniques. In: Bissonnette B, Dalens B., ed. *Pediatric Anesthesia: Principles and Practice.* New York: McGraw-Hill; 2002:141–166.

Lerman J, Coté CJ, Steward DJ. Regional analgesia techniques. In: Lerman J, Coté CJ, Steward DJ. *Manual of Pediatric Anesthesia.* New York: Springer; 2016:141–166.

Dadure C, Sola C, Dalens B, Capdevila X. Regional anesthesia in children. In: Miller, ed. Anesthesia. 7th ed. Philadelphia, PA: Elsevier/Saunders; 2010:2519–2557.

Rowney DA, Doyle E. Epidural and subarachnoid blockade in children. *Anaesthesia.* 1998;53(10):980–1001.

2.3. Indications and technical approaches to continuous catheter techniques

2.3.1. When would you consider placing a continuous catheter rather than a single-shot epidural?

When utilizing an epidural for analgesia or as an adjunct to intraoperative anesthesia, anesthesiologists most commonly opt to place an epidural catheter. Placing an epidural catheter is only slightly more arduous than performing a single-injection epidural, yet it affords the clinician much more flexibility with regard to the epidural blockade. Via the catheter, medication can be redosed for longer procedures, medication can be administered continuously for long procedures or postoperative pain control, and additional medication can be given for a block that is "too low" (not covering high enough dermatomes). Placement of an epidural catheter, rather than a single-injection epidural, should therefore be considered for procedures with the potential to outlast the duration of action of a single epidural bolus dose (variable depending on the choice of medication and additives), or in patients expected to have significant postoperative pain or who would benefit from decreased postoperative opioid requirements.

2.3.2. What are the risks of placing an indwelling catheter? How do we minimize them?

Similar to single-injection epidural placement, risks include epidural hematoma; epidural abscess or infection, lower extremity weakness; urinary retention; postdural puncture headache; sustained neurologic deficit or nerve injury; failed block; and inadvertent high epidural, subdural, or subarachnoid block. In addition, there is a risk of inadvertent catheter placement into an epidural vein (with additional risk of local anesthetic toxicity) or into the subarachnoid space.

Specific considerations when placing a catheter include the risk of catheter migration, potentially into an epidural vein, the subarachnoid space, or an intervertebral foramen. Catheter migration may result in an unintentional subarachnoid block, intravenous administration of local anesthetic (with risk of local anesthetic systemic toxicity), a failed block, or a unilateral block. Catheter migration should be suspected if the analgesic response to an epidural changes, is different than would be expected, or systemic side effects are seen. A unilateral block may also result from septum in the epidural space or the catheter tip lodging in the anterior epidural space. Other risks include inadvertent catheter removal, skin irritation from the adhesive or prep solution, disruption of the dressing with possible contamination of the catheter site (with risk of infection), catheter breakage, and leaking at the insertion site. All of these warrant reinspection of the patient and the epidural catheter, with consideration of catheter removal depending on the findings.

2.3.3. What techniques are available for confirming correct epidural catheter placement? How can we utilize them? (ultrasound, contrast injection, test dose, fluoroscopy, X-ray)

Because epidural catheters are usually placed through a Touhy or Hustead needle, the same needles are commonly used to access the epidural space for a single-injection epidural blockade. After identifying the ligamentum flavum and advancing the needle tip to the point of "loss of resistance," the catheter is threaded through the needle, with 3 to 4 cm of catheter beyond the tip of the needle. The placement of additional length increases the risks of catheter migration and increases the uncertainty of where the catheter tip lies and which dermatomes will be covered. It is important to note the depth to "loss of resistance," as well as the marking of the catheter at the insertion site for postoperative follow-up, in case there is a question of the catheter becoming dislodged.

Even following an uncomplicated catheter placement, it is important to confirm catheter position, which can be done in a variety of ways. The first step is always to aspirate on the catheter with a syringe, looking for return of blood or CSF (as a first measure of ruling out catheter placement into the subarachnoid space or an epidural vein). It is important to keep in mind that the incidence of false-negative aspirations is high, and thus this step should not be used as a sole measure of confirmation. Next, a test dose should be administered slowly through the catheter, again to check for placement into the subarachnoid space or an epidural vein prior to administering the full epidural dose. The consequence of inadvertent intravascular injection depends on the plasma level of the local anesthetic, as well as its rate of rise, making a slower injection safer. The most common test dose is a local anesthetic with epinephrine 1:200,000 (5 mcg/mL). However, it is important to recognize that the intravenous injection of epinephrine in a pediatric patient may not produce the same cardiovascular changes (increased heart rate and hypertension) that would be expected in an adult. Additionally, because many pediatric patients may be under general anesthesia during epidural placement, it is clear that there are limitations to the utility of the test dose in the pediatric population. However, while injecting the local anesthetic slowly, one should watch for peaked T-waves, arrhythmias, and tachycardia. Due to the risk of undetected catheter migration, it is advised to repeat these 2 steps prior to additional bolus doses.

In addition, other methods may be used to confirm epidural catheter placement and catheter tip location, which are especially important when threading a catheter into the lumbar or thoracic epidural space from the caudal approach. Fluoroscopy imaging of a radiopaque or styletted catheter may be used to confirm catheter tip location with respect to the vertebral bodies. The injection of a small dose of contrast into the catheter will identify the location of the catheter tip, as well as confirm the catheter's presence in the epidural space, rather than into a vein, subcutaneous space, or intervertebral foramen. Ultrasound imaging may also be utilized for confirmation of catheter location in neonates and infants, although this technique may be challenging in all patients and has limited utility in patients older than 3 months or weighing more than 10 to 12 kg. Finally, low electrical stimulation (Tsui test) can be used whereby an electrode is connected to the epidural catheter and stimulated with a current of 1 mA up to 10 mA. Elicited motor responses at very low current (<1 mA) indicate possible subarachnoid placement whereby motor responses at high currents (>10 mA) may suggest catheter placement in the subcutaneous tissue. Motor responses that occur within the reference current range and that diminish with local anesthetic injection suggest proper placement into the epidural space. However, intravascular placement may be present if motor responses remain following local anesthetic injection.

Further Reading

Bernards C, Hostetter L. Epidural and spinal anesthesia. In: Barash ed. *Clinical Anesthesia*. Philadelphia, PA: Lippincott; 2013: 905–934.

Maitra S, Baidya DK, Pawar DK, Arora MK, Khanna P. Epidural anesthesia and analgesia in the neonate: a review of current evidences. *J Anesth*. 2014;28:768–779.

Rowney DA, Doyle E. Epidural and subarachnoid blockade in children. *Anaesthesia*. 1998;53:980–1001.

Taenzer AH, Clark C 5th, Kovarik WD. Experience with 724 epidurograms for epidural catheter placement in pediatric anesthesia. *Reg Anesth Pain Med*. 2010 Sep–Oct;35(5):432–435.

Tsui BCH, Suresh S. Ultrasound imaging for regional anesthesia in infants, children and adults: a review of current literature and its application in the practice of neuraxial blocks. *Anesthesiology*. 2010;112:719–728.

3. Postoperative Pain Management

3.1. Advantages and limitations of patient-controlled and nurse-controlled analgesia in pediatric populations

3.1.1. When would you consider using a patient-controlled analgesia?

Patient-controlled analgesia (PCA) is the delivery of intravenous opioids for pain control through a computerized pump that is activated by the patient or nurse. In most cases, small boluses of opioid are delivered at short dosing intervals, depending on the pharmacokinetics of the medication. The pump is programmed to limit the total amount of opioid delivered over time. The pump records the patient's medication usage, which can drive the medical teams' decision-making. In pediatric pain control, most children older than 5 or 6 years can successfully use a PCA. The child should be sufficiently cognitively developed to know that pressing the button will result in drug delivery to help control pain. Limits of drug delivery are programmed into the pump to mitigate accidental overdose. All patients have cardiorespiratory monitoring at the initiation of the PCA for at least 24 hours and when any changes are made in the PCA programming.

3.1.2. Would you consider a continuous infusion?

The PCA has the ability to deliver continuous opioid infusions in addition to the bolus function. There is mixed literature on the utility of continuous infusions. On the one hand, a continuous infusion allows for less variability of in vivo drug levels, which will allow for better pain control during sleep when the PCA is not activated. On the other hand, a continuous infusion may lead to excessive dosing as the patient heals with systemic side effects like respiratory depression, pruritus, nausea, and vomiting even if the pain is under good control. In this scenario, the risks outweigh the benefits for providing a continuous infusion of opioids. In situations where the patient is unable to press the PCA due to cognitive delay or immaturity and he or she is expected to have severe acute pain, a continuous infusion may be warranted for 24 to 48 hours as the patient heals. In this second scenario, a nurse-controlled analgesia (NCA) pump could be employed instead of a continuous infusion.

3.1.3. What are the benefits of PCA use compared with nurse-administered bolus dosing?

The benefits of a PCA extend beyond the pharmacodynamics of the delivered drug. The PCA provides reliable, immediate pain relief that is controlled by the patient who is experiencing the pain. This reliability can alleviate anxiety about pain control, even to the point of some children asking to take the PCA home with them. Because pain is always subjective, the goal in using the PCA is to deliver medication when the patient has pain or expects pain. By using smaller doses and frequent dosing intervals of minutes, the patient can maintain appropriate blood levels depending on his or her unique metabolism of the medication. In contrast, a nurse-administered bolus is usually given based on the half-life, in hours, of the opioid medication and at higher doses than with a PCA. The administration of the dose can be highly variable from the initial request for the pain medication to the actual administration due to the many steps of acquiring the drug and the chance of nursing distraction to handle other patients' more pressing medical needs. This variability can cause anxiety in the patient and worsen the pain. The higher dosing can lead to more side effects due to higher peak blood levels.

3.1.4. Is it safe for a patient to have both a PCA and neuraxial anesthesia?

In a multimodal pain management plan, the PCA and neuraxial analgesia are primary components. When local anesthetics are given neuraxially, there can be times when supplemental analgesia is needed due to catheter problems or to pain that occurs outside of the dermatomal coverage. Intermittent opioids can provide supplemental analgesia. The inverse cannot be done when a PCA is the primary pain management tool. The placement of a neuraxial catheter carries rare but serious risks. Therefore, the neuraxial catheter should be used as the primary modality when possible in each clinical case and not as supplemental analgesia. Even single-shot neuraxial analgesia requires a sterile environment and a safe patient condition to avoid infection or needle trauma and is not performed as rescue pain control.

While it is possible to use both the PCA and neuraxial analgesia at the same time, this is a rare occurrence. A PCA can be used to provide supplemental analgesia if the neuraxial anesthesia is a failure. While neuraxial analgesia is often superior to intravenous opioids for major abdominal and thoracic surgical procedures, problems with the invasive catheter can lead to inadequate pain control, and a PCA is the next best option. Using a PCA in a situation where there is optimal pain control provided by neuraxial analgesia places the patient at undue risk of opioid side effects such as respiratory depression, sedation, gastrointestinal dysmotility, and urinary retention. These opioid side effects can also mask local anesthetic toxicity symptoms such as agitation and mimic late side effects such obtundation. Obviously, the treatment of opioid-induced respiratory depression in a somnolent, obtunded patient is much different than the treatment of local anesthesia systemic toxicity in an obtunded patient. The use of intravenous opioids can also slow down the transition time to enteral medication, which is recommended for acute postoperative pain over intravenous medication. The routine use of a PCA and neuraxial analgesia is not recommended.

Further Reading

Chou R, Gordon DB, de Leon Casasola OA, et al. Management of postoperative pain: a clinical practice guideline from the American Pain Society, the American Society of Regional Anesthesia and Pain Medicine, and the American Society of

Anesthesiologists' Committee on Regional Anesthesia, Executive Committee, and Administrative Council. *J Pain*. 2016 Feb;17(2):131–157.

Walker BJ, Polaner DM, Berde CB. Acute pain. In: Cote CJ, Lerman J, Anderson BJ , ed. *A Practice of Anesthesia for Infants and Children*. 5th ed. Philadelphia, PA: Elsevier; 2013:909–950.

Karl HW, Tyler DC, Miser AW. Controlled trial of morphine vs hydromorphone for patient-controlled analgesia in children with postoperative pain. *Pain Med*. 2012;13:1658–1659

Pediatric Orthopedic Surgery

Karen Boretskty

23

Case Scenario

A 10-year-old 36-kg boy suffers a fall while biking and presents for fixation of a distal radius fracture. His history is significant for attention deficit hyperactivity disorder, for which he takes methylphenidate extended release.

1. Preoperative Factors

1.1. What patient factors need to be taken into consideration when preparing a plan for the anesthesia and analgesia for this patient?

Forearm fractures are common injuries during childhood. When presenting for repair, both acute and chronic conditions need to be considered for purposes of perioperative planning. Elective surgery should be delayed for 2 hours following clear liquids and 6 hours following full liquids or a light meal. Heavy meals with a high fat content require 8 hours of digestion. The rate of gastric emptying, however, is slowed by both pain and opioid administration, and a conservative approach to induction and airway management, including a rapid-sequence induction with endotracheal intubation, may be prudent regardless of time from food intake to induction of anesthesia. Preinduction gastric imaging with ultrasound has recently been advocated as a more objective method of determining gastric volume and possible risk of aspiration.

Emergent surgery is indicated in the event of an open fracture, exposed bone, or neurovascular compromise (i.e., lack of perfusion and arterial pulses). Surgery should be planned as soon as feasible and gastric aspiration precautions observed. A mature and cooperative pediatric patient may have regional anesthesia (RA) in the form of a brachial plexus block with local anesthetic (LA) plus intravenous sedation. A rapid-sequence induction with endotracheal intubation is preferred if general anesthesia (GA) is indicated. Cuffed endotracheal tubes are recommended in children of this age. The use of succinylcholine in pediatric patients carries a black box warning from the Food and Drug Administration (FDA) due to potential hyperkalemic cardiac arrest in the presence of undiagnosed muscular dystrophy. Duchenne's muscular dystrophy is the most common of the muscular dystrophies, occurring predominantly in males, and the diagnosis is usually made in the first 5 years of life. Because the incidence of aspiration of gastric contents is more common than muscular dystrophy, and given the low probability that this patient has an undiagnosed myopathy, the use of succinylcholine may be justified. A modified rapid sequence using a nondepolarizing muscle relaxant is also acceptable.

This patient's medical history includes attention deficit hyperactivity disorder (ADHD) treated with extended-release methylphenidate, a form of amphetamine. ADHD occurs in 8% to 12% of pediatric patients and is an added risk factor for long bone fractures. Patients on chronic amphetamine treatment will have depleted endogenous catecholamine stores and may be more susceptible to intraoperative hypotension and bradycardia. These hemodynamic changes will not respond to indirect-acting catecholamine drugs like ephedrine, and patients will likely require direct-acting drugs such as epinephrine in the event of hypotension. The literature on patients having surgery without stopping chronic amphetamines is mixed; some patients have had dramatic episodes of refractory hypotension, and others have experienced no issues. For patients on these medications, the last dose administered should be confirmed and subsequent doses held pending surgery.

Further Reading

Cartabuke RS, Tobias JD, Rice J, Tumin D. Hemodynamic profile and behavioral characteristics during induction of anesthesia in pediatric patients with attention deficit hyperactivity disorder. *Paediatr Anaesth*. 2017;27:417–424.

Chou IC, Lin CC, Sung FC, Kao CH. Attention-deficit-hyperactivity disorder increases risk of bone fracture: a population-based cohort study. *Dev Med Child Neurol*. 2014;56:1111–1116.

Fischer SP, Healzer JM, Brook MW, Brock-Utne JG. General anesthesia in a patient on long-term amphetamine therapy: is there cause for concern? *Anesth Analg*. 2000;91:758–759.

Fischer SP, Schmiesing CA, Guta CG, Brock-Utne JG. General anesthesia and chronic amphetamine use. *Anesth Analg*. 2006;103:203–206.

Larach MG, Rosenberg H, Gronert GA, Allen GC. Hyperkalemic cardiac arrest during anesthesia in infants and children with occult myopathies. *Clin Pediatr*. 1997;36:916.

Mazurek AJ, Rae B, Hann S, Kim JI, Castro B, Coté CJ. Rocuronium versus succinylcholine: are they equally effective during rapid-sequence induction of anesthesia? *Anesth Analg*. 1998;87:1259–1262.

Schmitz A, Schmidt AR, Buehler PK, et al. Gastric ultrasound as a preoperative bedside test for residual gastric contents in children. *Paediatr Anaesth*. 2016;12:1157–1164.

Shi F, Xiao Y, Xiong W, Zhou Q, Huang X. Cuffed versus uncuffed endotracheal tubes in children: a meta-analysis. *J Anesth.* 2016;30:3–11.

1.2. What are the considerations for multimodal analgesia in the pediatric population?

Bone-related pain following open reduction internal fixation is often severe and difficult to treat. In children, acute pain is best managed by a multimodal approach in which nonpharmacologic methods, smaller doses of opioid and nonopioid analgesics, local anesthetic infiltration, and regional anesthetic techniques are combined to target multiple pain pathways. The result is better pain control with fewer drug-induced adverse effects. Such a multimodal technique advocates for opioids as a rescue therapy and no longer as first-line pain therapy.

The most commonly used nonopioid analgesic in pediatric practice is acetaminophen. While the exact mechanism of action is unclear, inhibition of prostaglandin synthesis in the central nervous system, activation of descending serotonergic pathways, cannabinoid agonism, and NMDA/Substance P antagonism are postulated pathways. Acetaminophen has minimal anti-inflammatory effect, lacks renal toxicity, and has not been implicated in antiplatelet activity or bone healing. Intravenous administration of acetaminophen avoids first-pass hepatic exposure, which may reduce the potential for hepatic injury, but acetaminophen should be used cautiously in patients with severe hepatic impairment or active liver disease. The recommended dose is 15 mg/kg PO or IV administered every 6 hours as needed. The daily maximum dose in children/adolescents is 75 mg/kg/d or 4 g, whichever is less. For preterm and term infants the daily maximum dose is 30 and 60 mg/kg/d, respectively.

Nonsteroidal anti-inflammatory drugs (NSAIDs) have established efficacy in children via anti-inflammatory and analgesic mechanisms through the blockade of prostaglandin and thromboxane synthesis by cyclooxygenase-1 (COX-1) and cyclooxygenase-2 (COX-2) enzymes. Nonselective NSAIDs such as ibuprofen, naproxen, and ketorolac, inhibit both COX-1 and COX-2. Of note, irritation of the gastric mucosa by COX nonselective NSAIDs is less common in children. The COX nonselective NSAIDs also reversibly inhibit platelet aggregation and cause small increases in bleeding time, rarely exceeding normal values. While there is no evidence that NSAIDs increase surgical bleeding complications, this may cause concern for some practitioners and should be individually considered. Selective COX-2 inhibitors such as celecoxib cause minimal gastric irritation or changes in platelet function. While NSAIDs have been linked to delayed bone healing in some animal models, they are widely considered appropriate in pediatrics, especially for short durations following surgery. Pediatric doses for the most common NSAIDs are shown in Table 23.1.

Nonopioid analgesics, when used alone, are best suited for mild to moderate pain. NSAIDs and acetaminophen are often combined for treating mild to moderate postoperative pain and result in superior analgesia to either drug alone. Nonopioid analgesics should be administered on a scheduled basis after an acute injury and not as needed in order to provide consistent basal analgesia and prevent analgesic gaps. Pediatric data on the perioperative value of ketamine and gabapentin are limited, but there are benefits in patients with chronic pain.

Table 23.1:
Dosing recommendations for common NSAIDs

Drug	COX-2 Specific	Route	Dose	Interval	Maximum Dose (Single)	Maximum Dose (24-hour)
Ibuprofen	No	PO/IV	10 mg/kg	q6–8h	400 mg	2400 mg
Ketorolac	No	IV/IM	0.5 mg/kg	q6–8h	30 mg	120 mg
Celecoxib	Yes	PO				
>10–25 kg			50 mg	q12h	50 mg	100 mg
>25 kg			100 mg	q12h	100 mg	200 mg

Further Reading

Anderson BJ. Paracetamol (acetaminophen): mechanisms of action. *Paediatr Anaesth.* 2008;18:915–921.

Bertolini A, Ferrari A, Ottani A, et al. Paracetamol: new vistas of an old drug. CNS Drug Rev. 2006;12:250–275.

Gazal G, Mackie IC. A comparison of paracetamol, ibuprofen or their combination for pain relief following extractions in children under general anaesthesia: a randomized controlled trial. *Int J Paediatr Dent.* 2007; 7:169–177.

Graham GG, Scott KF. Mechanism of action of paracetamol. *Am J Ther.* 2005;12:46–55.

Hartling L, Ali S, Dryden DM, et al. How safe are common analgesics for the treatment of acute pain for children? A systematic review. *Pain Res Manag.* 2016:5346819.

Jahr JS, Lee VK. Intravenous acetaminophen. *Anesthesiol Clin.* 2010;28:619–645.

Kokki H. Nonsteroidal anti-inflammatory drugs for postoperative pain: a focus on children. *Paedr Drugs.* 2003;5:103–123.

Munsterhjelm E, Niemi TT, Ylikorkala O, et al. Influence on platelet aggregation of i.v. parecoxib and acetaminophen in healthy volunteers. *Br J Anaesth.* 2006;97:226–231.

Niemi TT, Taxell C, Rosenberg PH. Comparison of the effect of intravenous ketoprofen, ketorolac and diclofenac on platelet function in volunteers. *Acta Anaesthesiol Scand.* 1997;41:1353–1358.

O'Connor JP, Lysz T. Celecoxib, NSAIDs and the skeleton. *Drugs Today.* 2008;44:693–709.

Wong I, St John-Green C, Walker SM. Opioid-sparing effects of perioperative paracetamol and nonsteroidal anti-inflammatory drugs (NSAIDs) in children. *Paediatr Anaesth.* 2013;23:475–495.

Yaster M. Multimodal analgesia in children. *Eur J Anaesthesthiol.* 2010;27:851–857.

1.3. What are considerations related to opioid administration in this patient?

In situations where opioid therapy is warranted, combination therapy with nonopioid and opioid medications (i.e., multimodal) results in a lower risk of serious and minor adverse events compared with opioid monotherapy. This reinforces the concept of adding opioid medications to, rather than replacing, nonopioid medication for moderate to severe pain. Opioid analgesics have the greatest risk of sedation, respiratory depression, nausea and vomiting, constipation, and pruritis. Similar to in adults, morphine, fentanyl, and hydromorphone are the most commonly administered IV opioid analgesics. Additionally, oxycodone, hydrocodone, and morphine are the most commonly administered oral opioids and can often be found in fixed combination with acetaminophen. In pediatric patients, it is recommended to administer the opioid and acetaminophen as separate medications and not as a combined formulation, to avoid potential acetaminophen over- and underdosing.

Codeine is no longer advocated for use in children. Codeine is a prodrug that has no intrinsic analgesic properties and must be metabolized into morphine. Large individual pharmacogenetic variation in the efficiency of conversion results in a subgroup of patients, hypermetabolizers, who produce excessive amounts of morphine when exposed to codeine. Hypermetabolism has been associated with inadvertent overdose, respiratory depression, and death. The FDA has issued a black box warning, and most pediatric hospitals in the United States have removed codeine from their formularies. Dosing for the most common opioids is shown in Table 23.2.

Sample calculations for the given case: 36-kg patient with a forearm fracture:

1. Acetaminophen: 15 mg/kg × 36 kg = 540 mg q6h. Start oral dosing upon arrival at hospital and continue q6. Convert to IV administration if a dose is due while patient is in the operating room. Convert back to PO when oral intake resumes.
2. Ketorolac: 0.50 mg/kg × 36 kg = 18 mg q6h IV; round to 15 mg q dose to avoid dilution errors. Utilize 15 mg q6h when IV access is first established, either in the emergency department or in the operating room. Continue for 24 hours total.

Table 23.2:
Guidelines for opioid dosing

Drug	Route	Dose	Maximum single Dose (opioid naive)	Interval
Morphine	IV	0.05–0.1 mg/kg		
	PO	0.15–0.3 mg/kg	30	q4–6h
Hydromorphone	IV	0.01–0.02 mg/kg		
	PO		4	q4–6h
Fentanyl	IV	0.5–1 mcg/kg		
Oxycodone	PO	0.05–0.1 mg/kg	10	q4–6h

3. Morphine sulphate (IV): 0.05 × 36 kg = 1.8 mg. Round to 1.5 mg q dose to avoid dilution errors. Titrate doses q 5 to 10 minutes to establish comfort in the emergency room, then order 1.8 mg IV q2–4h PRN breakthrough pain ≥4/10. Convert to oxycodone when oral intake resumes.
4. Oxycodone: 0.05 × 36 kg = 1.8 mg. Round to 1.5 mg q dose to avoid dilution errors. Order 1.5 mg PO q4–6h PRN breakthrough pain ≥4/10.

Further Reading

Hartling L, Ali S, Dryden DM, et al. How safe are common analgesics for the treatment of acute pain for children? A systematic review. *Pain Res Manag*. 2016:5346819.

Tobias JD, Green TP, Coté CJ. Codeine: time to say "no." *Pediatrics*. 2016;138:e1–e7.

Tobias JD, Green TP, Coté CJ, Racoosin JA. Death and respiratory arrest related to ultra-rapid metabolism of codeine to morphine. www.fda.gov/downloads/AdvisoryCommittees/CommitteesMeetingMaterials/PediatricAdvisoryCommittee/UCM343601.pdf. Accessed January 6, 2017.

2. Regional Anesthesia Considerations

2.1. Discuss how regional anesthesia use and timing differ in pediatric populations compared with adult populations

Peripheral nerve blocks (PNBs) offer safe and effective alternatives to GA and neuraxial anesthesia. A PNB may be used as the sole anesthetic (with or without sedation), as a supplement to GA, and/or for postoperative analgesia. In pediatric patients the latter 2 are most common. A brachial plexus block to provide analgesia should be considered for this patient and placed while in the operating room. In pediatrics, RA is most often used in combination with GA. Nerve block placement commonly occurs after anesthetic induction due to the safety concerns of performing RA in an awake and uncooperative child. Although this necessitates 2 anesthetics, RA adds benefit by decreasing dose exposure to GA and providing excellent control of postsurgical pain. Placement of RA may occur before or after the surgery, depending on the type of procedure, location of the nerve block, and expected placement of a perineural catheter. In small children, catheter dressings may approach the surgical field; therefore, placement of the catheter at the end of the surgery may be preferred.

Most PNBs utilized in adults have been used in children of all ages. Primary differences include the size and location of the nerves, as well as the proximity to adjacent critical structures. An infraclavicular brachial plexus block with a catheter is a good choice for this patient due to anticipated inpatient stay, affected bone distal to the midhumeral shaft, and incisions over the forearm. Supraclavicular or axillary blocks may also be acceptable choices, but catheter fixation and retention may be challenging. In the infraclavicular location, the brachial plexus lies deep to both pectoralis muscles, which provide better tethering to secure a catheter. In the case of lower extremity fracture, PNB, plexus block, or epidural analgesia can be used. However, recent large studies demonstrate a lower failure rate and more favorable risk profile for PNBs when compared with neuraxial blocks.

Further Reading

Coté C, Lerman J, Anderson B. A Practice of Anesthesia for Infants and Children. 5th ed. Philadelpa, PA: Elsevier; 2013.

Ecoffey C, Lacroix F, Giaufre E, et al. Association des Anesthesistes Reanimateurs Pediatriques d'Expression F. Epidemiology and morbidity of regional anesthesia in children: a follow-up one-year prospective survey of the French-Language Society of Paediatric Anaesthesiologists (ADARPEF). *Pediatr Anesth.* 2010;20:1061–1069.

Krane EJ, Dalens BJ, Murat I, Murrell D. The safety of epidurals placed during general anesthesia. *Reg Anesth Pain Med.* 1998;23:433–438.

Polaner D, Taenzer A, Walker B, et al. Pediatric Regional Anesthesia Network (PRAN): a multi-institutional study of the use and incidence of complications of pediatric regional anesthesia. *Anesth Analg.* 2012;115:1353–1364.

2.2. Evaluate the safety data of performing regional anesthesia in the unconscious pediatric patient

In adult populations, placement of RA under GA has been highly discouraged due to concerns of masking early warning signs of complications such as local anesthetic systemic toxicity (LAST) and nerve trauma. RA placement in awake children is often not feasible due to lack of cooperation; consequently, nerve block placement in children under GA has been accepted as the standard of care. In 2014, a multicenter analysis using the Pediatric Regional Anesthesia Network database demonstrated no difference in morbidity or mortality whether RA was administered in awake or anesthetized children. This is true for both neuraxial and PNBs. Similarly, the use of neuromuscular blocking drugs at the time of placement of regional anesthesia did not affect outcomes. LAST was more common in young children, and neurologic complications occurred most often in older children, yet both were rare events. When neurologic deficits did occur as the result of RA, they were most often transient and resolved within 6 months. Controversy still exists about the safety of performing interscalene blocks in children under GA or heavy sedation due to risk of catastrophic complications. American Society of Regional Anesthesia and Pain Medicine (ASRA) guidelines recommend placement of interscalene nerve blocks in awake or lightly sedated patients. However, a recent study of nearly 400 interscalene blocks placed under GA in pediatric patients reports no associated complications.

In adult populations, the use of ultrasound guidance has decreased the incidence of LAST without an appreciable difference in postblock nerve injury. Pediatric-specific data addressing changes in the incidence of infrequent complications as a result of increased ultrasound use are still lacking. However, ultrasound guidance does improve block efficacy and decrease required local anesthetic dose for select blocks in children.

Further Reading

Bernards CM, Hadzic, A, Suresh S, Neal JM. Regional anesthesia in anesthetized or heavily sedated patients. *Reg Anesth Pain Med.* 2008;33:449–460.

Ecoffey C, Oger E, Marchand-Maillet F, et al, SOS French Regional Anaesthesia Hotline. *Eur J Anaesthesiol.* 2014;31:606–610.

Krane EJ, Dalens BJ, Murat I, Murrell D. The safety of epidurals placed during general anesthesia. *Reg Anesth Pain Med.* 1998;23:433–438.

Neal JM, Bernards CM, et al. ASRA practice advisory on neurologic complications in regional anesthesia and pain medicine. *Reg Anesth Pain Med.* 2008;33:404–415.

Oberndorfer U, Marhofer P, Bosenberg A, et al. Ultrasound guidance for sciatic and femoral nerve blocks in children. *Br J Anaesth.* 2007;98:797–801.

Taenzer A, Walker BJ, et al. Asleep vs. awake: does it matter? Pediatric regional block complications by patient state: a report from the pediatric regional anesthesia network. *Reg Anesth Pain Med.* 2014;39:279–283.

Taenzer A, et al. Interscalene brachial plexus blocks under general anesthesia in children: is this safe practice? *Reg Anesth Pain Med.* 2014;39:502–505.

2.3. Discuss general indications and contraindications for regional anesthesia in pediatric patients

General considerations for the performance of RA include suitability for the proposed surgery, experience in performing the block, and patient/caregiver cooperation. RA has the advantage of improved patient satisfaction, superior analgesia, decreased incidence of postoperative nausea and vomiting, decreased exposure to GA medications (which may be especially important in younger children), and fewer postoperative cognitive changes. Risks of RA include seizures, cardiac arrest, temporary or chronic nerve damage, localized infection, and block failure.

Absolute contraindications to RA are the same in children as in adults and include patient refusal, infection at the needle insertion site, and true allergy to LA medication. True allergic reactions are rare and require further identification of the LA class as there is no cross-reactivity between amides and esters. Ester LA has a higher incidence of allergic reactions than amide LA.

Relative contraindications are more controversial. Placement of RA in the presence of coagulopathies depends on the degree of anticoagulation and the location of the nerve relative to the neuraxis. For neuraxial blocks (epidurals and spinals), the ASRA has published extensive evidence-based guidelines applicable to all patients of all ages. The evidence to direct decisions on deep plexus (lumbar plexus) and paraneuraxial (paravertebral) blocks in the anticoagulated patient is less clear, but most practitioners adhere closely to the ASRA guidelines for these blocks. In the case of the more peripheral PNBs, where the consequences of bleeding are less problematic, there is little evidence to support the same strict adherence to these guidelines, which many experts consider overly restrictive when applied to PNBs in the absence of data.

The placement of RA in patients with preexisting neuropathies also needs to be approached with caution. While PNB placement may hypothetically increase the risk of perineural injury in the setting of preexisting neuropathy, current data are unclear regarding the validity of such risk. Thus, an individualized risk-benefit analysis is suggested. When placing a PNB in a patient with a preexisting neuropathy, ultrasound for nerve localization will minimize the number of needle passes and help to accomplish a safe distance from the nerve. Additionally, using the lowest allowable dose of local anesthetic is advised.

The use of RA in patients at risk for acute compartment syndrome (ACS) is debated, with most surgeons taking a very conservative approach of avoidance. ACS occurs when pressure is increased in a closed muscle compartment secondary to bleeding and edema; it occurs most often following long bone fractures in the lower leg and forearm. Prophylactic fasciotomies are sometimes recommended for open reduction internal fixation of high-impact ulnar, radial, and tibial fractures at the time of repair, making ACS much less likely. Pediatric case series demonstrate the safe use of RA in ACS with timely recognition of neurovascular compromise. While there is no evidence that RA, especially PNBs, will mask the ischemic pain of ACS, this is still a cause for concern for some practitioners, and potential risks must be considered. Pediatric patients with ACS present with the "3 As," ***a***gitation, ***a***nxiety, and (increasing) ***a***nalgesic requirement, in contrast to adults, who present with the "6 Ps," ***p***ain, ***p***aresthesia, ***p***allor, ***p***aralysis, ***p***ulselessness, and ***p***oikilothermia. When a perineural catheter is used in a patient at risk for ACS, the lowest doses and concentrations of LA that provide relief are recommended. One suggested protocol is shown in Box 23.1. While block failure is a consideration, continued increases in pain should alert providers to the development of compartment syndrome.

Further Reading

Bae DS, Kadiyala RK, Waters PM. Acute compartment syndrome in children: contemporary diagnosis, treatment, and outcome. *J Pediatr Orthop.* 2001;21:680–688.

Benzon H. Regional anesthesia in the anticoagulated patient. www.nysora.com/mobile/regional-anesthesia/foundations-of-ra/3300-ra-in-anticoagulated-patient.html. Accessed January 17, 2017.

Box 23.1 Protocol for the Use of Regional Anesthesia in Patients at Risk for Compartment Syndrome

Identify: Identify patients at increased risk for development of compartment syndrome.

Awareness and planning: Discuss concerns with all members of the patient care team, including surgical, nursing, pain management, and anesthesia teams.

Regional anesthesia:

1. Bolus: 0.2% ropivacaine or 0.25% bupivacaine in minimum volume to accomplish nerve surround.
2. Infusion: Ropivacaine 0.1%. Initiate at three-fourths the usual infusion rate for the particular block.

Pain escalation:

1. First complaint: The nurse, resident, or fellow should see patient and triage and implement any indicated therapy, including assessment of bandages or casts that may need to be loosened. May increase infusion to full customary rate but not to exceed.
2. Second complaint: The anesthesia attending physician managing RA must evaluate the patient at the bedside and rule out/in any possibility of ACS. Notify and discuss findings with the attending surgeon.

Block failure: Any alleged block failure needs to be considered for possible ACS and discussed with the anesthesia attending physician managing the RA. If block failure is confirmed and ACS ruled out, the pain regimen should be escalated as indicated.

Chelly JE, Clark LD, Gebhard RE, Raw RM, Atchabahian A. Consensus of the Orthopedic Anesthesia, Pain, and Rehabilitation Society on the use of peripheral nerve blocks in patients receiving thromboprophylaxis. *J Clin Anesth*. 2014;26:69–74.

Horlocker TT, Vandermeuelen E, Kopp SL, Gogarten W, Leffert LR, Benzon HT. Regional anesthesia in the patient receiving antithrombotic or thrombolytic therapy: American Society of Regional Anesthesia and Pain Medicine Evidence-Based Guidelines (Fourth Edition). *Reg Anesth Pain Med*. 2018 Apr;43(3):263–309.

Neal JM, Bernards CM, et al. ASRA practice advisory on neurologic complications in regional anesthesia and pain Medicine. *Reg Anesth Pain Med*. 2008;33:404–415.

Noonan KJ, McCarthy JJ. Compartment syndromes in the pediatric patient. *J Pediatr Orthop*. 2010;30(2 suppl):S96–S101.

Walker BJ, Noonan KJ, Bosenberg AT. Evolving compartment syndrome not masked by a continuous peripheral nerve block: evidence-based case management. *Reg Anesth Pain Med*. 2012;37:393–397.

2.4. Review local anesthetic dosing guidelines for pediatric patients

Both amide and ester local anesthetics can be utilized for PNBs. Amides are most commonly used for single bolus injections, and choice of drug depends on desired speed of onset, duration of action, drug safety profile, and type of block to be performed). The LA dose for each block in children is calculated by weight, with dose being expressed as milliliters per kilogram (Table 23.3). Lean body mass is used for the weight when calculating the pediatric dose, and age-specific pharmacokinetics of local anesthetics must be considered when administering the drug. In general, children have a higher volume of distribution than adults, imparting some protection against LAST, although young infants and neonates have decreased plasma proteins, resulting in increased unbound plasma levels of LA. Additionally, adult hepatic function is not achieved until 3 to 6 months of age. Children with chronic disease and significant comorbidities may have hypoalbuminemia and resultant increases in the free fraction of LA. The maximum dose of local anesthetics should be calculated prior to placement of multiple nerve blocks in a single patient to avoid LAST.

Table 23.3:
Recommended single-injection/bolus local anesthetic doses for pediatric regional anesthetic technique

	Bupivacaine 0.25%, mL/kg	Ropivacaine 0.2% mL/kg
Femoral	0.20–0.25	0.20–0.25
Lumbar plexus	0.50	0.50
Fascia iliaca	0.50	0.50
Sciatic (gluteal or anterior)	0.20–0.25	0.20–0.25
Sciatic (popliteal)	0.20–0.25	0.20–0.25
Interscalene	0.15–0.20	0.15–0.20
Infraclavicular/supraclavicular	0.20–0.25	0.20–-0.25
Paravertebral	0.25–0.50	0.25–0.50
Quadratus lumborum	0.40–0.50	0.40–0.50
Rectus sheath	0.10–0.20	0.10–0.20

Meticulous attention to dosing of continuous infusions in children is essential due to concerns of drug accumulation. In particular, dosing by patient weight necessitates individual calculations and creates potential for mathematical errors. Ropivacaine, bupivacaine, chloroprocaine, and lidocaine have all been used for infusions in children. Lidocaine, however, has a theoretical risk of increased neurotoxicity in young children. Ropivacaine is often favored over bupivacaine due to decreased cardiotoxicity and increased motor-sparing properties. The maximum recommended infusion rate of ropivacaine for children is 0.4 to 0.5 mg/kg/h. Liver function and conjugation function of amide local anesthetics do not reach adult maturity until 4 to 6 months of age. Therefore, in children less than 4 to 6 months of age, infusions should not exceed 0.2 to 0.3 mg/kg/h. Some practitioners argue to use chloroprocaine infusions in infants less than 4 to 6 months of age, since chloroprocaine is metabolized by plasma esterases and theoretically is less likely to cause LAST in this group, but there currently are no studies to support this practice.

Dosing of perineural infusions depends also on the nerve to be blocked. Regional techniques involving direct visualization of the nerve, such as brachial plexus blocks, under ultrasound, usually require less volume per hour. This is in contrast to larger volume nerve blocks, such as epidural, paravertebral, and abdominal wall blocks, in which success may be dependent on larger volume for more extensive spread of LA. Recommended ropivacaine infusion rates for specific peripheral nerve blocks are presented in Table 23.4.

Calculations for case: infraclavicular approach to the brachial plexus in a 36-kg patient:

1. Bolus/single injection: 0.1 to 0.2 mg/kg or 4 to 7 mL of 0.2% ropivacaine or 0.25% bupivacaine (minimum volume to accomplish perineural surround is advised).
2. Infusion: 0.1% ropivacaine or bupivacaine can be used at a rate of 0.1 ml/kg/h. In this patient, the calculated rate is 3 to 3.6 mL/h. If compartment syndrome is a risk, follow the recommended protocol and start infusion at 2.5 mL/h.

Further Reading

Berde C. Convulsions associated with pediatric regional anesthesia. *Anesth Analg.* 1992;75:164–166.

Gunter JB. Benefit and risk of local anaesthetics in infants and children. *Paediatr Drugs.* 2002;4:649–672.

Mossetti V, Vicchio N, Ivani G. Local anesthetics and adjuncts in pediatric regional anesthesia. *Curr Drug Targets.* 2012;13:952–960.

Noonan KJ, McCarthy JJ. Compartment syndromes in the pediatric patient. *J Pediatr Orthop.* 2010;30(2 suppl):S96–S101.

Table 23.4:
Recommended continuous infusion starting rates for peripheral nerve catheters. Catheters may be titrated up to maximum dosage: 0.4–0.5 mg/kg/h. This may be achieved by increased rate (mL/h) or concentration of local anesthetic (i.e., 0.2% ropivacaine)

Nerve Catheter	Rate (mL/kg/h)	Maximum Rate (mL/h)	% Ropivacaine
Femoral	0.15	8	0.1
Lumbar plexus	0.25	15	0.1
Fascia iliaca	0.25	15	0.1
Sciatic (gluteal)	0.1	5	0.1
Sciatic (popliteal)	0.1	8	0.1
Interscalene	0.1	7	0.1
Infraclavicular/supraclavicular	0.15	10	0.1
Paravertebral (unilateral)	0.25	15	0.2
Paravertebral (per side for bilateral)	0.15	10	0.2
Quadratus Lumborum (per side for bilateral)	0.15	10	0.1 or 0.2
Rectus Sheath (per side for bilateral)	0.15	10	0.1 or 0.2

3. Postoperative Considerations

3.1. Should an opioid prescription be written at discharge? If so, is persistent postsurgical opioid use in this population a concern?

An adequate postoperative pain management plan is essential to facilitate a successful transition to the home environment. Inadequate pain relief and adverse drug effects are the 2 most common reasons for prolonged length of stay and hospital readmission. Due to the severity of pain following orthopedic procedures, a short course of opioid analgesics to supplement around-the-clock acetaminophen and NSAIDs is typically utilized.

While there is increasing concern over exposing pediatric patients to opioids with the potential for addiction and abuse, acute pain must be addressed to prevent unnecessary suffering and the possible transition to chronic pain. Prescription opioid abuse is not common in patients less than 12 years of age, and any increased incidence of opioid overdose presentations to emergency departments is predominantly the result of accidental ingestion of medications prescribed to family members. Adolescents are, however, an at-risk group, with increasing potential for opioid abuse and addiction. Preoperative risk factors in adolescents such as substance use disorder, chronic pain, preoperative opioid prescription filling, and female gender have recently been described as being associated with prolonged opioid use following surgery. Physicians and ancillary healthcare professional should be aware of risk factors for opioid abuse, which include a family history of substance abuse, psychiatric diagnosis, childhood trauma, sexual abuse, loss of a parent, violence, or an environment where prescription drug abuse is common. Adolescents should be screened for risk factors and monitored accordingly. Most states have drug monitoring programs that allow for and often mandate that physicians register opioid prescriptions and check for evidence of duplicate prescriptions. Massachusetts law limits opioid prescriptions for acute pain to minors to a 7-day supply, and other states such as North Carolina have instituted opioid prescribing limits for acute postsurgical pain. Ambulatory RA catheter programs are increasingly available for pediatric patients and allow the continued benefit of the RA at home, including opioid minimization in the immediate postdischarge time frame. Several pediatric studies have demonstrated the feasibility and safety of ambulatory catheters.

In summary, a multimodal approach to analgesia, including RA techniques, should be used to address pediatric pain for orthopedic surgery. Pain should be adequately addressed in both the hospital and home environments.

Further Reading

Bukstein O. Challenges and gaps in understanding substance use problems in transitional age youth. *Child Adolesc Psychiatr Clin North Am*. 2017;26:253–269.

Centers for Disease Control and Prevention. Opioid painkiller prescribing: where you live makes a difference. Atlanta, GA. www.cdc.gov/vitalsigns/opioid-prescribing/. Accessed March 8, 2017.

Dadure C, Pirat P, Raux O, Troncin R, Rochette A, Ricard C, Capdevila X. Perioperative continuous peripheral nerve blocks with disposable infusion pumps in children: a prospective descriptive study. *Anesth Analg*. 2003;97:687–690.

Gurnaney H, Kraemer FW, Maxwell L, Muhly WT, Schleelein L, Ganesh A. Ambulatory continuous nerve blocks in children and adolescents: a longitudinal 8-year single center study. *Anesth Analg*. 2014;118:621–627.

Harbaugh CM, Lee JS, Hu HM, McCabe SE, Voepel-Lewis T, Englesbe MJ, Brummett CM, Waljee JF. Persistent opioid use among pediatric patients after surgery. *Pediatrics*. 2018 Jan;141(1):e20172439.

24

Pediatrics: Scoliosis Repair

Jenna Sobey and Carrie Menser

Case Scenario

A 14-year-old girl presents for T2-L2 rod placement due to rapidly worsening scoliosis over the preceding 6 months. The patient is very active in sports, including swimming and track and field.

1. Patient Factors: Scoliosis in the Pediatric Population

1.1. *What are the types of idiopathic scoliosis in the pediatric patient population?*

There are 3 classifications of idiopathic scoliosis in pediatric patients defined by the age of onset. Infantile scoliosis is a curvature diagnosed in a child between birth and 3 years of age; it is the rarest form of idiopathic scoliosis, occurring in approximately 1% of all cases of pediatric idiopathic scoliosis. These patients are usually diagnosed within the first 6 months of life. Most of these cases resolve without treatment, but some do require bracing or surgical growth rods. Juvenile scoliosis includes those children diagnosed between the ages of 3 and 9 years and accounts for 12% to 20% of pediatric idiopathic cases. This type of scoliosis progresses more rapidly, rarely resolving without treatment. Adolescent idiopathic scoliosis is defined as that diagnosed between the ages of 10 and 16 years and occurs in 1% to 3% of adolescents. With these patients, curvatures generally worsen during growth spurts.

The severity of scoliosis is conventionally quantified using the Cobb angle, measured on standing coronal plain films. A Cobb angle of at least 10° defines scoliosis. An angle of 10° to 15° is usually mild and only requires observation, 20° to 40° may require bracing, and greater than 40° normally requires surgical correction. The risk of spinal curve progression increases with a higher Cobb angle and lower Risser grade. The Risser grade is used to measure ossification of the iliac apophysis (grade 1–4). The higher the Risser grade, the greater the skeletal ossification and less potential for growth and curve progression. An initial Cobb angle of 25° is an important threshold magnitude for long-term curve progression. Severe curvatures can result in respiratory and cardiovascular deterioration. Only 0.25% of patients will have curves that progress and require medical intervention of some kind, and only 0.1% will go on to warrant surgical correction. For curves greater than 21°, there is a 5.4-to-1 female-to-male ratio. The goal of surgical repair is correcting the current curvature and preventing further progression while preserving pulmonary function.

Back pain prevalence is significantly higher in patients with untreated scoliosis than in control populations; however, back pain severity and duration are not significantly increased compared with their peers. Pain severity does not correlate with curve size, but curve pattern may be associated with increased pain, and thoracolumbar curves seem to be the most related to pain. Pediatric scoliosis repair is one of the most painful operations performed in the pediatric population and therefore warrants all preventative techniques possible to reduce the incidence of chronic postoperative pain.

Further Reading

Asher MA, Burton DC. Adolescent idiopathic scoliosis: natural history and long term treatment effects. *Scoliosis.* 2006;1:2. doi:10.1186/1748-7161-1-2

Miller NH. Genetics of familial idiopathic scoliosis. *Clin Orthop Relat Res.* 2007;462:6–10.

Weinstein SL, Dolan LA, Cheng JCY, Danielsson A, Morcuende JA. Adolescent idiopathic scoliosis. *Lancet.* 2008;371:1527–1537.

Weinstein SL, Dolan LA, Spratt KF, Peterson KK, Spoonamore MJ, Ponseti IV. Health and function of patients with untreated idiopathic scoliosis: a 50-year natural history study. *JAMA.* 2003 Feb 5;289(5):559–567.

1.2. *Describe the challenges encountered when preparing pediatric patients for major surgery with a high nociceptive load*

A high level of anxiety is generated with the prospect of having surgery, be it a minor or major operation, and higher levels of anxiety have been linked to higher levels of postoperative pain in both adults and children. The surgical experience can be particularly anxiety producing in children due to the stressors of parental separation, pain/discomfort, and inability to resume their normal activities postoperatively. Pediatric patients also report higher pain intensity and more distress responses than adult cohorts. This anxiety in children can be intensified by parental anxiety, which can lead to even higher pain responses following surgery. Studies have also concluded that highly anxious parents have highly anxious children.

With this knowledge, it is highly important to adequately and realistically prepare not only pediatric patients but also their parents or guardians for what to expect perioperatively. This is best done by utilizing a multidisciplinary approach, incorporating a preoperative clinic visit with the surgical team, to provide insight and expectations regarding the surgery and postoperative limitations, as well as a visit with the anesthesia providers or perioperative clinic, to provide information regarding expectations for pain and analgesia. It is important to set realistic expectations for analgesic goals, focusing on pain control to a tolerable level to ensure maximum postoperative function, rather than on eliminating pain completely.

There is some evidence in the adult literature for various techniques of psychological preparation for patients undergoing surgery under general anesthesia to reduce postoperative pain, behavioral recovery, negative affect, and length of stay. Although implementation of these psychological techniques is unlikely to be harmful, the strength of the evidence to date is insufficient to reach firm conclusions on the success of these various techniques. No randomized controlled trials have been performed in the pediatric population regarding this hypothesis.

Further Reading

deGroot KI, Boeke S, van den Berge HJ, Duivenvoorden H, Bonke B, Passchier J. The influence of psychological variables on postoperative anxiety and physical complaints in patients undergoing lumbar surgery. *Pain.* 1997;69:19–25.

LaMontagne LL, Hepworth JT, Johnson BD, Cohen F. Children's preoperative coping and its effects on postoperative anxiety and return to normal activity. *Nurs Res.* 1996;45 (3):141–147.

Palermo T, Drotar D. Prediction of children's postoperative pain: the role of presurgical expectations and anticipatory emotions. *J Pediatr Psychol.* 1996;21:683–698.

Peterson L, Shigetomi C. The use of coping techniques to minimize anxiety in hospitalized children. *Behav Ther.* 1981;12:1–14.

Powell R, Scott NW, Manyande A, Bruce J, Vögele C, Byrne-Davis LMT, Unsworth M, Osmer C, Johnston M. Psychological preparation and postoperative outcomes for adults undergoing surgery under general anesthesia (Review). *Cochrane Database Syst Rev.* 2016 May 26;5:CD008646.

Redgeway V, Mathews A. Psychological preparation for surgery: a comparison of methods. *Br J Clin Psychol.* 1982;21:271–280.

Rhudy J, Meagher M. Fear and anxiety: divergent effects on human pain thresholds. *Pain.* 2000;84:65–75.

Schwartz BH, Albino JE, Tedesco LA. Effects of psychological preparation on children hospitalized for dental operations. *J Pediatr.* 1983;102:634–638.

2. Perioperative Pain Management

2.1. What are the preoperative analgesic methods utilized in pediatric patients presenting for scoliosis repair?

Preoperative preparation surrounding the child going for major scoliosis repair is important. Ensuring adequate optimization of medical conditions, including optimizing preexisting analgesic medications, is important. Most pediatric patients presenting for primary surgical intervention are not taking opioid medications. However, those who are taking opioids preoperatively should have their dose reduced to the lowest dose that maintains function weeks prior to surgery. This minimizes the proliferation of opioid receptors that expectedly occurs with chronic opioid use due to tolerance. If other analgesic adjunctive medications are being taken preoperatively, such as anticonvulsants, tricyclic antidepressants, or serotonin norepinephrine reuptake inhibitors, these medications should be maintained at their same dose, including on the day of surgery.

Preemptive and preventative analgesia has been shown to be important in reducing hypersensitive states related to the noxious stimulus from tissue injury. In the adult literature, studies have demonstrated the development of both peripheral and central sensitization due to the presence of significant inflammatory response that can occur in large surgical procedures. If this response is not adequately suppressed, injury to neural structures can result in alteration to dorsal horn neurons and increase the sensitivity of painful stimuli, as well as increase the size of the receptive field. Systematic reviews in the adult population have shown notable effect size with use of anticonvulsants, regional anesthesia, and nonsteroidal anti-inflammatory drugs (NSAIDs) administered prior to surgical incision.

Studies demonstrating the exclusive use of preoperative analgesics on outcomes in the pediatric scoliosis population are not well represented in the literature. Most trials examining preoperative analgesic regimens continued the regimen through the intra- and postoperative period. Thus, specific techniques and recommendations regarding analgesic medications are detailed in the following sections.

2.2. What intraoperative anesthetic and analgesic techniques are optimal for pediatric scoliosis repair?

The goals for management of patients undergoing scoliosis repair include an effective pain management regimen that is quick and easy to perform with a low failure rate. The methods chosen should not delay emergence or require an intensive care unit stay postoperatively for prolonged monitoring.

Pediatric scoliosis repairs are performed under general anesthesia and often require a total intravenous (IV) anesthetic due to somatosensory evoked potentials (SSEP) or motor evoked potentials (MEP) monitoring. This is usually accomplished utilizing a propofol infusion with an IV opioid infusion. A low-dose inhaled agent may also be utilized (<1 MAC) along with propofol, but one must be cautious due to potential for suppression of SSEP and MEP signals. Pediatric patients have a larger volume of distribution and increased clearance of propofol when compared with adults, and propofol dosing is approximately twice that in adults to achieve similar plasma concentrations. Dexmedetomidine can also be utilized along with propofol. It does not affect SSEP or MEP monitoring. One randomized controlled trial in 2015 found that when dexmedetomidine infusion was used versus remifentanil, there was superior efficacy in alleviating pain and in postoperative pain management for 48 hours after posterior lumbar spinal fusion.

Remifentanil and sufentanil are the 2 most commonly utilized opioids for analgesia during pediatric spine surgery. Remifentanil is an ultra-short-acting opioid eliminated by plasma esterases. It offers the advantage of potent intraoperative analgesia, with a rapid contact elimination half-life allowing for rapid emergence of patients following cessation of the infusion and immediate neurologic exam. This is also one of its disadvantages, in that the patients will often experience significant pain upon awakening due to lack of long-acting analgesia, if used as the primary analgesic. It has also been shown to cause acute opioid tolerance postoperatively, with patients in one study reporting higher pain scores and requiring higher doses of opioids for adequate analgesia in the postoperative period. Remifentanil can also be titrated easily for controlled hypotension intraoperatively. Sufentanil improves immediate postoperative pain control without a significant delay in tracheal extubation when compared with remifentanil in adult patients. Sufentanil can also be safely utilized in pediatric patients for spine surgery and can provide longer duration of analgesia compared with remifentanil. Alfentanil and fentanyl infusions can also be utilized; however, these agents take longer to wear off and can delay wake-up testing and postoperative extubation. Intraoperative methadone is another opioid that has some promise for utilization in pediatric scoliosis repair. In one adult study, a single dose of intraoperative IV methadone improved postoperative pain control and reduced opioid requirements in adult patients undergoing complex spine surgery without significant adverse events. Further evaluation is required in the pediatric population.

Ketamine, an NMDA receptor antagonist with weak mu and kappa opioid receptor agonism, is a promising analgesic agent to use in pediatric patients undergoing major spine surgery. Ketamine has potent analgesic properties and a low side effect profile, with reduced incidence of respiratory depression, nausea, vomiting, and ileus. Ketamine enhances the MEP amplitude and cortical SSEP signals without a change in latency, providing satisfactory monitoring conditions when used as an intraoperative infusion. In one study by Minoshima et al., an intraoperative and postoperative ketamine infusion was utilized for 48 hours postoperatively at 2 mcg/kg/h and had reduced overall morphine consumption versus placebo controls, as well as reduced antiemetic consumption in adolescent patients undergoing scoliosis repair.

Magnesium sulfate infusions are another consideration. They have been shown to reduce anesthetic requirements and can be helpful for controlled hypotension. In one large meta-analysis, IV magnesium was shown to reduce opioid use and pain scores. In another study, a magnesium bolus given at induction reduced postoperative opioid consumption, improved patient satisfaction scores, and improved the first night's sleep for patients undergoing major lumbar orthopedic surgery.

Further Reading

Absalom A, Kenny G. "Paedfusor" pharmacokinetic data set. *Br J Anaesth*. 2005;95(1):110.

Albrecht E, Kirkham KR, Liu SS, Brull R. Peri-operative intravenous administration of magnesium sulphate and postoperative pain: a meta-analysis. *Anaesthesia*. 2013 Jan;68(1):79–90.

Banoub M, Tetzlaff JE, Schubert A. Pharmacologic and physiologic influences affecting sensory evoked potentials: implications for perioperative monitoring. *Anesthesiology*. 2003;99(3):716–737.

Derrode N, Lebrun F, Levron JC, Chauvin M, Debaene B. Influence of perioperative opioid on postoperative pain after major abdominal surgery: sufentanil TCI versus remifentanil TCI. A randomized, controlled study. *Br J Anaesth*. 2003;91(6):842–849.

Hwang W, Lee J, Park J, Joo J. Dexmedetomidine versus remifentanil in postoperative pain control after spinal surgery: a randomized controlled study. *BMC Anesthesiol*. 2015;15:21.

Gottschalk A, Durieux ME, Nemergut EC. Intraoperative methadone improves postoperative pain control in patients undergoing complex spine surgery. *Anesth Analg*. 2011;112(1):218–223.

Kim SH, Stoicea N, Sogohomonyan S, Bergese SD. Intraoperative use of remifentanil and opioid induced hyperalgesia/acute opioid tolerance: systematic review. *Front Pharmacol*. 2014;5:108.

Levaux C, Bonhomme V, Dewandre PY, Brichant JF, Hans P. Effect of intra-operative magnesium sulfate on pain relief and patient comfort after major lumbar orthopaedic surgery. *Anaesthesia*. 2003 Feb;58(2):131–135.

Lotto ML, Banoub M, Schubert A. Effects of anesthetic agents and physiologic changes on intraoperative motor evoked potentials. *J Neurosurg Anesthesiol*. 2004 Jan;16(1):32–42.

Minoshima R, Kosugi S, Nishimura D, Ihara N, Seki H, Yamada T, Watanabe K, Katori N, Hashiguchi S, Morisaki H. Intra- and postoperative low-dose ketamine for adolescent idiopathic scoliosis surgery: a randomized controlled trial. Acta Anaesthesiologica Scandinavica 59(2015) 1260–1268

Ong CK, Lirk P, Seymour RA, Jenkins BJ. The efficacy of preemptive analgesia for acute postoperative pain management. *Anesth Analg*. 2005;100(3):757–773.

Straube S, Derry S, Moore RA, Wiffen PJ, McQuay HJ. Single dose oral gabapentin for established acute postoperative pain in adults. *Cochrane Database Syst Rev*. 2010 May 12;5:CD008183.

2.3. What postoperative analgesic regimens are optimal for pediatric patients undergoing scoliosis repair?

Maintaining adequate postoperative pain control in children undergoing scoliosis repair while not causing sedation from analgesic side effects can be a challenging prospect. Because the length of incisions required for scoliosis surgery is substantial and requires extensive bony and soft tissue dissection, postoperative pain can be quite significant. Therefore, adequate and effective analgesia in the postoperative period is paramount for providing an optimal postoperative course. Analgesia after scoliosis surgery is best achieved utilizing a multimodal approach, addressing not only nociceptive loads but also anxiety and muscle spasms.

2.3.1. Opioids

The most commonly utilized postoperative pain regimen normally begins with patient-controlled analgesia (PCA) with an opioid. Most adolescents can effectively utilize a PCA after being provided instruction, but if the patient has a developmental delay, nurse- or parent-controlled analgesia may be required. A PCA is normally started in the postanesthesia care unit (PACU) once an adequate level of analgesia has been established utilizing IV opioids titrated to effect, usually administered by a PACU nurse. This can be achieved with IV hydromorphone (10–20 mcg/kg/dose), morphine (10–20 mcg/kg/dose), or fentanyl (1–2 mcg/kg/dose). PCA opioid selection is normally based on the preference of the provider caring for the patient in the postoperative period and most often is morphine (.02 mg/kg demand q8–10min) or hydromorphone (4 mcg/kg demand q8–10min).

Some practitioners routinely utilize a basal infusion on the PCA in addition to demand dosing. While this technique is more commonly utilized in children than adults, we recommend caution with this approach, as it potentially poses significant risk of oversedation and respiratory depression, along with increased opioid exposure in a high-anxiety patient population. Nonetheless, if a patient is noting uncontrolled pain during times of rest, such as overnight, a low-dose basal infusion can assist with maintaining adequate analgesia without frequent awakenings to activate a demand bolus.

2.3.2. Nonopioid analgesic medications

Incorporating balanced analgesic regimens into postoperative care is key to reducing opioid side effects from escalating dose requirements.

Acetaminophen is often utilized in the postoperative period following pediatric scoliosis surgery in patients who are appropriate candidates. IV acetaminophen provides rapid and effective analgesia and is well tolerated. When given scheduled, it has been shown to improve overall analgesia; however, it has not been shown to reduce overall opioid requirement after major spine surgery in pediatric patients. It can be given IV or PO, at a dose of 10 to 15 mg/kg every 6 to 8 hours, not to exceed 3 g/d.

Gabapentin, the gamma amino butyric acid analog anticonvulsant, can also be utilized in the perioperative period. There remains conflicting evidence in the pediatric patient population. One study by Mayell et al. did not show any significant reduction of opioid consumption or pain scores in adolescent patients undergoing scoliosis repair with a single preoperative dose. However, in a randomized controlled trial by Rusy et al., 59 pediatric patients, aged 9 to 18, who were undergoing posterior spinal fusion were randomized to receive 15 mg/kg preoperatively and 5 mg/kg TID in the postoperative period. The gabapentin group received less total opioid and reduced pain scores in PACU and on the first postoperative day. Adult literature also suggests significant analgesic benefits and reduction of opioid consumption in the long-term postoperative period.

Muscle spasms can cause significant anxiety and discomfort in the postoperative period following scoliosis repair. It is important to provide pharmacologic relief, in addition to aggressive physical therapy. Due to its anxiolytic properties, diazepam is often an excellent choice in this setting. It is safest and most beneficial when offered on a PRN basis, usually 0.12 to 0.8 mg/kg/d PO, divided q6–8h. There have been no studies done separately in spine surgery for the use of diazepam, in either the pediatric or the adult population. Other alternative options are tizanidine, methocarbamol, and baclofen.

Nonsteroidal anti-inflammatory drugs are now commonly used for scoliosis repair, the most common being IV ketorolac. Intravenous ketorolac given intraoperatively to pediatric patients undergoing major orthopedic surgery has proven to reduce overall opioid consumption and pain scores in the postoperative period without significant increases in postoperative bleeding. There have been previous concerns regarding poor bone healing and pseudoarthrosis following spine surgery in adolescent patients with the use of ketorolac, yet recent evidence does not show any increased risk of this complication at standard dosing. Several studies examining the use of NSAIDs and complications with poor healing in orthopedic procedures have not revealed any association between this risk and the use of perioperative NSAIDs. Another potential risk related to the use of NSAIDs is increased risk of bleeding postoperatively. There has been some concern in the adult population for this risk, but a study by Vitale et al. did not show an increased risk of bleeding complications or reoperation with the utilization of ketorolac in the pediatric spine population. Normally ketorolac is dosed at 0.5 mg/kg/dose given intraoperative at surgical closure and can be continued in the postoperative period scheduled for up to 5 days.

Further Reading

Dodwell ER, Latorre JG, Parisini E, Swettler E, Chandra D, Mulpuri K, Snyder B. NSAID exposure and risk of nonunion: a meta-analysis of case control and cohort studies. *Calcif Tissue Int.* 2010 Sep;87(3):193–202.

Eberson CP, Pacicca DM, Ehrlich MG. The role of ketorolac in decreasing length of stay and narcotic complications in the postoperative pediatric orthopaedic patient. *J Pediatr Orthop.* 1999;19(5):688–692.

Hiller A, Helenius I, Nurmi E, et al. Acetaminophen improves analgesia but does not reduce opioid requirement after major spine surgery in children and adolescents. *Spine.* 2012;37(20):E1225–E1231.

Mayell A, Srinivasan I, Campbell F, Peliowski A. Analgesic effects of gabapentin after scoliosis surgery in children: a randomized controlled trial. *Paediatr Anaesth.* 2014;24(12):1239–1244.

Rusy LM, Hainsworth KR, Nelson TJ, et al. Gabapentin use in pediatric spinal fusion patients: a randomized, double-blind, controlled trial. *Anesth Analg.* 2010;110(5):1393–1398.

Sinatra RS, Jahr JS, Reynolds LW, Viscusi ER, Groudine SB, Payen-Champenois C. Efficacy and safety of single and repeated administration of 1 gram intravenous acetaminophen injection (paracetamol) for pain management after major orthopedic surgery. *Anesthesiology.* 2005;102(4):822–831.

Sucato DJ, Lovejoy JF, Agrawal S, Elerson E, Nelson T, McClung A. Postoperative ketorolac does not predispose to pseudoarthrosis following posterior spinal fusion and instrumentation for adolescent idiopathic scoliosis. *Spine.* 2008;33(10):1119–1124.

Sutters KA, Shaw BA, Gerardi JA, Hebert D. Comparison of morphine patient-controlled analgesia with and without ketorolac for postoperative analgesia in pediatric orthopedic surgery. *Am J Orthop.* 1999;28(6):351–358.

Vitale, M. G. et al. Use of ketorolac tromethamine in children undergoing scoliosis surgery. an analysis of complications. The Spine Journal 3, 55–62 (2003).

2.4. What is the role of regional anesthesia in pediatric patients undergoing scoliosis repair?

Regional techniques have also been utilized for postoperative analgesia following scoliosis repair in pediatric patients. Reports of success with regional techniques for this purpose are complicated by variation in techniques, dosing, and surgical procedures, and further studies are needed for definitive conclusion. Intrathecal (IT) morphine has been shown to prolong postoperative analgesia and decrease anesthetic agents used with limited effect on neuromonitoring. Tobias et al. performed a meta-analysis to evaluate the different regional techniques following spinal surgery and concluded IT morphine is effective at reducing postoperative pain scores and IV opioid requirements, without substantial negative effects. The IT dose utilized in the different studies was variable, but Gall et al. demonstrated improvements in the postoperative pain course and decreased intraoperative blood loss with a dose of 5 mg/kg of IT morphine. Effective doses of IT morphine range from 3 to 7 mcg/kg.

Epidural analgesia is also an option for regional analgesia, with techniques, agents, and doses utilized in the literature again demonstrating extreme variability. The studies do demonstrate epidural analgesia is effective for postoperative analgesia, although it is not necessarily superior to conventional IV PCA. The only randomized controlled trial comparing the two techniques by Amaranth et al. did not demonstrate a difference between epidural and IV PCA analgesia, but it did show more rapid return of gastrointestinal function in the epidural group. IT morphine with an epidural PCA was more effective than an IV PCA alone in one study by Ravish et al. Some providers choose to utilize a dual-catheter technique to allow the use of lipophilic opioids and avoid adverse effects of hydrophilic opioids. The decision to utilize regional techniques should take into consideration the cost to maintain the epidural infusion and the safe infrastructure in place for management, as well as the potential cost savings of reduced hospital or intensive care unit stay.

Some institutions utilize subcutaneous infusions of local anesthetics at the surgical site, but this technique has not shown superiority when compared with standard postoperative pain management techniques.

Further Reading

Gall O, Aubineau JV, Berniere J, Desjeux L, Murat I. Analgesic effect of low-dose intrathecal morphine after spinal fusion in children. *Anesthesiology*. 2001 Mar;94(3):447–452.

Goodarzi M. The advantages of intrathecal opioids for spinal fusion in children. *Paediatr Anaesth*. 1998;8(2):131–134.

Ravish M, Muldowney B, Becker A, Hetzel S, McCarthy JJ, Nemeth BA, Noonan KJ. Pain management in patients with adolescent idiopathic scoliosis undergoing posterior spinal fusion: combined intrathecal morphine and continuous epidural versus PCA. *J Pediatr Orthop*. 2012 Dec;32(8):799–804.

Taenzer AH, Clark C. Efficacy of postoperative epidural analgesia in adolescent scoliosis surgery: a meta-analysis. *Paediatr Anaesth*. 2010 Feb;20(2):135–143.

Tobias JD. A review of intrathecal and epidural analgesia after spinal surgery in children. *Anesth Analg*. 2004 Apr;98(4):956–965.

3. Persistent/Chronic Postoperative Pain

3.1. What qualifies as persistent postoperative pain or chronic postsurgical pain?

Persistent postoperative pain is often interchangeably described as chronic postsurgical pain. The International Association for the Study of Pain (IASP) defines chronic postsurgical pain as pain lasting longer than 2 months after surgery. Persistent postoperative pain is also defined as pain lasting longer than 2 months postsurgery. The definition does not take into account the complexity of the surgery performed or the expected recovery trajectory.

Further Reading

Macrae WA, Davies H. Chronic postsurgical pain. IK Crombie, S Linton, P Croft, M Von Korff, L LeResche (Eds.), Epidemiology of Pain, International Association for the Study of Pain, Seattle (1999), pp. 125–142

Sieberg CB, Simons LE, Edelstein MR, et al. Pain prevalence and trajectories following pediatric spinal fusion surgery. *J Pain*. 2013;14(12):1694–1702. doi:10.1016/j.jpain.2013.09.005

3.2. What is the incidence of persistent postoperative pain in major spine surgery in the pediatric population?

The reported incidence of persistent postoperative pain after major spine surgery in children is widely variable, ranging from 11% to 65%. Several studies have found the incidence of persistent pain or pain beyond the expected recovery time for major surgery to average about 20% in pediatric patients. Studies following pediatric patients after spinal surgery for idiopathic scoliosis identified the incidence of persistent pain to be 22% at 6 months (Connelly et al.) and 11% to 15% at 1 to 5 years (Sieberg et al.).

Further Reading

Connelly M, Fulmer RD, Prohaska J, et al. Predictors of postoperative pain trajectories in adolescent idiopathic scoliosis. *Spine*. 2014;39(3):E174–E181. doi:10.1097/BRS.0000000000000099

Rabbitts JA, Zhou C, Groenewald CB, Durkin L, Palermo TM. Trajectories of postsurgical pain in children: risk factors and impact of late pain recovery on long-term health outcomes after major surgery. *Pain*. 2015;156(11):2383–2389. doi:10.1097/j.pain.0000000000000281

Sieberg CB, Simons LE, Edelstein MR, et al. Pain prevalence and trajectories following pediatric spinal fusion surgery. *J Pain*. 2013;14(12):1694–1702. doi:10.1016/j.jpain.2013.09.005

Voepel-Lewis T, Caird MS, Tait AR, et al. A high preoperative pain and symptom profile predicts worse pain outcomes for children after spine fusion surgery. *Anesth Analg*. 2017 May;124(5):1594–1602. doi:10.1213/ANE.0000000000001963

3.3. What are risk factors for persistent pain after pediatric spine surgery?

Surprisingly to many, medical and biological factors (such as age and sex) have not been associated with persistent pain after spine surgery in the pediatric population. Rather, certain psychosocial factors and preoperative pain intensity have been the most consistent risk factors identified.

The presence of preoperative pain is a risk factor for persistent postoperative pain, with higher levels of baseline preoperative pain being predictive of persistent pain after surgery. Risk factors for persistent postoperative pain are similar to those associated with other chronic pain conditions and include multisite pain and somatic symptoms of depression, fatigue, anxiety, sleep difficulties, headache, and abdominal cramping. These are similar symptoms to those associated with central pain sensitization conditions in both pediatric and adult patients.

Psychosocial risk factors associated with persistent postsurgical pain have been identified as preoperative parental pain catastrophizing, preoperative patient pain catastrophizing, and high levels of preoperative anxiety.

Preoperative risk factors related to scoliosis, such as location of the preoperative curve and the severity of the scoliosis curve, do not significantly impact pain outcomes such as persistent postoperative pain. Surgical factors, such as surgical approach (anterior vs. posterior) and spinal fusion length, are not associated with an increased incidence of postoperative pain either.

Further Reading

Bastrom TP, Marks MC, Yaszay B, Newton PO, Harms Study Group. Prevalence of postoperative pain in adolescent idiopathic scoliosis and the association with preoperative pain. *Spine*. 2013;38(21):1848–1852. doi:10.1097/BRS.0b013e3182a4aa97

Connelly M, Fulmer RD, Prohaska J, et al. Predictors of postoperative pain trajectories in adolescent idiopathic scoliosis. *Spine*. 2014;39(3):E174–E181. doi:10.1097/BRS.0000000000000099

Rabbitts JA, Fisher E, Rosenbloom BN, Palermo TM. Prevalence and predictors of chronic postsurgical pain in children: a systematic review and meta-analysis. *J Pain*. 2017 Jun;18(6):605–614. doi:10.1016/j.jpain.2017.03.007

Rabbitts JA, Zhou C, Groenewald CB, Durkin L, Palermo TM. Trajectories of postsurgical pain in children: risk factors and impact of late pain recovery on long-term health outcomes after major surgery. *Pain*. 2015;156(11):2383–2389. doi:10.1097/j.pain.0000000000000281

Sieberg CB, Simons LE, Edelstein MR, et al. Pain prevalence and trajectories following pediatric spinal fusion surgery. *J Pain*. 2013;14(12):1694–1702. doi:10.1016/j.jpain.2013.09.005

Voepel-Lewis T, Caird MS, Tait AR, et al. A high preoperative pain and symptom profile predicts worse pain outcomes for children after spine fusion surgery. *Anesth Analg*. 2017 May;124(5):1594–1602. doi:10.1213/ANE.0000000000001963

3.4. Describe the mechanism for persistent pain after spine surgery

While the exact mechanisms underlying persistent pain after surgery are not known, theories have been postulated that long-term alterations in nociceptive pathways may play some role. Research in animal models has identified disruption in the descending modulation of nociceptive pathways and increased hyperalgesia as areas of particular interest as potential mechanisms in the development of persistent or chronic postsurgical pain. However, further research is needed to validate these theories.

Further Reading

Schwaller F, Beggs S, Walker SM. Targeting p38 mitogen-activated protein kinase to reduce the impact of neonatal microglial priming on incision-induced hyperalgesia in the adult rat. *Anesthesiology*. 2015;122(6):1377–1390. doi:10.1097/ALN.0000000000000659

Walker SM. Pain after surgery in children: clinical recommendations. *Curr Opin Anaesthesiol*. 2015;28(5):570–576. doi:10.1097/ACO.0000000000000227

Walker SM, Fitzgerald M, Hathway GJ. Surgical injury in the neonatal rat alters the adult pattern of descending modulation from the rostroventral medulla. *Anesthesiology*. 2015;122(6):1391–1400. doi:10.1097/ALN.0000000000000658

3.5. What treatment modalities are available for chronic postoperative pain following scoliosis repair?

Research on the efficacy of medication for the treatment of persistent postoperative pain is sparse. Studies by Rusy et al. and Mayell et al. found that multiple doses of gabapentin in the perioperative period reduced postoperative opioid requirements after surgery for idiopathic scoliosis, while a single perioperative dose did not. However, effects such as this one on the incidence of persistent postsurgical pain have not been described. Further studies are needed to delineate the long-term benefits of pharmacologic interventions.

Use of nonpharmacologic interventions such as cognitive-behavioral therapy, relaxation, and biofeedback has been successful in the treatment of pediatric chronic pain, but these interventions have not been studied specifically in persistent postoperative pain. Targeting good perioperative sleep hygiene may also provide some benefit for minimizing pain in children undergoing major surgery such as spine surgery, but its effect on persistent pain after surgery in children is not known.

Preoperative preparation may very well be the best "treatment" for reducing the incidence of persistent postoperative pain. Rabbits et al. found that families experienced surgeries as stressful and felt underprepared for the recovery process and pain after surgery. Therapies targeting preoperative pain, whether through pharmacologic or nonpharmacologic treatment to reduce preoperative pain, may improve long-term outcomes after pediatric spine surgery. Preoperative attention to baseline anxiety and pain coping skills is also critical to improving long-term outcomes. Rabbits et al. identified worry and anxiety, parental guilt, fear of pain, and fear of re-injury as potential targets for preoperative assessment and intervention. Adult studies after spine surgery have shown benefit from cognitive-behavioral interventions and structured meetings with other patients during the recovery phase postoperatively in reducing pain, catastrophizing, and functional disability. Web-based cognitive-behavioral therapy directed at families has shown promise in efficacy and feasibility for the management of pediatric chronic pain, but it has not been studied in the management of postoperative pain in children. Further research is needed to define specific efficacious preoperative interventions for the pediatric population.

Further Reading

Abbott AD, Tyni-Lenné R, Hedlund R. Early rehabilitation targeting cognition, behavior, and motor function after lumbar fusion: a randomized controlled trial. *Spine*. 2010;35(8):848–857. doi:10.1097/BRS.0b013e3181d1049f

Christensen FB, Laurberg I, Bünger CE. Importance of the back-café concept to rehabilitation after lumbar spinal fusion: a randomized clinical study with a 2-year follow-up. *Spine*. 2003;28(23):2561–2569. doi:10.1097/01.BRS.0000097890.96524.A1

Eccleston C, Palermo TM, Williams AC de C, Lewandowski A, Morley S. Psychological therapies for the management of chronic and recurrent pain in children and adolescents. Eccleston C, ed. *Cochrane Database Syst Rev*. 2009;36(2):CD003968. doi:10.1002/14651858.CD003968.pub2

Mayell A, Srinivasan I, Campbell F, Peliowski A. Analgesic effects of gabapentin after scoliosis surgery in children: a randomized controlled trial. Morton N, ed. *Paediatr Anaesth*. 2014;24(12):1239–1244. doi:10.1111/pan.12524

Monticone M, Ferrante S, Teli M, et al. Management of catastrophising and kinesiophobia improves rehabilitation after fusion for lumbar spondylolisthesis and stenosis: a randomised controlled trial. *Eur Spine J*. 2014;23(1):87–95. doi:10.1007/s00586-013-2889-z

Palermo TM, Eccleston C, Lewandowski AS, Williams AC de C, Morley S. Randomized controlled trials of psychological therapies for management of chronic pain in children and adolescents: an updated meta-analytic review. *Pain*. 2010;148(3):387–397. doi:10.1016/j.pain.2009.10.004

Palermo TM, Law EF, Fales J, Bromberg MH, Jessen-Fiddick T, Tai G. Internet-delivered cognitive-behavioral treatment for adolescents with chronic pain and their parents: a randomized controlled multicenter trial. *Pain*. 2016;157(1):174–185. doi:10.1097/j.pain.0000000000000348

Rabbitts JA, Aaron RV, Fisher E, et al. Long-term pain and recovery after major pediatric surgery: a qualitative study with teens, parents, and perioperative care providers. *J Pain.* 2017;0(0). doi:10.1016/j.jpain.2017.02.423

Rabbitts JA, Zhou C, Palermo T. Interrelationships between sleep and pain in children undergoing major surgery. *J Pain.* 2016;17(4S):S37. doi:10.1016/j.jpain.2016.01.153

Rusy LM, Hainsworth KR, Nelson TJ, et al. Gabapentin use in pediatric spinal fusion patients: a randomized, double-blind, controlled trial. *Anesth Analg.* 2010;110(5):1393–1398. doi:10.1213/ANE.0b013e3181d41dc2

Walker SM. Pain after surgery in children: clinical recommendations. *Curr Opin Anaesthesiol.* 2015;28(5):570–576. doi:10.1097/ACO.0000000000000227

3.6. What are the long-term consequences of persistent pain after spine surgery?

Chronic postsurgical pain after spine surgery has been associated with long-term consequences, including poorer health outcomes and greater functional disability. These long-term consequences include prolonged functional impairment, increased long-term use of both nonopioid and opioid analgesics, socioeconomic consequences, and long-term disability into adulthood. Persistent pain after surgery is also associated with decreased quality of life and functional disability.

Further Reading

Rabbitts JA, Fisher E, Rosenbloom BN, Palermo TM. Prevalence and predictors of chronic postsurgical pain in children: a systematic review and meta-analysis. *J Pain.* 2017 Jun;18(6):605–614. doi:10.1016/j.jpain.2017.03.007

Rabbitts JA, Zhou C, Groenewald CB, Durkin L, Palermo TM. Trajectories of postsurgical pain in children: risk factors and impact of late pain recovery on long-term health outcomes after major surgery. *Pain.* 2015;156(11):2383–2389. doi:10.1097/j.pain.0000000000000281

Pediatric Tonsillectomy

Andrew Franklin

25

Case Scenario

A 3-year-old child with a history of obesity, passive smoke exposure, and attention deficit hyperactivity disorder (ADHD) presents for outpatient adenotonsillectomy at an ambulatory surgery center due to severe sleep apnea. Parents report that the child is recovering from an upper respiratory tract infection, and a recent polysomnogram revealed an apnea-hypopnea index of 37 with mixed obstructive and central apneic episodes. Examination reveals a well-appearing active child with a BMI of 45, clear rhinorrhea, and no focal cardiopulmonary findings on physical examination. Parents are quite concerned about pain control after the procedure.

1. Pediatric Obstructive Sleep Apnea

1.1. Discuss the role of polysomnography (sleep study) in the diagnosis of pediatric obstructive sleep apnea and the data it provides

Pediatric obstructive sleep apnea (OSA) is functionally similar to adult OSA in that it results from partial or complete airway obstruction during sleep due to obstruction of airflow through the upper airways. Unlike in adult OSA, adenotonsillar hypertrophy is a major contributor to pediatric OSA, and adenotonsillectomy is one of the most common surgical procedures performed on children today. Though the cost-benefit relationship of the procedure has been questioned recently, the gold standard for diagnosis of pediatric OSA is nocturnal polysomnography (PSG), commonly referred to as a sleep study. During a PSG, an apneic episode is defined as 90% decrease in airflow from baseline, with further sensors determining whether the apneic event is central, obstructive, or mixed central/obstructive. In children, obstructive apneic episodes are far more common than central neurologic apneic episodes. Likewise, a hypopneic episode is defined as a 50% decrease in airflow from baseline. For the anesthesiologist, the most useful calculated metric from a PSG is the apnea-hypopnea index (AHI), which is the total number of hypopneic and apneic events that occur in an hour. The severity of OSA in the child can be summarized as follows:

Mild OSA: AHI 1–4.9
Moderate OSA: AHI 5–9.9
Severe OSA: AHI >10

The second most useful summary metric found in a PSG for the anesthesiologist is the oxygen saturation nadir, which is the lowest SpO_2 recorded by pulse oximetry during sleep. Mild cases of OSA may only have oxygen saturation nadirs of 90%, but severe cases of OSA may have nadirs as low as 70% during an apneic event. The anesthesiologist must review any available PSG data to gauge the severity of the child's OSA during the preoperative visit, as this will predict obstruction during inhalational induction and the physiologic status of the child in the recovery room after adenotonsillectomy.

Further Reading

Li Z, Celestin J, Lockey RF. Pediatric sleep apnea syndrome: an update. *J Allergy Clin Immunol Pract.* 2016 Sep–Oct;4(5):852–861.

Schwengel DA, Sterni LM, Tunkel DE, Heitmiller ES. Perioperative management of children with obstructive sleep apnea. *Anesth Analg*. 2009 Jul;109(1):60–75.

1.2. What are the implications of pediatric obesity on pediatric obstructive sleep apnea?

The growing epidemic of pediatric obesity in developed nations, particularly the United States, has major implications for nearly every aspect of pediatric medicine. The incidence and severity of OSA are significantly higher in obese children, and the magnitude of resultant multisystem dysfunction is greater. Adenotonsillectomy has been shown to reduce OSA symptoms in both lean and obese children, but surgery is far less likely to cure OSA in obese children. Only 28% of nonobese children display significant OSA symptoms after adenotonsillectomy, but 76% of obese children continue to suffer from OSA after adenotonsillectomy. These residual symptoms often require posttonsillectomy continuous positive airway pressure or even additional airway surgery to increase the cross-sectional area of the airway.

Further Reading

Lennon CJ, Wang RY, Wallace A, Chinnadurai S. Risk of failure of adenotonsillectomy for obstructive sleep apnea in obese pediatric patients. *Int J Pediatr Otorhinolaryngol*. 2017 Jan;92:7–10.

1.3. Discuss the important aspects that must be considered before scheduling a child for ambulatory adenotonsillectomy

Adenotonsillectomy for OSA and/or recurrent streptococcal pharyngitis remains one of the most common surgical procedures performed on children in the United States. Over the past decade, there has been an increasing push to move surgical procedures from an inpatient, hospital-based setting to outpatient settings such as freestanding ambulatory surgery centers due to significant cost savings, greater efficiency, and greater patient satisfaction. Pediatric adenotonsillectomy is usually considered an ambulatory surgical procedure today. Anesthesiologists are often called upon to assist pediatricians and surgeons in identifying those patients who cannot be treated safely in an outpatient setting due to significant risk of postoperative cardiopulmonary complications. Postoperative airway and respiratory complications such as stridor, laryngospasm, laryngeal edema, apnea, and persistent hypoxemia have consistently been shown to be higher in children younger than 3 years of age undergoing tonsillectomy. A clinical guideline endorsed by the American Academy of Pediatrics recommends overnight admission for this population. Despite these guidelines, dataset analysis of nearly 100,000 pediatric adenotonsillectomy procedures in the state of California show that one-third of children less than 3 years of age were discharged home after the surgical procedure.

Further Reading

Amoils M, Chang KW, Saynina O, Wise PH, Honkanen A. Postoperative complications in pediatric tonsillectomy and adenoidectomy in ambulatory vs inpatient settings. *JAMA Otolaryngol Head Neck Surg*. 2016 Apr;142(4):344–350.

Baugh RF, Archer SM, Mitchell RB, et al. American Academy of Otolaryngology–Head and Neck Surgery Foundation. Clinical practice guideline: tonsillectomy in children. *Otolaryngol Head Neck Surg*. 2011 Jan;144(1 Suppl):S1–30.

2. Preoperative Evaluation and Preparation

2.1. Discuss the routine use of preoperative gabapentinoids and their effect on postoperative analgesia for patients undergoing tonsillectomy

Gabapentin and pregabalin, calcium channel ligands originally used as antiepileptic agents, are first-line treatment agents in chronic pain with neuropathic features. However, these agents have become popular in the management of acute pain as well, particularly in multimodal opioid-sparing regimens, as they have shown some benefit in a variety of abdominal and orthopedic procedures. In a meta-analysis of both adult and pediatric patients, gabapentinoids taken orally prior to tonsillectomy provided lower resting pain scores during the first 12 hours after surgery as compared with control but did not provide significant benefit after 12 hours. Overall postoperative analgesic usage and incidence of postoperative nausea were lower for the first 24 hours after surgery when gabapentinoids were taken preoperatively. In addition, dizziness and headache, occasional side effects of these agents, were not observed to be higher in the treatment arms versus the control arms. There is no consensus regarding the appropriate preoperative dosage for either pregabalin or gabapentin for patients undergoing tonsillectomy to achieve these benefits, as a variety of dosages were used in different clinical studies. Gabapentin (5–10 mg/kg/dose) is available as a liquid suspension for young children, but a standard 300-mg capsule may be appropriate for adolescents or teenagers greater than 30 kg. Pregabalin is not commercially available as a liquid suspension, but 50 mg is appropriate for adolescent and teenage patients.

Further Reading

Hwang SH, Park IJ, Cho YJ, Jeong YM, Kang JM. The efficacy of gabapentin/pregabalin in improving pain after tonsillectomy: a meta-analysis. *Laryngoscope.* 2016 Feb;126(2):357–366.

2,2, What are the implications of preoperative fasting times on the perioperative course for children presenting for adenotonsillectomy?

A large body of evidence suggests that children who are permitted to consume clear liquids up to and until 2 hours prior to induction of anesthesia for surgery are happier and have better perioperative metrics. Interestingly, active counseling by members of the healthcare team regarding preoperative fasting strategies and liberal consumption of clear liquids may result in statistically significant reductions in postoperative visual analog pain scores (VAS) in the postanesthesia care unit (PACU). Pain is often difficult to differentiate from other sources of unhappiness in children; restless or crying children in the PACU are often thought to have pain and treated with analgesics. This finding likely reflects less overall irritability in the PACU in well-hydrated children, which could lead to less overall opioid administration.

Further Reading

Klemetti S, Kinnunen I, Suominen T, Antila H, Vahlberg T, Grenman R, Leino-Kilpi H. The effect of preoperative fasting on postoperative pain, nausea and vomiting in pediatric ambulatory tonsillectomy. *Int J Pediatr Otorhinolaryngol.* 2009 Feb;73(2):263–273.

2.3. Discuss the relationship between pediatric OSA-related hypoxemia and opioid receptors, focusing on postoperative opioid requirements

Most children undergoing tonsillectomy today have at least a mild component of upper airway obstruction due to tonsillar and adenoid hypertrophy. Moderate to severe airway obstruction may persist in the immediate postoperative period despite surgical removal of these tissues, leading to persistent hypoxemia, need for additional airway support, or even life-threatening apnea in the PACU. Accordingly, a major goal in the management of postoperative pain in children undergoing tonsillectomy is reducing overall opioid administration because the respiratory-depressant effects of opioids may magnify this problem in the postoperative period. Children with known preoperative hypoxemia, as noted by the oxygen saturation nadir reported on polysomnogram, require less morphine postoperatively to achieve similar pain scores. Most notably, children with an oxygen saturation nadir <85% required half the dosage of opioid to produce equivalent analgesia as compared with children with oxygen saturation nadirs ≥85%. Intermittent hypoxia has been shown to increase the quantity of opioid mu receptors in the brainstem of developing piglets. Children with intermittent hypoxia due to OSA may also express increased amounts of brainstem opioid receptors, explaining this finding. Clinically, children with moderate to severe OSA, particularly those with oxygen saturation nadirs <85%, should receive more judicious administration of opioid analgesics as standard weight-based dosing may lead to hypoxemia or apnea in the postoperative period.

Further Reading

Brown KA, Laferrière A, Lakheeram I, Moss IR. Recurrent hypoxemia in children is associated with increased analgesic sensitivity to opiates. *Anesthesiology*. 2006 Oct;105(4):665–669.

Brown KA, Laferrière A, Moss IR. Recurrent hypoxemia in young children with obstructive sleep apnea is associated with reduced opioid requirement for analgesia. *Anesthesiology*. 2004 Apr;100(4):806–810.

Moss IR, Laferrière A. Central neuropeptide systems and respiratory control during development. *Respir Physiol Neurobiol*. 2002 Jul;131(1–2):15–27.

3. Intraoperative Management

3.1. Discuss the efficacy and value of enteral or intravenous acetaminophen on the perioperative course of children undergoing adenotonsillectomy

Acetaminophen is an important component of many multimodal postoperative analgesic regimens that strive to reduce total opioid requirements. Acetaminophen alone has proven effective as a sole analgesic when adenoidectomy alone is performed, though pairing the agent with nonsteroidal anti-inflammatory drug (NSAID) is typically required when adenotonsillectomy is performed. Oral (15-mg/kg loading dose) and rectal (40-mg/kg loading dose) acetaminophen preparations have been important components of pediatric pain management strategies for decades, but intravenous (IV) acetaminophen (15-mg/kg loading dose) has recently gained popularity in routine perioperative care of the child undergoing adenotonsillectomy. Absorption of enteral acetaminophen may be delayed or incomplete, particularly during the intraoperative period, and the standard technique of suctioning the stomach with an orogastric tube just prior to extubation may remove much of the drug. These factors may lead to subtherapeutic plasma levels of acetaminophen and inadequate analgesia. Intravenous acetaminophen avoids these issues and also bypasses first-pass hepatic biotransformation. Acetaminophen has the ability to provide analgesia without added sedation, which may translate into earlier recovery room discharge in certain populations. The cost of IV acetaminophen is often considered by administrators as excessively high to be considered for routine usage, as no generic form of IV acetaminophen is currently available. Though this is a valid concern, the labor and facility costs of caring for a child who is excessively somnolent, nauseated, or hypoxemic from opioid administration must be weighed against the cost of IV acetaminophen and its beneficial opioid-sparing properties.

Further Reading

Alhashemi JA, Daghistani MF. Effects of intraoperative i.v. acetaminophen vs i.m. meperidine on post-tonsillectomy pain in children. *Br J Anaesth*. 2006 Jun;96(6):790–795.

Subramanyam R, Varughese A, Kurth CD, Eckman MH. Cost-effectiveness of intravenous acetaminophen for pediatric tonsillectomy. *Paediatr Anaesth*. 2014 May;24(5):467–475.

Vons KM, Bijker JB, Verwijs EW, Majoor MH, de Graaff JC. Postoperative pain during the first week after adenoidectomy and guillotine adenotonsillectomy in children. Paediatr Anaesth. 2014 May;24(5):476–482.

3.2. Discuss the controversy regarding the routine use of NSAIDs, particularly IV ketorolac, for pediatric adenotonsillectomy

The use of the IV NSAID ketorolac in the management of posttonsillectomy pain has been controversial for nearly 2 decades. Unlike acetaminophen, NSAIDs inhibit platelet aggregation and therefore may play a part in the development of clinically relevant postsurgical bleeding. A 2013 Cochrane Review studying this potential association concluded that there is "insufficient evidence to exclude an increased risk of bleeding" when NSAIDs were part of perioperative management of tonsillectomy. A few studies do show a greater association between posttonsillectomy bleeding and ketorolac (0.5 mg/kg IV q6h) as compared with other NSAIDs, while others show no association. Despite the mixed evidence, conservative management is to avoid ketorolac in children undergoing tonsillectomy. The NSAID ibuprofen (10 mg/kg PO q6h) is gaining greater popularity in standard posttonsillectomy pain management. In most studies, enteral ibuprofen does not contribute to the incidence of posttonsillectomy bleeding. Additionally, the use of enteral ibuprofen has been shown to be just as effective for analgesia as combination codeine with acetaminophen preparations. Intravenous ibuprofen is costly because no generic formulation is currently available, but it does seem to reduce the opioid requirement of children undergoing tonsillectomy.

Further Reading

Baugh RF, Archer SM, Mitchell RB, Rosenfeld RM, Amin R, Burns JJ, Darrow DH, Giordano T, Litman RS, Li KK, Mannix ME, Schwartz RH, Setzen G, Wald ER, Wall E, Sandberg G, Patel MM; American Academy of Otolaryngology-Head and Neck Surgery Foundation. Clinical practice guideline: tonsillectomy in children. *Otolaryngol Head Neck Surg*. 2011 Jan; 144 (1 Suppl): S1–30.

Lewis SR, Nicholson A, Cardwell ME, Siviter G, Smith AF. Nonsteroidal anti-inflammatory drugs and perioperative bleeding in paediatric tonsillectomy. *Cochrane Database Syst Rev*. 2013 Jul 18;(7). CD003591.

Moss JR, Watcha MF, Bendel LP, McCarthy DL, Witham SL, Glover CD. A multicenter, randomized, double-blind placebo-controlled, single dose trial of the safety and efficacy of intravenous ibuprofen for treatment of pain in pediatric patients undergoing tonsillectomy. *Paediatr Anaesth*. 2014 May;24(5):483–489.

Mudd PA, Thottathil P, Giordano T, Wetmore RF, Elden L, Jawad AF, Ahumada L, Gálvez JA. Association between ibuprofen use and severity of surgically managed posttonsillectomy hemorrhage. *JAMA Otolaryngol Head Neck Surg*. 2017 Jul 1;143(7):712–717.

3.3. Discuss the efficacy of surgical infiltration of local anesthetic or nerve blocks on perioperative analgesia for tonsillectomy

Though it seems intuitive that injection of local anesthetics into the tonsillar bed should provide reasonable analgesia, surgeons do not utilize this technique regularly because of variable efficacy. In addition, local anesthetic toxicity leading to cardiac arrhythmia has been implicated with local injection of amide local anesthetics for tonsillectomy. Glossopharyngeal nerve blocks may result in unacceptably high risks of upper airway obstruction due to inadvertent spread of local anesthetic to the recurrent laryngeal or hypoglossal nerves.

Further Reading

Bean-Lijewski JD. Glossopharyngeal nerve block for pain relief after pediatric tonsillectomy: retrospective analysis and two cases of life-threatening upper airway obstruction from an interrupted trial. *Anesth Analg*. 1997 Jun;84(6):1232–1238.

Hollis LJ, Burton MJ, Millar JM. Perioperative local anaesthesia for reducing pain following tonsillectomy. *Cochrane Database Syst Rev*. 2000;(2):CD001874.

Park AH, Pappas AL, Fluder E, Creech S, Lugo RA, Hotaling A. Effect of perioperative administration of ropivacaine with epinephrine on postoperative pediatric adenotonsillectomy recovery. *Arch Otolaryngol Head Neck Surg*. 2004 Apr;130(4):459–464.

3.4. Clonidine and ketamine have classically been used as adjuncts for perioperative analgesia for pediatric adenotonsillectomy. Review the medical evidence for these agents

The centrally acting alpha-2 agonist clonidine (0.3–3 mcg/kg PO) has classically been considered a reasonable adjunct in the perioperative care of the child undergoing tonsillectomy due to its potential efficacy at providing preoperative anxiolysis, reducing emergence delirium, and contributing to analgesia. Clonidine is known to contribute significantly to postoperative sedation, a feature that often leads to perioperative inefficiencies and greater hospital costs. The benefits of oral or rectal clonidine in pediatric perioperative care have not been consistently reported in the medical literature, and therefore the agent has largely been supplanted by the newer alpha-2 agonist dexmedetomidine.

Ketamine is a N-methyl-D-aspartate (NMDA) antagonist that has shown efficacy as an analgesic when used in subanesthetic dosages in multiple adult and pediatric surgical populations. Ketamine (0.5 mg/kg IV once intraoperatively) when compared with control groups has consistently been shown to reduce posttonsillectomy pain severity in children. The ability of ketamine to reduce total opioid consumption is less clear, and the medical evidence is split. Some studies cite association between ketamine and postoperative laryngospasm, likely due to ketamine-induced increases in salivary and respiratory tract secretions, but these side effects are typically offset with concomitant administration of an anti-sialogogue like glycopyrrolate.

Further Reading

Blackburn L, Ottaway K, Anderson BJ. The impact of clonidine on sedation after adenotonsillectomy: a prospective audit. *Paediatr Anaesth.* 2014 Dec;24(12):1268–1273.

DA Conceição MJ, Bruggemann DA, Conceição D, Carneiro Leão C. Effect of an intravenous single dose of ketamine on postoperative pain in tonsillectomy patients. Paediatr Anaesth. 2006 Sep;16(9):962–967.

Cho HK, Kim KW, Jeong YM, Lee HS, Lee YJ, Hwang SH. Efficacy of ketamine in improving pain after tonsillectomy in children: meta-analysis. PLoS One. 2014 Jun 30;9(6):e101259.

3.5. Dexmedetomidine has recently gained popularity in the routine care of the child presenting for pediatric adenotonsillectomy. Review the medical evidence for this agent in various phases of the perioperative period

The alpha-2 agonist dexmedetomidine has had a major impact on the routine practice of anesthesiology over the past decade. Dexmedetomidine is similar to clonidine in that both are alpha adrenoreceptor agonists, but dexmedetomidine has much greater affinity to the alpha-2 receptor, lending to its greater sedative and analgesic properties. Dexmedetomidine has become a valuable agent in pediatric anesthesiology, as it has found use in providing preoperative anxiolysis, reducing postoperative emergence delirium, and as an opioid-sparing adjunct. Dexmedetomidine (1–2 mcg/kg intranasal) is equivalent to the gold standard of midazolam (0.5–0.7 mg/kg PO) in its ability to provide preoperative anxiolysis to the fearful child without IV access. In many respects, perioperative dexmedetomidine is superior to preoperative midazolam in the pediatric patient with OSA undergoing tonsillectomy. Intranasal dexmedetomidine may take an additional 15 to 20 minutes to achieve adequate anxiolysis to facilitate parental separation and smooth inhalational induction compared with enteral midazolam. However, unlike benzodiazepines, dexmedetomidine does not augment the respiratory depressant activities of intraoperative IV opioids, an important factor to consider when caring for children with significant OSA.

Dexmedetomidine given either preoperatively or intraoperatively will also assist in reducing overall opioid requirement in the perioperative period. Indeed, dexmedetomidine reduces pain intensity while decreasing the opioid requirement and opioid-free interval for children in the recovery room after tonsillectomy but does tend to mildly increase the length of stay due to the additional sedative effects.

Emergence delirium is a very common occurrence in children 2 to 5 years of age undergoing adenotonsillectomy. Emergence delirium not only poses a safety hazard to the child in the recovery room but also may lead to the administration of additional opioids, sedatives, or hypnotics, contributing to respiratory depression in a child with moderate to severe OSA. Dexmedetomidine, along with propofol, has consistently been shown to prevent or reduce the severity of the incidence of emergence delirium without contributing significantly to respiratory depression.

Further Reading

Pestieau SR, Quezado ZM, Johnson YJ, Anderson JL, Cheng YI, McCarter RJ, Choi S, Finkel JC. High-dose dexmedetomidine increases the opioid-free interval and decreases opioid requirement after tonsillectomy in children. *Can J Anaesth.* 2011 Jun;58(6):540–550.

Sheta SA, Al-Sarheed MA, Abdelhalim AA. Intranasal dexmedetomidine vs midazolam for premedication in children undergoing complete dental rehabilitation: a double-blinded randomized controlled trial. *Paediatr Anaesth.* 2014 Feb;24(2):181–189.

Sottas CE, Anderson BJ. Dexmedetomidine: the new all-in-one drug in paediatric anaesthesia? *Curr Opin Anaesthesiol.* 2017 Aug;30(4):441–451.

3.6. Discuss the role of IV dexamethasone and IV antibiotics for routine pediatric adenotonsillectomy

Routine administration of IV dexamethasone (0.2–1 mg/kg IV, maximum dose 12 mg) is recommended for pediatric adenotonsillectomy due to its ability to reduce postoperative nausea/vomiting, contribute to postoperative analgesia, reduce airway edema, and promote earlier intake of food. Though the mechanism by which corticosteroids exert an antiemetic effect is unclear, several randomized controlled studies have shown that a single dose of IV dexamethasone reduces the incidence of nausea/vomiting for the first 24 hours after surgery.

Corticosteroids have potent anti-inflammatory effects leading to significant analgesia for children undergoing adenotonsillectomy.

Though dexamethasone for adenotonsillectomy has been largely touted for its beneficial effects, safety, and minimal side effects, it is important to note that there is some controversy regarding the contribution of perioperative dexamethasone to posttonsillectomy bleeding. A randomized, placebo-controlled trial that was designed to study the effect of dexamethasone on postoperative nausea and vomiting had to be terminated early due to concerns of excessive postoperative bleeding in children within the treatment arm. The results were published in a major journal and were met with significant controversy; subsequent trials have not found a dose-related increase in posttonsillectomy bleeding when dexamethasone was administered.

Further Reading

Czarnetzki C, Elia N, Lysakowski C, Dumont L, Landis BN, Giger R, Dulguerov P, Desmeules J, Tramèr MR. Dexamethasone and risk of nausea and vomiting and postoperative bleeding after tonsillectomy in children: a randomized trial. *JAMA.* 2008 Dec 10;300(22):2621–2630.

Steward DL, Grisel J, Meinzen-Derr J. Steroids for improving recovery following tonsillectomy in children. *Cochrane Database Syst Rev.* 2011 Aug 10;8:CD003997.

Yiu Y, Mahida JB, Cooper JN, Elsey NM, Deans KJ, Minneci PC, Merrill TB, Tobias JD, Elmaraghy CA. The effect of perioperative dexamethasone dosing on post-tonsillectomy hemorrhage risk. *Int J Pediatr Otorhinolaryngol.* 2017 Jul;98:19–24.

3.7. Surgical technique and the method by which the surgeon obtains surgical hemostasis both have a major impact on postoperative pain after pediatric tonsillectomy. Discuss various tonsillectomy surgical techniques and devices, focusing on the risks and benefits of each

Traditional tonsillectomy is performed by excising the entire palatine tonsil along with the surrounding capsule. Over the past decade, there has been growing interest in powered intracapsular tonsillotomy, also known as partial tonsillectomy, in which a special microdebrider device is utilized to remove tonsillar tissue while preserving the capsule and not violating surrounding peritonsillar vasculature and nerve fibers. Powered intracapsular tonsillotomy requires additional training and equipment but does cause less bleeding and less postoperative pain and allows earlier return to normal feeding. Tonsillotomy is typically performed with a carbon dioxide (CO_2) laser or argon plasma coagulation (APC), both more complex and expensive techniques but with proven safety and providing better postoperative conditions for the patient. Since tonsillotomy often does not remove all of the tonsillar tissue, regrowth of tonsillar tissue is a major drawback to this technique as regrowth rates as high as 16% have been cited.

Classical surgical tonsillectomy consisted of "cold" dissection with a scalpel, scissors, and other classical metal surgical instruments. Though cold dissection results in less overall pain during the immediate perioperative period, this technique is not commonly performed today in developed countries due to longer surgical times and greater blood loss. "Hot" dissection methods, specifically monopolar and bipolar electrocautery, are by far the most popular surgical technique today for pediatric tonsillectomy. Monopolar electrocautery is used more often than bipolar electrocautery. However, with bipolar cautery the dissipated heat is more controlled and less tissue damage occurs, leading to less inflammation and less pain.

A technique that is gaining popularity is cold-ablation (coblation) tonsillectomy, which utilizes a unique suction electrode device that resembles a high-temperature suction monopolar electrocautery unit. The key difference is that while electrocautery uses very high temperature (as high as 1200°C), coblation passes radiofrequency energy through a saline conducting medium to produce a plasma field that disrupts tissue at a much lower temperature (40–70°C). As expected, less tissue inflammation and less collateral damage to surrounding tissues lead to lower reported pain when coblation tonsillectomy or coblation intracapsular tonsillotomy is performed. Though these benefits of coblation tonsillectomy are significant, there are mixed results from studies that suggest that cauterizing tissue with coblation at lower temperatures may lead to a greater risk of posttonsillectomy bleeding.

Further Reading

Mostovych N, Holmes L, Ruszkay N, LaHurd A, Heinle R, Nardone H. Effectiveness of powered intracapsular tonsillectomy in children with severe obstructive sleep apnea. *JAMA Otolaryngol Head Neck Surg.* 2016 Feb;142(2):150–156.

Papaspyrou G, Linxweiler M, Knöbber D, Schick B, Al Kadah B. Laser CO(2) tonsillotomy versus argon plasma coagulation (APC) tonsillotomy: a retrospective study with 10-year follow-up. *Int J Pediatr Otorhinolaryngol.* 2017 Jan;92:56–60.

Metcalfe C, Muzaffar J, Daultrey C, Coulson C. Coblation tonsillectomy: a systematic review and descriptive analysis. *Eur Arch Otorhinolaryngol.* 2017 Jun;274(6):2637–2647.

4. Postoperative Management

4.1. What are the inherent risks of using opioid-acetaminophen combinations in the postoperative period?

The enteral opioids hydrocodone, oxycodone, and codeine are commonly sold in preparations that contain acetaminophen. In the United States, hydrocodone and codeine are most commonly delivered in combination preparations with acetaminophen. Though oxycodone is also available in an acetaminophen combination, it is much more readily available in a stand-alone opioid preparation. Though combining these weak enteral opioids with acetaminophen may theoretically provide additional analgesia and ease of administration, the risk of acetaminophen toxicity is elevated when these combination agents are administered. Children may potentially receive acetaminophen for pain or antipyresis at various points through the perioperative process, via various routes (enteral, IV, rectal) as prescribed by various providers (midlevel providers, anesthesiologists, surgeons). In addition, the primary caregiver or extended family members may inadvertently give supplemental acetaminophen despite the child already receiving a combination opioid + acetaminophen agent. It is advisable to utilize an acetaminophen-free opioid agent, such as oxycodone, for breakthrough pain while utilizing acetaminophen and/or an NSAID for primary control of postsurgical pain.

Further Reading

Amar PJ, Schiff ER. Acetaminophen safety and hepatotoxicity—where do we go from here? Expert Opin Drug Saf. 2007 Jul;6(4):341–55.

Martin DP, Bhalla T, Beltran R, Veneziano G, Tobias JD. The safety of prescribing opioids in pediatrics. Expert Opin Drug Saf. 2014 Jan;13(1):93–101.

George JA, Park PS, Hunsberger J, Shay JE, Lehmann CU, White ED, Lee BH, Yaster M. An Analysis of 34,218 Pediatric Outpatient Controlled Substance Prescriptions. Anesth Analg. 2016 Mar;122(3):807–13.

4.2. Discuss the risks implicit with routine use of codeine as an oral postoperative opioid in children

Codeine is an oral opioid that has been prescribed for decades to children undergoing tonsillectomy, dental rehabilitation, or even minor nonsurgical injuries. Codeine is a prodrug and is considered a weak opioid, as it must undergo hepatic biotransformation to morphine by CYP2D6, a hepatic cytochrome p-450 mixed oxidase enzyme complex. Only 10% of codeine normally undergoes O-demethylation to morphine by CYP2D6, with the majority of the drug undergoing glucuronidation to inactive metabolites. Due to the large number of polymorphisms of the CYP2D6 enzyme complex, the actual metabolism of codeine in various genetic populations is quite varied. Children who are "poor metabolizers" receive very little analgesia from codeine due to reduced CYP2D6 metabolism to morphine, while children who are "ultrarapid metabolizers" achieve very high morphine plasma levels in a relatively short period due to increased O-demethylation rates. Nearly 30% of children of Chinese ethnicity may be "poor metabolizers," while 30% of children of Ethiopian ethnicity may be "ultrarapid metabolizers." Several case reports exist of codeine-related morbidity and mortality when appropriate weight-based dosages of codeine were administered to children with CYP2D6 alleles associated with ultrarapid O-demethylation of codeine to morphine. Given these reports, multiple regulatory and patient safety organizations, including the US Food and Drug Administration (FDA), World Health Organization, and American Academy of Pediatrics, have all released statements warning against the use of codeine in children. The FDA issued a black box warning in 2013 that discouraged codeine use in patient less than 18 years of age.

Further Reading

Chidambaran V, Sadhasivam S, Mahmoud M. Codeine and opioid metabolism: implications and alternatives for pediatric pain management. *Curr Opin Anaesthesiol.* 2017 Jun;30(3):349–356.

Kelly LE, Rieder M, van den Anker J, et al. More codeine fatalities after tonsillectomy in North American children. *Pediatrics.* 2012;129:e1343–e1347.

Tobias JD, Green TP, Coté CJ; Section on Anesthesiology and Pain Medicine; Committee on Drugs. Codeine: time to say "no." *Pediatrics.* 2016 Oct;138(4): e1–e7.

4.3. Describe the metabolism of enteral hydrocodone and oxycodone, including important interactions when administered concomitantly with antibiotics and antiepileptic agents

Surgeons and anesthesiologists involved in the perioperative care of children undergoing tonsillectomy should make every effort to reduce the need for perioperative opioid. Reducing or eliminating postoperative opioid use after tonsillectomy significantly reduces the morbidity and mortality of this very common pediatric surgical procedure. Opioid-related respiratory depression in the setting of pediatric OSA, particularly when the child is unmonitored at home, is a major hazard to children in the postoperative period. Indeed, many surgeons and institutions rely solely on nonopioid analgesics such as acetaminophen and ibuprofen for postoperative analgesia and avoid prescribing postoperative opioids entirely after pediatric tonsillectomy. Given the major safety implications inherent with codeine administration to children, oxycodone or hydrocodone preparations are likely the best options for postoperative opioid therapy after pediatric tonsillectomy if an opioid is required.

In North America, enteral tablet or liquid hydrocodone is available only in combination with acetaminophen, which carries the additional risk of acetaminophen toxicity. Unlike codeine, hydrocodone (0.1–0.2 mg/kg/dose q6h as needed) is itself a weak opioid agonist, and its 2 primary active metabolites, hydromorphone and norhydromorphone, are also weak opioid agonists. Hydrocodone does not have the major variability in efficacy as does codeine, but there are also several case reports of hydrocodone deaths or major adverse effects when it is administered to children after tonsillectomy due to the general respiratory depressant effects of the opioid. In addition, the antibiotic clarithromycin (via CYP3A4 inhibition) and the antiepileptic valproic acid (via glucuronidation inhibition) may interfere with the breakdown of the active metabolites of hydrocodone, leading to the potential for persistently high plasma levels of active opioid metabolites.

Oxycodone, available in tablet or liquid preparations, is commercially available without concomitant acetaminophen and is considered a better postoperative analgesic when its side effect and metabolic profile is compared with those of hydrocodone and codeine. Despite this, several case reports also exist about opioid-related toxicity when oxycodone is administered to children. Oxycodone (0.1–0.2 mg/kg/dose q6h as needed) is a weak opioid agonist, and its major metabolites, noroxycodone, noroxymorphone, and oxymorphone, are also metabolically active opioid agonists. Oxymorphone is more than 10 times as potent as oxycodone, but for most patients only 10% of oxycodone is converted to oxymorphone by most CYP2D6 variants. Ultrarapid metabolizers with certain CYP2D6 alleles may convert a larger proportion of oxycodone to oxymorphone causing greater oxymorphone plasma levels and greater risk of opioid toxicity.

Further Reading

Balyan R, Mecoli M, Venkatasubramanian R, Chidambaran V, Kamos N, Clay S, Moore DL, Mavi J, Glover CD, Szmuk P, Vinks A, Sadhasivam S. CYP2D6 pharmacogenetic and oxycodone pharmacokinetic association study in pediatric surgical patients. *Pharmacogenomics*. 2017 Mar;18(4):337–348.

Hutchinson MR, Menelaou A, Foster DJ, Coller JK, Somogyi AA. CYP2D6 and CYP3A4 involvement in the primary oxidative metabolism of hydrocodone by human liver microsomes. *Br J Clin Pharmacol*. 2004 Mar;57(3):287–297.

Madadi P, Hildebrandt D, Gong IY, Schwarz UI, Ciszkowski C, Ross CJ, Sistonen J, Carleton BC, Hayden MR, Lauwers AE, Koren G. Fatal hydrocodone overdose in a child: pharmacogenetics and drug interactions. *Pediatrics*. 2010 Oct;126(4):e986–e989.

Section III

Advanced Regional Anesthesia and Analgesia

Military Advanced Regional Anesthesia and Analgesia (MARAA)

Foreword to the Military Advanced Regional Anesthesia and Analgesia 1st edition

Regional anesthesia and specifically peripheral nerve blocks have been part of our practice for many decades, but lately a combination of factors has made these techniques increasingly more relevant, even crucial, in how we approach and treat acute pain. We continue to consider anatomy as the foundation of a sound regional anesthesia practice, but within this field, we have become increasingly more aware of the importance of myofascial compartments and fascial planes, and at the same time, we have developed a better practical understanding of nerve architecture. In terms of how we perform these techniques, we have incorporated, relatively recently, ultrasound-imaging technology, which has given us not only the ability to visualize, in real time, the desired anatomical targets but also the capacity to determine spread of local anesthetic in relationship to them. The image of spread provide us, for the first time in the history of our specialty, with a tool that has the ability, albeit potential, to predict success by associating patterns of local anesthetic spread with technique success. Lately we also have developed an increased awareness of the role that successful acute pain management plays in the pathophysiology and prevention of chronic pain syndromes. What makes all these advances all the more important is that they are taking place in the midst of what has been denominated the "opioid epidemics." This crisis, and its impact on patients, families, society, and economics, has made us reevaluate the strategies used in acute pain management and forced us to develop new and better techniques, with emphasis on narcotic-spearing modalities. In this context, a manual dedicated to the techniques of peripheral nerve blocks with emphasis on multimodal approach to acute pain is certainly welcome.

The first edition of the Military Advanced Regional Anesthesia and Analgesia (MARAA) manual was enriched by a preface written by the late Alon P Winnie, a giant in our field and a visionary in pain management, who with much foresight understood that treating acute pain goes beyond the basic and noble cause of alleviating pain in the short term.

This second edition of the MARAA manual is an improved effort to describe the relevant anatomy and procedural details of the most common techniques of regional anesthesia, within a context of modern multimodal analgesia. Although written by, and aimed primarily for the military anesthesiologist, its importance transcends any boundaries for its descriptions and recommendations are applicable to any busy center in the United States and around the world. It is, in other words, a practical tool for the modern and busy anesthesiologist looking for practical and straightforward guidelines on how to approach acute pain management. The manual itself, and the military pain initiative behind it, are the creative efforts of Dr. Chester "Trip" Buckenmaier III, a practicing anesthesiologist and a retired colonel in the Unites States Army. Dr. Buckenmaier has been a leader in the field of acute pain management and was a pioneer of military pain initiatives that have benefited our wounded soldiers in the field and during their evacuation from it. The importance of these initiatives transcends the military for they apply as well to the civilian environment. His vision, knowledge of the subject, and relentless dedication in pursuit of his goals have made him a great warrior in the noble cause of relieving our patients' pain and suffering.

I am honored to have been invited by Dr. Buckenmaier to write this foreword, and I salute the efforts that went into writing this manual. I am sure that it will be an invaluable tool for anesthesia practitioners, military and civilian, everywhere. In a time when traditional ways of alleviating pain are being questioned, and we struggle to devise newer and better ways of dealing with acute pain and its chronic implications, the MARAA book is certainly a great tool in that fight.

Carlo Franco

Foreword to Military Advanced Regional Anesthesia and Analgesia 1st edition

Almost 50 years ago a seminal observation in the renaissance and subsequent explosive development of regional anesthesia was made by a resident prosector preparing a cadaver for a nerve block course taught by the resident's chairman. Although the dissection was primarily focused on the nerves, the resident noted a consistent relationship between the nerves, muscles, and fascia: the brachial plexus, for example, was surrounded by a fascial sheath, provided in large part by the surrounding muscles, throughout its development and distribution to the upper extremity. As the dissection continued, he noted a similar fascial envelope surrounding the other major plexuses, cervical, lumbar, and sacral. As a result, the resident theorized that it might be possible to block an entire plexus by injecting local anesthetic through a needle inserted into its sheath, just as in producing epidural anesthesia. He tried it clinically and it worked. After his first few successful single-injection blocks, he commented to his fellow residents how useful such single injection techniques would be on the battlefield, especially since the use of a catheter would allow analgesia to last as long as necessary.

Over the subsequent half century, many (perhaps too many!) approaches to these "fascial envelopes" have been described, and many of them have become popular throughout the world. Furthermore, technological advances have kept pace with the increasing use of regional anesthesia, making all the techniques simpler to learn, safe to administer, and much more successful. Although regional anesthesia was being utilized frequently in hospital clinical practice, it took the Military Advanced Regional Anesthesia and Analgesia (MARAA) group's vision to recognize the unique value of these techniques during wartime; for centuries, morphine has been the traditional painkiller on the battlefield, despite producing a high incidence of nausea and vomiting, bringing the possibility of abuse and dependence, and never completely abolishing the pain. Continuous plexus or peripheral blocks can relieve pain completely and can maintain relief as long as necessary. Colonel Chester C. Buckenmaier III, the founder of MARAA, personally provided the first successful application of a continuous peripheral nerve block on the battlefield: he placed a continuous catheter in the leg of a soldier who had sustained a severe shrapnel injury to his left calf from a rocket-propelled grenade. This one catheter with a continuous infusion of local anesthetic provided complete pain relief during this soldier's entire evacuation, the initial surgery at the combat support hospital in Iraq, transport to Germany, a second surgical procedure there, transport home to Walter Reed Army Medical Center, and four additional surgical procedures there, the last being amputation. The catheter was finally removed after the last procedure, 16 days after its insertion!

As impressive as this approach is to the management of the acute pain of battlefield injuries and subsequent surgical procedures, its advantages may go even further: evidence is accumulating that neural blockade of acute pain may prevent the subsequent development of chronic pain (complex regional pain syndrome I and II, phantom limb pain, etc.); researchers are even predicting that the absence of excruciating pain following devastating injuries could prevent the development of posttraumatic stress syndrome. Only time and the data being obtained by MARAA will tell.

Military anesthesiologists should be proficient in regional anesthesia techniques, which will undoubtedly play an increasingly important role in providing pain relief and recovery during wartime. MARAA hopes to make this possible by providing this excellent, brief but complete synopsis of regional anesthesia as a resource for anesthesiologists serving in the armed forces. Not intended for the beginner or trainee, this book is carefully structured to provide a quick review of the anatomy and technique of each nerve block, formatted for easy reference on the battlefield or in the operating room. Because of the variable circumstances under which a block may be carried out on the battlefield, each technique is described using paresthesia, nerve stimulation, and ultrasound. I am certain not only that this book will go a long way toward integrating continuous plexus and peripheral nerve blocks into military medicine but also, ultimately (because soldiers aren't soldiers forever), that both the manual and MARAA will have a positive impact on civilian medicine and, in particular, the way we manage painful trauma in large-scale civilian disasters.

Alon P. Winnie

Prologue

The Military Advanced Regional Anesthesia and Analgesia (MARAA) Handbook was originally developed as a supplement to Emergency War Surgery, Third United States Revision. In Emergency War Surgery, regional anesthesia is described as "a 'field friendly' anesthetic requiring minimal logistical support while providing quality anesthesia and analgesia on the battlefield." The first MARAA text has become a popular standard for military healthcare personnel deploying in support of the past 18 years of conflict. This popularity has, in part, been due to the general realization of the importance of aggressive acute pain management following trauma for the successful recovery and rehabilitation of wounded warriors. Although the MARAA text was conceived and executed in support of military healthcare providers caring for combat wounded, the lessons and techniques herein are no less effective or important for civilian trauma. The contributors to this MARAA handbook 2nd edition and the original text have collaborated to provide a useful resource for managing the pain of battlefield and civilian trauma.

Rapid advancement in medical science has been the hallmark of US military medicine throughout the nation's history. The recent wars in Iraq and Afghanistan are no exception. Life-saving advances in body armor, rapid medical evacuation from point of injury, availability of blood products, improved far-forward surgical and critical care capability, and rapid air evacuation of casualties to level IV medical facilities have contributed to a less than 10 percent died-of-wounds rate in the current conflicts. The military medical triumph represented by this statistic is undeniable, although the achievement has resulted in other problems, particularly in the management of acute pain. Since the US Civil War, morphine has been the accepted standard for battlefield pain control because options for pain management in previous conflicts were limited, comprehension of pain mechanisms nascent, and casualties, when they survived, tended to remain near the battlefield while they recovered. Modern combat casualty care now emphasizes rapid evacuation to progressively higher levels of medical care with critical care support provided at all times (including transport). Casualties who earlier were kept in a war zone for days to weeks until they were stable for transport are now transported by plane from Iraq to Germany within eight to 72 hours of injury. The environment of evacuation aircraft—crowded, deafening, jolting, poorly lit, with limited monitoring capabilities—only magnifies the difficulties of using opioid-only pain control therapy. Healthcare providers placed in this situation are less likely to use adequate doses of morphine because of valid patient safety concerns. The large numbers of healthcare providers in the evacuation chain and long evacuation distances further complicate opioid use in these patients. Furthermore, the need for advanced techniques in the management of trauma pain is heightened with the realities of the ongoing opioid crisis in the United States that impacts all Americans both civilian and military.

Fortunately, among the medical advances arising from the current conflicts are improved understanding and management of pain in war casualties. Through the MARAA and later DVCIPM (Defense and Veterans Center for Integrative Pain Management) organizations (see Chapter 1), like-minded pain management providers from the Air Force, Army, Navy, Veterans Administration, and civilian medicine have greatly improved the management of pain in combat wounded through the application of modern pain treatment medications and technologies, including advanced regional anesthesia. In the US military, chronic pain is now recognized as a disease process of the nervous system, not just a symptom of trauma. This text celebrates this advancement, preserving what has been learned to serve as a new, higher standard for pain management in this and forthcoming conflicts.

The primary goal of this handbook is to assist with the education of anesthesiology residents, fellows, and other allied medical professionals (Special Forces' medics, nurse anesthetists, emergency room physicians, and others) in the art and science of acute pain medicine and regional anesthesia. As John J. Bonica stated in *The Management of Pain*, "The proper management of pain remains, after all, the most important obligation, the main objective, and the crowning achievement of every physician." This handbook is dedicated to the US military professionals who have been wounded in the service of this country. It is our hope that the knowledge within this text will be used to ease the burden of their wounds.

Chester C. Buckenmaier III

The Military Advanced Regional Anesthesia and Analgesia Initiative: A Brief History

26

> He who would become a surgeon should join the army and follow it.
>
> —Hippocrates

The history of warfare parallels the history of medical advances. In the field of anesthesia, wars have resulted in marked technical, chemical, and procedural advances, including the first battlefield use of inhalational anesthesia (Mexican-American War), first widespread use of anesthetics and inhalers for the application of inhaled anesthetics (US Civil War), use of the eye signs chart for safe monitoring by lay practitioners (World War I), development of specific short-course training centers for predeployment anesthesia training (World War II), and the establishment of military anesthesia residency programs in response to shortages of specialty trained doctors (Korean War). The medical advances arising from the wars in Iraq and Afghanistan continued this historical trend (Figure 26.1), as evidenced by the establishment of the Military Advanced Regional Anesthesia and Analgesia Initiative (MARAA), which later became the Defense and Veterans Center for Integrative Pain Management (DVCIPM).

MARAA was formed in 2003 as a collaborative effort of like-minded military anesthesiologists who perceived a need for improvement in battlefield pain management. Deployed military anesthesiologists recognized a disconnect between battlefield and civilian analgesic care that needed to be bridged. As one provider put it, "Pain control in Baghdad, 2003, was the same as in the Civil War—a nurse with a syringe of morphine." Colonel (Retired) John Chiles was the first to voice the potential benefit of increasing the use of regional anesthesia in the Iraq War. Chiles, along with Lieutenant Colonel Chester Buckenmaier, established the Army Regional Anesthesia and Pain Management Initiative in 2000. Dr Buckenmaier administered the first continuous peripheral nerve block in Operation Iraqi Freedom on October 7, 2003. Upon his return to the United States, Buckenmaier, Chiles, Lieutenant Colonel Todd Carter, and Colonel (Retired) Ann Virtis created MARAA, following in the tradition of the Anesthesia Travel Club created by John Lundy to rapidly disseminate research advances to practitioners. The importance of MARAA was recognized by the legendary anesthesiologist Alon P. Winnie, who often attended MARAA educational workshops (Figure 26.2).

MARAA's initial purpose was to develop consensus recommendations from the US Air Force, Army, and Navy anesthesia services to implement improvements in medical practice and technology to promote regional anesthesia and analgesia in the care of military beneficiaries. The organization also served as an advisory board to the individual

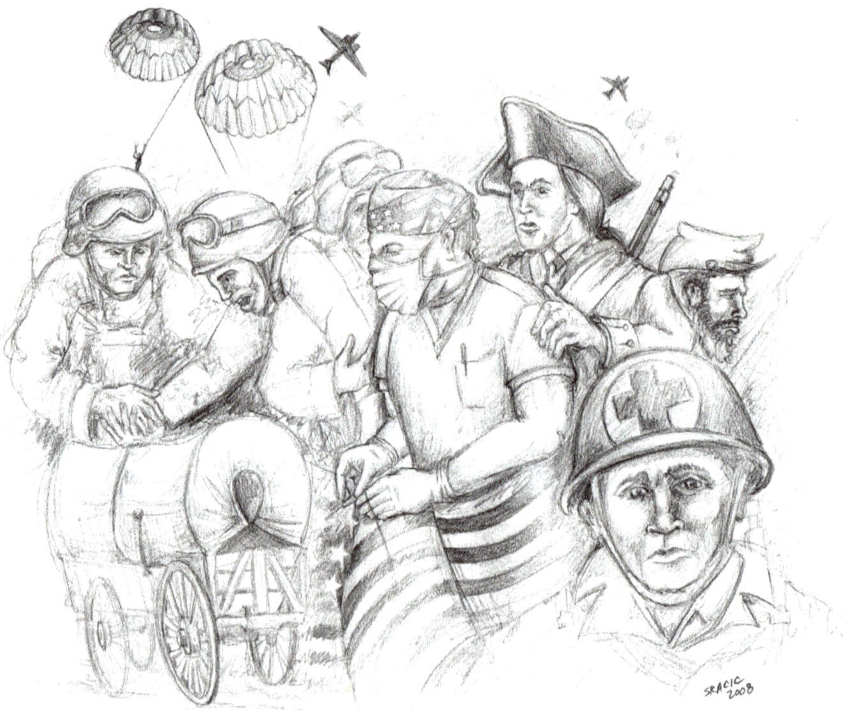

Figure 26.1 *As Long As There Is War, There Will Be Wounded*, by Lieutenant Michael K. Sracic, MD, MC, US Navy, 2008.

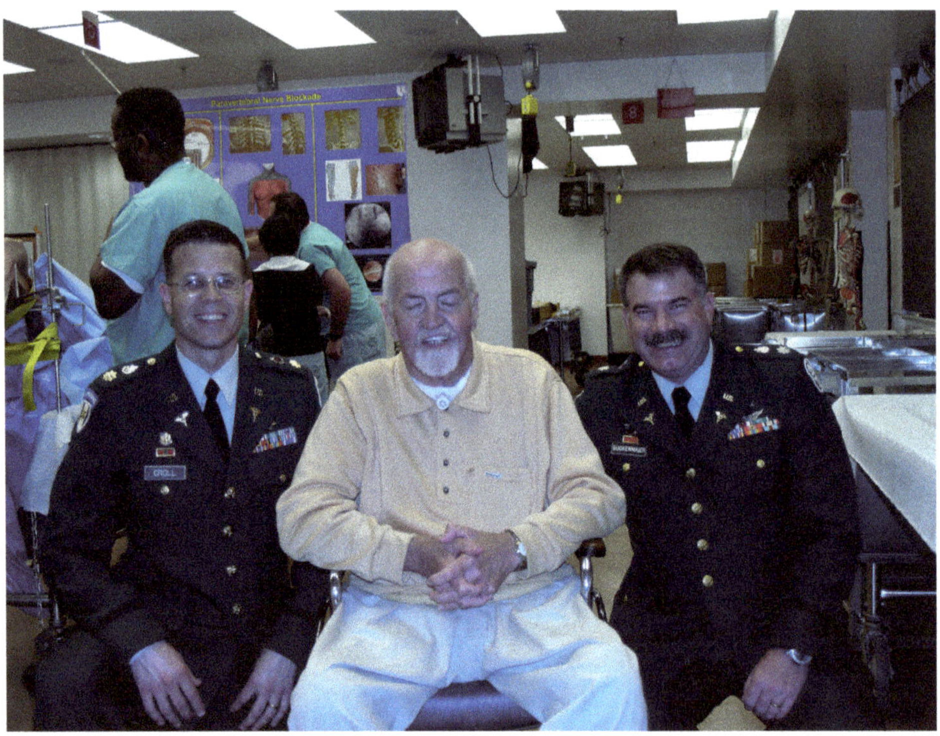

Figure 26.2 MAARA Annual Workshop faculty; left to right: Scott M. Croll, Alon P. Winnie, Chester Buckenmaier.

Table 26.1:
Attendees at the first meeting of the Military Advanced Regional Anesthesia and Analgesia Initiative

Colonel John Chiles, Army	Service Consultant
LTC Chester Buckenmaier, Army	Service consultant designee; MARAA president
Lt Col Todd Carter, Air Force	Service consultant
Captain Ivan Lesnik, Navy	Service consultant
CDR Dean Giacobbe, Navy	Service consultant designee
Major Peter Baek, Air Force	Service consultant designee

service anesthesia consultants to the surgeons general. Initial support of MARAA resulted from the public's demand for better pain control for wounded service members, which later led to congressional funding through the John P. Murtha Neuroscience and Pain Institute, the Telemedicine and Advanced Technology Research Center, and the Henry M. Jackson Foundation.

The first MARAA meeting was held in February 2005 (Table 26.1). By October 2006, MARAA participants had grown to include more than 30 senior military anesthesiologists. Acknowledging the importance of nursing support of anesthesia, the MARAA board expanded to include a certified registered nurse anesthetist from each uniformed service in April 2006. In the beginning, the MARAA meetings focused on securing approval of the Stryker PainPump 2 (Stryker; Kalamazoo, Mich) for use on Air Force military aircraft and establishing the need for patient-controlled analgesia pumps on the battlefield and on evacuation aircraft. MARAA later developed a series of training modules and consensus recommendations on pain management for anesthesiologists preparing for deployment. The Air Force, having primary responsibility for evacuating wounded service members from Iraq and Afghanistan to Germany and the United States, quickly recognized the value of this initiative and promptly issued a memorandum outlining specific directives to Air Force providers based on MARAA recommendations. As the MARAA products began to improve pain control for wounded service members, their impact was recognized in professional and lay journals ranging from *Pain Medicine* to *Newsweek* and *Wired* magazine.

Following the 2009 publication of the first MARAA book, a rapid evolution of pain management continued both inside and outside of the Department of Defense (DoD). The Centers for Disease Control and Prevention (CDC) was just beginning to understand the consequences arising from the nation's overreliance on opioids for pain management. Notably, the DoD and the Veterans Administration's (VA) health systems played significant roles in shaping the nation's pain strategy. Driven by their common desire to optimize pain care for the cumulative number of wounded, ill, and injured service members, the DoD, and VA health systems were among the first large organizations to begin shifting toward team-based pain care that emphasized the need for nonmedication pain treatments and coordination of pain care across multiple medical specialties. The 2009 VHA Pain Directive introduced the Stepped Care Model of pain management that defined how VA pain care should be coordinated as pain increased in complexity and chronicity. The Army Surgeon General chartered the Tri-Service Pain Management Task Force in 2009 to develop a DoD comprehensive pain management strategy that was holistic, multidisciplinary, and multimodal in its approach; that utilized state-of-the-art/science modalities and technologies; and that focused on optimizing function and quality of life for patients with acute and chronic pain. In 2011, the Institute of Medicine (IOM) of the National Academies released the "Pain in America" report, which essentially called for the nation to pursue a pain strategy that paralleled what was being undertaken in the DoD and VA. The Department of Health and Human Services later codified the IOM report's recommendations in the HHS National Pain Strategy (2016). The urgency to implement each of these pain strategies became even more clear when, in 2016, the CDC published guidelines with sweeping changes to what would be considered appropriate use of opioids. The DoD and VA followed shortly with their joint clinical practice guideline for opioid therapy for chronic pain (Table 26.2).

Table 26.2:
Federal pain management publications

Date Published	Document	Proponent Organization(s)
2009	VHA Pain Management Directive	Veterans Health Administration
2010	DoD Pain Management Task Force Report	United States Army, Office of the Surgeon General
2011	Relieving Pain in America; A Blueprint for Transforming Prevention, Care Education and Research	Institute of Medicine of the National Academies
2015	National Pain Strategy	NIH Interagency Pain Research Coordinating Committee
2016	CDC Guideline for Prescribing Opioids for Chronic Pain	Centers for Disease Control and Prevention
2017	Clinical Practice Guideline for Opioid Therapy for Chronic Pain	Departments of Defense and Veterans Affairs

The structure and focus of what was once known as MARAA has continued to adapt in order to maintain a position on the leading edge of pain medicine. What was once an organization consisting of anesthesiologists focused almost exclusively on regional anesthesia has evolved over the years to a multidisciplinary group of clinicians and researchers focused on promoting comprehensive and integrative pain management. MARAA was renamed the Defense and Veterans Center for Integrative Pain Management in 2011 and designated the DoD's Center for Excellence for pain management in 2016.

This second edition of the MARAA text continues to expand and refine the lessons learned through military conflict on the improved pain management of war casualties. The information will be of interest to any provider involved in the management of acute pain.

Regional Anesthesia Equipment

27

1. Introduction

The safe and successful application of regional anesthesia requires specialized training and equipment. The primary purpose of this chapter is to serve as a guide for resident and fellow anesthesiologists during their regional anesthesia and acute pain medicine rotations. The facility, equipment, and staffing solutions described here may not be entirely workable at other institutions; however, the editor is confident that other clinicians can benefit from this systematic approach to regional anesthesia and acute pain medicine. Contemporary regional anesthesia relies on sophisticated equipment, allowing clinicians to provide safe and accurate needle placement and anesthetic delivery. This chapter will review the equipment used at institutions such as Duke University Medical Center (DUMC) and Walter Reed National Military Medical Center (WRNMMC) and also on the modern battlefield.

(Note: The equipment displayed in this chapter is for illustration purposes only and should not be considered an endorsement of any product.)

2. Regional Anesthesia Area (Preoperative Block Area)

Regardless of the practice environment (military care roles 3 through 4), a key component to the successful practice of regional anesthesia includes the use of a designated area outside of the operating room to perform regional anesthesia techniques (peripheral nerve blocks [PNBs] and neuraxial techniques). Having a designated preoperative block area will improve block success and decrease costs by preventing unnecessary operating room delays, providing additional time for long-acting local anesthetics to "set up," and allowing providers time to assess the quality of the nerve block prior to surgery and to intervene if necessary. Additionally, a preoperative block area will enhance resident/fellow education by providing an instructional environment free from the pressures and distractions of a busy operating room environment. The preoperative block area should include standard monitors, oxygen delivery, suction, airway equipment, emergency hemodynamic medication and supplies, ultrasound machines, peripheral nerve stimulators, and a rolling block cart (Figure 27.1).

The block cart contains the supplies and drugs necessary to perform regional anesthesia techniques and manage block-related complications and emergencies, including (Figure 27.2):

- Various needle types and lengths, including single-injection and continuous peripheral nerve block needles, neuraxial block needles

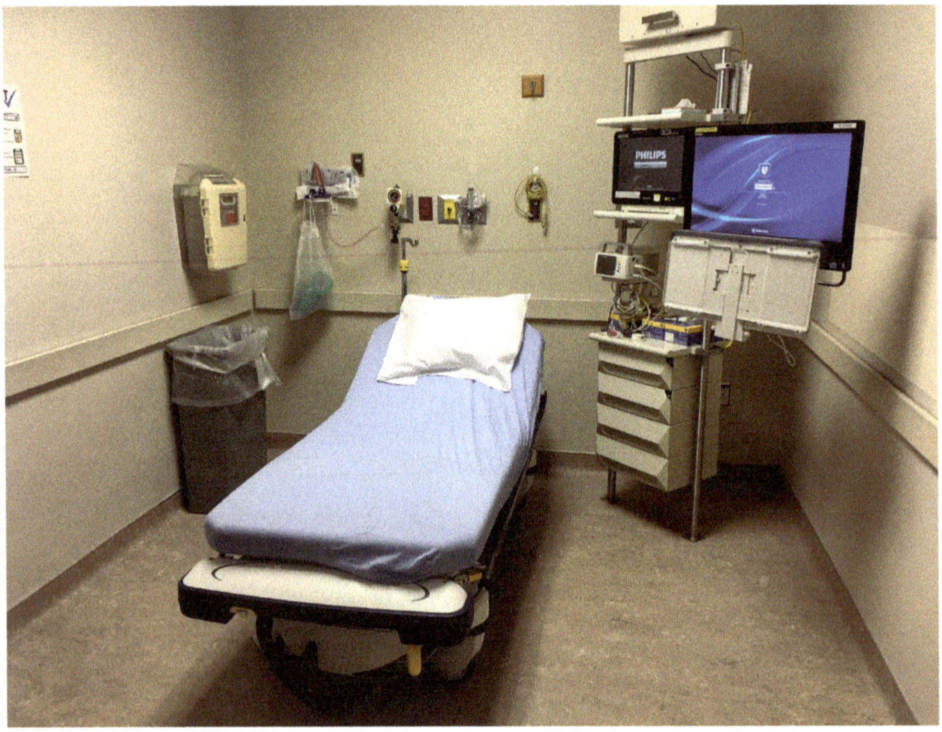

Figure 27.1 Preoperative block area.

- Various syringe sizes
- Gloves
- Peripheral nerve stimulators
- Antiseptic solutions (e.g., chlorhexidine, iodine)
- Ultrasound gel
- Ultrasound probe covers
- Continuous peripheral nerve block trays, spinal/epidural trays
- Topical skin adhesive solutions (e.g., DERMABOND ADVANCED® Topical Skin Adhesive, Hollister® Medical Adhesive Spray)
- Clear occlusive dressings (e.g., 3M™ Tegaderm™)
- Adhesive skin closure products (e.g., Steri-Strip™ Skin Closure)
- Local anesthetics
- Resuscitation drugs
- Emergency airway equipment
- Lipid emulsion 20%
- Sharp container attached to the cart

Certain military practice environments will necessitate adjustments or alternatives to this equipment list.

3. Patient Consent for Regional Anesthesia

As with any medical procedure, proper written consent for the regional anesthetic procedure should be obtained. Counseling should include information on the risks of regional anesthesia, including but not limited to intravascular injection, local anesthetic toxicity, and potential nerve injury or other injury. Patients receiving a regional anesthetic block of the extremity should be reminded to avoid using the blocked extremity (particularly ambulating on a blocked lower

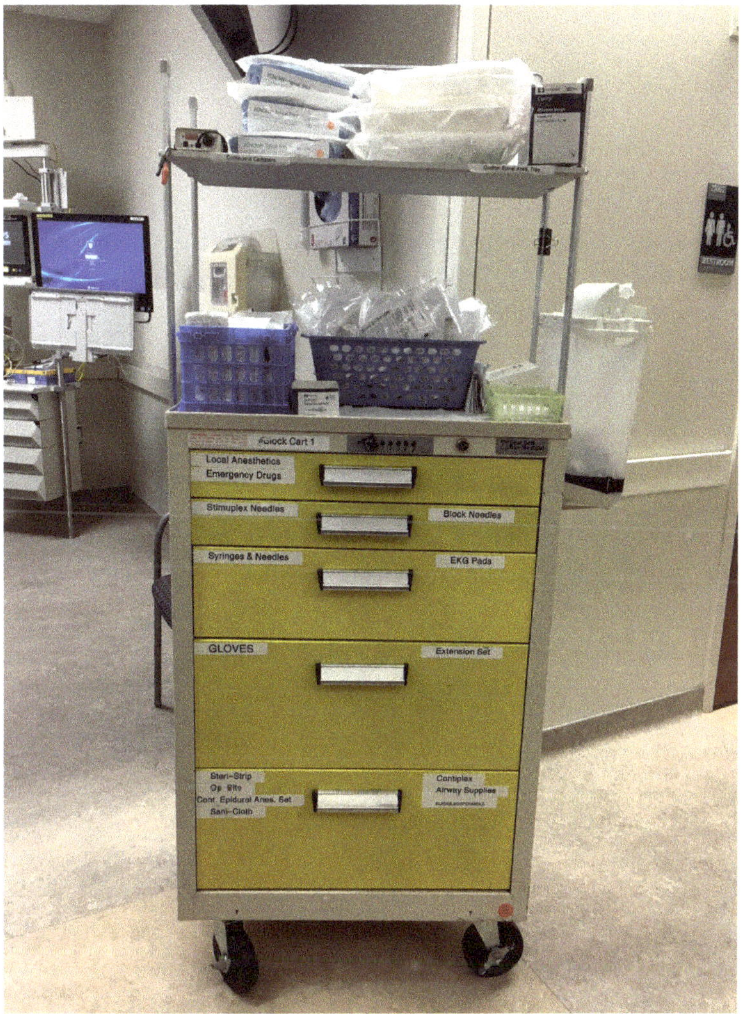

Figure 27.2 Block cart.

extremity without assistance) until complete block resolution. In addition, patients should be warned that protective reflexes and proprioception for the blocked extremity may be diminished or absent for 24 hours.

A process for site verification prior to nerve block procedures must be implemented. Prior to block placement, sidedness should be verbally confirmed with the patient and visually confirmed on the operative consent. The provider should initial the extremity to be blocked. If another anesthesia provider manages the patient in the operating room, details of the block procedure must be communicated during the handoff.

4. Regional Anesthesia Documentation

The regional anesthesia procedure must be appropriately documented, including details of any difficulties and/or complications that may have occurred. Essential information should include the following:

- Location of block performance (e.g., preoperative block area, operating room, postanesthesia care unit)
- Block indication (e.g., surgical, postoperative pain management)
- Time out performed prior to block placement
- Monitors used (e.g., blood pressure, pulse oximetry, electrocardiogram)
- Oxygen (e.g., liters/min, face mask)

- Patient positioning
- Laterality of block
- Type of block
- Approach
- Single-injection versus continuous technique
- Technique used (e.g., combined ultrasound and nerve stimulator technique)
- Minimal current in milliamperes (mA) and type of motor response if peripheral nerve stimulator is used
- Sterile technique used (e.g., solution, drapes)
- Needle used, including length, gauge, brand, and model
- Catheter type (e.g., nonstimulating or stimulating, single or multi-orifice)
- Needle insertion depth in centimeters
- Catheter information—centimeters beyond needle tip and depth at skin
- Number of block placement attempts
- Local anesthetic used, including concentration and volume
- Local anesthetic additives used (e.g., epinephrine 1:400,000 as an intravascular marker)
- Local anesthetic injection details, including multiple aspiration for heme, incremental injection, pain on injection, etc.
- Level of sedation
- If applicable, details surrounding difficulties that may have occurred during the procedure, including but not limited to complications and/or inability to perform the block

5. Equipment

5.1. Needles

A variety of regional anesthesia needles are available. Qualities of a good PNB needle include the following:

- Stimulating PNB needles should be insulated along the shaft, with only the tip exposed to deliver current.
- Stimulating PNB needles should allow for appropriate peripheral nerve stimulator connection.
- PNB needles should have a comfortable finger grip at the proximal end of the needle.
- PNB needles should include, or provide the ability to connect, long, clear extension tubing to facilitate aspiration and local anesthetic injection.
- PNB needles are typically beveled at 45° (as compared with traditional needles, which are beveled at 17°) to enhance tactile sensation of the needle passing through tissue planes and to reduce the possibility of neural trauma.
- PNB needles with centimeter markings on the needle shaft are helpful in determining needle depth.

Centimeter markings on the needle shaft are beneficial when correlating needle depth with predetermined skin-to-nerve distance measured on ultrasound (Figure 27.3). A typical PNB setup is illustrated in Figure 27.4. Figure 27.5 provides the preferred method for all local anesthetic injections.

New echogenic needles are designed to optimize needle visibility during ultrasound-guided PNBs (Table 27.1). These needles have engraved patterns designed to maximize ultrasound wave reflections back toward the ultrasound probe. The 3 most common patterns are dihedral grooves, tetrahedral grooves, and Xx-pattern with clear coating. Echogenic needles, however, are more expensive, and not all designs consistently improve needle visualization.

5.2. Peripheral nerve stimulators

When performing PNBs utilizing a nerve stimulation technique, an appropriate motor response achieved at a current of 0.5 to 0.2 mA suggests accurate needle placement for local anesthetic injection. As such, peripheral nerve stimulators allow for objective evidence of needle-to-nerve proximity, as compared with the subjective evidence of a paresthesia technique.

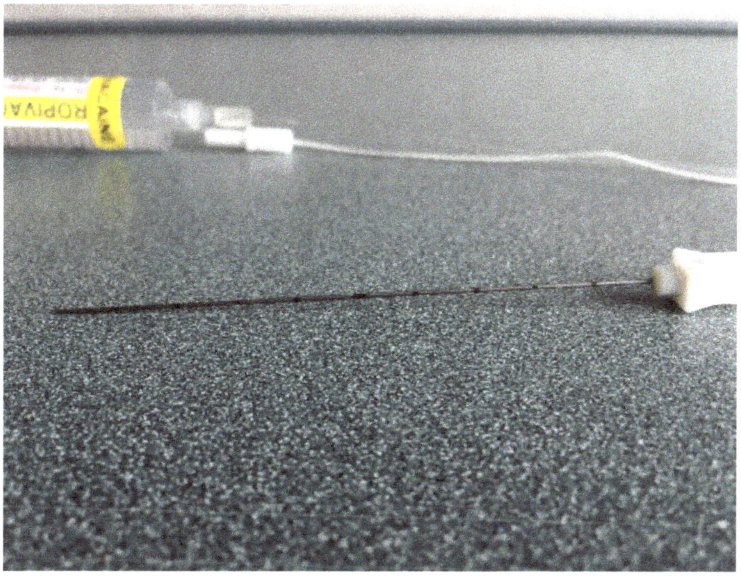

Figure 27.3 Stimulating 100-mm, 21-gauge single injection peripheral nerve block needle with centimeter markings.

Chapter 29, "Physics of Ultrasound and Nerve Stimulation Ultrasonography," discusses peripheral nerve stimulation in detail. A variety of peripheral nerve stimulators are available on the market (Table 27.2). A good peripheral nerve stimulator has the following characteristics:

- light, compact, battery-operated design with adjustable current from 0 to 5 mA in 0.01-mA increments at 2 Hz impulse frequency;

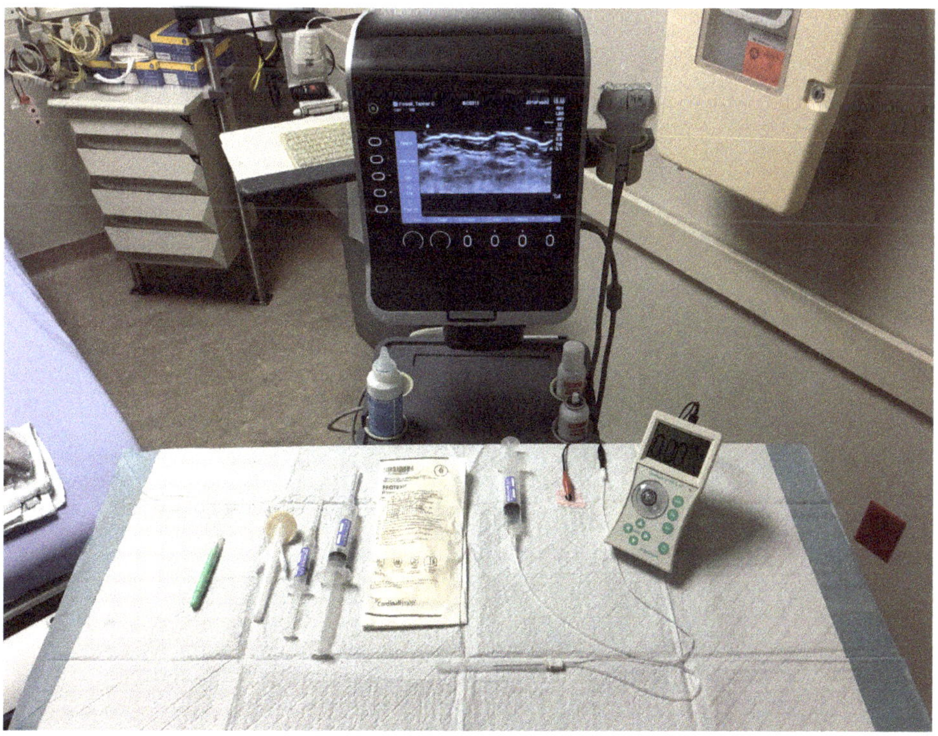

Figure 27.4 Setup for a single-injection peripheral nerve block.

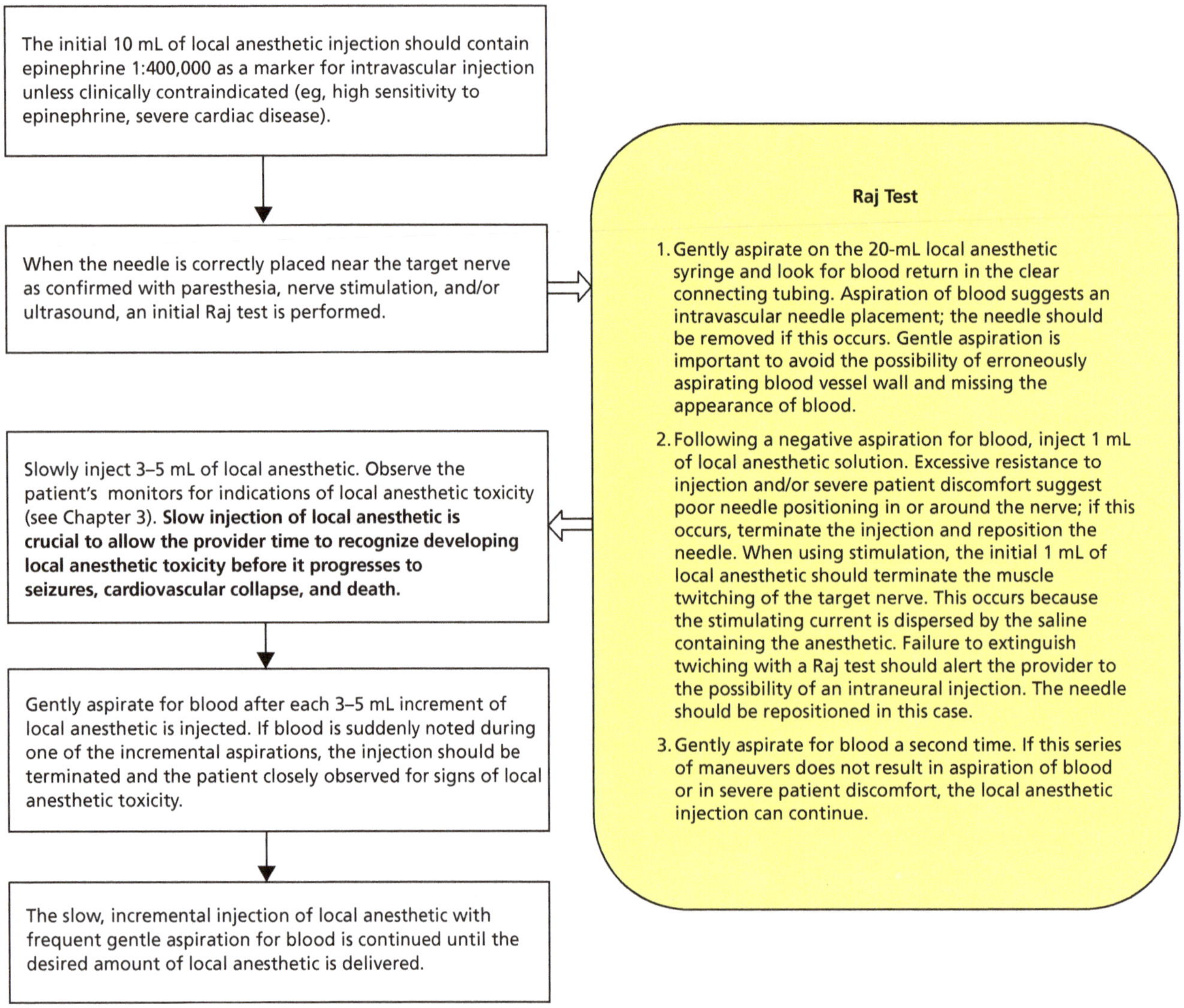

Figure 27.5 Procedure for injection of local anesthetic solutions.

Table 27.1:
Sample of echogenic needles available on the market

Brand	Etched Pattern on Needle	Description
EchoBright (Halyard™, Life-Tech, Halyard Health Inc.)	Dihedral V-shaped grooves	Produces a constant, even intensity of reflection when angle of insonation varies over a range from 0° to 80°. Can be connected to nerve stimulator.
SonoPlex (PAJUNK® GmbH Medizintechnologie PAJUNK™, Germany, GmbH Medizintechnologie)	Tetrahedral reflectors spaced out circumferentially around needle shaft	Allows reflection and imaging at wide range of insertion angles and bevel orientations. Can be connected to nerve stimulator.
Stimuplex Ultra (B. Braun Melsungen AG, Melsungen, Germany)	X pattern with clear coating	Reflects more ultrasound waves back to the probe than previous Stimuplex designs.

Table 27.2:
Sample of available on-the-market peripheral nerve stimulators

Peripheral Nerve Stimulator	Brand	Characteristics
Stimuplex® HNS12 Nerve Stimulator with SENSe (HNS12)	B. Braun Melsungen AG, Melsungen, Germany	User-friendly; Sequential Electrical Nerve Stimulation (SENSe) technology available, which allows to find the nerve in a shorter period of time with a prolonged motor response
MultiStim ECO	PAJUNK® GmbH Medizintechnologie	User-friendly for combined nerve stimulation and ultrasound techniques.
MultiStim SENSOR	PAJUNK® GmbH Medizintechnologie	Stimulation handle allows painless percutaneous stimulation.
MultiStim SWITCH	PAJUNK® GmbH Medizintechnologie	One function indicates patient's tissue resistance (e.g., intraneural, intravascular). There is a switchover function that allows the selection of catheter-through-the needle vs. catheter-over-the needle techniques.

- bright and easily visualized digital display;
- both a visual and an audible signal of an open or closed circuit between the stimulator, needle, and patient; and
- an impulse duration adjustable between 0.1 millisecond (ms) and 1 ms.

5.3. Continuous peripheral nerve blockade

Chapter 53, "Continuous Peripheral Nerve Blocks," provides details on WRNMMC procedures for placing and securing continuous peripheral nerve block (CPNB) catheters. The majority of catheters placed at WRNMMC and in military deployed settings are nonstimulating catheters because of how long the catheters remain in situ (1 to 2 weeks on average). Some available stimulating catheter systems with coiled tips (e.g., Arrow® SmithCath® Stimulating cPNB) recommend removal after 72 hours. In the pain management of combat-wounded soldiers, hundreds of nonstimulating CPNB catheters have been placed, some of which have remained in place for as long as a month, without catheter-related complications

Desirable characteristics of a long-term CPNB catheter are listed in Table 27.3. The Contiplex® Tuohy (B. Braun Melsungen AG, Melsungen, Germany) CPNB nonstimulating catheter system used at WRNMMC has had years of successful long-term use in combat casualties and remains the recommended CPNB system for use in the field.

5.4. Ultrasound

While peripheral nerve stimulation provides objective evidence of needle-to-nerve proximity, ultrasound-guided regional anesthesia provides real-time, direct visualization of needle-to-nerve distance and provides information on local anatomy at the block site.

Improvements in ultrasound technology allow for high image resolution with smaller, portable, and less expensive ultrasound machines (Figure 27.6).

Elements of a superior ultrasound machine for regional anesthesia include high image quality, compact/rugged design, simple/intuitive controls, easy image storage/retrieval, and ease of portability. Ultrasound for PNBs is discussed in chapter 29.

5.5. Infusion pumps

Recent improvements in acute pain management on the battlefield would have been impossible without improvements in microprocessor-driven infusion technology. The use of CPNB and other pain management techniques during casualty evacuation depends on this technology.

Infusion pumps for the austere military environment should have the attributes listed in Table 27.4. The pain infusion pump currently used during casualty evacuation for patient-controlled analgesia (PCA), epidural catheters, and CPNB is the ambIT® PCA pump (Summit Medical Products Inc, Sandy, Utah [Figure 27.7]). In addition, a

Table 27.3:
Desirable characteristics of a long-term continuous peripheral nerve block catheter

• Easily placed through a standard 18-gauge Tuohy needle
• Composed of inert, noninflammatory material
• Centimeter markings to estimate depth/catheter migration
• Colored tip to confirm complete removal from patient
• Flexible, multi-orifice tip
• Hyperechoic on ultrasound
• Radiopaque
• Secure injection port
• Capable of stimulation
• Nonadherent within weeks of use
• High resistance to breaking or kinking
• Low resistance to infusion
• Bacteriostatic
• System to secure the catheter to patient's skin

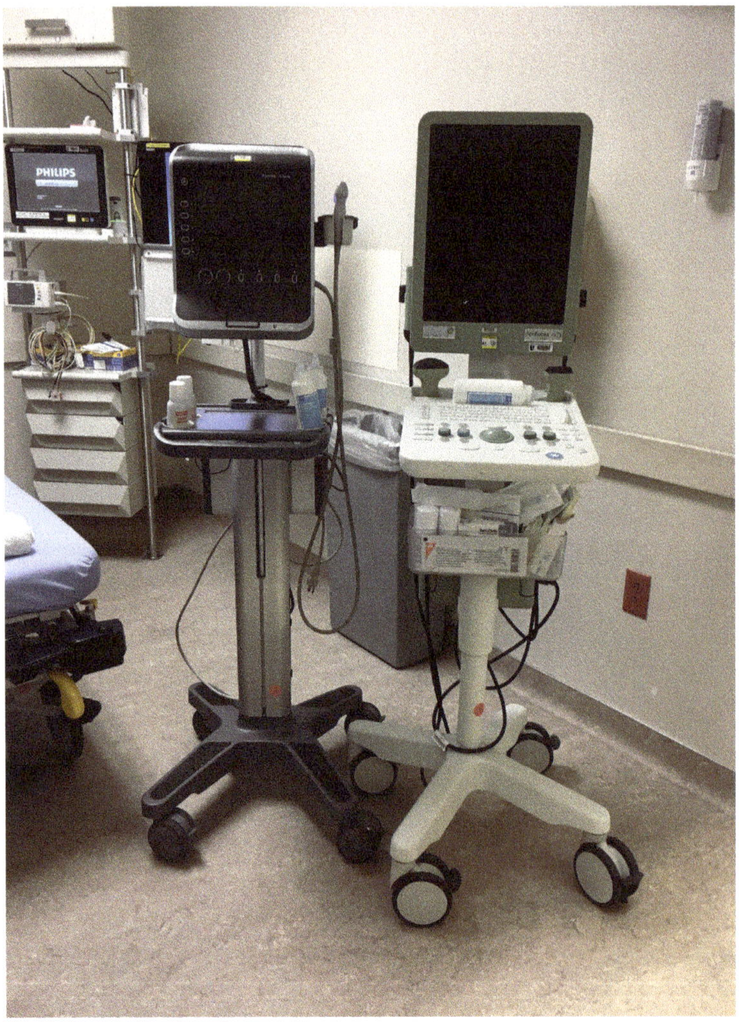

Figure 27.6 Ultrasound machines.

Table 27.4:
Desirable characteristics of a military infusion pump

- Easily identifiable by shape and color
- Used only for pain service infusions
- Lightweight and compact
- Reprogrammable for basal rate, bolus amount, lockout interval, and infusion volume
- Battery operated with long battery life
- Program lockout to prevent program tampering
- Simple and intuitive operation
- Medication free-flow protection
- Latex free
- Visual and audible alarms
- Stable infusion rate at extremes of temperature and pressure
- Inexpensive
- Durable for long service life without needing maintenance
- Certified for use in US military aircraft

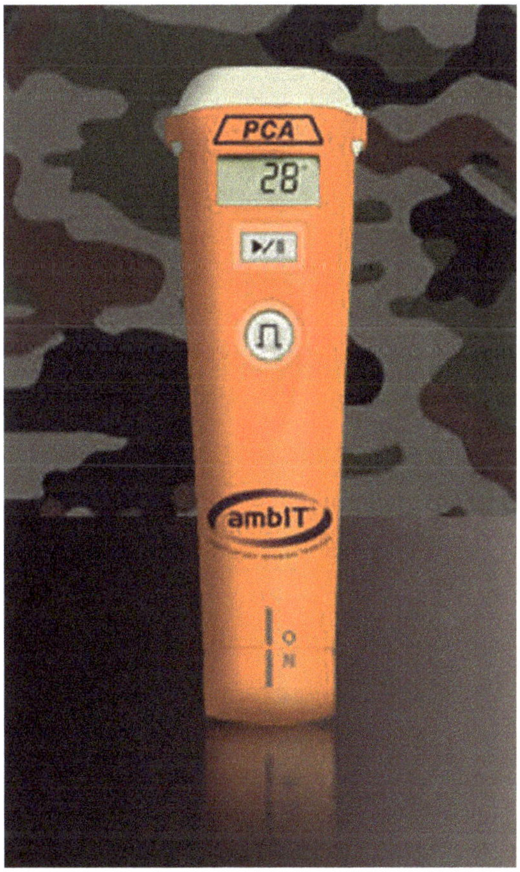

Figure 27.7 Casualty evacuation acute pain management pump (ambIT® PCA pump [Summit Medical Products Inc., Sandy, Utah; used with permission]) in current military use.

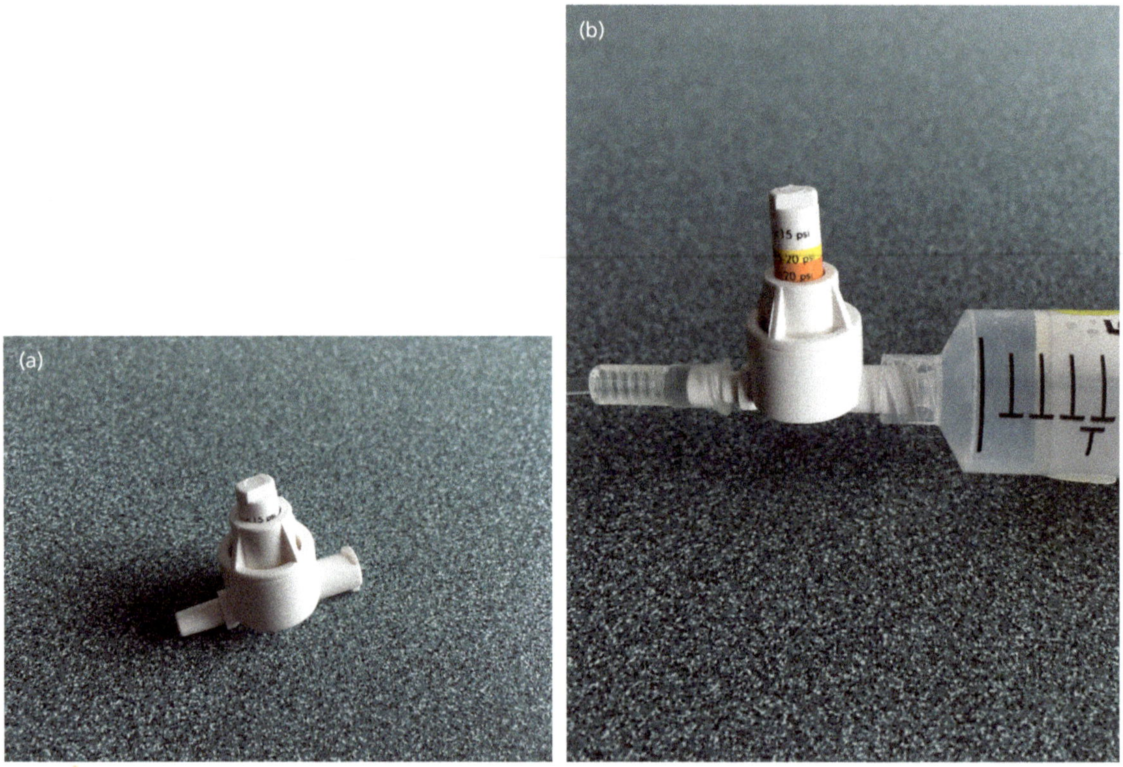

Figure 27.8 (a) Injection pressure monitor; (b) injection pressure monitor.

wide variety of elastomeric pumps are available on the market. These pumps are disposable and usually very user-friendly. However, they are nonrefillable and have fixed-volume reservoirs, limiting the duration of perineural infusion.

5.6. Injection pressure monitor

A pressure monitor is a manometer used to objectively assess injection pressure during the placement of PNBs. Monitoring opening injection pressure with this equipment can help identify potentially unsafe injection prior to depositing a full volume of local anesthetic solution. High injection pressures (>15 psi) at the onset of injection may indicate intraneural needle placement, leading to severe fascicular injury and even persistent neurologic deficits. The injection pressure monitor (B-Smart™, B. Braun Melsungen AG, Medical Inc, Melsungen, Germany) is available on the market (Figures 27.8A and 27.8B).

Local Anesthetics and Additives

28

1. Introduction

Regional anesthesia allows for myriad benefits over general anesthesia alone, such as superior pain control with decreased opioid requirements, earlier return of ambulation and bowel function, and earlier readiness for discharge. Many of these benefits are the direct result of the properties of local anesthetics (LAs). This chapter will serve as a review of the characteristics of LAs and the different LAs commonly used in peripheral nerve blocks. It also discusses nerve block adjuvants that can be utilized to augment the LA effect.

2. Basic Review of Local Anesthetics

The main mechanism of action of LAs is on an intracellular binding site found in nerve fiber transmembrane sodium channels. Binding at this site ultimately blocks sodium movement through the channel, thus preventing membrane depolarization and effectively blocking a nerve's action potential and signal transduction (Figure 28.1). Nerve fibers with different functions have unique physical properties that affect the way they respond to LAs. Fortuitously, nociceptive nerves fibers (A delta: fast, sharp pain; C: slow, throbbing pain) are more susceptible to LA blockade than larger motor nerve fibers (A alpha). The reason for this dose-dependent response is multifactorial and has to do with resistance to LA of unmyelinated fibers, faster blockade of smaller fibers, and the anatomic positioning of nerve fibers within larger bundles. In general, pain and autonomic nerves are blocked before those for temperature and light touch, followed by proprioception, deep pressure, and finally motor function.

2.1. Physicochemical properties

All LAs have similar structural components (Figure 28.2), a lipophilic and a hydrophilic end connected by an amide or ester linkage, which determine the site of metabolism (liver and plasma, respectively). Local anesthetics are weak bases with pKa between 7.5 and 9. Thus, at a normal physiologic pH of 7.4, the protonated or ionized form of LAs is favored in extravascular environments.

Speed of Onset. The balance between the neutral and ionized forms of LAs has clinical significance. The neutral form must traverse the cell membrane to ultimately reach the site of action, but it is the ionized form that then binds the sodium channel. In general, the lower the pKa (closer to physiologic pH), the more the balance is shifted to the neutral form and the faster the onset.

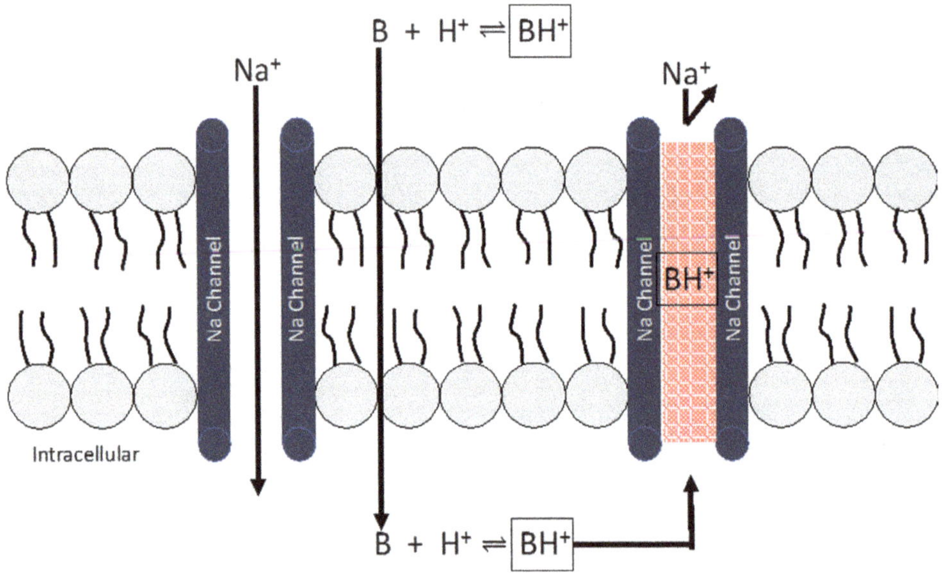

Figure 28.1 Local anesthetic binding site. LAs penetrate the cell membrane in the neutral form but are active in the protonated form where they bind and inactivate the neuronal sodium channel.

Potency. Local anesthetic potency is related to lipid solubility or, more accurately, hydrophobicity. Local anesthetics that are more hydrophobic more easily penetrate the lipid cell membrane and reach the intracellular site of action.

Duration of Effect. Duration of LAs is multifactorial but is commonly thought to be related to protein binding. Local anesthetics bind readily to albumin and α-1-acid glycoprotein. Highly bound drugs will stay bound to the site of action and have a longer duration. Duration has also been shown to be related to hydrophobicity, as more hydrophobic molecules take longer to clear from the local tissue. Clearance is also affected by the vascularity of the surrounding tissue as ultimately it is the vascular system that carries unbound LA away from the site of injection and target nerve.

Block outcomes and characteristics are highly dependent on which LA is chosen and also on the volume and concentration used. Volume for single-injection blocks should be partially determined by injection site and block technique. Typical volumes for usual blocks can be found in the dedicated block chapters. Concentration of LA also has significant

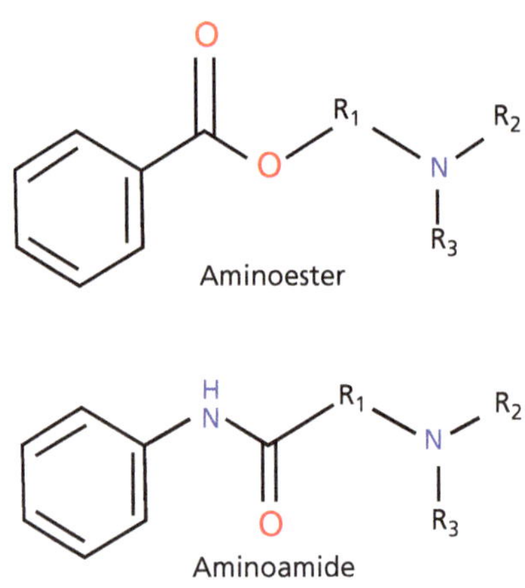

Figure 28.2 Local anesthetic structure. Basic structure of LAs with either an ester linkage metabolized by plasma esterases or an amide linkage metabolized by hepatic enzymes.

effect on block outcomes. Because LAs must pass through multiple fascial and fibrous layers of the epi-, peri-, and endoneurium as well as the cell membrane itself, a diffusion gradient is necessary for block onset. Increasing drug concentration thus can hasten onset. Also, it will allow for a greater effect on the larger myelinated motor fibers, allowing for motor blockade in addition to a dense sensory block. Increased concentration similarly increases block duration as it will take a longer time for local blood flow to clear more LA. It is imperative, however, to consider the maximum allowable dose as one increases drug concentration, especially for high-volume blocks or when performing multiple blocks in smaller patients because toxic plasma levels can quickly be reached.

3. Local Anesthetic Toxicity

Local anesthetics, like all drugs, have systemic effects that can be toxic and even lethal when plasma concentrations exceed the therapeutic range. Although doses causing local anesthetic systemic toxicity (LAST) have been described, it is important to note that similar toxic effects can be caused by a small dose injected directly intravascularly. Nevertheless, one should always strive to use the minimum amount of LA necessary to achieve a successful block in order to minimize the risk of LAST. Interestingly, even at a perineural level, LAs themselves have been shown in vitro to be neurotoxic and even myotoxic. In vitro studies have shown that LAs cause cell damage and death in a concentration-dependent fashion. This remains as a hypothetical concern as numerous studies and clinical experience have proven the safety of LA at clinical doses.

3.1. Signs and symptoms

At toxic doses LAs have an excitatory effect in the central nervous system (CNS) by blocking inhibitory pathways, especially in the amygdala. This can manifest as clonus, visual disturbances, tinnitus, perioral numbness or paresthesia, generalized anxiety, agitation, or disinhibition. Patients often express feelings of impending doom. Untreated, these symptoms can progress to seizure, respiratory arrest, and death. Cardiovascular symptoms generally follow CNS symptoms as the cardiovascular system is more resistant to the effects of LAs. Symptoms include cardiac arrhythmias, hypotension, and cardiovascular arrest.

3.2. LA absorption

Toxicity is related to systemic absorption and, ultimately, plasma concentration of LA. Absorption is related to the site of injection, with the greatest plasma concentrations achieved by direct intravascular injection. Absorption by site of injection from greatest to least is as follows: intercostal > caudal > epidural > brachial plexus > femoral/sciatic > subcutaneous > intra-articular > spinal. While this can help guide drug dosing, even a small, subtoxic dose of LA can result in immediate onset of toxicity when injected directly into a vessel such as the carotid artery during an interscalene block. It should also be understood that just as it is the unbound free fraction of LA that has action on the neuronal sodium channels, similarly it is the unbound drug that is responsible for systemic toxicity. Low protein states such as malnutrition or liver failure will increase the portion of unbound LA and thus increase the risk for systemic toxicity.

3.3. Prevention and treatment

Because toxicity from LA is one of the most dangerous risks of a regional anesthetic technique, great caution must be used during block placement, with every precaution taken to aid in rapid detection and treatment of toxicity. During block placement, all standard American Society of Anesthesiologists (ASA) monitors must be utilized. Supplemental oxygen should be delivered especially if sedation is used. Incremental injection of LA should be slow and preceded by gentle aspiration after every 5 mL of injectate. The use of sedation is a topic of some debate. Even mild sedation can mask symptoms of both LA toxicity and nerve injury. The use of benzodiazepines, however, can also be protective by raising the seizure threshold. Most important, all emergency equipment and personnel must be immediately available for Advanced Cardiac Life Support (ACLS), intubation, and resuscitation. This includes immediate availability of lipid emulsion and instructions for use. Because this is the only available reversal agent for LAST, regionalists must be familiar with its indication and dosage:

- Intralipid, the most commonly available lipid emulsion therapy, is a 20% lipid emulsion that is indicated for the treatment of LA-induced cardiac arrhythmia.
- It is given intravenously (IV) 1 mL/kg every 3 to 5 minutes up to 3 mL/kg.
- This is followed by a 0.25-mL/kg/min infusion for 2.5 hours.

Guidelines for treatment of LAST can be found on the American Society of Regional Anesthesia and Pain Medicine (ASRA) website. Propofol, while also a lipid emulsion, is not appropriate for LA toxicity reversal as any therapeutic dosing would far exceed that which would first cause cardiovascular collapse.

4. Local Anesthetics Commonly Used for Regional Anesthesia

A summary of this content can be found in Table 28.1.

4.1. Ropivacaine

Ropivacaine is the most commonly used LA for both single-injection and continuous peripheral nerve blocks. Its favorable safety profile makes it the drug of choice for many regionalists. Ropivacaine has a pKa of 8.2. As a direct product of the drug design, being a pure levorotatory stereoisomer, it has a very favorable toxicity profile, especially compared with other long-acting LAs. It has a mild vasoconstrictive effect and is considered significantly less cardiotoxic than bupivacaine, with a quicker onset time though a slightly shorter duration. While considered a long-acting LA like bupivacaine, it is slightly less potent than bupivacaine, which may explain both its shorter duration and its higher toxic dose. At large doses, it too can cause severe systemic toxicity.

Table 28.1:
Local anesthetics: basic overview

Adjuvant	pKa	Max Dose Plain/ epinephrine (mg/kg)	Onset (min) (hr)	Duration	Concentrations	Special Considerations
Lidocaine	7.7	4.5/7	1–2	0.5–1.5	1%–2%	Concern for TNS in spinals, safe for epidurals
Mepivacaine	7.6	5/7	5–10	1–2	1.5%	Dense motor block, ideal for surgical blocks
Bupivacaine	8.1	2.5/7	5–10	4–10+	0.25, 0.5%	Concern for toxicity, not ideal for high-volume blocks
Ropivacaine	8.2	3/4	10–30	4–8	0.2, 0.5%	LA of choice for most blocks, including CPNB
Chloroprocaine	8.7	10/15	5–10	0.5–1.5	1%	Fast onset and recovery, used for ambulatory spinals

4.2. Bupivacaine

Bupivacaine is a long-acting LA commonly used for peripheral nerve blocks and neuraxial techniques. It has a pKa of 8.1, and has a longer duration of action, around 4 to 12 or even 24 hours, though a slightly longer onset time compared with ropivacaine. Bupivacaine has a less favorable therapeutic index than ropivacaine especially concerning risk for cardiotoxicity at high doses. It is still commonly used, with effective and safe outcomes. A single-enantiomer version, levobupivacaine, has been developed that has been shown to have a slightly safer toxicity profile, allowing for a larger subtoxic dose. Concern still exists with levobupivacaine for drastic cardiovascular and CNS toxic effects at high doses.

4.3. Mepivacaine

Mepivacaine is an intermediate-acting LA. It causes a relatively dense motor block and thus is ideal as a single injection for surgical blocks in shorter procedures with little or no postoperative pain. It has a pKa of 7.6 and a rapid onset time. For this reason it is commonly employed when rapid onset time is necessary. It has a favorable therapeutic index and pharmacokinetics similar to those of lidocaine. Mepivacaine has a slightly longer duration of action than lidocaine because of both its vasoconstrictive effect and significant protein binding. It does have a shorter duration than long-acting LAs such as ropivacaine.

4.4. Lidocaine

Lidocaine has a pKa of 7.7, allowing for a relatively rapid onset time. It is more commonly employed for epidural anesthesia than peripheral nerve blocks, though it has a favorable therapeutic index and intermediate duration. Concern for transient neurologic syndrome (TNS) has caused it to fall out of favor for use in spinal anesthetics.

4.5. 2-chloroprocaine

2-Chloroprocaine was withdrawn from the market in the 1980s because of concerns of increased neurotoxicity. This risk was thought to be from the included preservative, and a new preservative-free version has been introduced. It has been successfully and safely used for decades, especially for spinal and epidural anesthesia. Uniquely, the metabolism of 2-chloroprocaine by plasma esterases is extremely rapid. Its rapid onset time of 5 to 10 minutes and rapid recovery of 70 to 150 minutes makes it ideal for ambulatory surgery, where quick recovery of function is necessary. This characteristic also lends a theoretical safety benefit as toxicity may be harder to reach.

4.6. Mixing of local anesthetics

When considering the need for quick onset and prolonged duration of action, many regionalists will use an injectate mixture of LAs such as lidocaine and bupivacaine. Studies have shown mixed results with this practice, which in general may minimally speed onset time while simultaneously decreasing duration. Because LA toxicity is additive, smaller doses of both drugs must be used, which may help explain the effect on block onset and duration.

4.7. Use in continuous peripheral nerve block catheters

When one is considering an LA for use with a continuous peripheral nerve block catheter (CPNB), the ideal drug has a favorable safety profile, is easily titratable, and is motor sparing. For this reason, ropivacaine 0.2% is most commonly employed for both inpatient and ambulatory peripheral nerve block catheters.

5. Peripheral nerve block and adjuvants

Many adjuvants have been added to LAs to manipulate the characteristics of single-injection peripheral nerve blocks with varying success. Discussed in the following are the commonly implemented adjuvants with documented and proven

Table 28.2:
Suggested adjuvant dosing for adult single-injection nerve blocks

Adjuvant	Dosing	Special Considerations
Epinephrine	1:200,000 or 1:400,000	Prolongs short-acting LAs, caution in patients with neuropathy, contraindicated with 2-chloroprocaine.
Clonidine	100–150 mcg	Usually dosed 1 mcg/kg. Hypotension, bradycardia, and sedation may be more pronounced at higher doses.
Dexamethasone	1–8 mg	May have similar effect when given systemically.
Buprenorphine	100–300 mcg	Usually dosed 1.5 mcg/kg rounded to 100, 150, 200 mcg, etc. Concern for nausea and vomiting.

reliable outcomes. A summary can be found in Table 28.2. Not discussed are the many adjuvants that either have not been shown to have beneficial effect (opioids) or that have debatable therapeutic benefit (midazolam, magnesium, ketamine). It is important to emphasize that the use of these medications in peripheral nerve blocks, while clinically accepted and supported by the literature, is not approved by the Food and Drug Administration. Most adjuvants are injected perineurally in a mixture with LAs; however, medications given IV at the time of block placement can also be considered block adjuvants. Fentanyl and midazolam are commonly given as sedation for block placement but, as discussed earlier, may mask symptoms of toxicity or nerve injury even at low doses.

5.1. Epinephrine

Epinephrine is a commonly employed adjuvant for single-injection peripheral nerve blocks. When injected as a mixture with LAs, it can have a number of beneficial effects. At concentrations of 1:200,000 (5 mcg/mL) to 1:400,000 (2.5 mcg/mL), it may aid in detection of intravascular injection. This may be especially useful in blocks that are high-risk for intravascular injection or done without ultrasound guidance. At concentrations of 1:400,000, it has been shown to prolong block duration and decrease plasma concentration levels of drug by causing local vasoconstriction at the site of injection. Prolongation of block has been shown to more significantly benefit short-acting LAs and may have a negligible effect on long-acting LAs, especially ropivacaine. The decrease in systemic absorption may be significant when concern for toxicity with large-volume doses is present. While epinephrine has a proven safety record when given perineurally, there is concern for neurotoxicity from decreased neuronal perfusion, which may be magnified when combined with LAs. This risk should be taken into consideration in patients with diagnoses of or have a high risk for neuropathy. Epinephrine is contraindicated as an adjuvant to spinal 2-chloroprocaine as the combination has uniquely been shown to cause flulike symptoms.

5.2. Clonidine

Clonidine is an alpha-2 receptor agonist commonly given systemically for treatment of refractory hypertension. Its effect of membrane hyperpolarization on C- and A-fibers gives it analgesic properties when given both systemically and locally. It also has been shown to inhibit LA clearance. When given perineurally as a mixture with LAs, clonidine has been shown to significantly prolong analgesic time by approximately 2 hours. While rare, side effects when it is given as an adjuvant are similar to those when given systemically (i.e., hypotension, bradycardia, and sedation). The side effects are more pronounced at doses higher than 100 to 150 mcg. It has not been shown to be neurotoxic in animal studies.

5.3. Dexamethasone

Dexamethasone is a corticosteroid with minimal mineralocorticoid effect. It has multiple beneficial effects when given systemically, including analgesia. It has a well-documented beneficial effect when given perineurally as a mixture with LAs. When injected perineurally, it can increase analgesic time by multiple hours even with long-acting LAs. Its proposed mechanism of action is its inhibitory effect on C-fibers. It has been shown to have a very favorable side effect and safety profile. Interestingly, recent evidence has suggested that its effect on block prolongation may similarly be achieved when given systemically instead of perineurally. This may have clinical significance as it is commonly given IV intraoperatively as part of prophylaxis against postoperative nausea and vomiting.

5.4. Buprenorphine

Buprenorphine is a partial opioid agonist commonly given systemically as part of treatment for chronic pain and opioid addiction management. It has an inhibitory effect on voltage gated sodium channels similar to that of LAs. When given perineurally in mixture with LAs, it has been shown to increase analgesic time of nerve blocks by multiple hours. It has been safely used to enhance single-injection nerve blocks with little to no systemic opioid side effects but may still cause nausea and vomiting. It has not been shown to be neurotoxic in animal studies.

29

Physics of Ultrasound and Nerve Stimulation

1. Ultrasonography

Ultrasound guidance has become the principal tool for the placement of peripheral nerve blocks since the beginning of this century. The evolution of point-of-care ultrasound imaging systems has made these systems more affordable, easy to use, and ubiquitous in the clinical environment. In the US military, point-of-care ultrasound systems are organic to role 2 and above levels of care, and new handheld devices are finding their way to the most austere areas of medical care.

As with any device or instrument, an understanding of the fundamentals of how ultrasound systems work and how they can be optimized affords the operator the greatest likelihood of safe, efficient, and successful placement of a needle adjacent to the target of interest.

2. Physics of Ultrasound

2.1. Properties of sound

Sound is a form of oscillating mechanical energy transmitted through a medium by the compression (condensation) and expansion (rarefication) of particles of matter. Ultrasound is emitted at frequencies above the threshold of human hearing (>20 kHz). The frequencies used for medical ultrasound imaging range between 1 MHz and 20 MHz. The wavelength (λ) of a sound wave is the quotient of the speed of sound (v) and frequency (f).

$$\lambda = \frac{v}{f}$$

The speed of sound (v) is defined as the square root of the quotient of elasticity (or bulk modulus, B) and density (ρ).

$$v = \sqrt[2]{B/\rho}$$

It is thus related to the characteristics of the conductive media and unrelated to frequency or amplitude. Harder materials (greater bulk modulus) conduct sound at greater velocity. However, in practice the speed of sound in solid is not exactly described by the equation above as it is also related to the geometry of the substance and the interactions of longitudinal and transverse waves.

Table 29.1:
Speed of sound and acoustic impedance in various media.

Substance	Speed of Sound (m / s)	Acoustic Impedance (g / [cm² · s])
Water (20°C)	1480	1.48×10^5
Blood	1570	1.61×10^5
Bone	3500	7.80×10^5
Fat	1450	1.38×10^5
Liver	1550	1.65×10^5
Muscle	1580	1.70×10^5
Polythene	2000	1.84×10^5
Air	330	0.0004×10^5
Soft tissue (average)	1540	1.63×10^5
Aluminum	6320	17.1×10^5
Steel (434)	5850	45.63×10^5

Adapted from Allan, P. (2006). Clinical Doppler ultrasound. Oxford: Churchill Livingstone/Elsevier.

Acoustic impedance (Z) is the resistance of a substance to conduct sound and is defined as the product of the velocity (v) of sound in and density (ρ) of a substance.

$$Z = v \cdot \rho$$

Air and lung have low acoustic impedance, while bone and metal have high acoustic impedance. The difference between the acoustic impedance of 2 substances dictates how much sound energy is transmitted or reflected at their interface. Air-tissue and tissue-bone interfaces reflect nearly all the incident sound wave. Table 29.1 lists the velocity of sound and acoustic impedance of several biologic and man-made materials.

2.2. Piezoelectric effect

Piezoelectricity is the fundamental principle driving the operation of ultrasound transducers. The prefix *piezo* is derived from the Greek "to compress," and refers to the properties of some crystals to emit an electric impulse when deformed. This piezoelectric effect has 2 components: direct piezoelectric effect, which is the ability of a crystalline structure to emit an electric impulse following deformation, and the reverse piezoelectric effect, where the deformation of a crystalline structure occurs with the input of electrical energy to the material.

2.3. Attenuation, power, and intensity

Attenuation is the loss of sound energy within a medium. This lost energy represents information that cannot be processed or used in the imaging process. Such losses can be from absorption of the energy (conversion to heat) by the material, reflection and scattering as the sound wave encounters interfaces within the substance, and transmission through the medium (Figure 29.1). The coefficient of attenuation (a_c) is the attenuation that occurs through each centimeter of a substance expressed as decibels per centimeter (dB/cm); as the attenuation coefficient and the length the sound wave travels through the substance increase, so will attenuation. For soft tissues, the attenuation coefficient is between 0.3 and 0.7 dB/cm. The most significant source of attenuation is through absorption of sound energy by a substance.

Attenuation is also related to the frequency of the sound wave. As frequency of the wave increases, attenuation increases. The practical result is that as the frequency gets higher, more of the sound energy is lost to the tissue, diminishing the tissue penetration at a given amplitude.

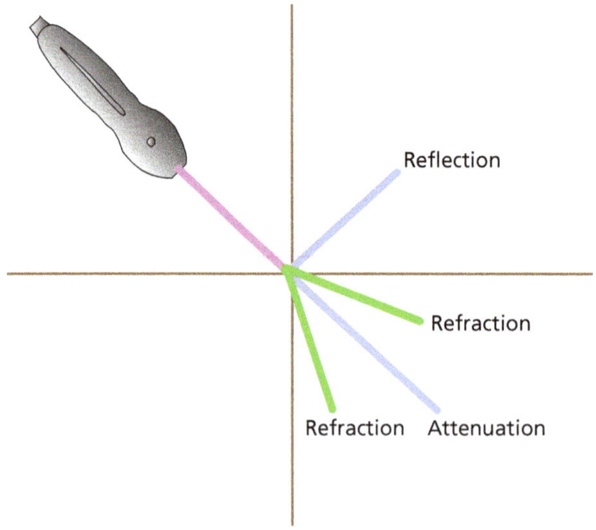

Figure 29.1 Causes of ultrasound dispersion in a medium.

Adjustments to both the power and the intensity of a sound wave can be used to overcome attenuation losses within a substance, providing more information for image processing. Power (*P*) is the rate at which energy is being delivered to a system described as units of energy over time and expressed as watts (*W*).

Intensity is the rate at which energy is delivered over a given area. For a point energy source, intensity (*I*) is expressed as:

$$I = \frac{P}{4\pi r^2}$$

Thus, as a sound wave travels through a substance, the intensity decreases with the square of the distance from the source (*r*) (Figure 29.2). Increasing power will increase the intensity of the sound wave at a given distance from the source; however, this is at the price of a greater amount of heat imparted to the tissue through attenuation.

2.4. Frequency, resolution, and penetration

As was touched upon earlier, the attenuation through a medium (in dB) is related to frequency:

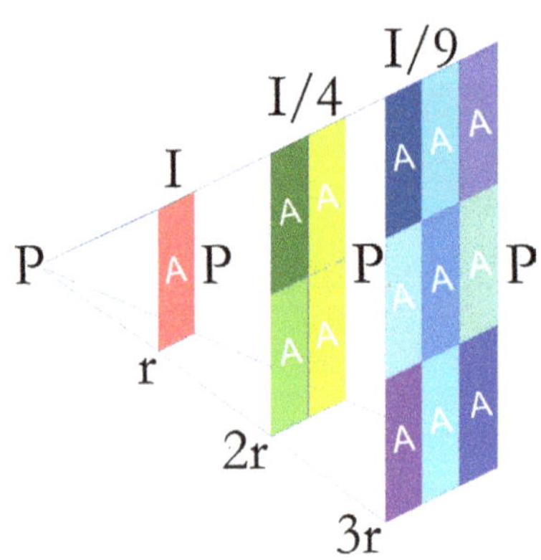

Figure 29.2 Power versus intensity. Power (*P*) is the amount of energy applied to a substance per unit time and is constant as the wave travels through the medium. Intensity (*I*) is the amount of energy delivered per unit area (*A*) and decreases with the square of the radius (*r*).

Table 29.2:
Penetration and attenuation of sound at different frequencies.

Frequency (MHz)	Penetration (cm)	Attenuation (dB)
15.0	4	7.5
10.0	6	5
7.5	8	3.8
5.0	12	2.5
3.5	17	1.8
2.0	30	1.0

Adapted from Kremkau, F., & Forsberg, F. (2016). Sonography: principles and instruments. St. Louis, MO: Elsevier.

$$a_{(dB)} = a_c \cdot f \cdot L$$

where f is frequency and L is the depth traveled through the substance. Thus, lower frequency sound energy has lower attenuation and therefore better penetration into a medium. This has implications with regard to transducer selection; over a given power range, the lower the frequency, the greater the penetration of the sound wave into a tissue, allowing the imaging of deeper structures. Table 29.2 provides average tissue penetration (assuming an average soft tissue attenuation coefficient of 0.5 dB/cm) and attenuation relative to transducer frequency.

However, with the greater penetration that comes with lower frequencies, there is a loss of resolution for objects within the tissue being imaged. Lateral resolution (LR) is the minimum distance 2 echogenic structures must be separated to be imaged as 2 distinct echo returns. It is directly related to the beam width (w_b). Thus a 15 MHz wave has a lateral resolution of 0.1 mm while a 2 MHz wave has a lateral resolution of 0.8 mm. Axial resolution determines the minimum depth 2 echogenic structures must be separated to be resolved as discrete objects. Like lateral resolution, it is related to wavelength but also includes the spatial pulse length. Spatial pulse length (SPL) is the size of the pulse measured in millimeters as a factor of wave cycles:

$$SPL = n \cdot \lambda$$

Where n is the number of cycles and λ is wavelength. Axial resolution relates to frequency through the following equation (in mm):

$$AR = \frac{SPL}{2}$$

Most point-of-care ultrasounds emit a 2- to 3-cycle pulse; thus a 2 MHz transducer will have an axial resolution of 1.2 mm, and a 15 MHz transducer will have a resolution of 0.2 mm.

2.5. Reflection, refraction, and transmission

In the ultrasound transducer, the piezoelectric crystal array acts as both the emitter and the detector of ultrasound waves; as a result, only the energy from the echo return that reaches the probe can be processed for imaging. The strength of the ultrasound wave return depends on the nature of the reflective surface and the amount of energy lost to the tissue through attenuation.

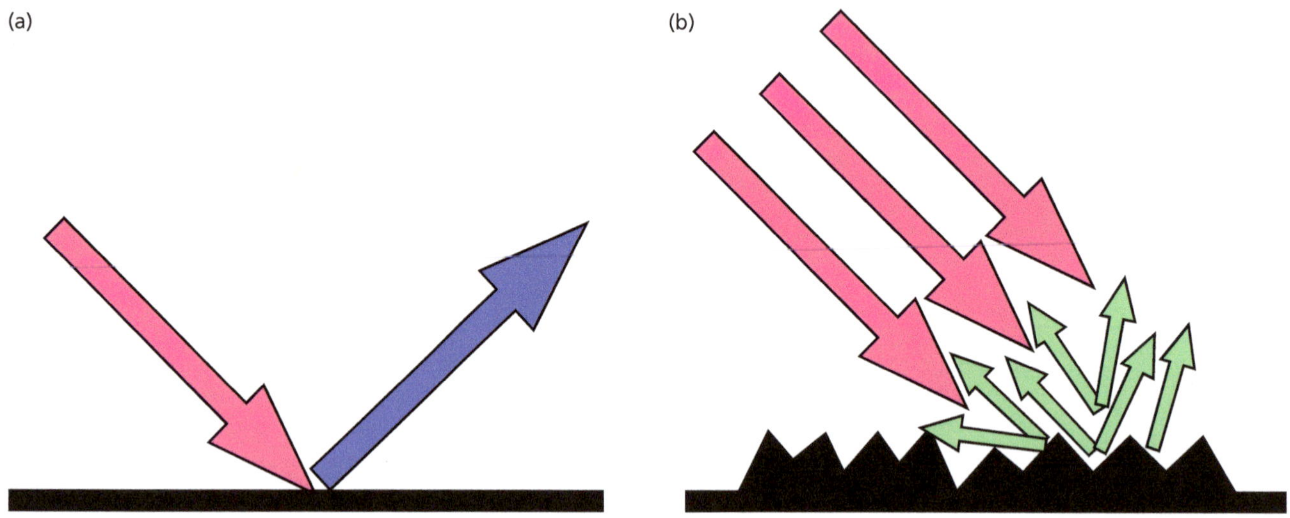

Figure 29.3 Specular reflection (a) and scatter (b).

Reflected waves are the echoes generated by the tissue; these are directed toward the transducer (perpendicular incidence), or at angles other than perpendicular to the incident wave (oblique incidence). The greater the component of perpendicular incidence, the better the quality of the image; thus optimal resolution of in-plane objects such as needles occurs at incident angles between 90° and 45° to the face of the object. Beyond 45° most of the ultrasound energy is reflected away from the probe face and is lost. Along a smooth echogenic boundary such as fascial sheaths, the diaphragm, walls of major vessels, and block needles, the reflected waves travel parallel to one another (Figure 29.3a) in a process called specular reflection. Irregular boundaries such as pleura and visceral organs, incident waves are reflected at variable angles, creating scatter (Figure 29.3b). This scatter directs energy away from the transducer, reducing image quality. This scattering may also result in signal noise that creates a hazy appearance to the structure and tissue beyond it known as backscatter.

Transmission is the incident wave energy that passes into and through a media. Refraction is the change in the path taken by the sound wave when transiting a boundary between 2 dissimilar substances (see Figure 29.1). If the propagation speed of the deeper medium is higher than the superficial medium, then the transmitted wave will refract at an angle greater than the incident wave at the interface. Refraction may impact on image quality if the change in direction results in reflection of the transmitted wave obliquely to the incident wave.

2.6. Doppler ultrasound

The Doppler effect describes the change in frequency of a wave caused by motion of the reflector or emitter. The difference in the received (f_R) versus emitted frequency (f_O) is called the Doppler shift (f_D) and is expressed using the following equation, where v is the velocity of the reflected wave and c is the speed of sound through the media:

$$f_D = f_O \cdot \frac{2 \cdot v}{c}$$

As the reflector moves toward the source, the received echo will increase in frequency, and then as the reflector moves away from the source, the frequency of the received wave will decrease.

The Doppler angle (θ) impacts on the degree of Doppler shift observed for a given emitter and reflector. The Doppler shift (f_D) is related to the cosine of Doppler angle by the following equation, where v is the velocity of the reflected wave, c is the speed of sound in substance, and f_O is the emitted frequency:

$$f_D = \frac{f_O \cdot v \cdot \cos\theta}{c}$$

Thus, the ideal Doppler angle for maximum detection of the flow of a substance (maximum Doppler shift) would be 0° or parallel to the direction of flow. At 90° the Doppler shift would be 0; thus placement of a transducer should be 60° or less to the direction of flow for best assessment of fluid flow. However, at angles less than 30° the ultrasound wave is reflected almost completely at the vessel wall-blood interface, preventing detection of blood flow.

By convention, color Doppler modes display the relative velocities of blood flow using a color scale, with blue hues indicating a negative Doppler shift (blood moving away) and red hues indicating a positive Doppler shift (blood moving toward) from the receiver. This can be remembered using the mnemonic **BART** (**B**lue **A**way, **R**ed **T**oward). The numeric portion of the scale indicates the maximum velocity range that can be displayed.

3. The Ultrasound Machine

Point-of-care ultrasound machines are computerized instruments consisting of a transducer, pulsed beam generator, signal processor, and display. The transducer emits and detects the ultrasound energy used in tissue imaging. The pulsed beam generator drives the transducer, times the pulse and receive phases, sets the wave frequency, amplifies the return signal, and digitizes the data for the signal processor. The signal processor filters and analyzes the data from the pulse generator and then creates and stores the image for display. The display presents the processed information in a format usable by the ultrasound operator.

3.1. Transducers

The transducer both emits ultrasound waves and detects their echo returns using an array of piezoelectric crystals. Modern devices use synthetic lead zirconate titanate ceramics. These composite materials are imparted with specific piezoelectric properties during manufacture that determine its resonant frequency. An assembly of these piezo-composites is arranged in a linear or curved array of varying frequencies that dictate the resolution and penetration properties of the probe.

The ultrasound beam can be focused, allowing the sound energy to be concentrated over a narrow region. This results in a reduction in the beam width, improving lateral resolution. This can be accomplished through curvature of the array, placement of an acoustic lens, or electronically through phased arrays.

Coupling medium (ultrasound gel) is used as an interface between the probe and the skin. This layer fills gaps between the skin and the probe, eliminating air/probe and air/skin interfaces. The low acoustic impedance of air would result in total reflection of the ultrasound wave at the air/skin interface.

3.2. Pulsed beam generator

The pulsed beam generator is responsible for creating the specific ultrasound wave emitted by the transducer. Most manipulations performed by the operator to optimize the ultrasound image are effected through adjustments to the behavior of the pulsed beam generator. This includes gain, phased arrays, and compound spatial imaging.

3.3. Image formation

The ultrasound machine creates an image by correlating the depth of an echo return with the time taken for the signal to reach the detector following the pulse:

$$d = \frac{c \cdot t}{2}$$

where *c* is the propagation speed of sound through a substance and *t* is the pulse-return transit time. A pixel corresponding to a reflected wave is illuminated on a display, corresponding to the calculated depth of the reflected wave. Though this process is fundamental to the function of the ultrasound machine, it is also a source of error. The processing software must make specific assumptions with regard to the behavior of sound within the medium and the reflected waves:

1. Sound waves propagate linearly from the source.
2. The amplitude of the echo is directly related to the echogenic properties of the reflector.
3. Echoes represent reflections from objects in the path of the wave.
4. The distance to the imaged target correlates to the round-trip travel time of the pulse.
5. The propagation speed is uniform through the tissue.

When any of these assumptions are inaccurate, improper representations of tissues or structures occur. These artifacts may confuse or mislead the operator if they are not recognized. One of the more common sources of artifact relates to the uniform propagation velocity of sound through tissues: most manufacturers use a soft tissue average of 1540 m/s as the propagation speed; however, tissues often contain a mixture of adipose, muscle, and connective tissues. Examples of specific artifacts will be detailed later in the chapter.

3.4. Gain and time gain compensation

Amplification of a signal is a form of processing that increases the amplitude of the input waveform without altering the frequency or pulse length. The signal processor receives the amplified signal and filters background noise from the data. In effect, waves below a certain amplitude are filtered from the processed image to provide the necessary contrast to identify structures. When significant attenuation occurs, the return echo may be weak and the default amplification fails to meet the threshold for display of the data. Gain on the ultrasound machine is the ratio of voltage of the amplified output wave to the original input wave and is expressed in decibels (dB). Gain adjustments increase the amplification of the input signal, bringing more of the waveform above the filter threshold of the signal processor, thereby improving resolution. This, however, occurs at the price of increased displayed noise or speckling, creating a grainy image and loss of contrast.

Time gain compensation takes advantage of the increased attenuation that occurs the deeper an ultrasound wave travels in a substance. It allows for progressively increased amplification of reflections from deeper structures. This is achieved by boosting the amplification of signals that arrive to the transducer later during the detection phase of the transmit/receive cycle. Manufacturers accomplish this by dividing the image into depth zones that correspond to return signals with greater transit times. User adjustment of these zones is accomplished through sliders, knobs, or keys, depending on the number of regions programmed by the instrument manufacturer (Figure 29.4).

3.5. Spatial compound imaging

Phased array transducers are capable of selectively triggering individual piezoelectric elements. The array can be fired simultaneously, creating a beam wave front parallel to the transducer face, or can be fired sequentially with a small (<1 μs) delay between each element, creating a directed wave front that propagates at an angle tangential to the array. These directed tangential waves image the tissue at differing angles, allowing visualization of structures that would otherwise be obscured by overlying objects. Compound spatial imaging combines a sequence of angled wave fronts to create a single image that can impart improved resolution and dimensionality to the target tissues (Figures 29.5a and 29.5b).

3.6. Exam modes and user-adjustable parameters

Most point-of-care ultrasound systems have preprogrammed examination modes designed to optimize the image to suit the specific procedure to be performed. These modes have preset gain adjustments, transducer frequency ranges, focal points, and postprocessing algorithms that are applied to the input signals to create the desired effects. For example, modes

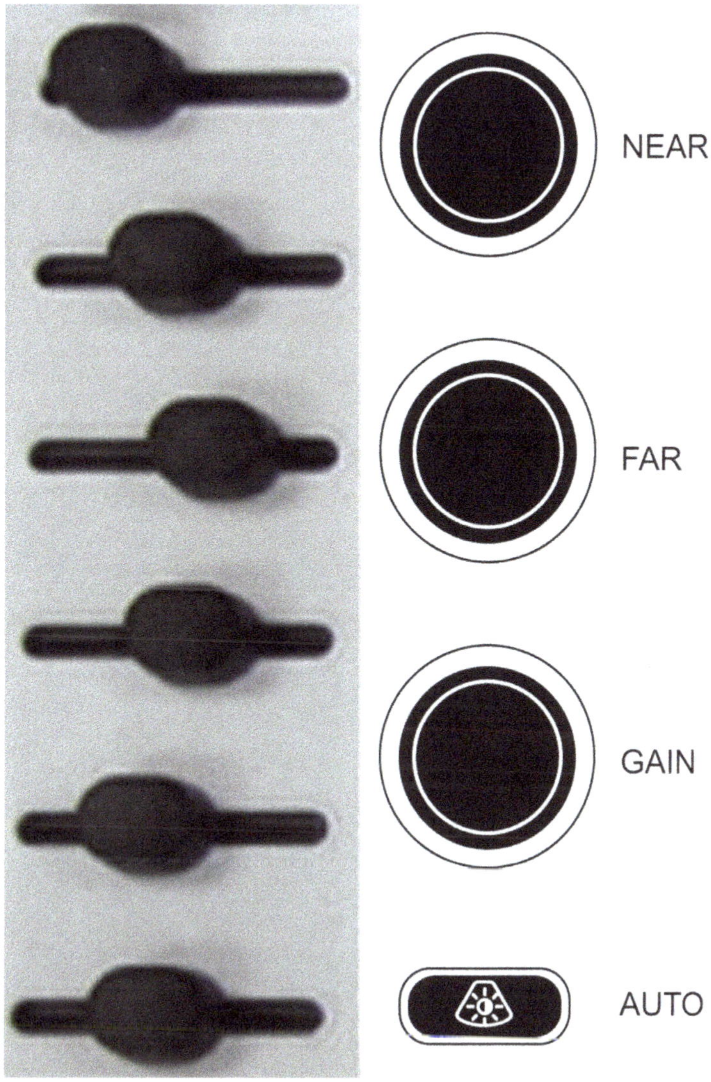

Figure 29.4 Examples of time gain compensation adjustment buttons and sliders.

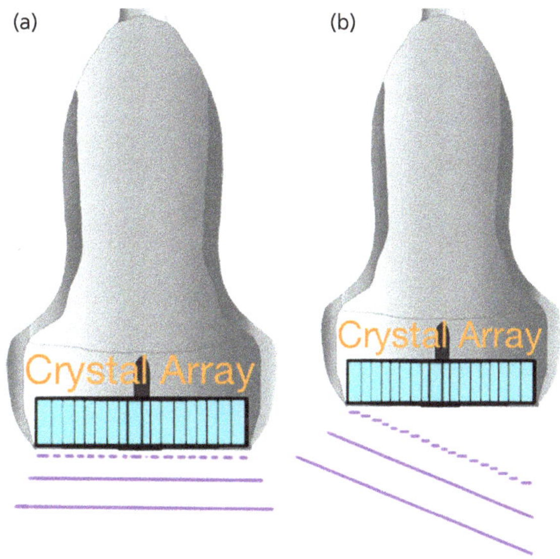

Figure 29.5 Compound spatial imaging. When the crystal array fires simultaneously (a), a wave front is generated that is parallel to the face of the probe. When the timing of the firing of the individual crystals of the array is offset (b), a wave tangential to the face of the probe is generated.

designed for nerve exams and block placement are designed to improve the contrast at interfaces of similar acoustic impedance and maximize resolution, while modes used for vascular access are designed to highlight vascular wall/blood interfaces with decreased affinity for small structures. Selecting the proper exam mode for the desired tissue and procedure is a significant determinant for the ease and precision of image acquisition.

Some manufacturers allow user selection of electronic focal points. Electronic focusing takes advantage of phased array systems to create an ultrasound wave front that converges to concentration point in much the same way a physical acoustic lens focuses the sound energy. However, unlike a fixed acoustic lens, the wave generated by the phased array can be adjusted so that the depth of the convergence point can be changed. Through the use of submenus or hot keys, operators can adjust the depth of the convergence point on these machines to maximize the resolution of specific structures.

3.7. Contrast agents

Differentiation of tissues with comparable echogenic properties, such as nerves within adipose containing connective tissue or highly vascularized organs, is difficult as the sound will tend to propagate through the various tissues without significant reflection at the interfaces. The use of injectable media with differing acoustic properties than the target tissues can create the necessary interfaces between tissue planes to allow echogenic reflection between the tissues, enhancing differentiation of the anatomic structures. To aid in the identification of nerves, injection of saline or local anesthetic can create such an interface where reflection rather than transmission occurs between the solution and surrounding structures, improving image quality.

For vascular tissues, the use of engineered injectable encapsulated microbubble contrast agents improves the resolution of the vessels and detection of flow using Doppler due to the high difference in acoustic impedance between the air-filled spheroids and the surrounding blood.

4. Transducer Manipulation

There are 4 cardinal transducer movements used in image acquisition embodied by the mnemonic **PART**: **P**ressure, **A**lignment, **R**otation, and **T**ilt.

4.1. Pressure

Pressure movements (Figure 29.6a) are the axial forces applied to the patient through the transducer used to improve coupling of the transducer to the tissue surface, compress structures, and improve resolution of objects at the limit of the transducer's penetration range. These movements may be quite forceful and can lead to patient discomfort. Furthermore, these manipulations can lead to compression of structures such as veins, obscuring them from view. Two variations on pressure movements are often used to optimize imaging of objects: heel-toe and roll. Heel-toe (or press) manipulations

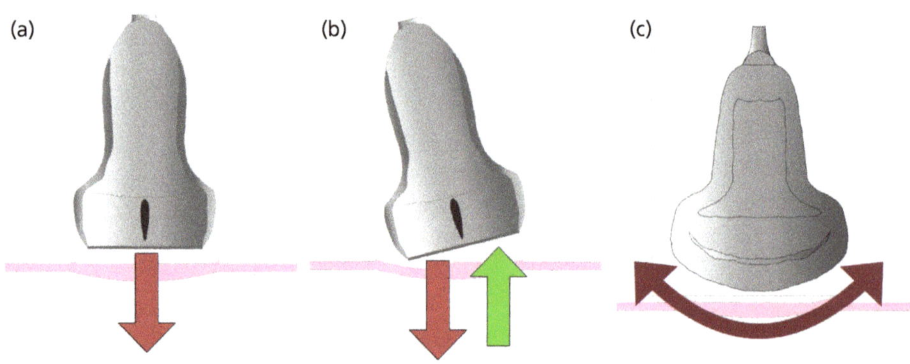

Figure 29.6 (a) Pressure; (b) press or heel-toe; (c) roll.

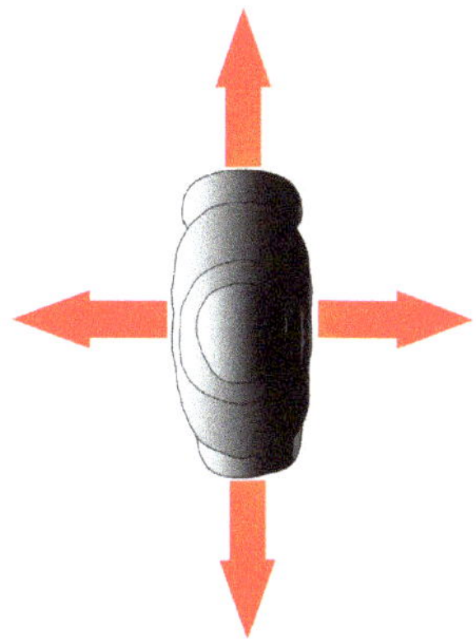

Figure 29.7 Alignment.

(Figure 29.6b) apply distal pressure while relaxing the proximal side of the probe face. This, in effect, aligns the probe face tangentially to the skin surface, angling the wave front so that it better aligns with the reflective surface of the target structure. Roll is a similar maneuver performed using the curved edge of a curvilinear probe (Figure 29.6c). Roll and heel-toe can also be used to image structures deep to tissues of high acoustic impedance such as bone by angling the incident beam to a plane where the target structures are no longer obscured.

4.2. Alignment

Alignment movements are longitudinal and transverse movements (Figure 29.7) of the transducer along the body surface. These are the primary movements used in performance of the ultrasound examination and in aligning a nerve block needle with the target structure. The operator glides the transducer along the skin to image the underlying structures and acquire the desired objects.

4.3. Rotation

Rotation movements are clockwise and counterclockwise movements along the long axis of the probe (Figure 29.8). These manipulations are used to optimize the orientation of the probe to the desired imaging plane (transverse or longitudinal) of the target structure. They fine-tune the alignment maneuvers during in-plane procedural techniques. Rotational alignment errors are the most common source of improper needle placement during in-plane approaches. It is for this reason that the "bevel-up" (Figure 29.9) or bevel oriented toward the probe orientation of the needle is emphasized during needle advancement. With the "bevel-up" orientation the classic step appearance of the needle is

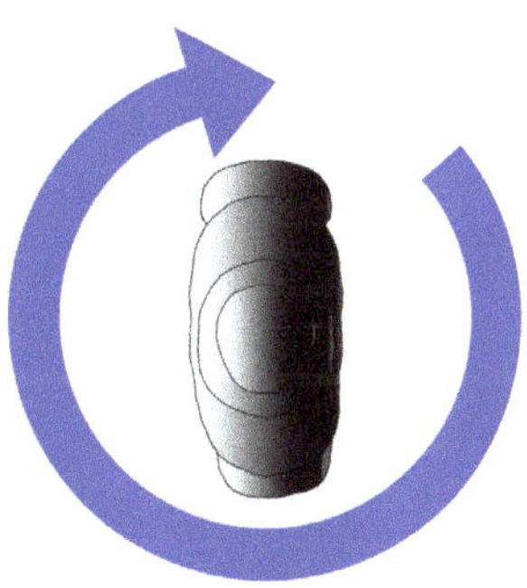

Figure 29.8 Rotation.

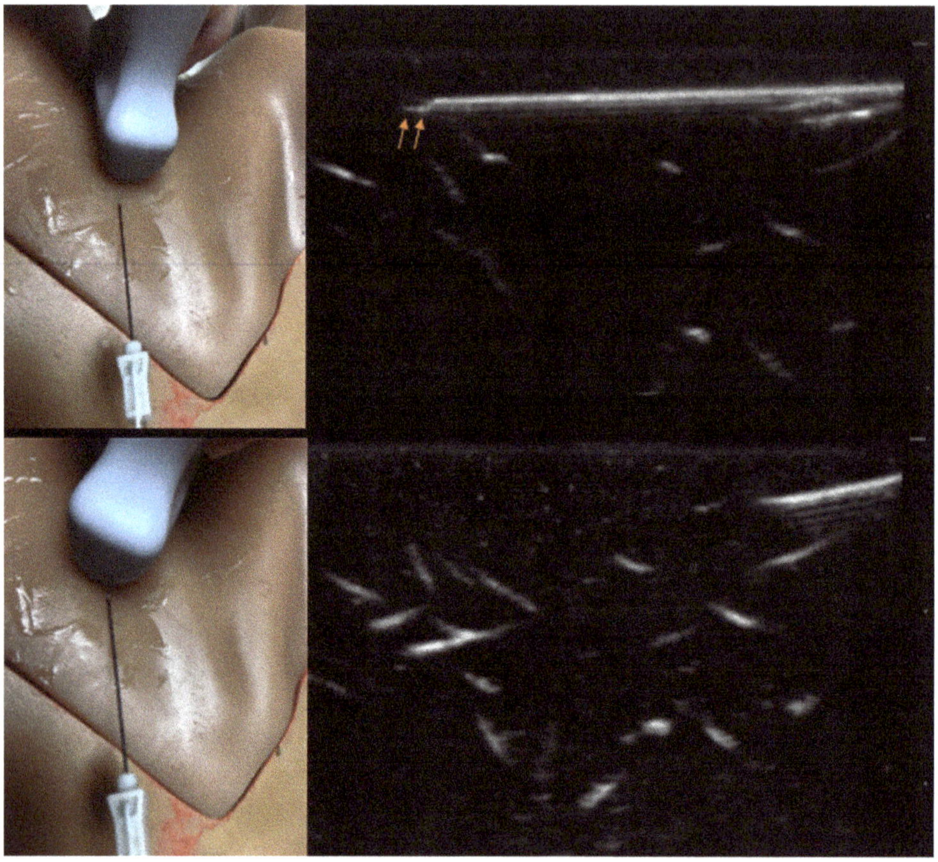

Figure 29.9 Bevel-up orientation (top figure) with classic step-down appearance of the needle bevel (arrows). With the bevel down (bottom figure), the bevel is not visible and the shaft can be confused with the needle tip.

visualized. This appearance is due to the length difference between the front and back walls of the needle due to the slope of the bevel. Other orientations may mask the front wall due to shadowing by the back wall, making determination of the needle tip unreliable.

4.4. Tilt

Tilt manipulations change the angle of the ultrasound beam relative to the probe face (Figure 29.10). Much like pressure movements, these adjustments can be used to image structures obscured by other echogenic objects or to align the ultrasound beam with multiple target structures so that they are viewed in the same plane. Tilt maneuvers also allow the operator to take advantage of a property of specular reflective objects called anisotropy. Anisotropy is the difference in the reflective properties of a material due to changes in the incident angle of the wave source. The optimal reflective angle for nerves lie within 10 degrees from perpendicular to the fascia; thus the transducer must be within this 20 degree band, otherwise the signal will be lost to attenuation. When tracing a structure along its course, the path it takes may be altered and deviate from the plane of the skin. As the path the probe advances along the skin diverges from that taken by the target, the angle of incidence will deviate as the plane of the skin is no longer parallel to the tissue plane. Tilting the probe realigns the incident beam with the target plane. The degree of anisotropy can also be used to differentiate among tissue types: tendons have an anisotropy of about 2 degrees; thus, by titling the probe one can distinguish nerve from tendon using the difference in reflective behavior.

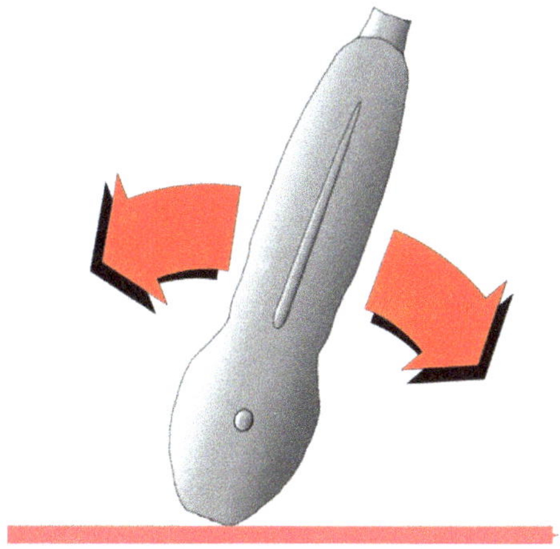

Figure 29.10 Tilt.

5. Artifacts

Artifacts are false displays of anatomy due to errors or distortions in echo signal processing and display. These errors result in incorrect display of structures that are nonexistent, missing, distorted, or in the incorrect anatomic location. Artifacts can be due to operator error and misconfiguration of the machine for the exam to be performed, resulting in poor resolution of the desired anatomic structures. Most artifacts that result in anatomic distortions or misrepresentations are due to the behavior of the incident and reflected ultrasound waves in the differing tissues and the consequence of the computational assumptions made by the engineers who designed the system discussed earlier in the chapter. The following artifacts are due either to differences in the actual propagation speed of sound from the assumed propagation speed for tissues, or to delays in echo returns as the return echo meets interfaces of differing acoustic impedance.

5.1. Bayonet sign

The bayonet sign is an apparent kink and step-off of the needle shaft, giving the impression of a bayonet under the barrel of a rifle (Figure 29.11). This is due to the needle transiting between 2 tissues of dramatically different propagation speeds. In the instance where the tip of the needle looks to have kinked deep to the needle, the segment of the needle that appears to be more superficial is in a substance with faster propagation velocity, such as muscle, while the segment that appears deeper has a slower propagation speed, such as a fluid-filled space.

5.2. Refraction error

Refraction error occurs when the reflected wave transits between tissues of differing acoustic impedance, resulting in a shift in the path of the wave off its initial axis. This causes the machine to interpret the source of the echo to be along the deviated path rather than from its actual origin.

5.3. Reverberation artifact

Reverberation artifacts (Figure 29.12) occur when the incident wave strikes 2 strong reflectors or between the transducer and reflector. These artifacts are the result of 2 possible acoustical interactions.

In the first mechanism, the incident beam strikes the strong reflector and the typical reflection occurs; however, the reflected beam then strikes a surface with greater acoustic impedance, causing a portion of the energy to be transmitted to the transducer and a reflection occurs back into the tissue toward the first highly reflective surface. This process repeats until attenuation results in the loss of detectable echo, or the next pulse cycle begins.

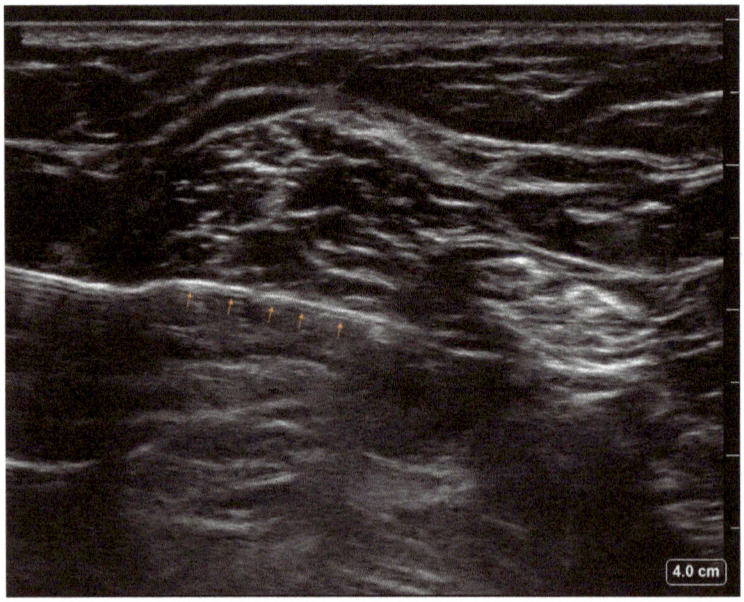

Figure 29.11 Bayonet sign. Apparent bend in a needle (arrows) due to change in acoustic properties between different tissues.

The second process involves reflections of sound waves between 2 highly echogenic surfaces such as the walls of a needle. The incident beam reflects off the shallower reflective surface, with transmission through the first surface followed by reflection by the deeper surface, resulting in repeated echoes of the same structure, the extent of which is determined by the extent of attenuation and the length of the pulse-return cycle.

In both cases, each return echo occurs at a later time point than the one before. This causes the machine to interpret the reverberations as having taken a longer transit time, which is falsely displayed as a deeper object.

Comet tail artifact (Figure 29.13) is a form of reverberation artifact that occurs along an irregular reflective plane such as pleura, diaphragm, and lung. A significant amount of the reflected energy is scattered; however, some of the planes will

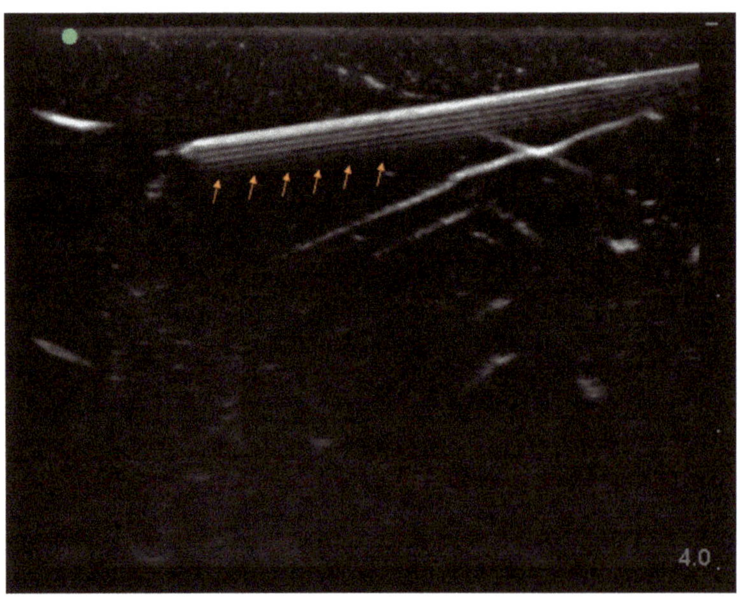

Figure 29.12 Reverberation artifact (arrows).

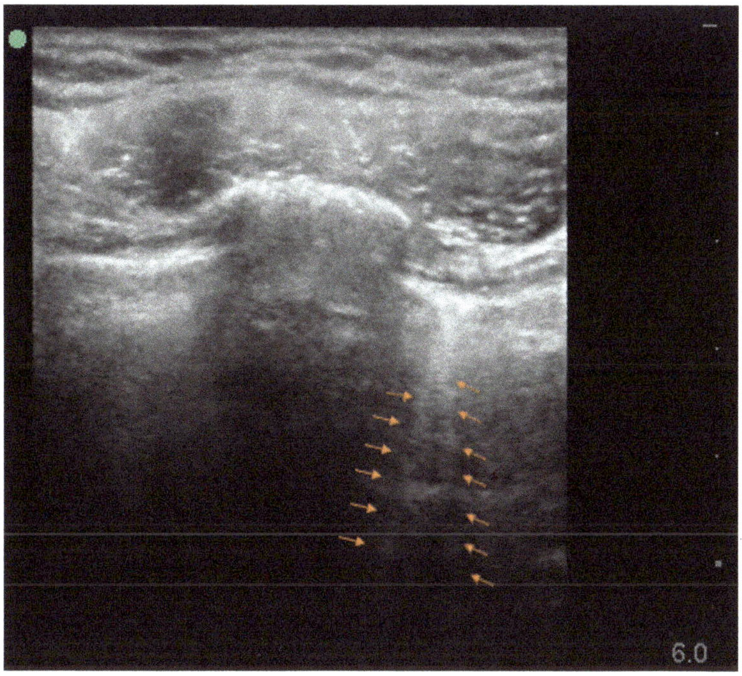

Figure 29.13 Comet tail artifact (arrows).

be perpendicular to the incident wave. Since the interface between the pleura and underlying lung represents a transition between an area of relatively high acoustic impedance (the pleura, diaphragm, and lung tissue) and low acoustic impedance (air within the alveoli), alternating reflection and transmission occurs, leading to the reverberation. Since only certain portions of the echoes are reflected back to the transducer, the reverberations are restricted to a limited area. This artifact can be used to aid in the identification of pleura or diaphragm and may appear to shift position with ventilation as the reflective surface changes with movement of the structures.

Posterior acoustic enhancement (Figure 29.14) is a reverberation artifact observed in cystic structures or vessels. The vascular or cystic walls are specular reflectors with high acoustic impedance, while the fluids within have a low acoustic impedance. This creates a system where reverberations occur between the walls of the structures, creating false echoes of the back wall deep to the object.

These reverberation artifacts can obscure the ability to identify deeper structures as the reflections may overwhelm any echoes from those tissues that lie within the path of the reverberations. This is why advancing a needle superior to a target structure may lead to obscuring of the target due to reverberations. This may also be observed in imaging the radial nerve at the level of the axilla, due to its lying behind the artery in relation to the transducer, and may thus be masked by any posterior acoustic enhancement that may occur. One means of differentiating posterior acoustic enhancement artifacts from actual structures is to observe the behavior of the sonographic image: if it pulses in synchrony with the vessel, this likely represents reflection of the vessel wall; if it is static, it is likely the nerve, since it is not adherent to the vessel and would not oscillate with pulsations.

5.4. Acoustic shadowing

Acoustic shadowing (Figure 29.15) artifacts occur at the interface between media of significantly differing acoustic impedance such as muscle and bone or air and tissue, with the tissue of higher acoustic impedance deep to the lesser. This results in near-total reflection of incident energy at the interface with minimal transmission, causing an image dropout deep to the reflective surface. Any objects deep to the shadow will be unresolvable.

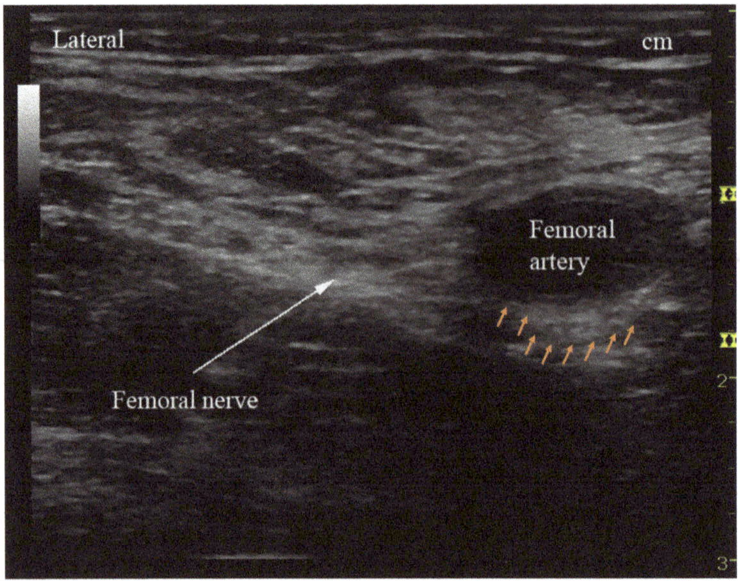

Figure 29.14 Posterior acoustic enhancement (arrows).

6. Nerve Stimulation

Prior to nerve stimulation–guided blockade techniques, block placement was guided by external or palpable anatomy and paresthesia. These methods were relatively unreliable and placed the patient at risk for injury during the performance of the nerve block. The development of techniques utilizing electrical stimulation of motor and sensory nerves to confirm needle localization in the late 1970s greatly improved the safety and reliability of nerve blockade and led to wide adoption of regional anesthetic procedures for surgical and postoperative analgesia.

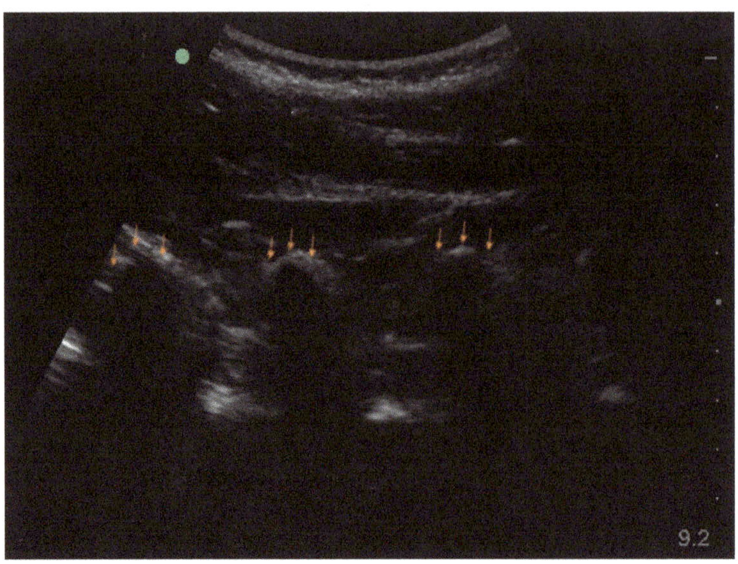

Figure 29.15 Acoustic shadowing (arrows) resulting from near-total reflection of ultrasound waves at the interface between the paraspinous muscles and lamina of the vertebral bodies.

7. Physics of Nerve Stimulation

Peripheral nerve stimulators generate a pulsed electrical current that triggers depolarization of the target nerve. This depolarization results in muscle stimulation along the distribution of the targeted motor nerve or electrical tingling referred to the cutaneous distribution of sensory nerves. To accomplish this nerve stimulation, the device must be designed such that the characteristics of the electrical waveform will trigger depolarization and can be adjusted to allow detection of the minimal stimulation threshold. The user observes the strength of the motor or sensory reaction to impulses at a set intensity (current). The needle is advanced until brisk response is noted. The current is reduced until the motor or sensory twitch is lost. If the loss occurs at the desired threshold current, the needle is at the target location. If the loss occurs at a current lower than the threshold, then the needle is too close to the nerve and should be withdrawn. If the loss is at a higher than desired current, then the needle is advanced until reaction to the stimulus is observed. This process is repeated until the needle placement is optimized to the desired current level. The nature of the waveform and current required is dictated by the physical properties of the nerve, such as degree of myelination or density of ion channels. These histologic features determine the rebase and chronaxie for a nerve type.

7.1. Rebase and chronaxie

Rebase is the minimum amount of continuous current required to depolarize a nerve, and chronaxie is the minimum duration of a current impulse to stimulate a nerve at 2 times the rebase. The current (*I*) required to stimulate a nerve is related to rebase (*P*), chonaxie (κ), and duration of the impulse (*t*) through the following equation:

$$I = P \cdot \left(1 + \kappa/t\right)$$

Each nerve type has a distinct rebase and chronaxie, which influence the current required to stimulate depolarization. Large A-alpha motor fibers have the lowest chonaxie (0.05–0.1 ms), while smaller A-delta sensory and C-fibers have higher chonaxie (0.150 ms and 0.4 ms, respectively); thus it is possible to selectively stimulate motor fibers using pulse lengths of 50 to 100 ms and minimize or prevent stimulation-related pain as it is below the threshold for sensory A-delta (140 ms) and C-fibers (400 ms). Adjustments to impulse duration allow for selective nerve stimulation or stimulation of physiologically deranged nerves; for example, glycosylation of nerves in diabetic patients alters the chonaxie; by increasing pulse duration, stimulation of these nerves may be possible without the need for excess current.

7.2. Cathodic versus anodic stimulation

The polarity of the nerve tip dictates the way in which the current behaves as the needle is passed through tissue and the current/distance relationship with the target nerve. In nerve stimulation, the cathode is the negative terminal and acts as the electron donor; the anode (or grounding lead) is the positive terminal and acts as the electron acceptor. Current thus flows from the cathode to the anode, counter to electron flow. In anodic stimulation, the cations are discharged from the anode on the skin and flow through the body to the needle cathode, where stimulation occurs.

Conventional peripheral nerve stimulators make use of cathodic stimulation for 2 principal reasons: (1) anodic stimulation results in an increase in the concentration of cations under the anode, resulting in a hyperpolarization of the nerve under the anode, placing the nerve in a refractory state and thus resistant to depolarization; and (2) significantly higher current (3–4 times) is required to depolarize a nerve using anodic stimulation.

7.3. Peripheral nerve stimulator

The peripheral nerve stimulator (Figure 29.16) consists of a needle lead, a grounding lead, microprocessor controller, timing clock, display system, and controls. Modern nerve stimulators are capable of delivering a constant current by adjusting output voltage to accommodate for differences in impedance as the needle advances through different tissue planes.

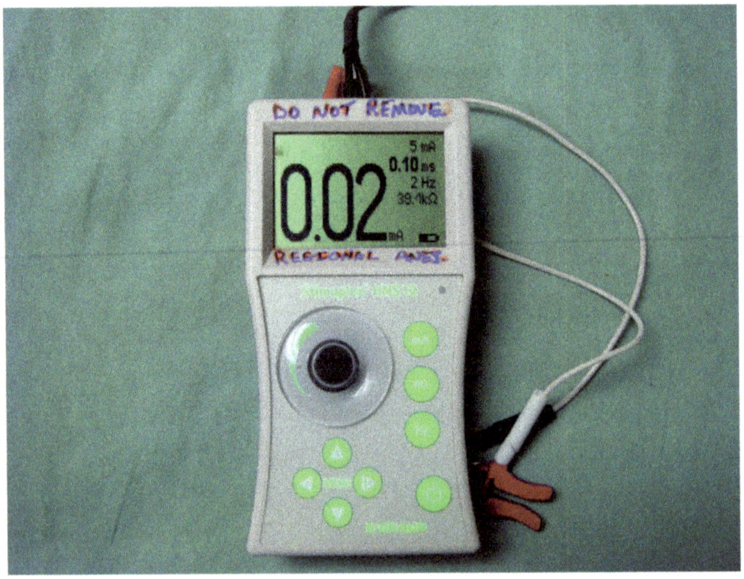

Figure 29.16 Nerve stimulator.

Using timing inputs from the clock, the microprocessor controller creates the stimulating impulse at the desired pulse width dictated by the rebase and chronaxie of the target nerve type.

The user adjusts the delivered current to the patient using an analog or digitally controlled potentiometer. Many peripheral nerve stimulators also allow the user to adjust the pulse width to allow stimulation of motor or sensory fibers. Users are also able to set the rate at which the machine produces a pulse wave. This frequency adjustment is typically between 1 Hz and 2.5 Hz. The higher the frequency, the more pulses are generated per second, and the easier it is to detect changes in response to movement of the needle. However, higher frequency pulses may lead to greater discomfort in patients with fractures or other musculoskeletal injury due to more frequent contracture of traumatized tissue. In cases of injury along the motor distribution of the target nerve, a lower frequency is used to decrease the amount of stimulation, but slower and more cautious needle manipulations should be performed so as not to miss the desired stimulation.

7.4. Insulated needles

The energy density at the needle tip is the current that stimulates the target nerve. Uninsulated needles suffer from greater current dispersion as the entire needle shaft is in contact with potentially conductive body tissues. This may lead to alternate electrical paths that draw current away from the target area, necessitating increasing current to overcome these losses. Insulated needles have a nonconductive covering along the shaft. This prevents loss of energy to surrounding tissue through dispersion currents and concentrates the energy at the needle tip. This concentration effect restricts dispersion to the tip alone and greatly reduces the current necessary to depolarize the target nerve.

7.5. Needle tip to nerve distance estimation

Nerve stimulation–guided techniques rely on correlation between the amount of current necessary to achieve the threshold for stimulation and the distance the needle tip is from the nerve. The greater the distance from the nerve, the more current is required for depolarization. This current/distance relationship is described by Coulomb's law:

$$E = K\frac{Q}{r^2}$$

Where E is the threshold depolarization current, K is Coulomb's constant, Q is the needle tip current, and r is the distance of the needle tip from the nerve. Expressed in terms of the needle tip current:

$$Q = E\frac{r^2}{K}$$

Thus, the amount of emitted current necessary to attain the threshold depolarization current is proportional to the square of the needle distance from the nerve. The needle tip requires 16 times more current when it is 4 mm from the nerve than when it is 1 mm from the nerve to achieve depolarization.

In practice, for peripheral nerve localization, depolarization currents of 0.2 to 0.5 mA correspond to needle tip placement adjacent to the nerve; at current less than 0.2 mA there is significant risk for intraneural placement.

7.6. Limitations of peripheral nerve stimulation

There are several factors that impact on the reliability and utility of nerve stimulation–based block techniques. Anatomic derangements may impact on the ability to use such techniques. For example, an amputee may no longer have a limb distal to the point of stimulation to observe response; in such cases a sensory stimulator could be used, with the patient describing the perceived location of the stimulus; this perceived stimulation is known as *phantom stimulation*. Patients with contractures may also not demonstrate motor responses at the desired threshold for determination of needle tip proximity to the nerve.

Patients with neurologic pathology such as glycosylation of nerves in diabetics, demyelination disorders, or nerve trauma may not respond to nerve stimulation or may require significantly higher current to achieve the same degree of motor response as would a nonaffected individual.

Because this is a stimulating procedure, patients traditionally received moderate sedation in the performance of these techniques. Furthermore, patients with trauma along the distribution of the stimulated nerve may not tolerate the motor contractions and might require significantly more sedation to perform the procedure. Use of these techniques is limited when the patient is under general anesthesia with motor blockade.

In vivo and in vitro study of cathodic stimulation demonstrated biphasic variability in intensity of motor stimulation with increasing current as the needle approached the nerve. In a rat sciatic model, at currents over 0.5 mA the intensity of the muscle twitch decreased by 60%, and at >1.0 mA complete conduction block occurred in vitro. In vivo a 10% to 30% conduction block was observed as current was increased beyond 1.0 mA. This paradoxical decrease in nerve conduction with closer proximity to the nerve began to manifest at about 2 to 4 cm from the nerve depending on the current. Intraneural needle placement demonstrated an expected return in nerve stimulation and a threefold decrease in threshold activation current. Anodic stimulation showed a linear relationship between nerve distance and current with nerve response and was proportionate to increasing current. This biphasic behavior of cathodic stimulation may explain the relatively high incidence of intraneural injections using nerve stimulation techniques when evaluated using ultrasound.

8. Conclusion

A sound understanding of the basic physical principles that underlie the instruments used to aid in the performance of nerve blocks provides the clinician with the tools to safely guide the needle to the target nerve. Whether nerve stimulators, ultrasound machines, or both are used to perform regional anesthesia, this basic understanding of how these technologies function when used on a patient is an important addition to, but not a substitute for, detailed anatomic knowledge. This technology can only confirm and refine correct needle placement for regional blocks; it should never be considered a substitute for the physician's understanding of the anatomic basis for each block.

30

Upper Extremity Neuroanatomy

1. Introduction

Regional anesthesia of the upper extremity involves appreciating the respective contributions of 2 major nerve plexuses, the cervical plexus and the brachial plexus (Figure 30.1). A detailed understanding of the anatomy of these plexuses and their relationship to other surrounding structures is essential for the safe and successful practice of regional anesthesia of the upper extremity. An overview of the cervical and brachial plexus blocks is included in Table 30.1.

2. Cervical Plexus

The cervical plexus is formed from a series of nerve loops between adjacent anterior primary rami of cervical nerve roots C1 through C4. The cervical plexus is located deep to the sternocleidomastoid muscle and lies medial to the scalene muscles. The

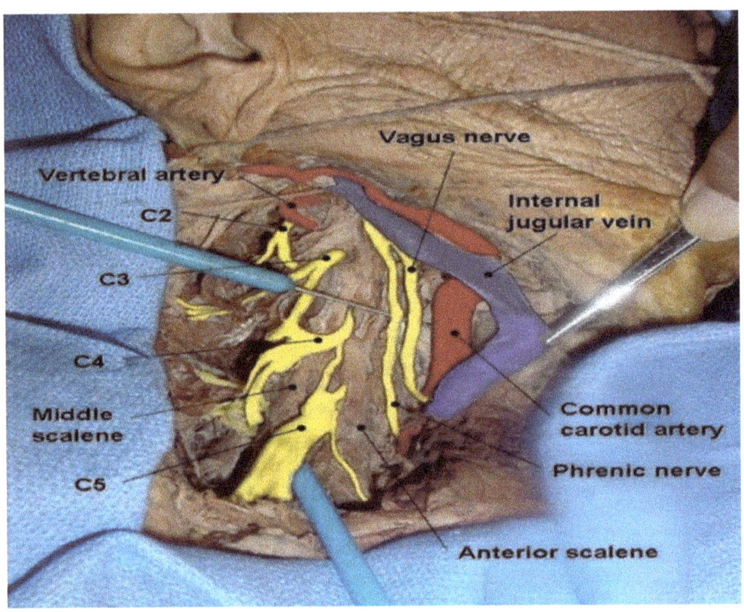

Figure. 30.1 Cadaver dissection demonstrating brachial and cervical plexus with their neurovascular relationship.

Table 30.1: Overview of the cervical and brachial plexus blocks

Upper Extremity Proximal Blocks			
	Indications	Side Effects	Complications
Cervical Plexus Block	Surgeries involving the head, anterior and lateral neck, and the shoulder areas; carotid endarterectomy; internal jugular and subclavian vein cannulation; transvenous cardiac pacemaker insertion	• Hemidiaphragmatic paralysis (phrenic nerve block) • Aspiration (block of the glossopharyngeal nerve) • Horner's syndrome • Hoarseness • Coughing • Hypotension • Bradycardia	• Systemic toxicity (local anesthetic overdose, intravascular injection) • Neurologic injury (traumatic: needle; ischemic: epinephrine; toxic: local anesthestic) • Subarachnoid/epidural injection • Spinal cord injury
Brachial Plexus Block	***Interscalene***: surgery at the shoulder ***Supraclavicular***: surgery distal to the shoulder ***Infraclavicular***: surgery at or distal to the elbow ***Axillary block***: surgery at or distal to the elbow	• Hemidiaphragmatic paralysis (phrenic nerve block) • Horner's syndrome • Hoarseness • Coughing • Hypotension • Bradycardia	• Systemic toxicity (local anesthetic overdose, intravascular injection) • Neurologic injury (traumatic: needle; ischemic: epinephrine; toxic: local anesthetic) • Pneumothorax (mostly with supraclavicular block) • Subarachnoid/epidural injection • Spinal cord injury

deep branches of the plexus are motor nerves, which include the phrenic nerve (C3, C4, C5 roots which innervates the diaphragm) and the ansa cervicalis nerve (innervates the omohyoid, sternothyroid, and sternohyoid muscles). The superficial nerves of the cervical plexus emerge from the middle of the sternocleidomastoid muscle and include the following (Figure 30.2):

- *Lesser occipital nerve (C2)*: innervates the skin posterior to the ear.
- *Great auricular nerve (C2-C3)*: innervates the ear and angle of the mandible to the mastoid process.
- *Transverse cervical nerve (C2-C3)*: innervates the anterior neck.
- *Supraclavicular nerve (C3-C4)*: innervates the area over the clavicle and shoulder.

3. Brachial Plexus

The brachial plexus is formed from the anterior primary rami of cervical nerves (C5-C8) and the first thoracic (T1) nerve roots, for a total of 5 originating nerve roots. Occasionally, contributions to the brachial plexus arise from the C4 nerve root (prefixed plexus) or from the T2 nerve root (postfixed plexus). The roots of the plexus travel between the anterior and posterior tubercles of the transverse processes of the cervical vertebrae posterior to the vertebral artery, which is housed by the foramen transversarium. They are contained within the posterior fascia of the anterior scalene and anterior fascia of the middle scalene muscles forming the interscalene space. The principal components of the brachial plexus include the following (Figure 30.3):

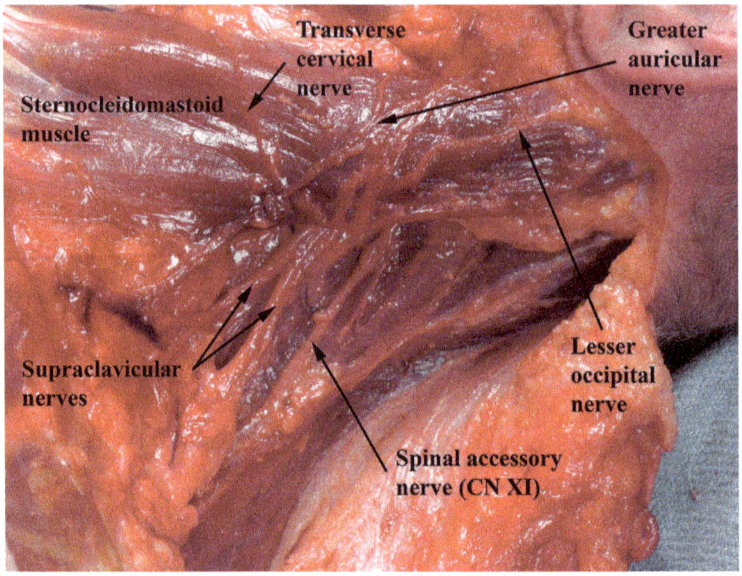

Figure 30.2 Dissection of the cervical plexus in the posterior triangle.

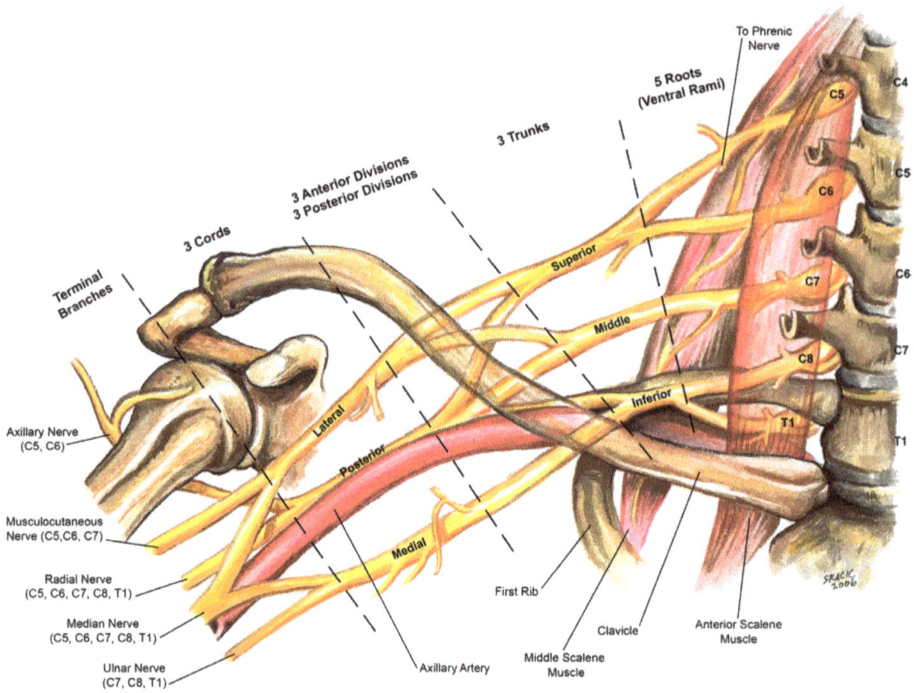

Figure 30.3 Principal components of the brachial plexus.

- **Three trunks.** Formed by the union of the nerve roots; superior (C5 and C6), middle (C7), and inferior (C8 and T1). The trunks pass between the anterior and middle scalene muscles, lying slightly closer to the middle than the anterior scalene. They pass over the first rib and under the clavicle.
- **Six divisions.** Formed as the trunks pass between the first rib and the clavicle, and divide into an anterior division (destined to become the anterior or flexor compartment muscles of the arm) and a posterior division (posterior extensor muscle compartments of the arm).
- **Three cords.** The divisions recombine as they emerge from beneath the clavicle to form 3 cords: lateral cord (anterior divisions of the superior and middle trunk), medial cord (anterior continuation division of the inferior trunk), and posterior cord (posterior divisions of all 3 trunks). The cords are named based on their relationship to the axillary artery. The lateral and medial cords give rise to the nerves supplying the flexor surface of the upper extremity, and the posterior cord to the nerves supplying the extensor surface of the upper extremity.
- **Five terminal branches.** The cords give rise to 5 terminal branches. The musculocutaneous nerve (C5-C7) arises from the lateral cord and innervates the coracobrachialis, biceps brachii, and brachialis muscles, and the skin to the lateral forearm. The median nerve is a compilation of the lateral cord (C6-C7) and the medial cord (C8, T1). It innervates muscles of the anterior forearm and the thenar half of the muscles and skin of the palm. The ulnar nerve is a branch of the medial cord (C7-T1) and innervates the forearm and hand medial to the midpoint of digit 4. The axillary nerve (C5-C6) is a branch of the posterior cord and innervates the shoulder joint and lateral skin over the deltoid muscle. The radial nerve (C5-T1), which is also a branch of the posterior cord, innervates all of the muscles of the posterior compartments of the arm and forearm and most of the posterior skin of the upper extremity.

Anatomic dissections of the brachial plexus consistently reveal a distinguishable sheath of fibrous tissue surrounding the brachial plexus, vasculature, and loose investing connective tissue, which passes from the paravertebral fascia of the cervical vertebra distally to the clavicle. The practice of the interscalene, supraclavicular, and infraclavicular brachial plexus block techniques relies upon the anatomic reality of this continuous fascial compartment. The sheath concept theoretically improves the success of single-injection blocks and continuous peripheral nerve catheters by offering an enclosed compartment containing the local anesthetic solution near nerve tissue targets and allowing the predetermined volume of local anesthetic to surround and bathe the targeted nerves (Figures 30.4 and 30.5).

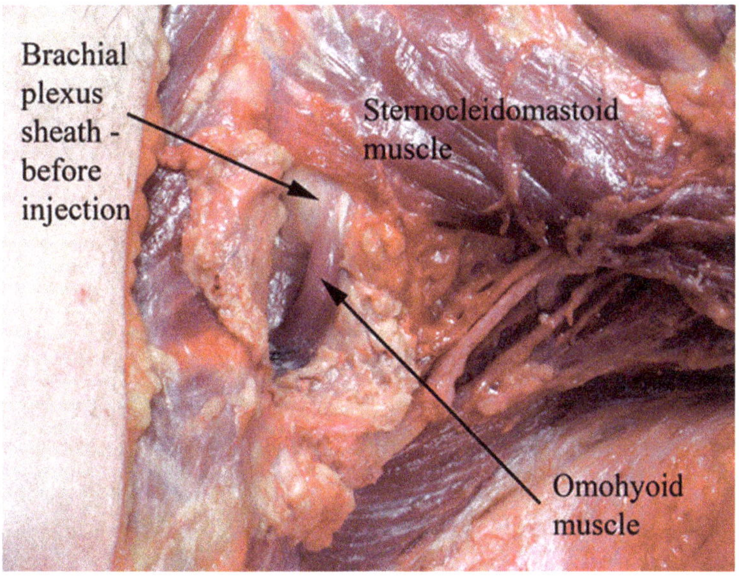

Figure 30.4 Continuous fascial sheath prior to injection of saline.

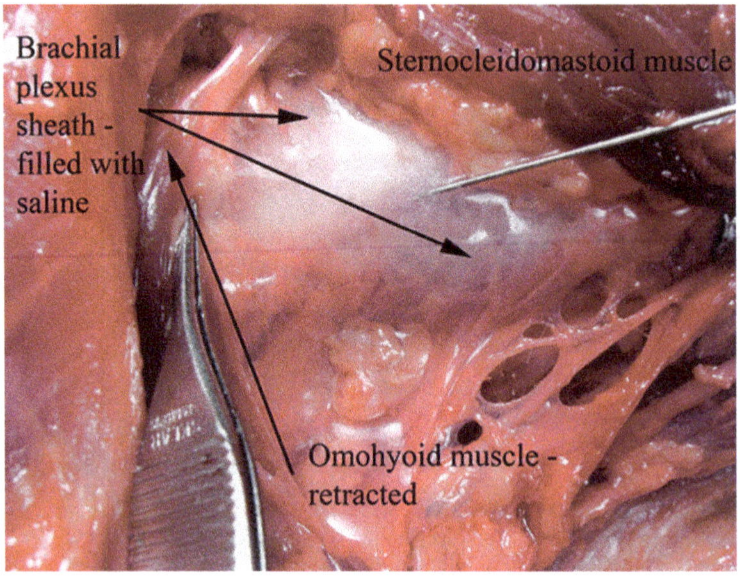

Figure 30.5 Continuous fascial sheath injected with normal saline.

While the concept of a continuous perivascular sheath has withstood careful anatomical scrutiny, and has contributed to high rates of success using single injection techniques, there are some who would question the veracity of a single contiguous "envelope" surrounding the roots and trunks of the cervical and brachial plexuses and who would instead consider that each individual neural element has its own unique, identifiable fascial compartment. Regardless, it is undeniable that single-injection techniques performed using either neural stimulation or ultrasound guidance result in clinically significantly high success rates somewhat independent on absolute volumes of injected local anesthetic solutions above 5–10 mL.

Cervical Plexus Block

31

1. Introduction

The cervical plexus block provides anesthesia and analgesia to the head and neck region. Depending on the type of intended surgery, the plexus can be blocked at either a superficial or a deep level. The superficial branches (Figure 31.1) of the cervical plexus innervate the skin and superficial structures of the head, neck, and shoulder. The deep

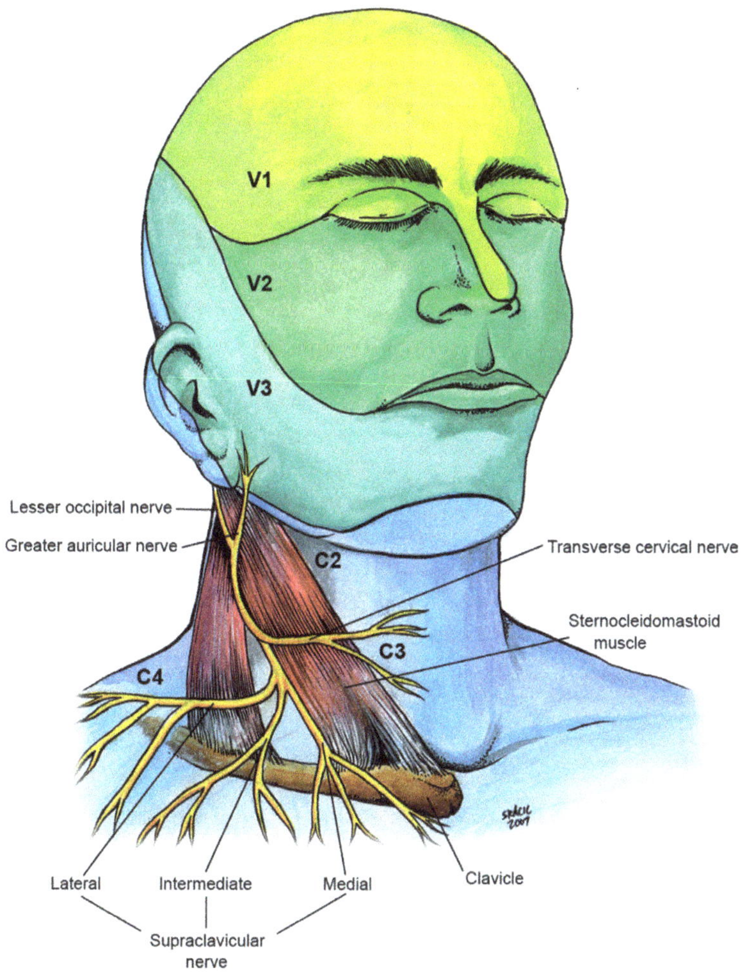

Figure 31.1 Superficial cervical plexus.

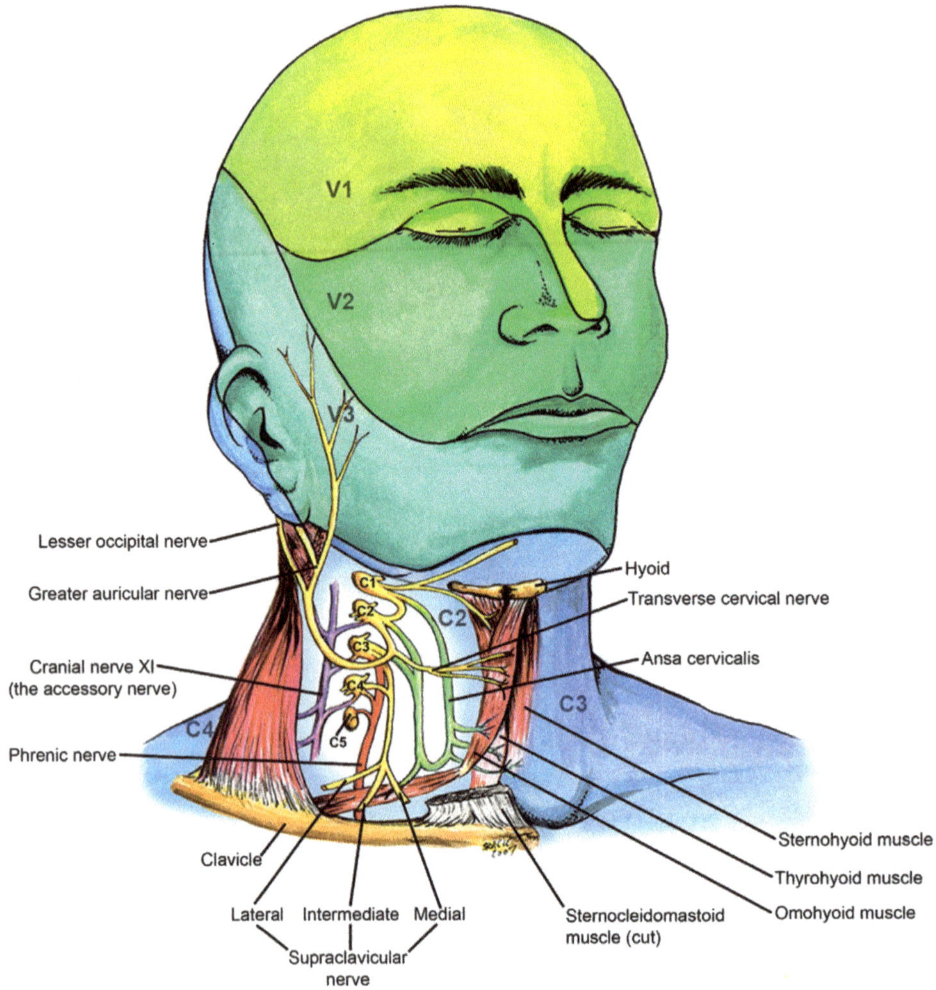

Figure 31.2 Deep cervical plexus.

branches (Figure 31.2) innervate the muscles of the deep anterior neck and the diaphragm. The deep cervical plexus block is used for deeper surgeries of the neck, such as carotid artery or thyroid surgery, and the superficial cervical plexus block is used for superficial cutaneous surgeries of the head and neck. This block is also useful as a supplement to other regional techniques of the upper torso.

2. Anatomy

The cervical plexus is formed from the anterior primary rami of the C1 through C4 nerve roots; it lies anterior to the cervical vertebrae and posterior to the sternocleidomastoid muscle. It includes 5 main components: (1) the cutaneous branches, which supply the lesser occipital, greater auricular, transverse cervical, and supraclavicular nerves; (2) the ansa cervicalis, which innervates the infrahyoid and geniohyoid muscles; (3) the phrenic nerve, which is the only motor nerve to innervate the diaphragm; (4) contributions to the accessory nerve (CN XI), which innervates the sternocleidomastoid and trapezius muscles; and (5) direct muscular branches, which supply prevertebral muscles of the neck.

Bilateral deep cervical plexus blocks, which would result in complete diaphragmatic paresis, should not be performed. Also, patients with chronic pulmonary conditions such as unilateral pneumonectomy surgery in the past may not be suitable candidates for an contralateral deep cervical plexus block. Caution must be taken when placing a deep cervical plexus block because of the close proximity of the vertebral artery in the foramen transversarium and the dural sleeve

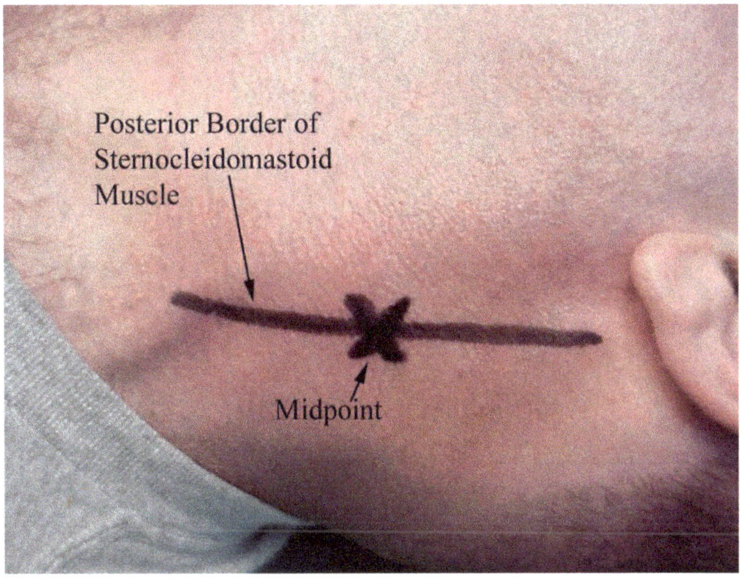

Figure 31.3 Landmarks for the superficial cervical plexus.

in the intervertebral foramen. Placing the block too close to the vertebral artery may result in an intravascular injection; placing it too close to the dural sleeve may result in an epidural or subarachnoid injection.

3. Procedure

3.1. Landmarks

Superficial cervical plexus (Figure 31.3)**.** Identify and mark the posterior border of the sternocleidomastoid muscle, as well as the midpoint of the muscle.

Deep cervical plexus (Figure 31.4)**.** Position the patient supine with the head turned toward the nonoperative side. Palpate the transverse process of C6 (Chassaignac's tubercle) at the level of the cricoid cartilage. Palpate the mastoid

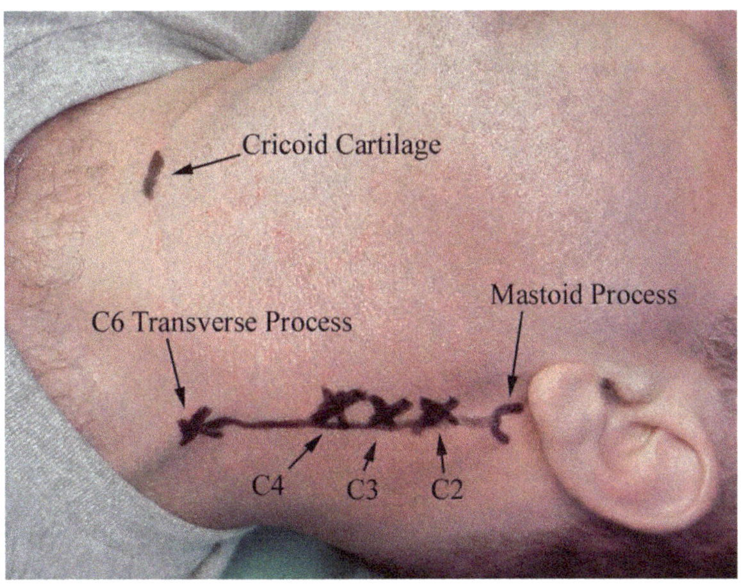

Figure 31.4 Landmarks for the deep cervical plexus.

process behind the ear. Draw a line between the mastoid process and Chassaignac's tubercle. The transverse processes of the other cervical vertebrae will lie on or near this line. The first palpable transverse process below the mastoid process is C2. Palpate and mark the transverse processes of C2 to C4 (the C4 transverse process lies approximately at the level of the mandible). Insert the needle medially and caudally so that the needle tip is resting on the transverse process. Ultrasound guidance is useful to determine bony and muscular anatomical landmarks.

3.2. Needles

- 22-gauge, 5-cm, short-bevel needle.

3.3. Injection

Superficial Cervical Plexus. Insert the needle at the midpoint of the posterior border of the sternocleidomastoid muscle to approximately half the depth of the muscle, and inject 3 to 4 mL of local anesthetic. Also perform a subcutaneous injection of additional local anesthetic cephalad and caudad along the length of the sternocleidomastoid muscle posterior border.

Deep Cervical Plexus. Attach a 10-mL control syringe to the needle so that one individual can both aspirate as well as inject the local anesthetic solution; an alternative is to use clear extension tubing bridging the needle and syringe if control syringes are not readily available. Once the transverse process is contacted, withdraw the needle 1 to 2 mm. Inject the local anesthetic slowly with frequent aspirations. After completing the injection, remove the needle and repeat the block at the next level. (Many clinicians perform only a superficial cervical plexus block, and the surgeon infiltrates deeper structures as required.)

Local Anesthetic

Superficial Cervical Plexus. 5 to 10 mL.
Deep Cervical Plexus. 3 to 5 mL at each level or 15 mL at C3 only.

Teaching Points. Caution should be exercised in patients receiving a deep cervical plexus block for carotid endarterectomy surgery. These patients will likely have atheromatous plaques that could be dislodged with excessive head hyperextension or which might cause cerebral ischemia with head rotation. For carotid endarterectomies, the surgeon must infiltrate the carotid body with local anesthetic because the cervical plexus does not innervate this structure.

Interscalene Block

32

1. Introduction

The interscalene approach blocks the brachial plexus at the root level (Figure 32.1). It is particularly well suited for operations on the shoulder, clavicle, or upper arm. Cervical nerve roots (C5-C8) are preferentially blocked, with variable proximal spread to the cervical plexus (C1-C4), while usually sparing the ulnar nerve (originates from C8-T1). The entry point is the omotrapezoid triangle formed by the lateral edge of the sternocleidomastoid muscle (SCM), the anterior edge of the trapezius muscle, and the superior border of the omohyoid muscle. The interscalene block is characterized by the shortest latency of onset of action and injection of the smallest volume of local anesthetic among all the approaches to the brachial plexus owing to the proximity of the injected volume of local anesthetic to the central neuraxis.

2. Anatomy

The nerves of the brachial plexus emerge from their respective intervertebral foramina and course posterior to the vertebral artery. They then pass between the anterior and (slightly closer to the) middle scalene muscles as the trunks (superior C5-C6, middle C7, inferior C8-T1) of the brachial plexus. The interscalene block (ISB) is performed at the level of the C6 vertebral body, which corresponds to the cricoid cartilage of the neck. By blocking the plexus at this level, the local anesthetic is deposited around the upper roots (C5, C6) that innervate the muscles of the shoulder, specifically the deltoid, supraspinatus, infraspinatus, and teres major (Figure 32.1 through 32.4). Occasionally, there may be proximal spread to the cervical plexus (C2, C3, C4) and cervical sympathetic chain, which can result in Horner's syndrome and hoarseness postblock. The ISB was formerly thought to always result in hemidiaphragmatic paresis because of the close proximity of the phrenic nerve to the interscalene groove when larger volumes of local anesthetic were injected (30–50 mL). More recently, with use of ultrasound guidance and smaller volumes (10 mL to 20 mL), however, it has been identified that this is no longer the case. However, in light of a possible hemidiaphragmatic paralysis resulting from the ISB, the block should not be given to a patient who is unable to tolerate a reduction in pulmonary function greater than 30%. The block typically spares the ulnar nerve, making it unsuitable for hand and forearm surgeries.

3. Procedure

3.1. Landmarks

Place the patient supine with the head turned toward the opposite side, while relaxing the shoulders and having the patient reach toward the ipsilateral knee with the hand.

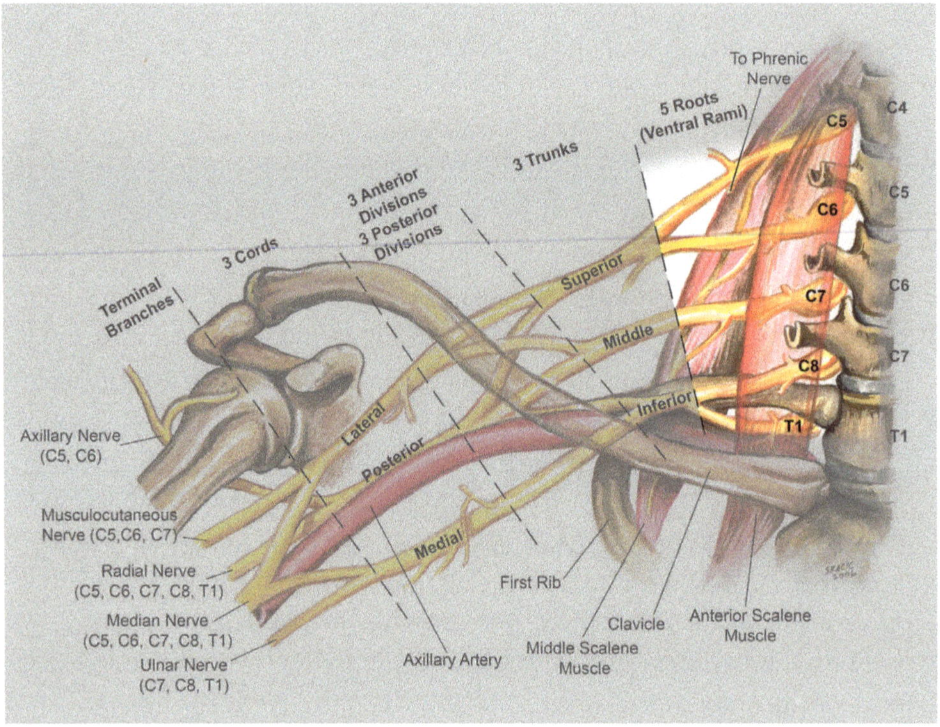

Figure 32.1 External anatomy for the interscalene block.

Identify the cricoid cartilage and palpate the interscalene groove located at the C6 level. Palpate the lateral border of the SCM, and move your fingers laterally into the interscalene groove (between the anterior and middle scalene muscles). The external jugular vein often crosses the border of the SCM at this point. If this is the case, the initial needle insertion should be posterior to the vessel (see Figure 32.2). Initial needle insertion (at the level of C6) is indicated by an "X" (Figure 32.5 and 32.6).

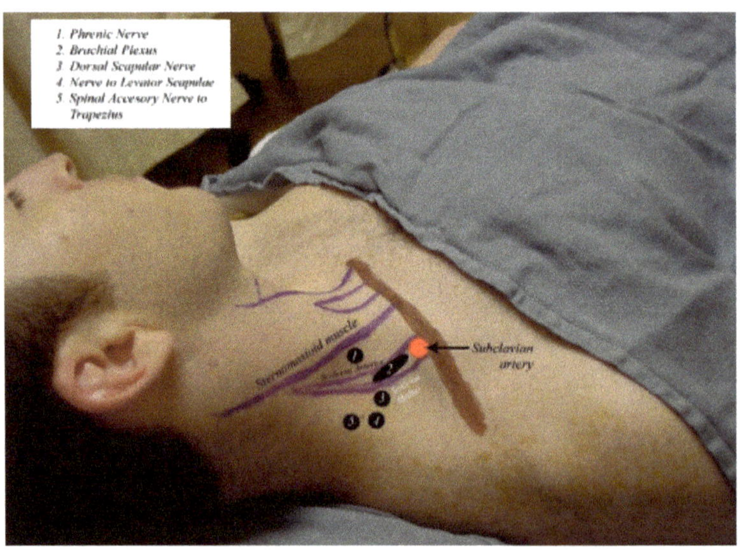

Figure 32.2 Interscalene block external anatomy.

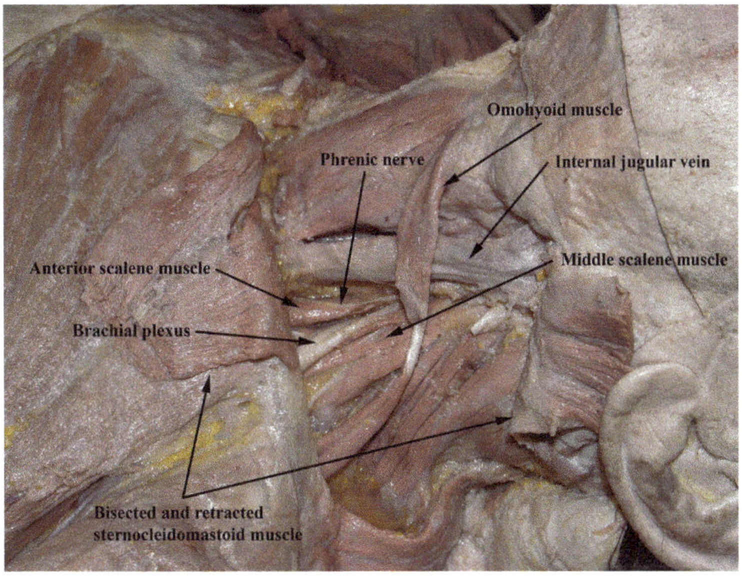

Figure 32.3 Interscalene block dissection.

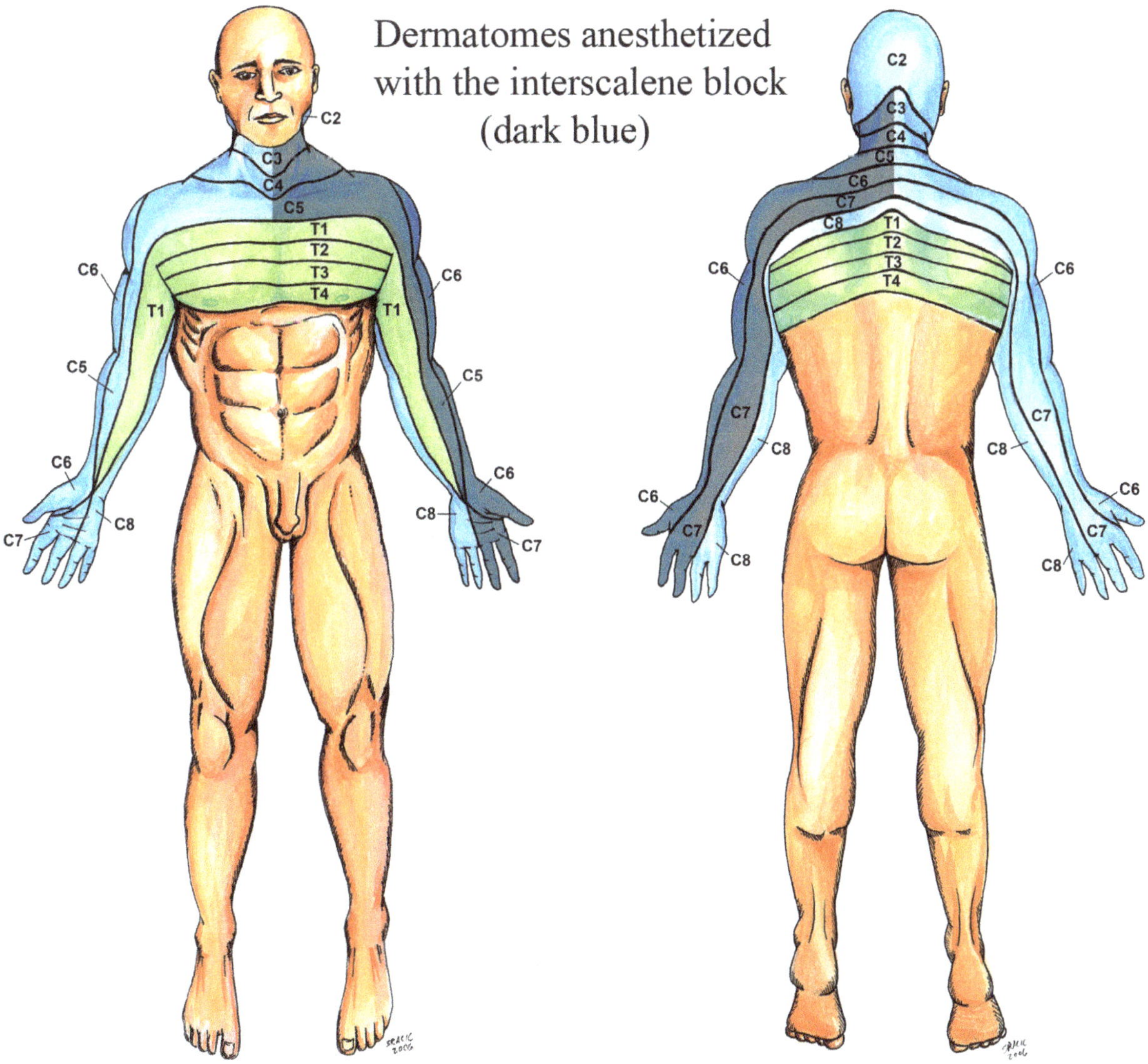

Figure 32.4 Dermatomes anesthetized with the interscalene block (dark blue).

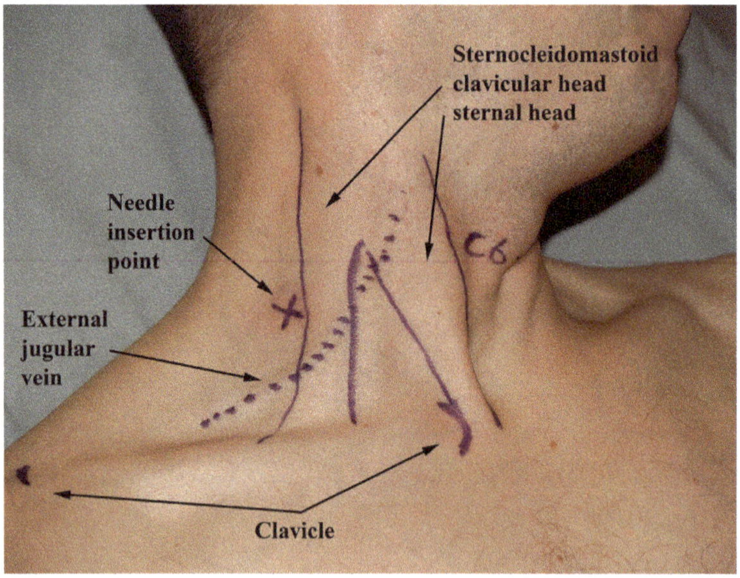

Figure 32.5 External anatomy for the interscalene block.

3.2. Needles

- 22-gauge, 5-cm, insulated needle
- 18-gauge, 5-cm insulated Tuohy needle for catheter placement; catheters introduced 3 cm beyond needle tip

3.3. Stimulation

The nerve stimulator is initially set at 1.0 to 1.2 mA. Muscle twitch in the shoulder, biceps, or triceps at 0.5 mA or less indicates adequate proximity of the uninsulated tip of an insulated Teflon-coated block needle to the brachial plexus for

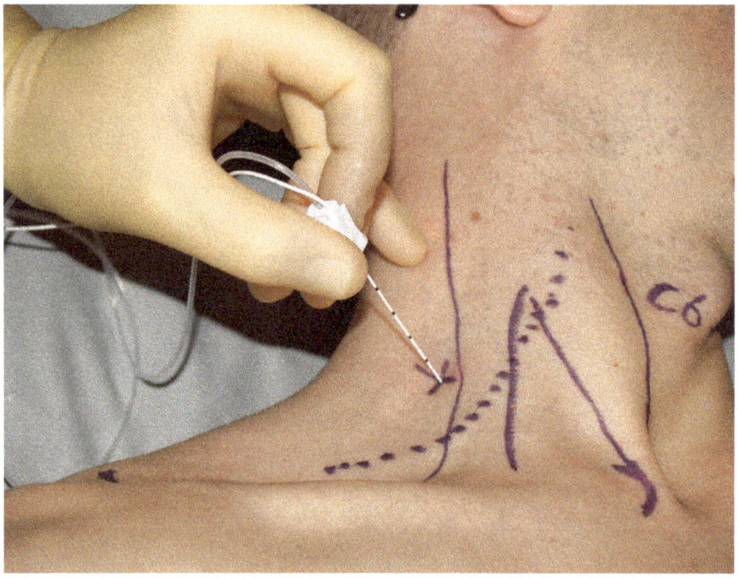

Figure 32.6 Needle position for the interscalene block.

local anesthetic injection. Stimulation below the elbow suggests a needle position that is too caudal in the brachial plexus for shoulder surgery. In most adults, the brachial plexus is rarely deeper than 1 to 2 cm below the skin. Stimulation of the trapezius muscle suggests that the needle tip is too posterior to the plexus. Conversely, stimulation of the diaphragm indicates phrenic nerve stimulation, and the needle tip sits anterior to the plexus on the belly of the anterior scalene muscle.

Motor Response Predicting Accurate Needle Placement
Acceptable Responses: Twitch of the pectoralis, deltoid, triceps, biceps or any forearm or hand muscles.

Unacceptable Responses: Trapezius twitch/shoulder shrug (due to stimulation of the spinal accessory nerve, not the brachial plexus). Shoulder paresthesia should not be used as an indication, since it is due to the stimulation of the suprascapular nerve.

3.4. Local Anesthetic

In most adults, 20 to 30 mL of local anesthetic is sufficient to block the plexus.

3.5. Additional Procedures

An intercostobrachial nerve (T1, T2) block (10 mL subcutaneous injection of local anesthetic from mid-biceps muscle to the inferior axilla) should be performed for major shoulder procedures where there is the expectation of involvement of the medial upper arm. Paravertebral nerve blocks of T1-T2 may supplement the interscalene block for procedures involving significant posterior dissections.

Teaching Points. Injection of local anesthetic into the neighboring vertebral artery can result in devastating complications, including seizures, motor paralysis, respiratory depression, and death. Proper injection technique with frequent, gentle aspiration for blood is critical for safe block placement.

4. Block with Ultrasound Probe

4.1. Probe

High frequency (5–12 MHz), linear.

4.2. Probe Position

The oblique plane gives the best transverse view of the brachial plexus; a cross-sectional (axial) view displays the nerves as hypoechoic circles with hyperechoic surrounding rings. Position the probe on the neck at the level of C6 (Figures 32.7 through 32.9).

4.3. Approach

The plexus can be approached from either a posterior or an anterior position. To use the posterior approach, begin the needle insertion at the lateral aspect of the probe in-plane or in-line; short-axis view of relevant anatomy; the needle will

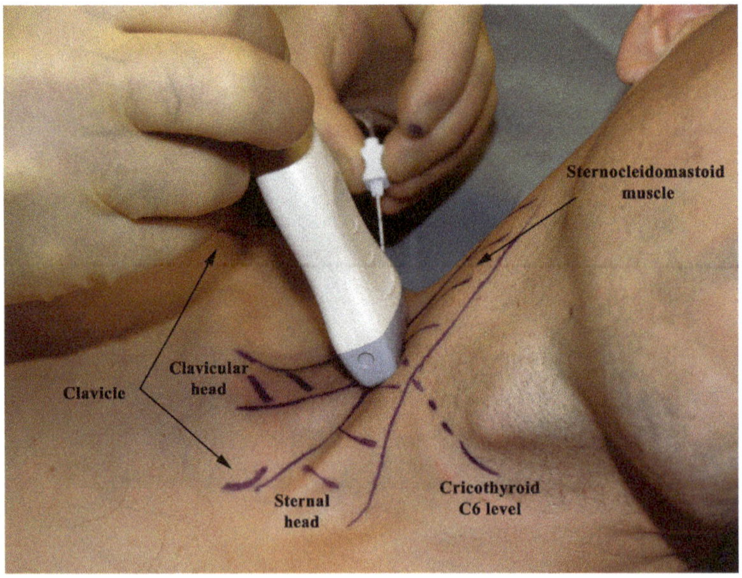

Figure 32.7 Ultrasound probe positioned at the level of C6.

traverse the middle scalene muscle as the plexus is reached. For the anterior (out-of-plane) approach, insert the needle at the medial aspect of the probe, taking care to avoid the carotid artery and internal jugular vein; the needle will traverse the anterior scalene muscle on the way to the plexus.

4.4. Injection

Once the needle is adjacent to the nerve trunks, injection of local anesthetic may begin. The "donut sign" (created by the local anesthetic surrounding the nerves) is a positive indicator that the anesthetic is being properly distributed. Dynamic

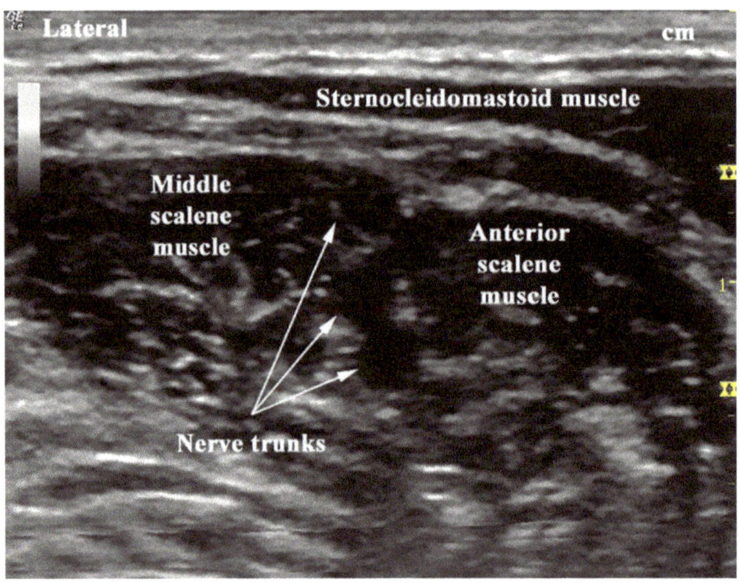

Figure 32.8 Ultrasound anatomy for the interscalene block.

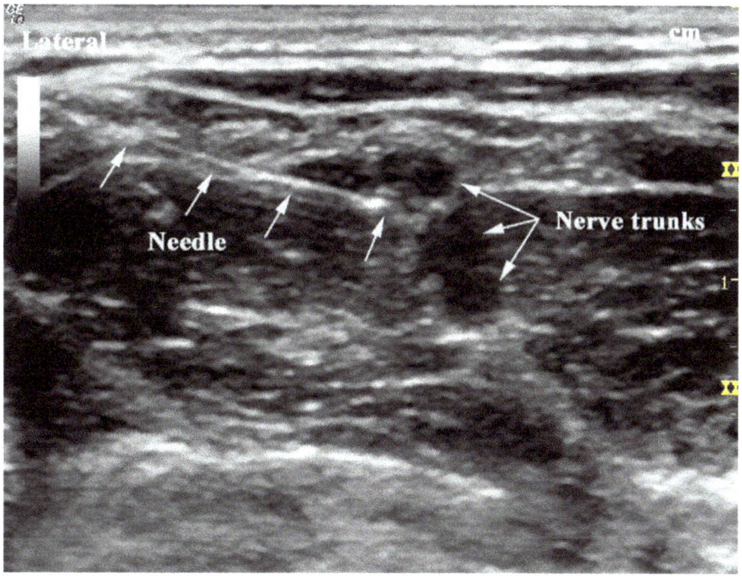

Figure 32.9 Ultrasound image with needle for an interscalene block.

needle repositioning should ensure local anesthetic spread around the superior and middle trunks. Occasionally the nerve will expand if the epineurium has been breached. This is typically of little consequence unless forceful injection is undertaken (> 20 psi) using larger volumes of local anesthetic solution.

Teaching Points. For ease of anatomic identification, locate the plexus at the level of a supraclavicular block (identify the subclavian artery, and the plexus will be just lateral to it). Once the plexus is located, slowly move the probe cephalad to observe the bundled nerve structures coalescing into major trunks, aligned superior to inferior. This is the transition from the more caudad divisions to the more cephalad trunks. Injection of local anesthetic should be directed toward the superior trunk of the plexus.

33

Supraclavicular Block

1. Introduction

The supraclavicular approach blocks the plexus at the level of the three trunks (superior, middle, inferior) and is ideal for procedures of the upper arm, from the midhumeral level down to the hand (Figure 33.1). The brachial plexus is most compact at the level of the trunks formed by confluence of elements of the C5-T1 nerve roots, so blockade here has the greatest likelihood of blocking all of the five terminal branches of the brachial plexus. This results in rapid onset times and, ultimately, high success rates for surgery and analgesia of the upper extremity (excluding the shoulder). In fact, the supraclavicular block was sometimes referred to as the "spinal" of the arm due to the analogy of using smaller volumes of local anesthetic compared to interscalene and axillary approaches. With the popularity of ultrasound guided approaches, however, and markedly reduced volumes of local anesthetic being used to achieve high success rates with interscalene and multiple-injection axillary brachial plexus blocks, this is no longer a truism.

2. Anatomy

At the trunk level of the brachial plexus, the C5 and C6 nerve roots join to form the superior trunk, the C7 nerve root forms the middle trunk, and the C8 and T1 nerve roots join to form the inferior trunk (the C4 and T2 nerve roots may also contribute significantly at these points) (Figures 33.2 and 33.3). Because the plexus is compactly arranged at this location, local anesthesia readily covers all the plexus nerves, which results in a rapid, dense block. Note that the interscalene groove can occasionally be obscured near the clavicle by the omohyoid muscle. Palpation or ultrasound visualization of the subclavian artery just superior to the clavicle provides a useful anatomic landmark for locating the brachial plexus, which is lateral to the artery at this level.

The complication most often associated with this block is pneumothorax, although its incidence has been markedly reduced from a reported high of 6% down to less than 0.06% since the introduction of ultrasound guidance. When manipulating the needle in this region, remember that the apex of the lung is just medial and posterior to the brachial plexus, as well as deep to the first rib. Using a shorter needle (5 cm) and directing the needle from lateral to medial can potentially decrease the incidence of pneumothorax. Unlike an interscalene block, the supraclavicular block causes diaphragmatic hemiparesis in approximately 50% of patients, with minimal accompanying reduction in forced vital capacity. Signs and symptoms of a large pneumothorax include sudden cough and shortness of breath, although more typically the onset of clinical signs may be delayed for some hours.

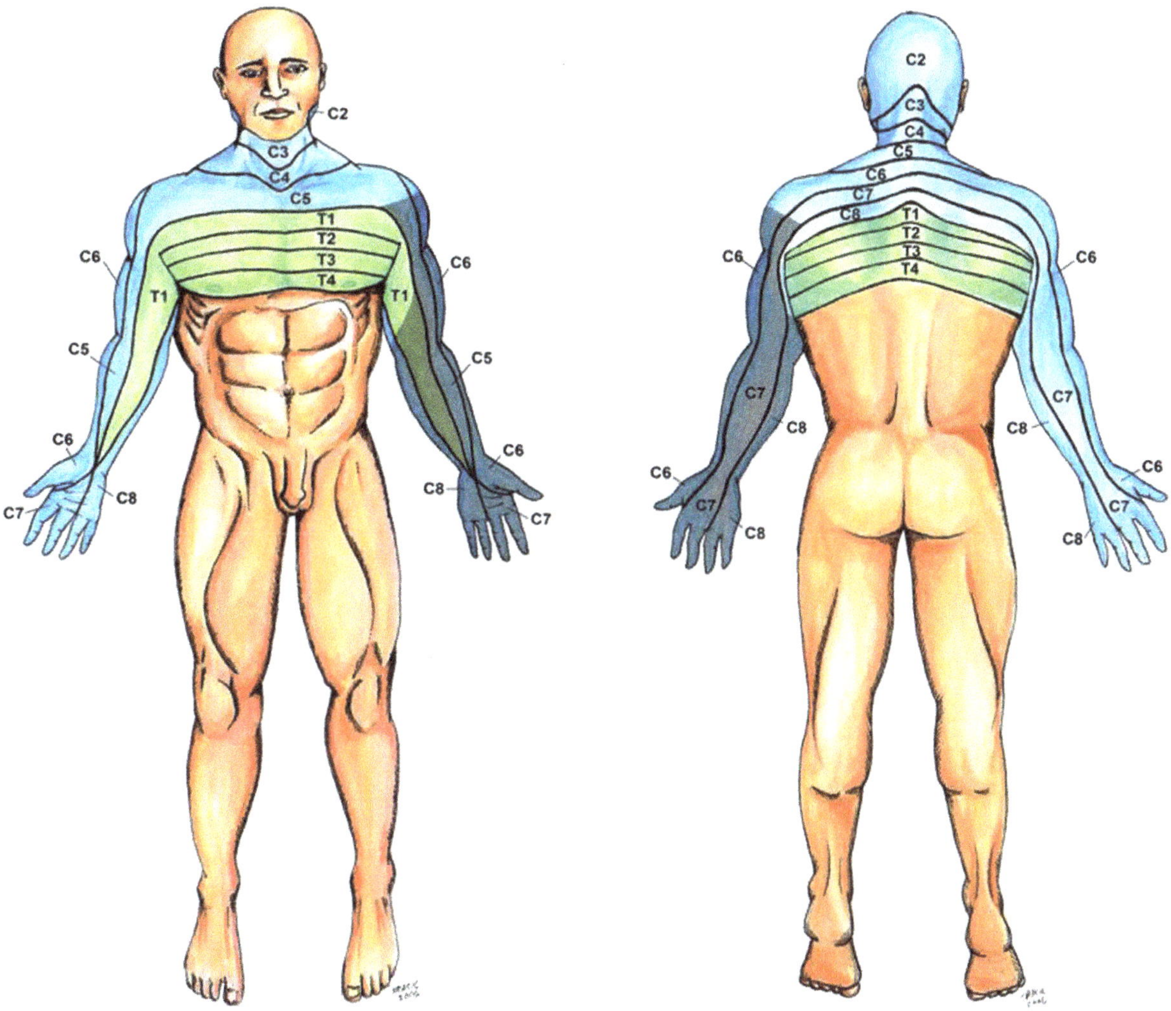

Figure 33.1 Dermatomes anesthetized with the supraclavicular block (dark blue).

3. Procedure

3.1. Landmarks

Place the patient in a supine position with the head turned toward the nonoperative side. Palpate the posterior border of the sternocleidomastoid muscle at the C6 level and roll your fingers laterally over the anterior scalene muscle until they lie in the interscalene groove (the groove may be harder to identify below the C6 level because of the overlying omohyoid muscle). Then move your fingers laterally down the interscalene groove until they are approximately 1 centimeter from the midclavicle. This location is the initial insertion site for the needle (Figure 33.4). The clinician stands at the patient's head and directs the needle toward the axilla using the classic approach with a nerve stimulator. (Figure 33.5).

3.2. Needles

- 22-gauge, 5-cm, insulated needle.
- 18-gauge, 5-cm, insulated Tuohy needle for catheter placement. Catheters introduced 3 to 5 cm beyond needle tip.

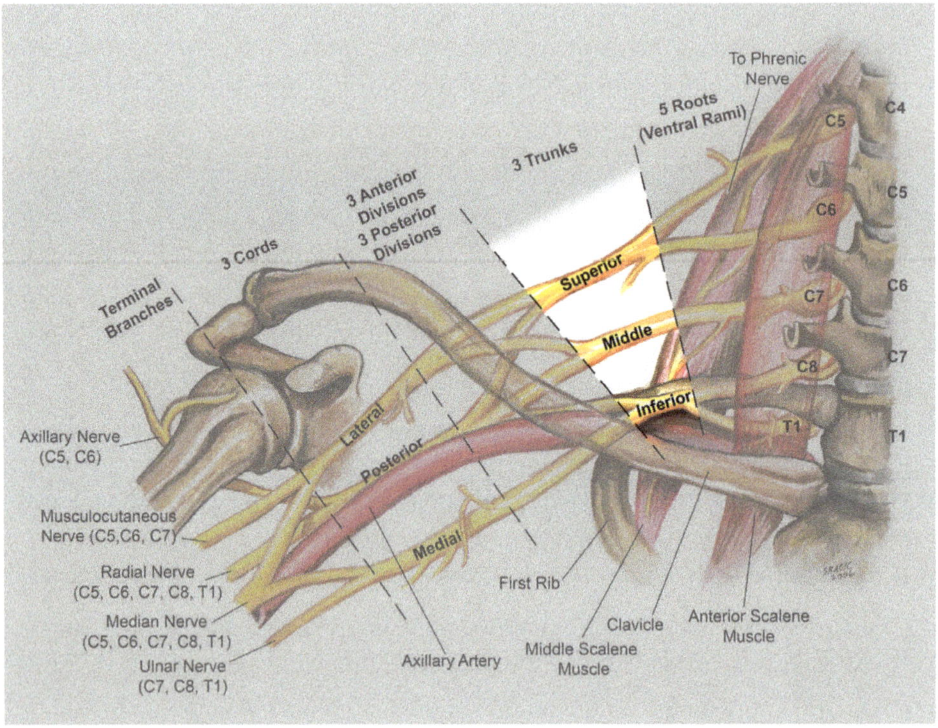

Figure 33.2 Brachial Plexus—Trunks

3.3. Stimulation

The nerve stimulator is initially set at 1.0 to 1.2 mA. Proper needle placement is indicated by flexion or extension of the digits at 0.5 mA or less. The brachial plexus can be deeply situated at this location but is often reached at a depth of 2 to 4 cm. Aspiration of bright red blood suggests subclavian artery penetration, indicating the needle is too medial. Stimulation of the musculocutaneous nerve (biceps contractions) usually indicates the needle is too lateral. Pectoralis muscle contraction indicates the needle is anterior, and scapular movement indicates the needle is posterior to the plexus.

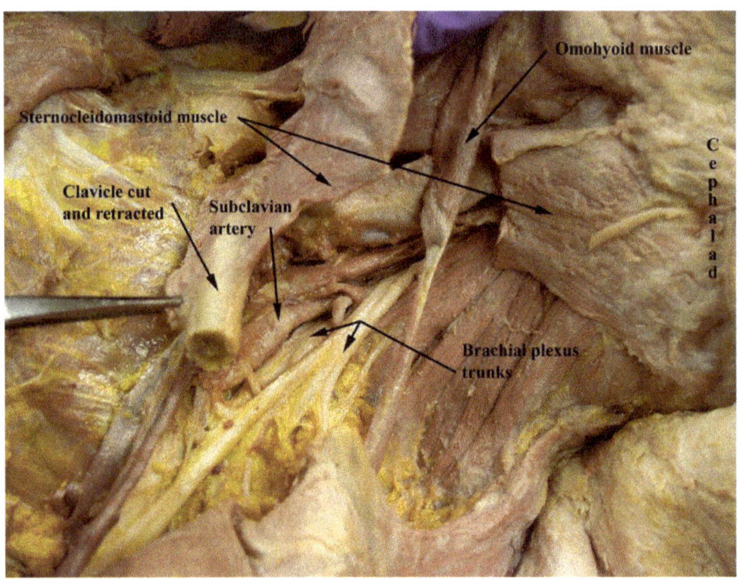

Figure 33.3 Dissection of the brachial plexus cephalad to the clavicle.

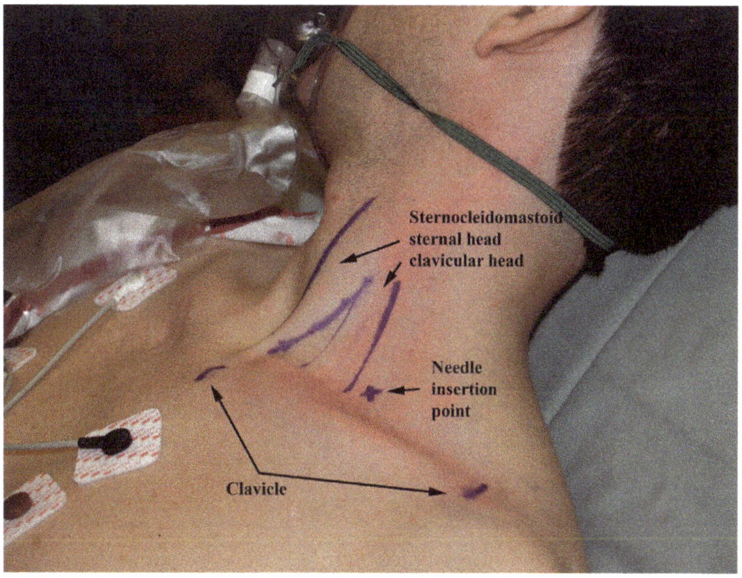

Figure 33.4 External anatomy for the supraclavicular block.

> **Motor Response Predicting Accurate Needle Placement:**
>
> **Acceptable Responses:** Finger twitch (flexion or extension).
>
> **Unacceptable Responses:** Trapezius twitch/shoulder shrug (due to stimulation of the spinal accessory nerve, not the brachial plexus).

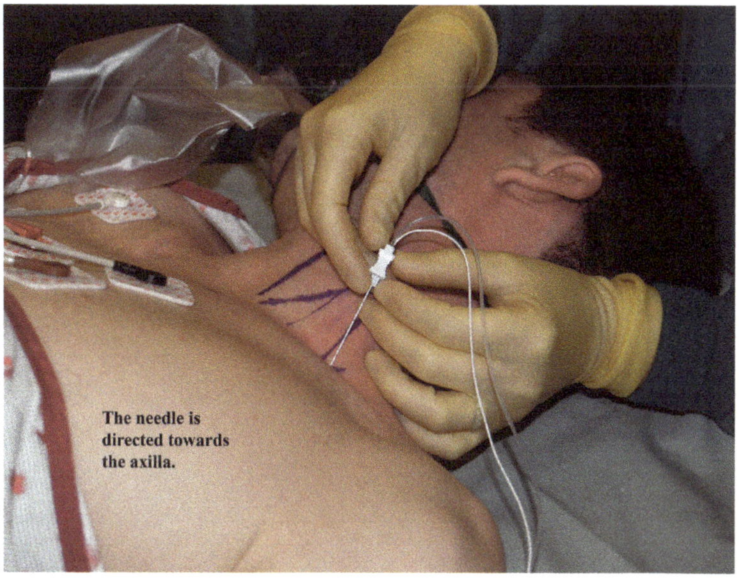

Figure 33.5 Needle position for the supraclavicular block.

3.4. Local Anesthetic

In most adults, 20 to 30 mL of local anesthetic is sufficient to block the plexus.

3.5. Additional Procedures

The intercostobrachial nerve lies anterior and slightly superior to the axillary artery; it innervates the skin along the upper medial border of the arm. To block this nerve, place a subcutaneous "wheal" of local anesthetic from the border of the pectoralis muscle insertion on the humerus to the inferior border of the axilla. The skin wheal should be placed as proximal on the arm as possible.

Teaching Points. Because of the close proximity of the lung, the needle should never be directed medially. If a tourniquet is being used for surgery, consider adding the intercostobrachial nerve block.

4. Block with Ultrasound Probe

4.1. Probe

- High frequency (5–12 MHz), linear.

4.2. Probe Position

The coronal oblique plane gives the best transverse view of the brachial plexus; again, a cross-sectional (axial) view displays the nerves as hypoechoic circles with hyperechoic rings ("bundle of grapes"). Position the probe on the neck directly above the clavicle in the supraclavicular fossa. At this level, the plexus will be configured as trunks or divisions and is typically located lateral and slightly superior to the subclavian artery at a depth of 2 to 4 cm (Figure 33.6).

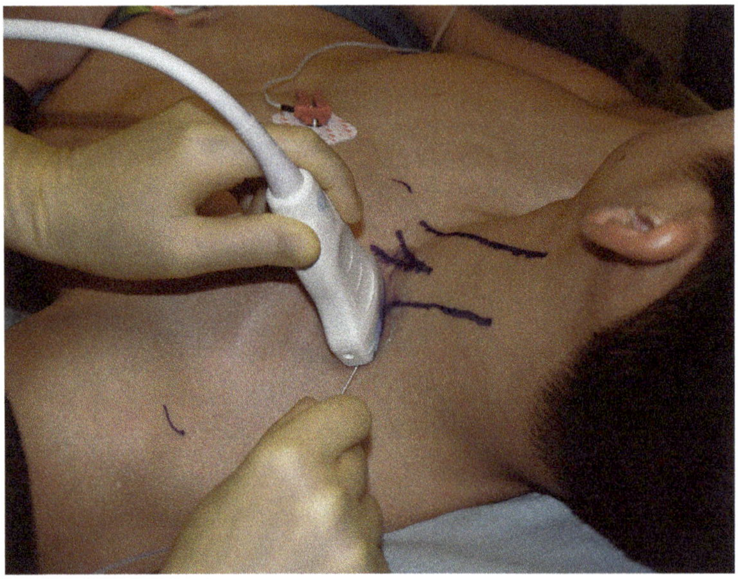

Figure 33.6 Ultrasound probe positioned directly above the clavicle in the supraclavicular fossa.

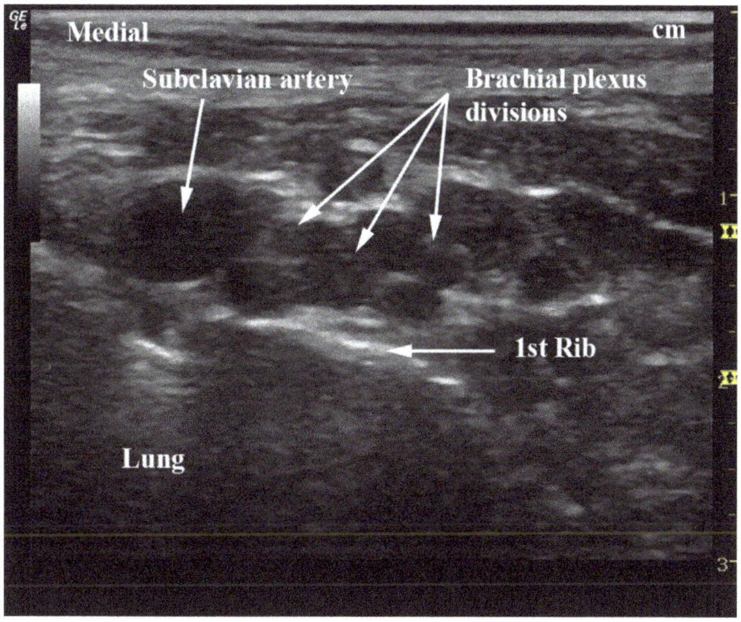

Figure 33.7 Ultrasound anatomy for the supraclavicular block.

4.3. Approach

Insert the needle at the lateral end of the ultrasound probe and advance it parallel to the ultrasound beam until it approaches the plexus. Take care to maintain the needle within the ultrasound beam plane which is only 1 mm, or about as thick as a sheet of paper; this maneuver helps ensure that you can constantly visualize the entire needle length from the proximal shaft to the tip. If the image of the needle is lost during the block procedure, cease advancing the needle until it can be revisualized through probe manipulation (Figure 33.7).

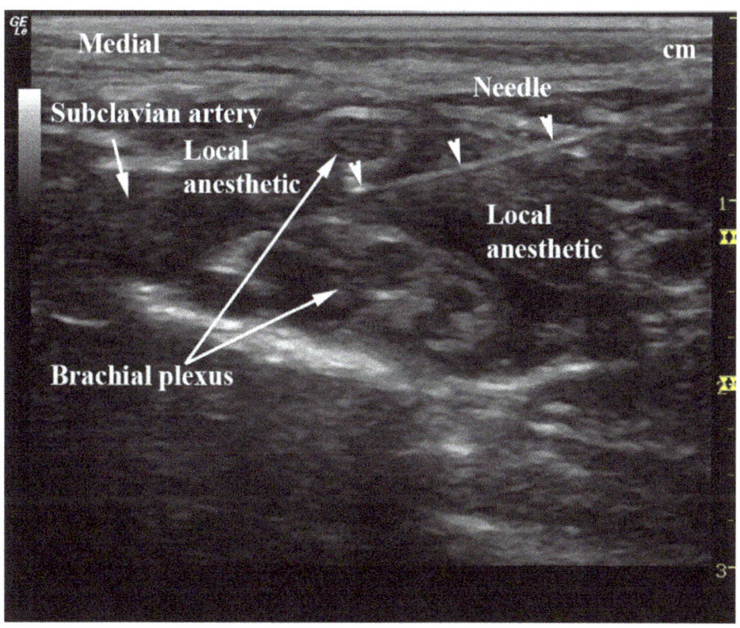

Figure 33.8 Ultrasound image of the supraclavicular block with needle and local anesthetic injected.

4.4. Injection

It is important to observe the spread of the local anesthetic during the injection, allowing real-time readjustment of the needle tip position if the spread is not appropriate. The "donut sign" (created by the local anesthetic surrounding the nerves) is a positive indicator that the anesthetic is being properly distributed (see section on interscalene ultrasound injection). Precise application of the local anesthetic can be achieved by injecting small aliquots (5 mL) and observing the local anesthetic spread (Figure 33.8).

Teaching Points. Be aware that this block is performed with the needle passing from a lateral to medial direction. It is very important to always keep the tip and shaft of the needle in clear view to ensure that the needle is not penetrating too deep into the supraclavicular fossa; deep penetration can result in an inadvertent pneumothorax or vascular puncture. If the needle image is maintained above the level of the first rib and pleura, the risk of pneumothorax is minimal.

Infraclavicular Block

34

1. Introduction

The infraclavicular brachial plexus block is ideal for operations distal to the elbow. Adequate time (approximately 20 minutes) should be allowed after the block placement to achieve a surgical level of anesthesia. Although there are multiple approaches to the infraclavicular block, success depends on where the needle tip contacts the cords of the brachial plexus. Caution must be taken to ensure that the needle tip is maintained within the infraclavicular fossa at the level of the cords and not directed distally toward the terminal branches located in the axilla. The latter erroneous position usually results from excessive angulation of the needle toward the axilla and may result in inadequate blockade of the musculocutaneous and axillary nerves.

2. Anatomy

The infraclavicular block is performed at the level of the cords of the brachial plexus. The cords are named according to their relation to the axillary artery: lateral, medial, and posterior. The lateral cord is formed from the anterior divisions of the superior and middle trunks, the medial cord is formed from the anterior division of the inferior trunk, and the posterior cord is formed from the posterior divisions of all 3 trunks. The plexus, which begins to spread around the axillary artery at this level, is not as compact as the more proximal trunks (Figures 34.1 through 34.3). Therefore, this block typically has a longer latency of onset of local anesthetic activity , and may not be as dense as, a supraclavicular nerve block. Compared with the supraclavicular block, an advantage of the infraclavicular block is the reduced possibility of pneumothorax, hemidiaphragmatic paralysis, and avoidance of cervical vascular structures. This block does not produce a reduction in respiratory function. Additionally, it has been shown to be superior to the axillary nerve block for anesthetizing the axillary and musculocutaneous nerves, making a supplemental musculocutaneous nerve block unnecessary. Acceptable muscle stimulation patterns when using neural stimulation are either extension (radial nerve) or flexion (median nerve) of the digits. A biceps twitch (musculocutaneous nerve) suggests that the needle placement is too lateral. The axillary vessels can be punctured using this approach, and vessel compression in this area is difficult.

3. Procedure

3.1. Landmarks

Externally rotate and abduct the operative arm. Palpate the coracoid process. Make a mark 2 cm medial and 2 cm caudad from the coracoid process (Figure 34.4). This is the

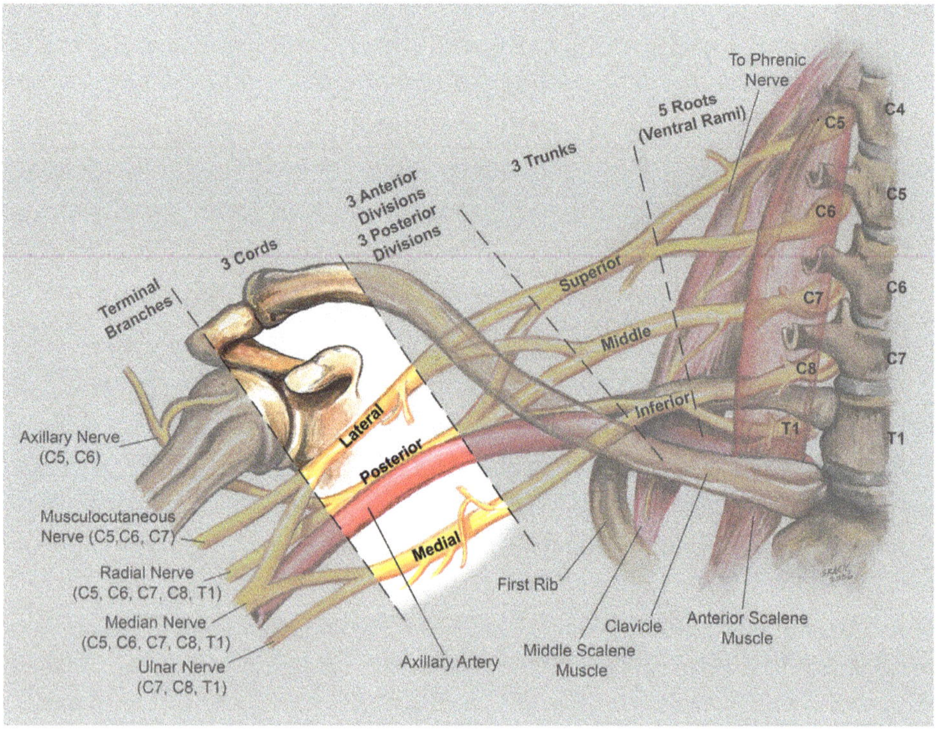

Figure 34.1 Cords of the brachial plexus.

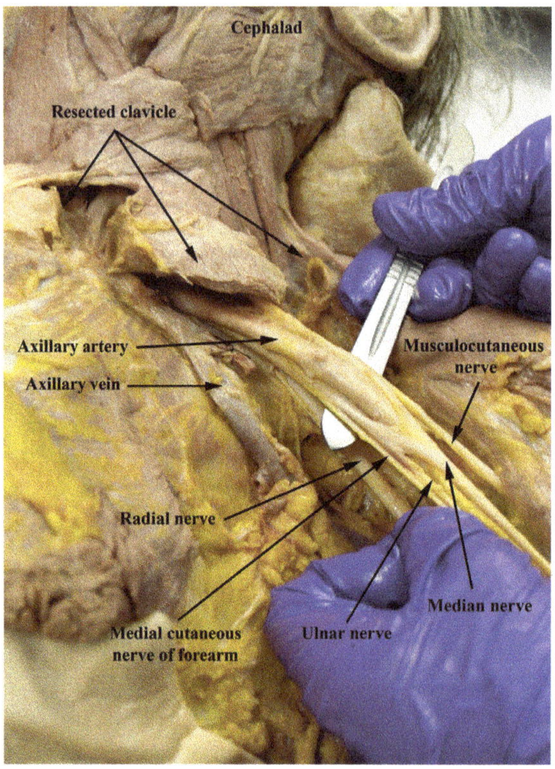

Figure 34.2 Dissection of the brachial plexus cords.

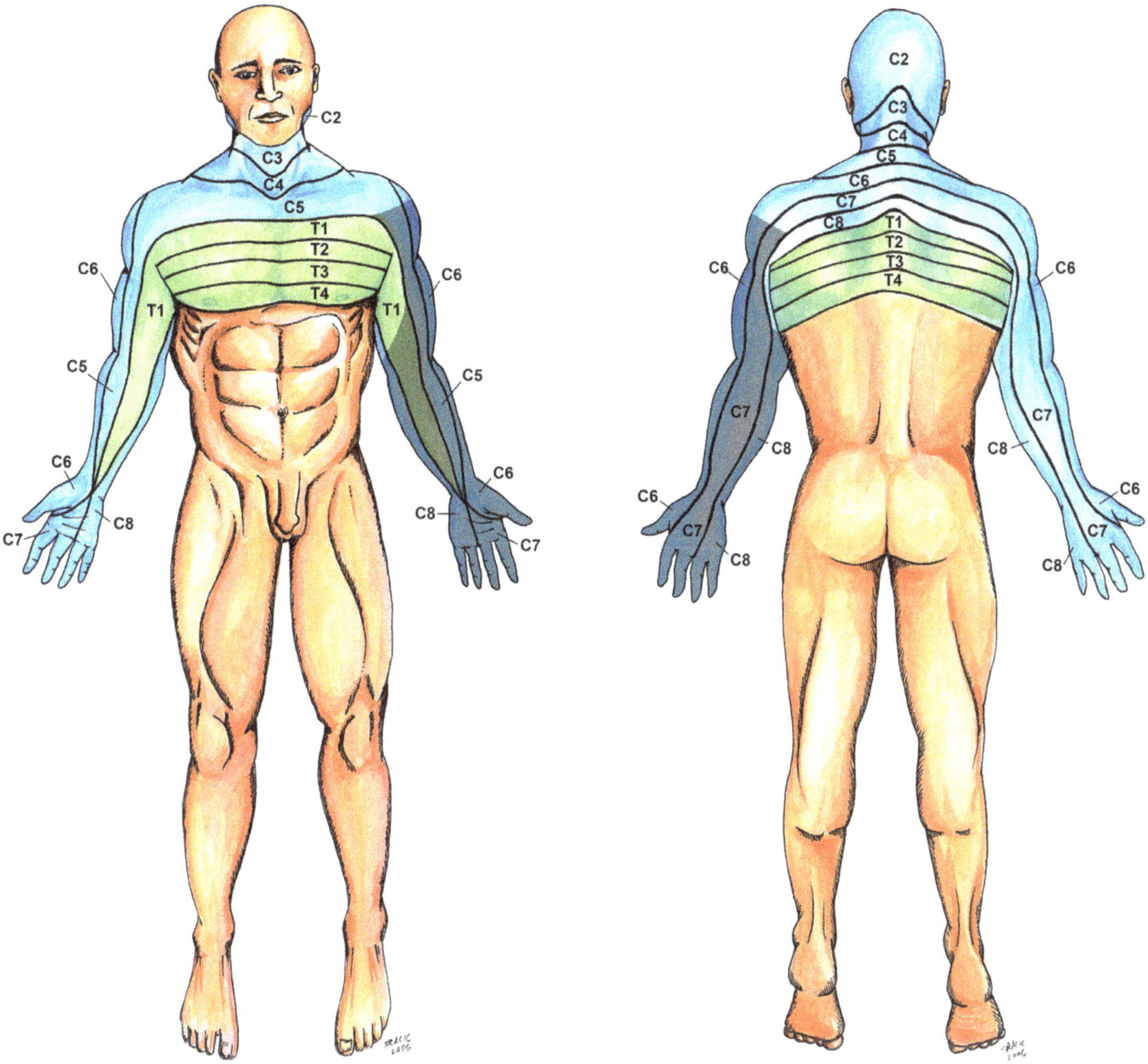

Figure 34.3 Dermatomes anesthetized with the infraclavicular block (dark blue).

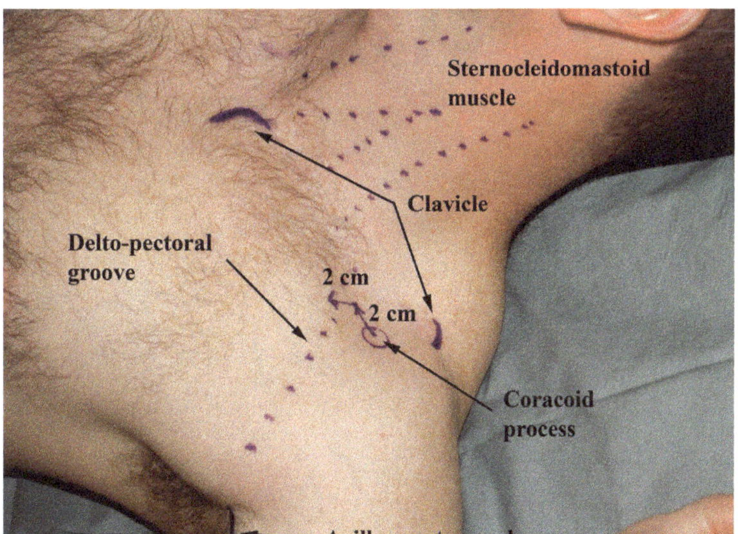

Figure 34.4 External anatomy for the infraclavicular block.

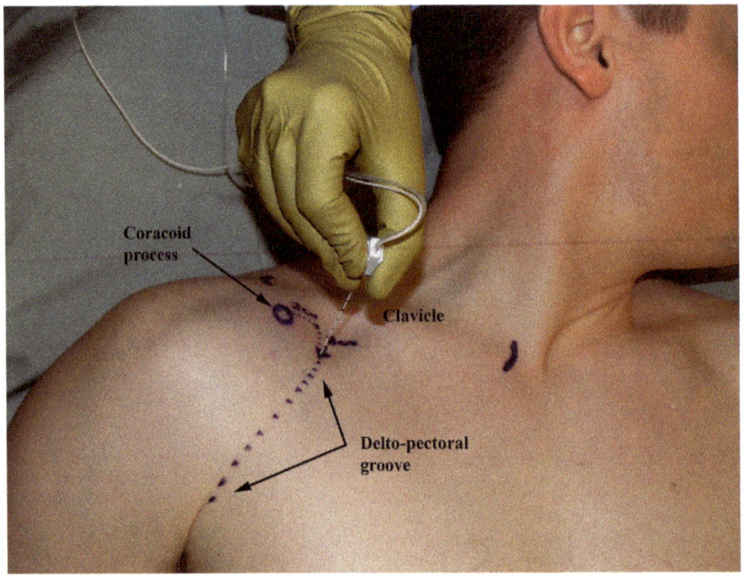

Figure 34.5 Needle position for the infraclavicular block.

insertion point. Palpate the axillary artery as proximal as possible in the axilla. This is the direction of initial insertion. Insert the needle at an approximately 60° angle from the horizontal (Figure 34.5).

3.2. Needles

- 21-gauge, 10-cm, insulated needle.
- 18-gauge, 10-cm, insulated Tuohy needle for catheter placement. Catheters inserted 3 cm.

3.3. Stimulation

The nerve stimulator is initially set between 1.0 and 1.2 mA. Finger and/or thumb flexion at 0.5 mA or less indicates adequate needle placement for local anesthetic injection. Finger extension with stimulation is also acceptable.

3.4. Local anesthetic

In most adults, 30 to 40 mL of local anesthetic will block the plexus at this level. Ultrasound use has not been demonstrated to be associated with significantly lower volumes of anesthetic solution for successful block.

Motor Response Predicting Accurate Needle Placement

Acceptable Responses: hand twitch

Unacceptable Responses: deltoid (axillary), biceps (musculocutaneous), subscapularis muscle, pectoralis muscle (direct muscle stimulation)

4. Alternative Approach

A simple alternative to the coracoid approach is the deltopectoral groove approach (see Figure 34.5). With the patient's arm at the side, mark the base of the clavicle and palpate the deltopectoral groove from the axilla up to the clavicle. At approximately 1 cm below the clavicle, place the needle in the deltopectoral groove (perpendicular to the bed), and then redirect it 10° toward the axilla. Advance the needle until the plexus is encountered. Compared with the coracoid approach, this approach will block the plexus at a more proximal location, which is desirable because the plexus is more compact and is easier to block proximally.

5. Block with Ultrasound Probe

5.1. Probe

- High frequency (5–12 MHz), linear.

5.2. Probe Position

The parasagittal plane gives the best transverse view of the brachial plexus; below the level of the clavicle, the nerves appear hyperechoic. Position the probe beneath the clavicle and medial to the coracoid process (Figure 34.6).

5.3. Approach

The needle is typically inserted in plane at the cephalad (lateral) aspect of the probe and will be visualized at the lateral border of the axillary artery the nerves and axillary artery and vein will be seen in short-axis views. The hyperechoic structure lateral to the artery is the lateral cord; the needle should pass lateral to this cord and progress farther to the posterior cord. The posterior cord is the hyperechoic structure located at the base of the axillary artery (Figure 34.7). Recent evidence suggests that deposition of local anesthetic around the posterior cord will result in improved block success. Another approach to the posterior cord is via the inferior aspect of the probe (still in the parasagittal plane). With this

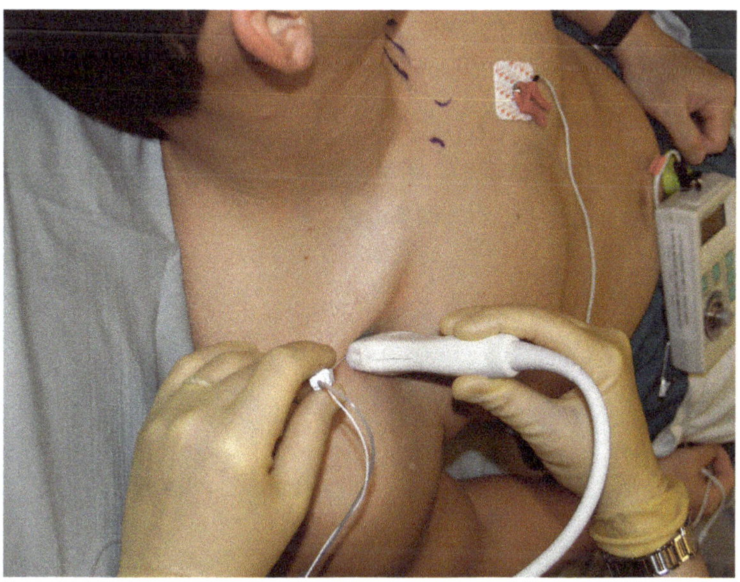

Figure 34.6 Ultrasound probe and needle position for the infraclavicular block.

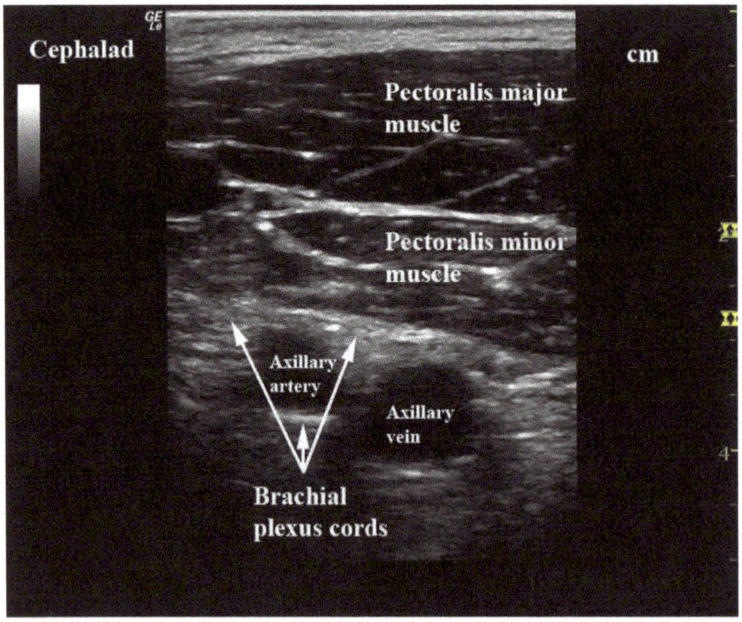

Figure 34.7 Ultrasound anatomy of the brachial plexus cords.

technique, the needle is visualized at the medial border of the axillary artery, and between the axillary artery and vein. The needle must travel along the lateral aspect of the medial cord to reach the posterior cord. This approach is technically more difficult because of the close proximity of the axillary artery to the needle path; however, it allows catheters to be threaded with less difficulty.

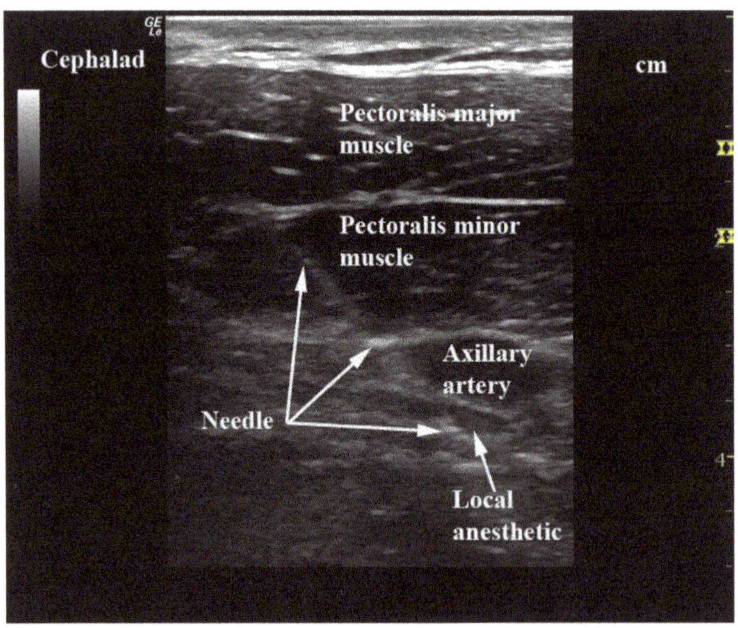

Figure 34.8 Ultrasound image of the infraclavicular block with needle and local anesthetic injection.

5.4. Injection

It is important to observe the spread of the local anesthetic during the injection, which allows readjustment of the needle position if the spread is not appropriate. Spread should appear around the posterior cord; any spread above the artery in the area of the pectoralis muscles will likely result in block failure (Figure 34.8).

Teaching Points. As with the nerve stimulator technique, care must be taken to avoid vascular puncture because compression for bleeding in this area can be difficult. Always keep the axillary artery and vein in view during needle guidance, and always ensure that the full length of the needle to the tip in the longitudinal (in-plane) view is clear.

35

Axillary Block

1. Introduction

Except for single-nerve blocks in the arm and forearm, the axillary block is the most distal block performed on the brachial plexus. Because of the distal location (in contrast to other brachial plexus approaches), the axillary block has negligible risks of respiratory compromise secondary to pneumothorax or phrenic nerve blockade. In addition, the peripheral location permits adequate arterial tamponade to be applied if an unintentional puncture occurs.

2. Anatomy

At this level, the plexus has divided into its 5 terminal nerve branches, with 2 major nerves originating from each cord. The lateral cord divides into the musculocutaneous nerve and the lateral portion of the median nerve, the medial cord divides into the ulnar nerve and the medial portion of the median nerve, and the posterior cord divides into the radial nerve and axillary nerve (Figures 35.1 and 35.2). The median, ulnar, and radial nerves all travel with the axillary artery within the axillary perivascular sheath; however, the musculocutaneous nerve travels separately within the belly of the coracobrachialis muscle. For this reason, the musculocutaneous nerve must be blocked separately during an axillary nerve block. This block should only be performed for surgeries involving the hand or forearm (Figure 35.3). A supraclavicular or infraclavicular nerve block should be used for surgeries involving the upper arm or elbow to obtain more complete coverage of the upper extremity. Any patient who is unable to abduct his or her arm more than 45° at the shoulder is not an appropriate candidate for the axillary block.

3. Procedure

3.1. Landmarks

There are multiple approaches to the axillary block, including paresthesia-seeking, nerve-stimulating, ultrasound, perivascular, and transarterial techniques. With the paresthesia-seeking and nerve-stimulating approaches, all 4 nerves (median, ulnar, radial, and musculocutaneous) can be individually identified and anesthetized; both of these methods seem to be equally successful. However, in procedures using the nerve- stimulation technique, studies have shown that actual stimulation of the musculocutaneous nerve leads to a more successful outcome than a simple injection into the coracobrachialis

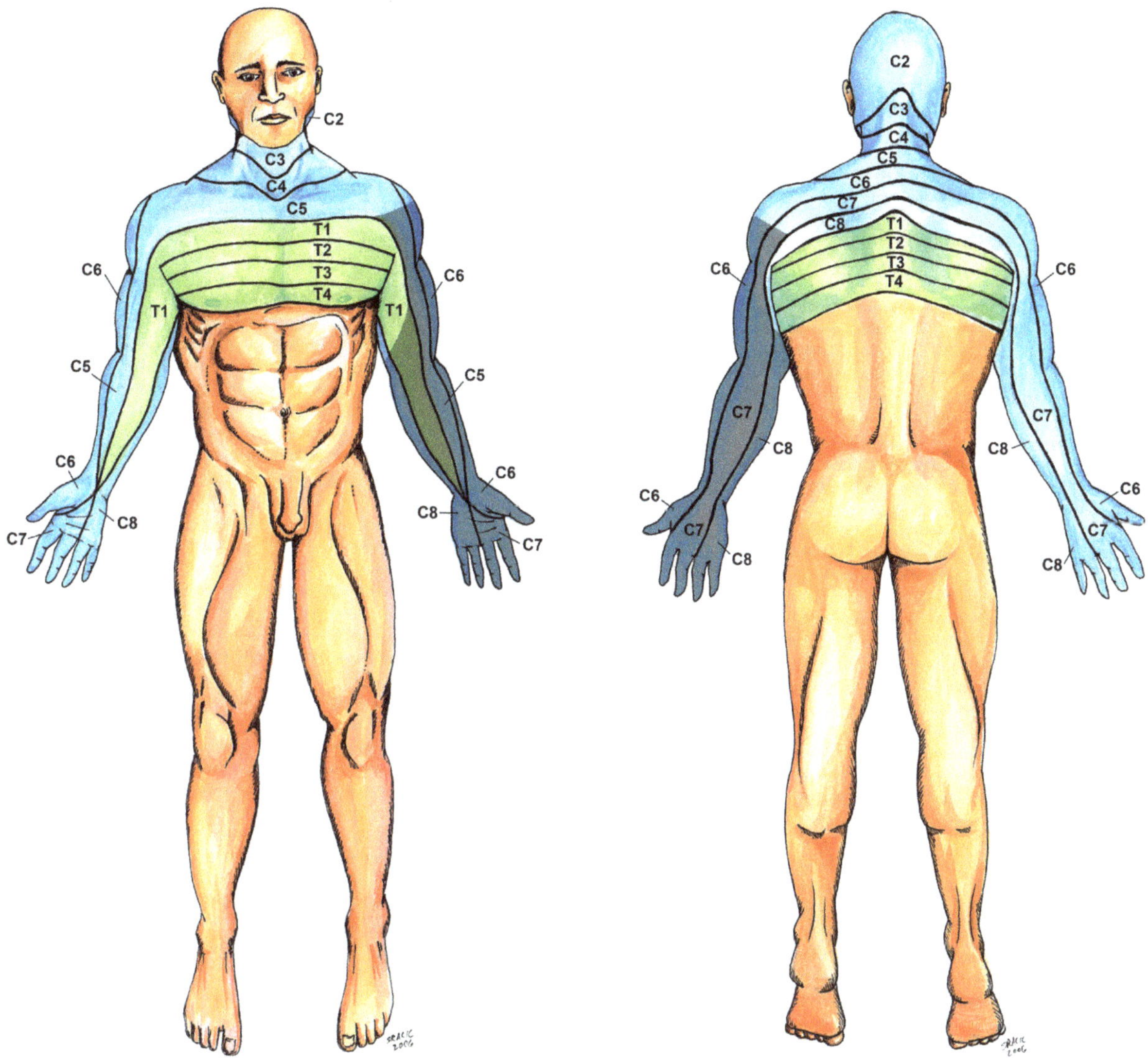

Figure 35.1 Dermatomes anesthetized with the axillary block (dark blue).

muscle. It is important to note that although a true axillary sheath may exist, it may not be a tubular structure that neatly houses the terminal branches of the plexus. Instead, it may be a collection of connective tissues that surround the nerves and vessels, creating individual fascial compartments that can inhibit spread of the local anesthetic. The patient is positioned supine with the operative arm abducted and externally rotated (Figure 35.4). The axillary artery is palpated as high in the axilla as possible. The needle is inserted superior to the axillary artery, entering at a 45° angle. To identify the coracobrachialis muscle for the musculocutaneous block, the biceps muscle is displaced laterally, and the coracobrachialis muscle is palpated just medial to it. At the level of the upper half of the humerus, the needle is inserted into the substance of the coracobrachialis muscle.

3.2. Needles

- 22-gauge, 3.8-cm, insulated b-bevel needle.
- 18-gauge, 3.8-cm insulated Tuohy needle for catheter placement. Catheters introduced 3 to 5 cm.

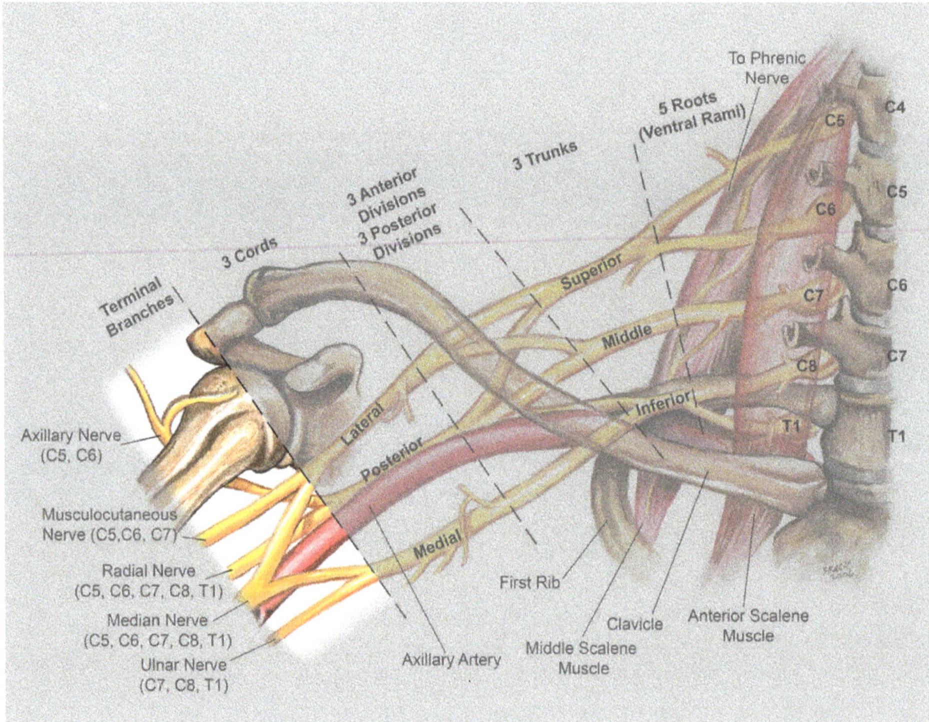

Figure 35.2 Brachial Plexus—Terminal Branches

3.3. Stimulation

Median, ulnar, and radial nerves may be stimulated. The nerve stimulator is initially set between 1.0 and 1.2 mA. Finger flexion and/or thumb opposition at 0.5 mA or less indicates proper needle placement (Figure 35.5).

Aspiration of bright red blood means the needle has entered the axillary artery. If this occurs, the transarterial technique for axillary block can be selected: in this case, advance the needle until blood aspiration stops, and deposit half of the local anesthetic volume deep to the artery. Then withdraw the needle until blood aspiration ceases again, and deposit the remaining local anesthetic at this more superficial location.

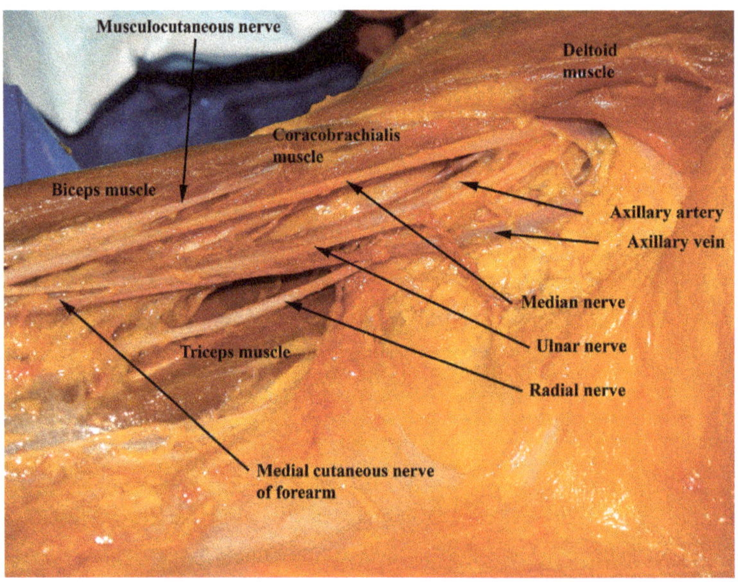

Figure 35.3 Axillary dissection.

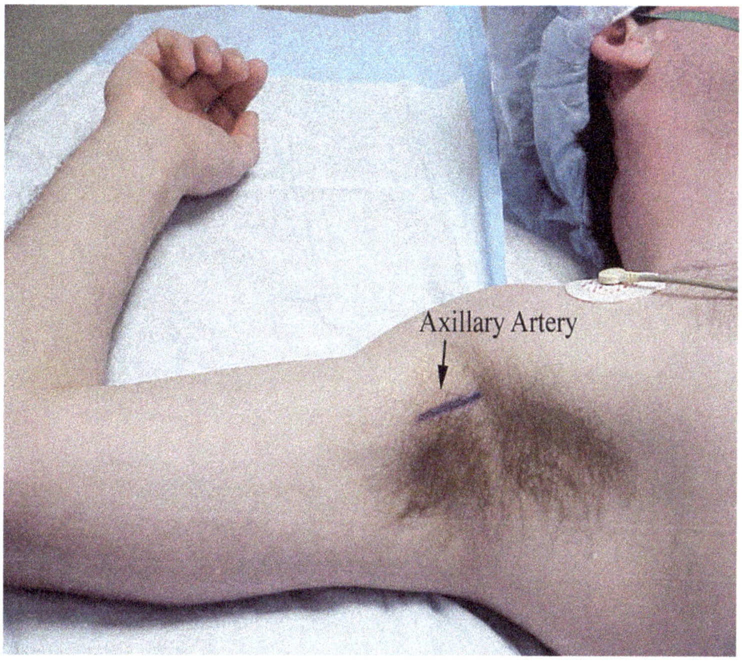

Figure 35.4 External anatomy of the axillary block.

Musculocutaneous Nerve. The nerve stimulator is set to approximately 2.0 mA. Fan the needle through the coracobrachialis muscle until vigorous biceps contraction is elicited (ensure that biceps contraction is not secondary to direct stimulation of the biceps muscle).

3.4. Local anesthetic

Median, Ulnar, and Radial Nerves. In most adults, 30 to 40 mL of local anesthetic will block these nerves using a nerve stimulator or transarterial approach for the axillary block; much smaller volumes suffice for ultrasound guided approaches.

Musculocutaneous Nerve. In most adults, 10 mL of local anesthetic will block this nerve.

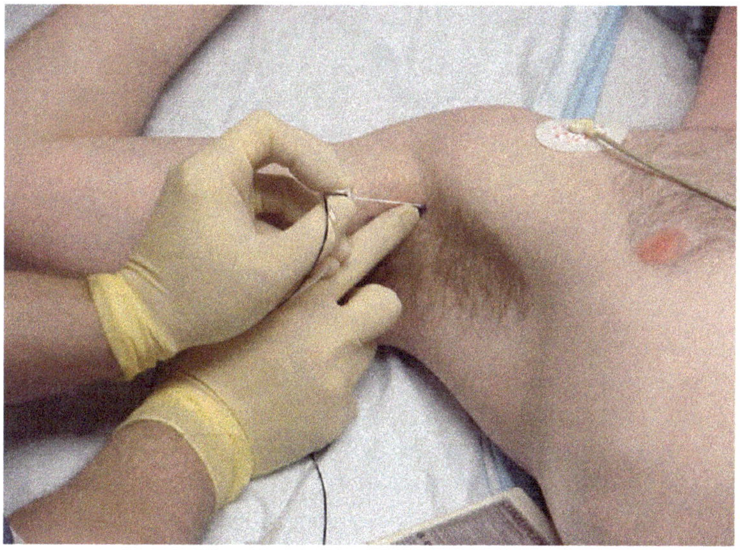

Figure 35.5 Needle position for the axillary block.

Teaching Points. Application of distal pressure during injection can help push the local anesthetic in a more proximal direction. Adducting the arm immediately after injection can also help with proximal spread of local anesthetic. If an arm tourniquet is used during the surgical procedure, blockade of the intercostobrachial nerve is required (see chapter 33, "Supraclavicular Block").

4. Block with Ultrasound Probe

4.1. Probe

- High frequency (5–12 MHz), linear.

4.2. Probe Position

The transverse plane gives the best view of the brachial plexus at this level; nerves will appear as hyperechoic roundish structures with hyperechoic borders.

4.3. Approach

The patient is supine, with the arm abducted 90° and externally rotated so the dorsum of the hand rests on the bed. The probe should be placed high in the axilla, at the intersection of the pectoralis major muscle with the biceps muscle (Figure 35.6). At this level, the axillary artery and all 3 main nerves to be blocked (median, ulnar, radial) should be in view (Figure 35.7). Typical anatomic relations of the nerve to the artery are as follows: the median nerve is located superficial and slightly cephalad to the artery, the radial nerve is located deep to the artery, and the ulnar nerve is located

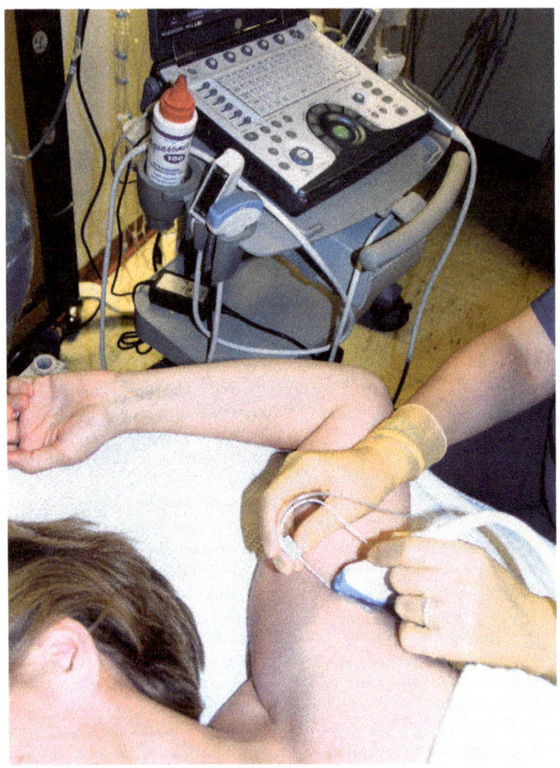

Figure 35.6 Probe placement at the intersection of the pectoralis major muscle with the biceps muscle.

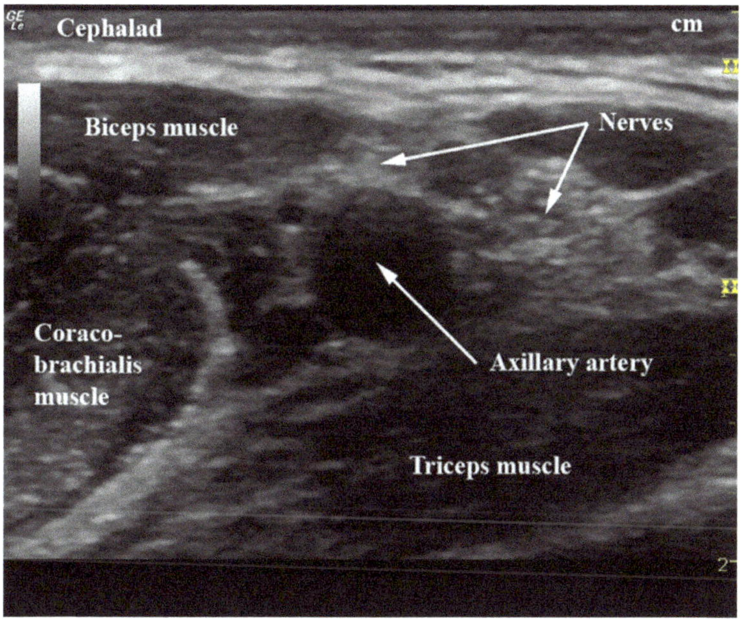

Figure 35.7 Ultrasound anatomy for the axillary block.

caudad to the artery. If all 3 nerves are not visualized at the same time, sliding the probe from a medial to lateral direction should help identify the missing nerve. Individual nerves can be confirmed by stimulation. Once each nerve is identified, 1-10 mL of local anesthetic should be injected around each nerve (Figure 35.8). (Note: axillary veins are often not seen while performing this block under ultrasound guidance because they are easily compressed by the ultrasound probe.)

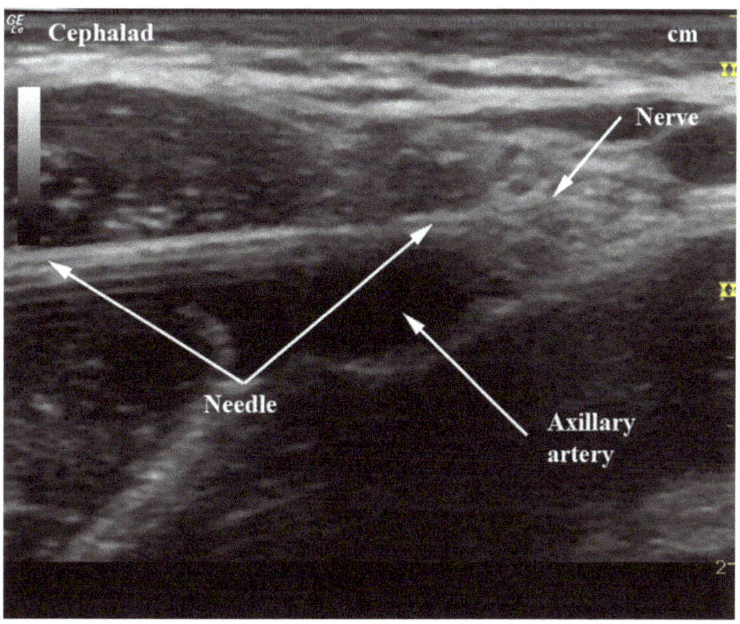

Figure 35.8 Ultrasound image with needle placement for an axillary block.

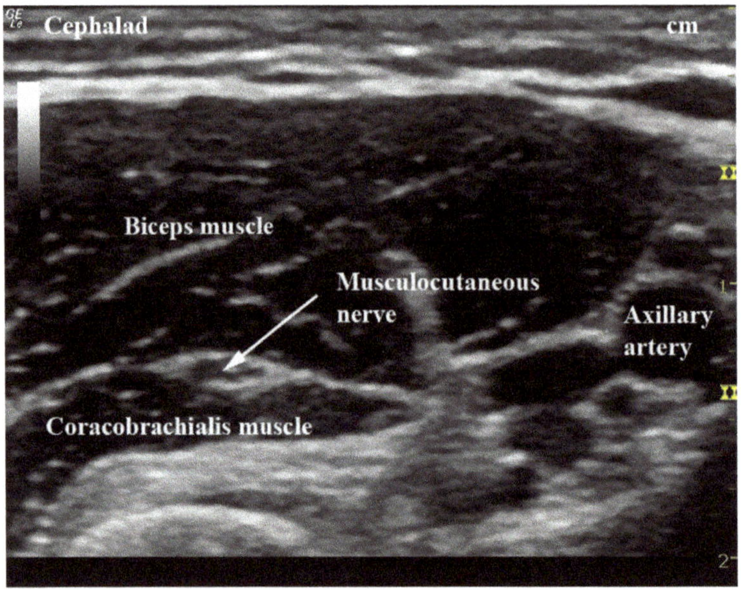

Figure 35.9 Ultrasound image of the musculocutaneous nerve.

Teaching Points. As opposed to a field block or stimulation technique, blockade of the musculocutaneous nerve under ultrasound guidance is more precise. The patient's arm remains abducted and externally rotated while the probe is positioned at the junction between the pectoralis major and biceps muscles with the axillary artery in view. While the probe is slowly brought toward the biceps muscle, the musculocutaneous nerve should come into view, either between the biceps and coracobrachialis muscles or within the body of the coracobrachialis muscle (Figure 35.9). Local anesthetic should be injected when the needle tip is visualized near the nerve or if stimulation of the biceps muscle is noted.

Upper Extremity Peripheral Nerve Blocks

36

1. Introduction

Terminal branches of the brachial plexus may be blocked to enable minor surgical procedures involving a territory within a single nerve distribution. Individual terminal nerves may also need to be blocked to supplement less than adequate brachial plexus block. Additionally, these distal injections may be of value in situations precluding more proximal approaches, such as preexisting infections or history of coagulopathy due to the proximity of major vascular structures to the needle entry site.

2. Anatomy

The 3 major peripheral nerves of the upper extremity (radial, median, and ulnar) may all be blocked at the level of the elbow (Figure 36.1). The ulnar nerve can be localized by palpating the ulnar groove between the medial epicondyle of the humerus and the olecranon process. Blockade of the ulnar nerve at this level abolishes sensation to the medial aspect of the hand, including the fifth digit and the medial half of the fourth digit.

The median nerve is situated medial to the brachial artery, which is thus used as the landmark for the median nerve blockade. Median nerve block results in sensory loss along the anterolateral surface of the hand, including the thumb through middle finger.

The radial nerve lies between the brachialis and brachioradialis muscles about 1 to 2 cm lateral to the biceps tendon. The radial nerve block at this level provides sensory anesthesia to the dorsolateral aspect of the hand, including thumb, index, middle, and lateral half of the ring finger, up to the distal interphalangeal joint.

More distal blockade of the upper extremity may be accomplished at the level of the wrist. The median nerve lies between the palmaris longus and flexor carpi radialis tendons. The ulnar nerve is located lateral to the flexor carpi ulnaris and just medial to the ulnar artery. It is important to note that the radial nerve has already branched at the level of the wrist, thus requiring field block over the radial aspect of the wrist to achieve successful blockade of this nerve.

3. Technique

3.1. Landmarks

Pertinent landmarks at the level of the elbow include the ulnar groove, median and lateral condyles of the humerus (ulnar nerve); brachial artery pulsation (median nerve); and tendon of the biceps muscle (radial nerve). At the level of the wrist, key landmarks

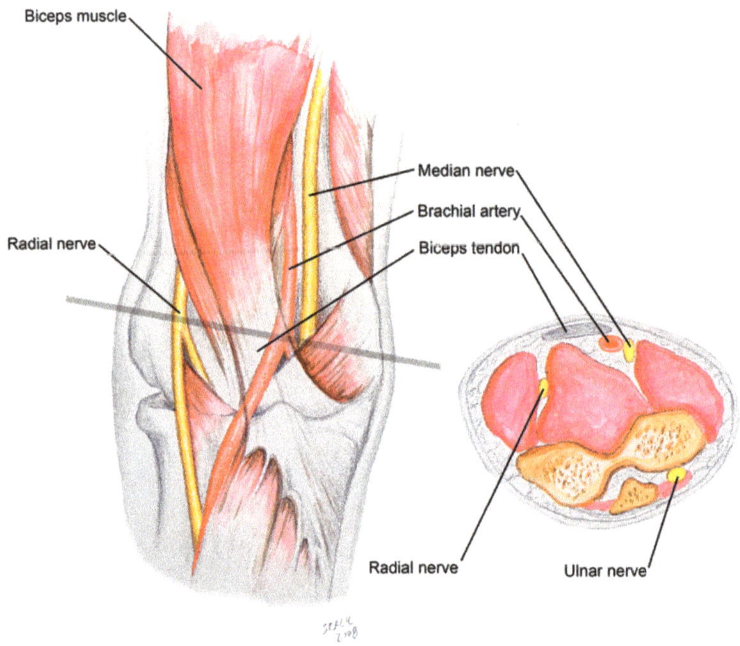

Figure 36.1 Peripheral nerve anatomy at the elbow.

include the tendons of the flexor palmaris longus and flexor carpi radialis (median nerve), anatomic snuffbox (radial nerve), and ulnar styloid (ulnar nerve).

3.2. Needles

- 22-gauge, 5-cm, insulated needle for nerve stimulation techniques.
- 22-gauge, 5-cm regional needle or 25-gauge, 1- to 1.5-inch bevel needle.

3.3. Local Anesthetic

The choice of the local anesthetic is determined by the clinician's preference and the desired duration of the block. The use of local anesthetic with epinephrine adjunct is advisable when injecting at the level of the elbow, but it is not recommended for the wrist or digit blocks.Volumes between 3 and 7 mL may be required depending on the location of needle placement.

3.4. Stimulation

Nerve stimulation is useful in defining peripheral nerve branches at the elbow level; minimal utility is gained from stimulation at the wrist level. The presence of muscle twitches with 0.5 mA or less suggests adequate proximity of the stimulating needle to the corresponding peripheral nerve and should be appreciated prior to injection of local anesthetic.

3.5. Additional procedures

When performing an elbow block, an additional 5 mL of subcutaneous local anesthetic injected laterally from the biceps tendon to the brachioradialis muscle will provide anesthesia for the lateral cutaneous nerve of the forearm.

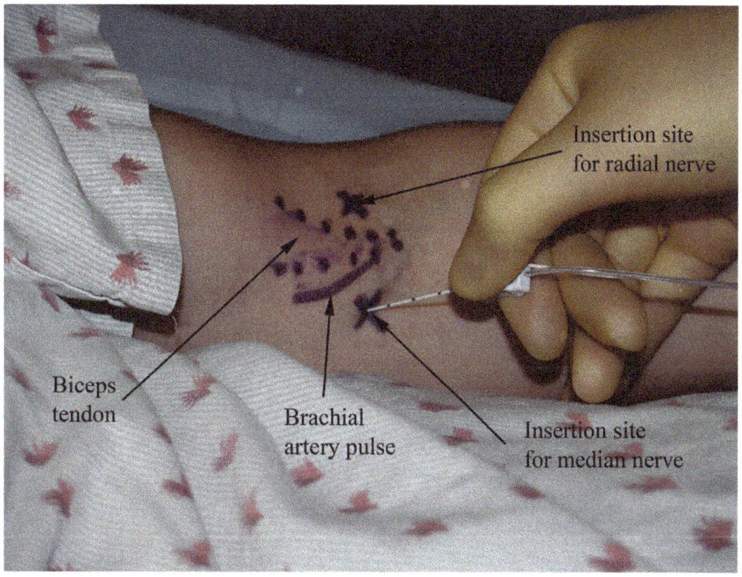

Figure 36.2 External anatomy for the radial nerve and median nerve blocks with needle position for the radial nerve block.

3.6. Ultrasound guidance

High-frequency (5–12 MHz), linear probe, and the in-plane approach are recommended due to the proximity of vascular structures and the smaller size of nerves. The pertinent neural and vascular structures must be clearly visualized prior to injection of local anesthetic.

3.7. At the elbow

Radial Nerve. The needle is inserted lateral to the biceps tendon above the antecubital crease (the line bisecting medial and lateral epicondyles). The nerve lies within the groove between the tendon and the brachioradialis muscle (Figure 36.2). The proper location can be confirmed with ultrasound **(Figure 36.3),** by eliciting paresthesias, and/or from an expected motor response (finger/wrist extension) with use of a nerve stimulator.

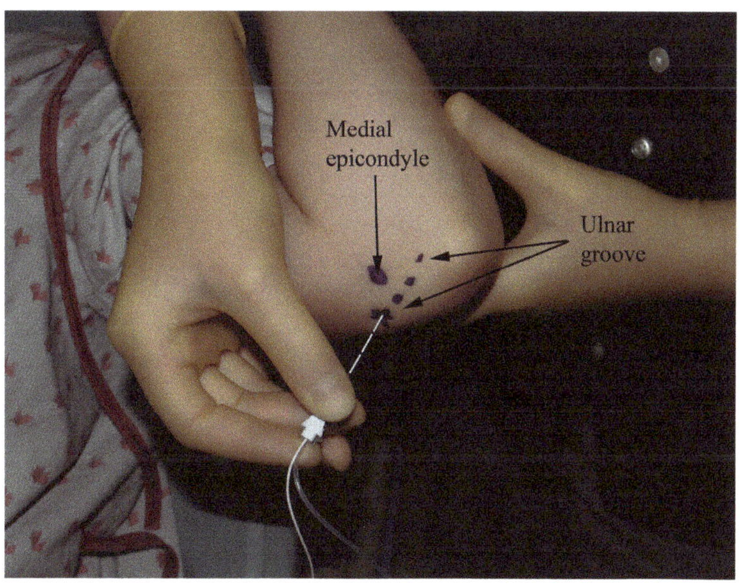

Figure 36.3 Radial nerve of the right arm at elbow level.

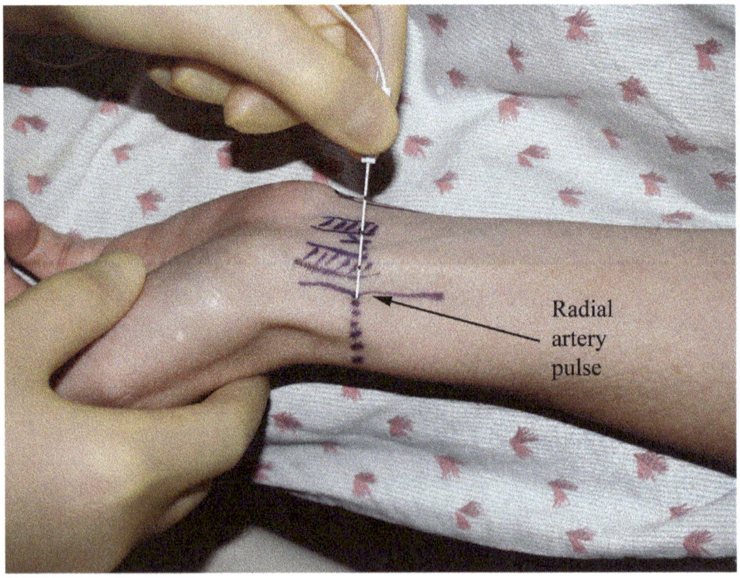

Figure 36.4 Brachial artery and median nerve of the right arm at elbow level.

Median Nerve. Needle is placed at the antecubital crease medial to the palpated brachial pulse (see Figure 36.2). The final position can be confirmed with ultrasound, (Figure 36.4) by evoking paresthesias, or from an evoked motor response (finger/wrist flexion or hand pronation), usually at 1- to 2-cm depth, with nerve stimulation.

Ulnar Nerve. With the elbow flexed at midrange, insert the needle into the ulnar groove 1 to 3 cm proximal to the medial epicondyle (see Figure 36.5). Care should be taken to avoid excessive injection pressure or intraneural injection in this relatively tight space, and local anesthetic injection should be limited to 4 or 5 mL. Confirm needle placement with ultrasound prior to injecting (Figure 36.6).

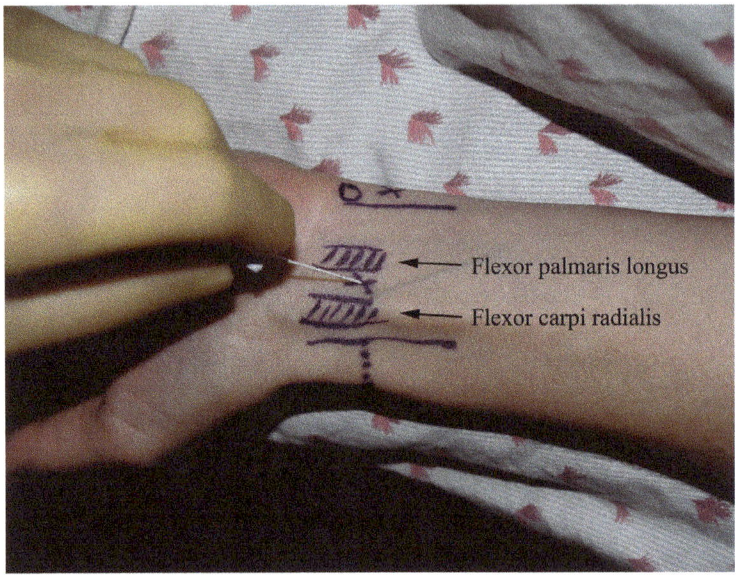

Figure 36.5 External anatomy and needle position for the ulnar nerve block.

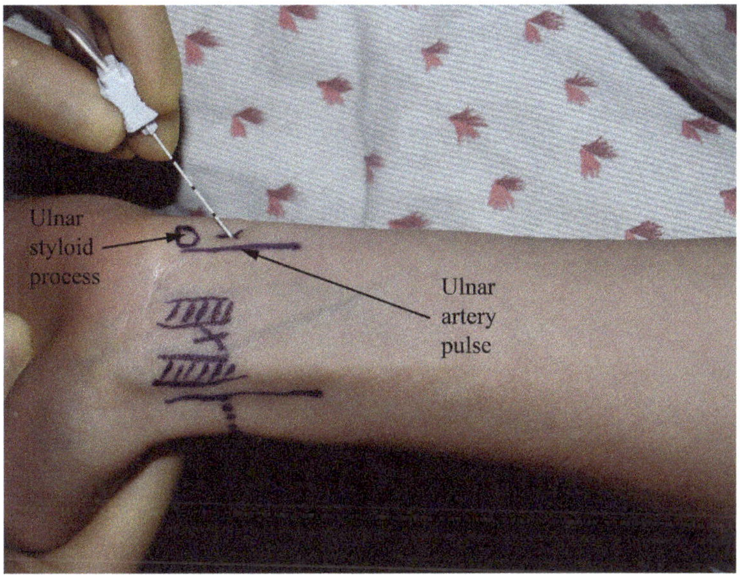

Figure 36.6 Ulnar nerve within the olecranon fossa, right arm.

3.8. At the wrist

Radial Nerve. To block the branches of the radial nerve, make an injection along the radial artery's lateral border 2 cm proximal to the wrist (see Figure 36.7). Then extend the injection dorsally over the border of the wrist, covering the anatomic snuffbox.

Median Nerve. Flex the wrist to palpate the target structures. Insert the needle between the tendons of flexor palmaris longus and flexor carpi radialis, 2 cm proximal to the wrist flexor crease and posteriorly toward the deep fascia (see Figure 36.8).

Ulnar Nerve. While the ulnar artery pulsation may be used as a landmark, it is frequently difficult to appreciate it in many patients. A more practical approach is to insert the needle proximal to the ulnar styloid process (see Figure 36.9).

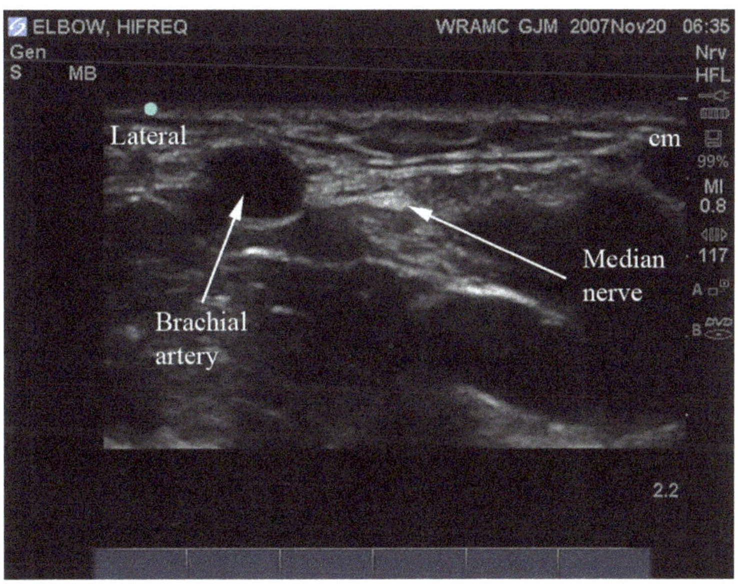

Figure 36.7 External anatomy and needle position for radial nerve block at the wrist.

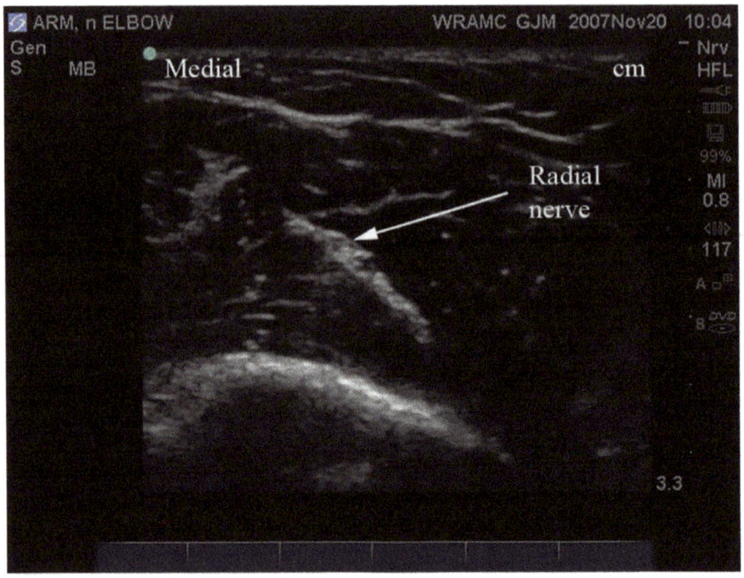

Figure 36.8 External anatomy and needle position for median nerve block at the wrist.

Teaching Points. Follow proper injection technique, which includes frequent aspiration for blood, incremental injection, consideration of injection pressure, and avoidance of "pinning" nerves against underlying bone with the injection needle.

Use caution when injecting local anesthetic into the olecranon fossa for the ulnar nerve block, as the nerve is "trapped" in a confined space at this location. Ensure that injection pressure is not too high, use smaller volume of the injectate, and avoid overflexing the elbow to prevent "pinning" of the nerve in the fossa.

When performing an elbow block, an additional local anesthetic injected laterally from the biceps tendon to the brachioradialis muscle will provide anesthesia for the lateral cutaneous nerve of the forearm.

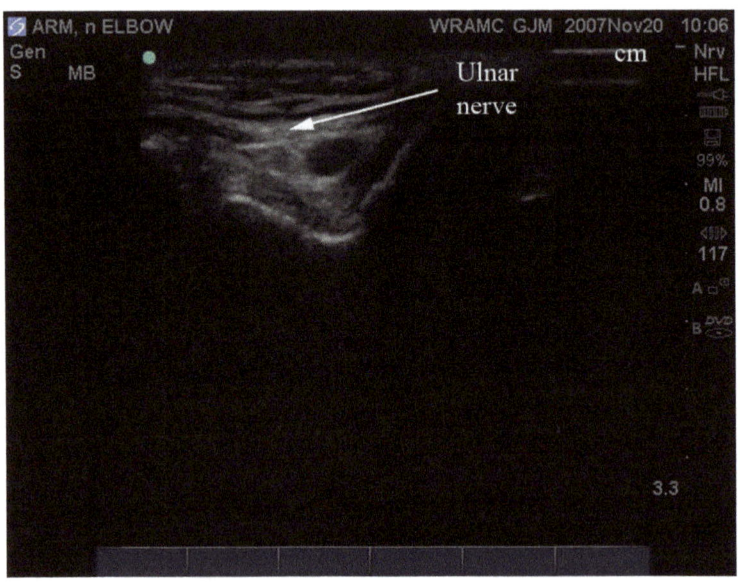

Figure 36.9 External anatomy and needle position for ulnar nerve block at the wrist.

4. Intravenous Regional Block (IVRA)

4.1. Introduction

Intravenous regional anesthesia (IVRA), or "Bier block" is an effective alternative to brachial plexus block for brief surgical procedures or manipulations of the upper extremity in the acutely injured patient. It is most suitable for peripheral procedures, such as ganglionectomies, carpal tunnel release, Dupuytren's contractures, laceration repair, or reduction of fractures. Most frequently, IVRA is used for procedures limited to 1 hour's duration, but occasionally it is utilized for surgeries lasting more than 1 hour; however, this approach requires a mandatory tourniquet deflation for at least 1 minute prior to reestablishing the analgesia.

IVRA entails injecting local anesthetic solutions into the venous system of an upper extremity, which has been exsanguinated by compression or gravity, and isolated with a tourniquet from the central circulation. It obviates the requirement for the use of a peripheral nerve stimulator or ultrasound machine, making it a user-friendly and cost-effective option, specifically valuable in the areas with scarce resources. One of the disadvantages is the very finite duration of the block, which is usually limited only to the operative period. Manipulations of the peripheral nerves may produce paresthesias, which may necessitate the use of adjuvant parenteral analgesic or sedative agents. Potential complications are outlined in Table 36.1.

4.2. Anatomy

The relevant anatomy involves the distribution of the venous system of the upper extremity and location of the antecubital fossa.

4.3. Contraindications

The only absolute contraindication to IVRA is patient refusal. Relative contraindications include the following:

- Crush injuries, vascular injuries or compound fractures of an extremity
- Inability to locate peripheral veins
- Local skin infections
- History of allergy to local anesthetics
- Preexisting vascular arteriovenous shunts and patients in whom a tourniquet is unsuitable (such as patients with severe peripheral vascular disease)
- Sickle cell disease

Table 36.1:
Potential complications from intravenous regional anesthesia of the upper extremity

Complications	
Drug-Related	Equipment-Related
Lidocaine: peripheral vasodilation and diminished cardiac contractility (hypotension); local anesthetic toxicity (CNS-related events: tinnitus, perioral numbness, seizures; or cardiovascular collapse)	Tourniquet failure or inadvertent deflation
Opioids: nausea, vomiting, and mild sedation	Ischemic pain and discomfort
	Systemic hypertension with prolonged inflation
	Sudden increase in venous pressure within the occluded tissue to a level higher than cuff pressure
	Leakage of drugs from the isolated extremity into the systemic circulation (due to intact interosseous circulation)
	Compartment syndrome

4.4. Equipment

- Local anesthetic: lidocaine HCl, 0.25% to 0.5% (alternative is prilocaine, 0.5%)
- One rubber tourniquet (Penrose drain) 12 to 18 in. in length (30–45 cm) and 7/8 in. wide (2.3 cm)
- One 18- or 20-gauge intravenous (IV) extracatheter (catheter over needle)
- One 500-mL or 1-L bag of IV solution connected to an infusion set (may substitute a saline-flushed IV port instead)
- Standard American Society of Anesthesiologists (ASA) monitors (electrocardiograph, blood pressure, pulse oximeter)
- Resuscitation equipment (IV catheter, crystalloid solution, and infusion set for the contralateral upper extremity)
- Two pneumatic tourniquets of appropriate size for the selected extremity
- One Esmarch bandage 60 in. in length (152 cm) and 4 in. wide (10 cm) for exsanguinating the arm
- Sterile skin preparatory set
- 30- or 50-mL Luer-lock syringe
- One graduated measuring cup for mixing of solution, preferably with a 100-mL capacity
- Adhesive tape: various sizes

4.5. Technique

1. A double-pneumatic tourniquet is placed on the proximal cuff high on the upper arm (biceps) or forearm (Figure 36.10).
2. An indwelling plastic extracatheter is inserted into a peripheral vein as far distally as possible (Figure 36.11).
3. The arm is elevated, and a rubber Esmarch bandage is wrapped around it spirally from the fingertips to the distal cuff of the double tourniquet to exsanguinate the arm (Figure 36.12).
4. The axillary artery is digitally occluded, and the proximal pneumatic cuff is inflated to 50 to 100 mm Hg above the systolic arterial blood pressure while maintaining pressure on the axillary artery; the Esmarch bandage is removed.
5. Lidocaine HCl 0.5% (30–50 mL) is injected via the indwelling plastic catheter (Figure 36.13).
6. The arm is brought down to the level of the procedure table, the IV cannula is withdrawn, and pressure is quickly applied over the site using sterile gauze.
7. About 25 to 30 minutes after the onset of anesthesia or when a patient complains of tourniquet pain, the distal cuff is inflated, and the proximal cuff is deflated, to minimize the development of tourniquet pain (Figure 36.14).

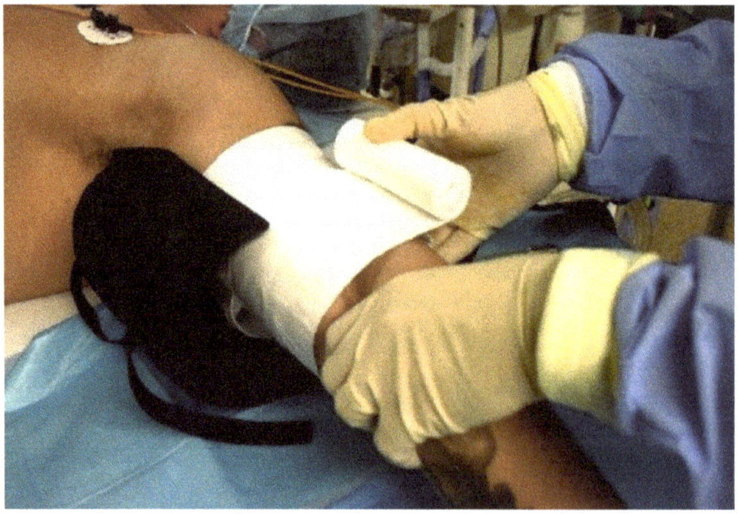

Figure 36.10 Placement of a double-pneumatic arm tourniquet.

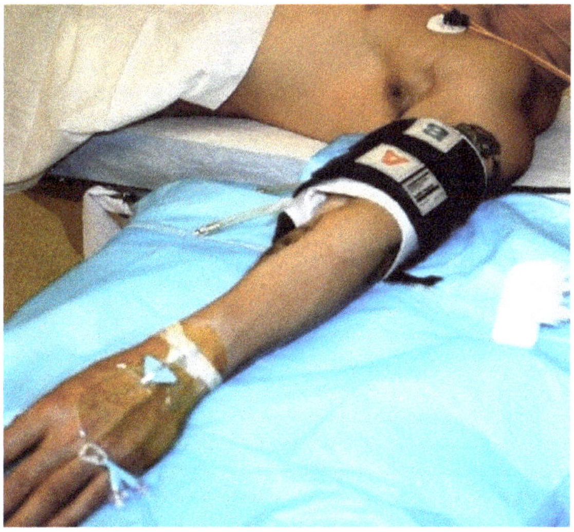

Figure 36.11 Placement of a distal intravenous catheter.

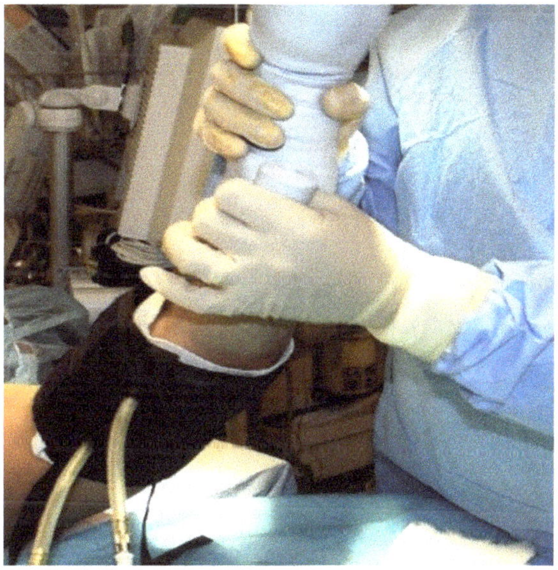

Figure 36.12 Exsanguination of the extremity with elevation and an Esmarch bandage.

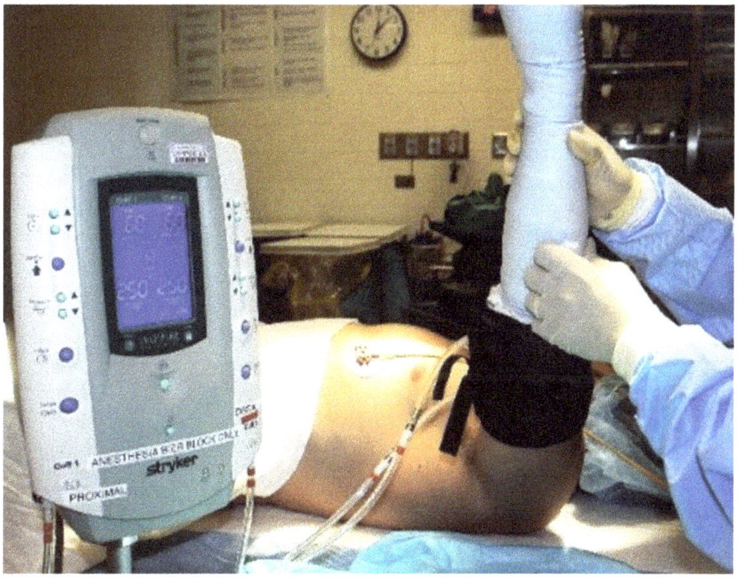

Figure 36.13 Injection of local anesthetic.

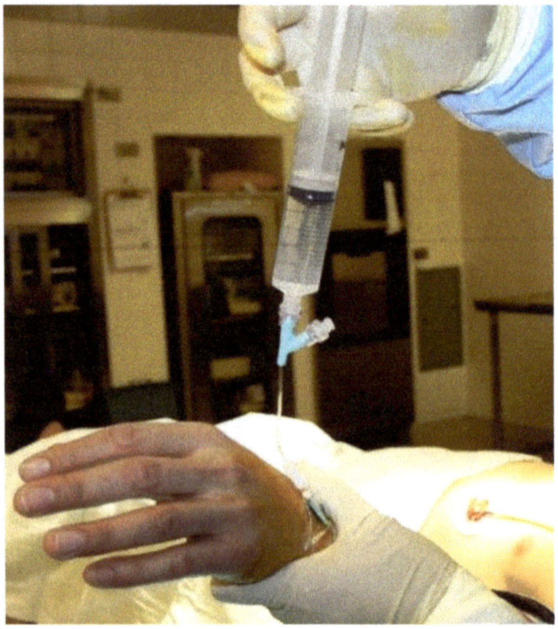

Figure 36.14 Double-pneumatic tourniquet inflation.

Teaching Points: An intact tourniquet system is absolutely essential for the successful and safe performance of IVRA. An unintentional deflation of the tourniquet or the presence of a vascular communication even with an intact, functioning tourniquet may result in serious toxic sequelae due to IVRA. Deflate the tourniquet in a cyclical fashion while assessing for signs of toxicity. Intermittent cuff deflation may effectively prolong the time to achieve peak arterial concentrations of the local anesthetic but may not be entirely reliable in minimizing toxicity due to release of local anesthetic into the circulation. The tourniquet should not be deflated until at least 30 minutes have elapsed from the time local anesthetic (and adjuvants, if used) is injected into the isolated venous system.

Pectoralis and Serratus Plane Blocks

37

1. Introduction

The pectoralis (Pecs) blocks are fascial plane blocks developed by Rafael Blanco. These blocks consist of the Pecs 1, Pecs 2, and serratus plane blocks (Table 37.1). The Pecs 1 block is an effective block for breast surgery and various other surgeries of the chest wall lateral to the nipple line. The Pecs 2 block provides axillary analgesic coverage. The Pecs 1 and 2 blocks are often performed in combination for extensive breast surgeries involving axillary lymph node dissections. The serratus plane block provides even more extensive axillary coverage extending to the upper abdomen.

2. Anatomy

The pectoralis major muscle inserts superiorly into the inferior clavicle, superolaterally into the proximal humerus, and medially into the sternum, and extends inferiorly to the level of the seventh rib. The pectoralis minor muscle inserts superolaterally into the coracoid process and inferomedially into the the third, fourth, and fifth ribs. The clavipectoral fascia is the fascial layer overlying the superficial aspect of the pectoralis minor muscle, separating it from the pectoralis major muscle. The pectoral nerves originate from the brachial plexus to innervate the pectoral muscles. The pectoral nerves are both motor and sensory nerves.

The lateral pectoral nerve most commonly arises from C5, C6, and C7. It most frequently arises with 2 branches from the anterior divisions of the upper and middle trunks (33.8%) or as a single root from the lateral cord (23.4%). It is the larger of the 2 pectoral nerves and runs between the major and minor pectoral muscles adjacent to the pectoral branch of the thoracoacromial artery to innervate the pectoralis minor muscle. The pectoral branch of the thoracoacromial artery runs under the upper part of the pectoralis minor. The lateral pectoral nerve is consistently adjacent to the thoracoacromial artery, and this can serve as a reliable landmark for fascial plane identification.

The median pectoral nerve most commonly arises from C8 and T1. It usually arises from the medial cord (49.3%), anterior division of the lower trunk (43.8%), or lower trunk (4.7%). It runs under the pectoralis minor muscle (crosses the pectoralis minor muscle in 62% of patients, and in the remaining 38% is located at the lateral border of the pectoralis minor muscle), traverses the 2 layers of the clavipectoral fascia, and reaches the lower one-third of the pectoralis major muscle. The anterior divisions of the T2-T6 intercostal nerves run between the pleura and the posterior intercostal membrane and traverse in a plane within the intercostal muscles toward the sternum.

Table 37.1: Pectoralis blocks

Type of Block	Benefits	Cons	Dermatomal Coverage
Pecs 1	Truncal coverage without anticoagulation risk of a paraneuraxial block	Spares the medial aspect to the breast (medial to the nipple line)	Lateral and median pectoral nerves
Pecs 2	Truncal coverage without anticoagulation risk of a paraneuraxial block	Spares the medial aspect to the breast; blocks the thoracodorsal and long thoracic nerves, which are purely motor nerves	T2–T6 (lateral cutaneous branches of the intercostal nerves)
Serratus plane	Truncal coverage without anticoagulation risk of a paraneuraxial block	Inadvertent blockade of the thoracodorsal and long thoracic nerves, which are purely motor nerves	T2–T9 (the lateral cutaneous branches of the intercostal nerves)

These branch into lateral and anterior branches. The lateral branches of the T3-T6 intercostal nerves pierce the external intercostal and serratus anterior muscles at the midaxillary line, and further branch into anterior and posterior terminal branches that innervate the mammary gland and skin from T3 to T6. The lateral branch of the T2 intercostal nerve does not form terminal branches but instead innervates the skin of the upper thoracic chest wall and the medial aspect of the upper arm as the intercostobrachial nerve. The anterior branches cross in front of the internal mammary artery and pierce the internal intercostal muscle, intercostal membranes, and the pectoralis major muscles to innervate the medial aspect of the breast.

The long thoracic nerve originates from C5 to C7, enters the axilla with the brachial plexus, and traverses along the superficial aspect of the serratus anterior muscle. It innervates the serratus anterior muscle. It is a purely motor nerve, and injury to this nerve results in winged scapula.

The thoracodorsal nerve originates from the posterior cord, travels with the thoracodorsal artery, and innervates the latissimus dorsi in the posterior wall of the axilla. Gerdy's ligament, or the suspensory ligament of the axilla, is a tough connective tissue layer that maintains the concave shape of the axilla.

Sensory innervation of the thorax is primarily from the thoracic intercostal nerves, via the ventral rami of the thoracic spinal nerves. The thoracic nerve roots also provide motor and sympathetic innervation of the thorax. The thoracic intercostal nerves travel along the inferior aspect of each thoracic rib between the innermost and internal intercostal muscles. Just posterior to the angle of the rib, they give off collateral and lateral cutaneous branches; the lateral cutaneous branches pierce the intercostal muscles and, in a plane between the serratus anterior muscle and the external intercostal muscle, divide into anterior and posterior branches. The anterior cutaneous branches emerge just laterally to the sternum to innervate the anterior thorax from the midline to the midclavicular line. The lateral branches of the lateral cutaneous branch of the intercostal nerve innervate the thorax lateral to the midclavicular line. Each intercostal nerve innervates its own rib.

The muscles of the shoulder girdle are innervated by the brachial plexus: the pectoralis muscles by the median and lateral pectoral nerves, the latissimus dorsi by the thoracodorsal nerve, and the serratus anterior muscle by the long thoracic nerve.

3. Procedure

3.1. Equipment

- High frequency (6–15 MHz), linear
- 21- or 22-gauge, 9- to 10-cm echogenic needle

Please refer to Figures 37.1 and 37.2 for Pecs 1 and 2 and serratus plane block.

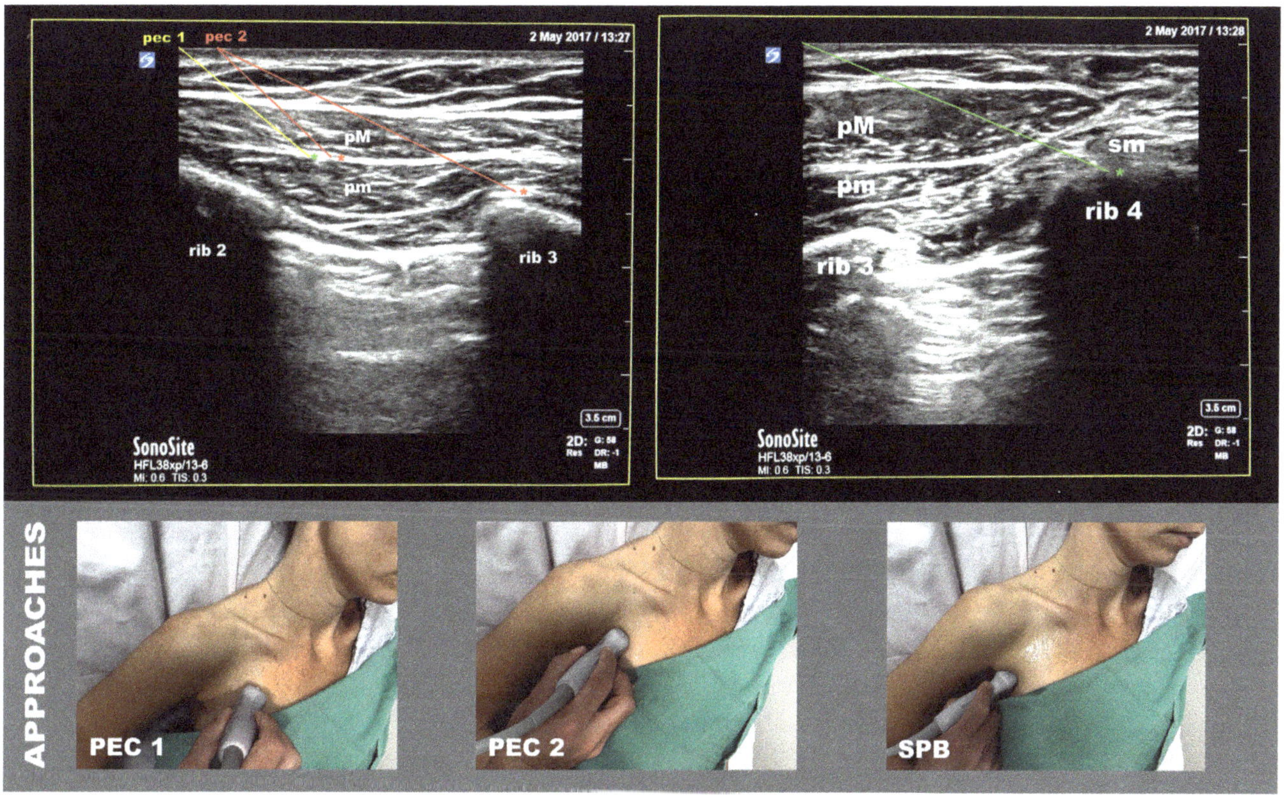

Figure 37.1 Pectoralis 1 and pectoralis 2 and serratus plane blocks.

Legend: pec 1: pectoralis block 1; pec 2: pectoralis block 2; pM: pectoralis major muscle; pm: pectoralis minor muscle; sm: serratus muscle. Colored lines represent needle trajectories for the block approaches described.

Pecs 1 Block. The patient can be positioned in either the supine or the semirecumbent position. The arm should be abducted at the shoulder and flexed at the elbow, as with positioning for an axillary brachial plexus block. The ultrasound probe is placed under the lateral third of the clavicle, in a parasagittal orientation similar to that of an infraclavicular block. Identify the subclavian muscle, axillary artery, and axillary vein at this level. Next, slide the probe caudally and laterally, with an oblique angulation, toward the axilla. Aim the transducer beam toward the lung. Begin counting the ribs, with the first rib under the axillary artery, and slide the ultrasound probe distally and laterally to the lateral border of the pectoralis minor muscle at the level of the third rib, bringing Gerdy's ligament and the serratus anterior muscle into view. The final

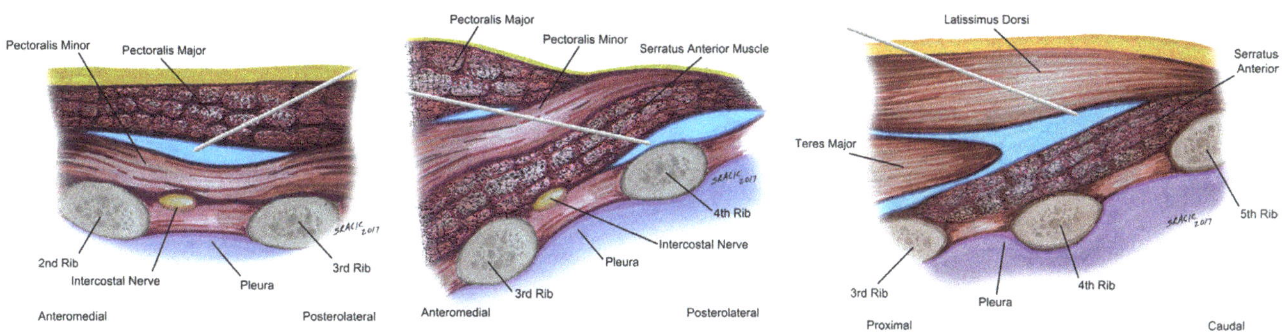

Figure 37.2 Local anesthetic deposition for Pecs 1 and 2 and serratus plane block.

ultrasound probe position should be at the level of the third rib. Check the location of the thoracoacromial artery with Doppler. Insert the needle in plane to the probe in a superomedial to inferolateral direction to place the needle tip in the interfascial plane between the pectoralis major and minor muscles. After negative aspiration for blood or air, inject the local anesthetic in 5-mL aliquots, visualizing the spread within this plane.

Pecs 2 Block. There are several different approaches to the Pecs 2 block. In the first approach, patient positioning and technique are exactly the same as those used in the Pecs 1 block (final probe position at the level of the third rib). The desired plane of injection is different, however. Insert the needle in plane to the probe in a superomedial to inferolateral direction to place the needle tip in the interfascial plane between the pectoralis minor and serratus anterior muscle. After negative aspiration for blood or air, inject the local anesthetic in 5-mL aliquots, visualizing the spread within this plane.

In the second approach, the technique is similar to that described previously, except that the local anesthetic is injected deep to the serratus anterior muscle, between the serratus anterior muscle and the rib. This may more effectively block the intercostal nerves, while sparing the thoracodorsal nerve, which is a purely motor nerve.

A third approach has also been described. The ultrasound probe is placed at the outer third of the clavicle at the level of second rib. The needle is advanced in a medial-to-lateral direction directly toward the second rib. When bone contact has been made, the needle is withdrawn slightly to inject local anesthetic between the external intercostal muscle and the serratus anterior muscle. This approach may block the intercostobrachial nerve as well as the lateral branches of the third through sixth intercostal nerves, while avoiding blockade of the long thoracic nerve.

Serratus Plane Block. The patient is positioned in the supine or semirecumbent position, with the arm on the side to be blocked slightly abducted to provide access to the ipsilateral chest wall. The ultrasound probe is placed over the anterior chest in the midclavicular line in the sagittal plane. Move the ultrasound probe caudally and laterally, counting ribs until the fifth rib is identified in the midaxillary line. Identify the latissimus dorsi muscle (superficial and posterior), teres major muscle (superior), and serratus anterior muscle (deep and inferior). Identify the thoracodorsal artery, which may help to identify the plane superficial to the serratus anterior muscle. Advance the needle in plane with ultrasound probe, in a superoanterior to inferoposterior direction toward the fifth rib, to place the needle tip in one of two possible locations: the interfascial plane between the latissimus dorsi and the serratus anterior muscle, or beneath the serratus anterior muscle and above the intercostal muscles. Inject local anesthetic, visualizing spread within either plane. Blanco has suggested that the superficial plane of injection may be more effective, though research is lacking.

Local Anesthetic. Ten to 20 mL of local anesthetic is sufficient volume for the Pecs 1 and Pecs 2 blocks. More volume may be required for the serratus plane block (0.4 mL/kg).

Contraindications and Risks. The Pecs 1, Pecs 2, and serratus plane blocks all risk pneumothorax. Additionally, the Pecs 1 and Pecs 2 blocks at the level of the second or third rib risk intravascular injection into the thoracoacromial artery or cephalic vein.

Teaching Points. To cover incisions over the medial aspect of the breast, the anterior branches of the anterior divisions of the intercostal nerves must be covered. The Pecs blocks can be supplemented by infiltration between the pectoralis major muscle and external intercostal muscle fascia medial to the nipple for medial dermatomal coverage.

Erector Spinae Plane Block

38

1. Introduction

The erector spinae plane block was first described by Forero et al. as a truncal interfascial plane block capable of producing unilateral analgesia over the anterior and posterior thorax, sparing the sternum and the spinous processes. Its successful use has been described for chronic pain conditions of the thorax as well as postoperative analgesia. Continuous erector spinae plane block has been described for multiple rib fractures. Forero et al. observed that the analgesia produced by the erector spinae plane block extends beyond its effect of cutaneous anesthesia; they proposed that this effect may be attributable to spread into the thoracic paravertebral space.

2. Anatomy

The innervation of the thorax is derived from the upper thoracic spinal nerves. At each spinal level, the upper thoracic spinal nerve splits into a dorsal and ventral ramus at the intervertebral foramen. The dorsal ramus courses posteriorly through the paravertebral space, the costotransverse foramen, and into the erector spinae muscle. Within the body of the erector spinae muscle, the dorsal ramus divides into a medial branch that ascends through the rhomboid major and trapezius muscles, and ends in a posterior cutaneous branch and a lateral branch.

The ventral ramus courses laterally as the intercostal nerve. The intercostal nerve runs deep to the internal intercostal membrane early in its course, and it ultimately emerges between the innermost intercostal and internal intercostal muscles. The intercostal nerve gives off a lateral cutaneous branch, which ascends superficially at the midaxillary line and divides into anterior and posterior branches supplying the lateral thoracic wall. The intercostal nerve continues anteriorly until its termination as the anterior cutaneous branch, innervating the anterior chest wall and upper abdomen (Figure 38.1).

3. Procedure

3.1. Equipment

- High-frequency (6–15 MHz) linear ultrasound probe transducer
- 21- or 22-gauge, 9- to 10-cm echogenic needle

Technique. The patient is placed in the sitting position or lateral decubitus position. The ultrasound probe is placed 3 cm lateral to the T5 spinous process in a longitudinal orientation, parasagittal plane, on the side of the thorax to be blocked. The trapezius

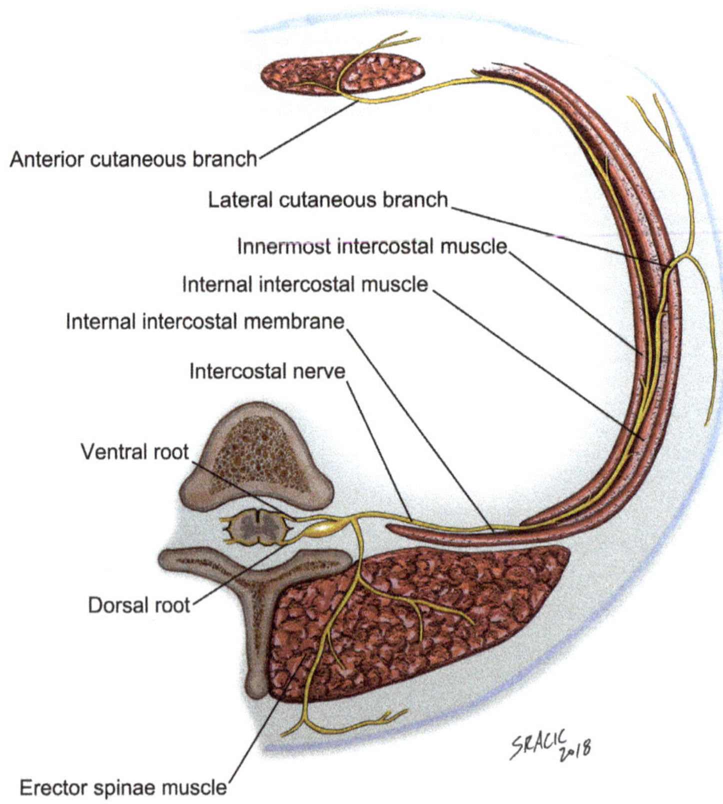

Figure 38.1 Thoracic neuroanatomy.

muscle is identified superficially, the rhomboid major underneath, the erector spinae muscle deep to the rhomboid, and the transverse process of T5. Insert the needle in plane to the ultrasound probe in a cephalad-to-caudad direction to place the needle tip in the interfascial plane between the rhomboid major and the erector spinae muscles (Figure 38.2). Alternatively, the tip may be placed deep to the erector spinae muscle to contact the transverse process of T5; injection in this plane between the erector spinae muscle and the transverse process deposits local anesthetic in closer proximity to the dorsal and ventral rami of the spinal nerve roots. Once properly positioned, and after negative aspiration for heme, inject local anesthetic, visualizing spread in both the cranial and caudal directions (Figure 38.3).

Local Anesthetic. Twenty milliliters of local anesthetic (bupivacaine or ropivacaine 0.2%–0.5%) is appropriate for adult patients.

Contraindications and Risks. The typical contraindications to regional anesthesia (patient refusal, active infection at the site of injection, coagulopathy, lack of patient cooperation) apply. Some providers consider the erector spinae plane block to be "less invasive" than neuraxial and paravertebral blocks, thereby avoiding their attendant risks. Despite the more superficial location of injection, cadaveric studies and clinical reports suggest that the injectate diffuses into the paravertebral space; therefore, epidural and intrathecal spread by secondary intent or inadvertent needle tip malpositioning should be considered a potential risk associated with this approach. It can be argued that the same ASRA anticoagulation guidelines that apply to all neuraxial and paraneuraxial deep blocks should be considered for the erector spinae plane block.

Anatomic Coverage. The erector spinae plane block produces unilateral anterior and posterior thoracic cutaneous sensory loss. Forero et al. described dermatomal coverage in the cephalocaudad dimension from T2-T9 in one case and, in another case, T3-T9 over the posterior thorax and T3-T6 over the anterior thorax. In the anterior-to-posterior direction, sensory blockade spanned from the midclavicular line to a line 3 cm lateral to the spinous process. Cutaneous sparing was seen in the skin overlying the sternum as well as the skin overlying the spinous processes.

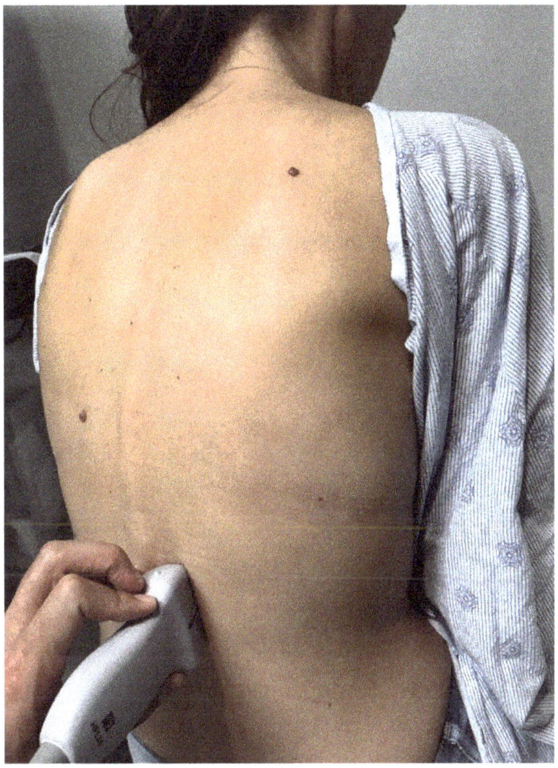

Figure 38.2 Ultrasound probe positioning for the erector spinae plane block.

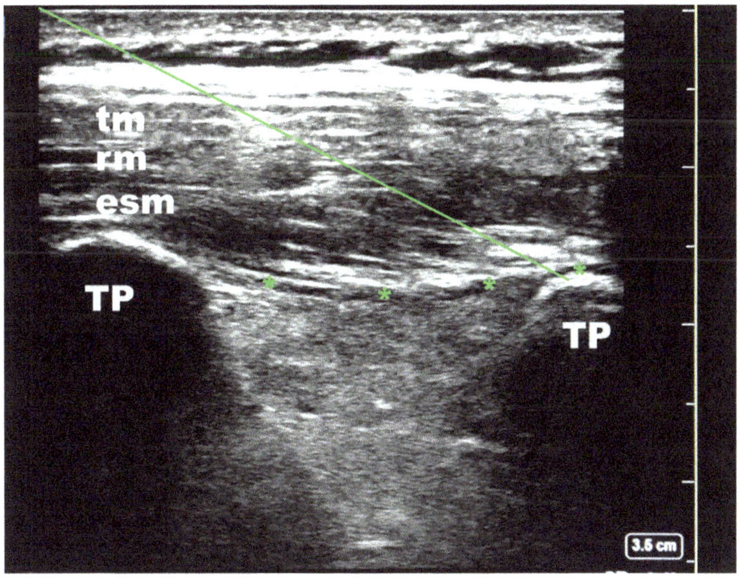

Figure 38.3 Erector spinae plane block ultrasound anatomy.

Legend: tm: trapezius muscle; rm: rhomboid major muscle; esm: erector spinae muscle; TP: transverse process. The green line represents the needle trajectory, with the green asterisk representing local anesthetic spread in the erector spinae plane.

If the interfascial plane between the rhomboid major and the erector spinae are injected with local anesthetic, this coverage extends to include the axilla and the medial upper arm. Forero et al. propose that the optimal plane of injection is deep to the erector spinae (between erector spinae and transverse process of T5), which deposits local anesthesia closer to the dorsal and ventral rami of the spinal nerve roots. This plane of injection, however, will spare the axilla and medial upper arm.

In cadaver studies using both methylene blue and CT contrast dye, Forero et al. found that injectate spread to an upper extent of T1, a lower extent of T11, and medial spread toward the midline, with limited lateral spread. Dissection of cadavers injected with dye superficial to the erector spinae muscle revealed staining of the dorsal rami of the spinal nerve roots; in cadavers injected with dye deep to the erector spinae muscle, CT revealed craniocaudal spread within a "paraspinous gutter" between the transverse processes anteriorly and erector spinae muscle posteriorly, as well as spread laterally to the tips of the transverse processes. Dissection of these cadavers revealed staining of the intercostal muscles, as well as staining deep to the intercostal muscles near the ventral and dorsal rami of the spinal roots.

Teaching Points. Local anesthetic distribution into the paravertebral space is by diffusion; hence, local anesthetic concentration may influence the speed and extent of the block. Local anesthetic spread into the thoracic paravertebral space may block the rami communicantes containing sympathetic fibers, and visceral abdominal analgesia has been suggested with erector spinae plane blocks at the T7 level bilaterally. Although initial reports concerning this approach are encouraging, considerable additional research is needed to better define and characterize this block.

Lower Extremity Neuroanatomy

39

1. Introduction

The safe practice of lower extremity regional anesthesia depends on a comprehensive understanding of neuroanatomy in this region of the body. Regional anesthesia of the lower extremity involves the lumbar plexus and the sacral plexus.

2. Lumbar Plexus

Lumbar spinal nerves exit caudad to their numbered vertebrae. They then divide into posterior and anterior rami. The lumbar plexus (Figure 39.1) consists of the anterior rami of L1-L4; these form anterior to the lumbar transverse processes within the proximal body of the psoas muscle. The posterior rami of L1-L5 supply the muscles and skin of the back. Major nerves of the lumbar plexus are as follows (Figure 39.2):

- Ilioinguinal and iliohypogastric nerves (L1): These pass anterior to the quadratus lumborum and emerge near the anterior superior iliac spine (ASIS). They innervate abdominal muscles as well as the skin of the inguinal and pubic areas.
- Lateral femoral cutaneous nerve (L2, L3): Emerges medial to the ASIS, passing deep to the inguinal ligament to supply sensation to the anterolateral surface of the thigh.
- Femoral nerve (L2-L4): Passes deep to the inguinal ligament to innervate the iliacus, hip flexors, and knee extensors of the thigh. This nerve continues on below the knee as the saphenous nerve to supply sensation to the medial lower leg.
- Obturator nerve (L2-L4): Passes medial to the psoas muscle, into the pelvis, and then through the obturator foramen to innervate the medial thigh adductor muscles.
- Lumbosacral trunk (L4, L5): Passes over the sacrum into the pelvis and joins the formation of the sacral plexus from the anterior rami of S1-S4.

3. Sacral Plexus

Found within the lesser pelvis on the anterior surface of the piriformis muscle. It is formed from the anterior spinal nerve rami of L4-S4. Most nerves originating from the sacral plexus leave the pelvis via the greater sciatic foramen. Major nerves of the sacral plexus are as follows (Figure 39.2):

- Sciatic nerve (L4-S3): Travels in the posterior thigh and provides motor and sensory innervation to the posterior thigh and the majority of the lower leg (with the exception of the medial lower leg). It is the single largest nerve in the body. It is composed

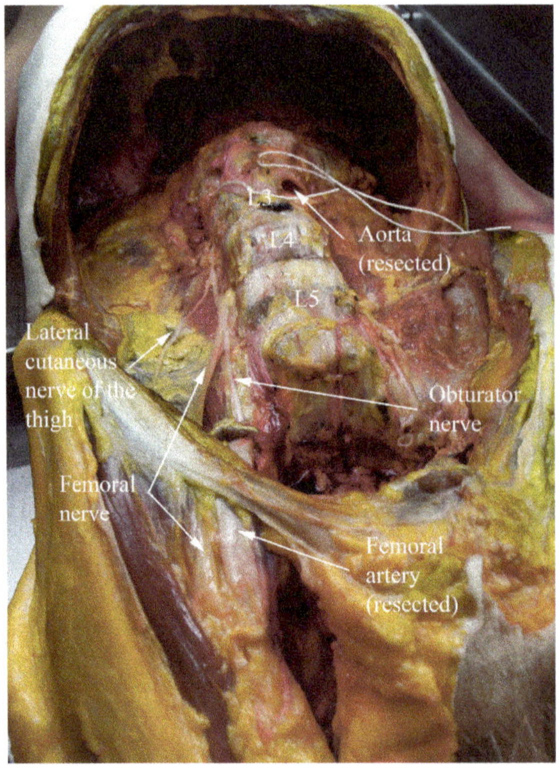

Figure 39.1 Dissected right lumbar plexus. The exposed nerves have been dissected from the substance of the psoas muscle, which has been removed.

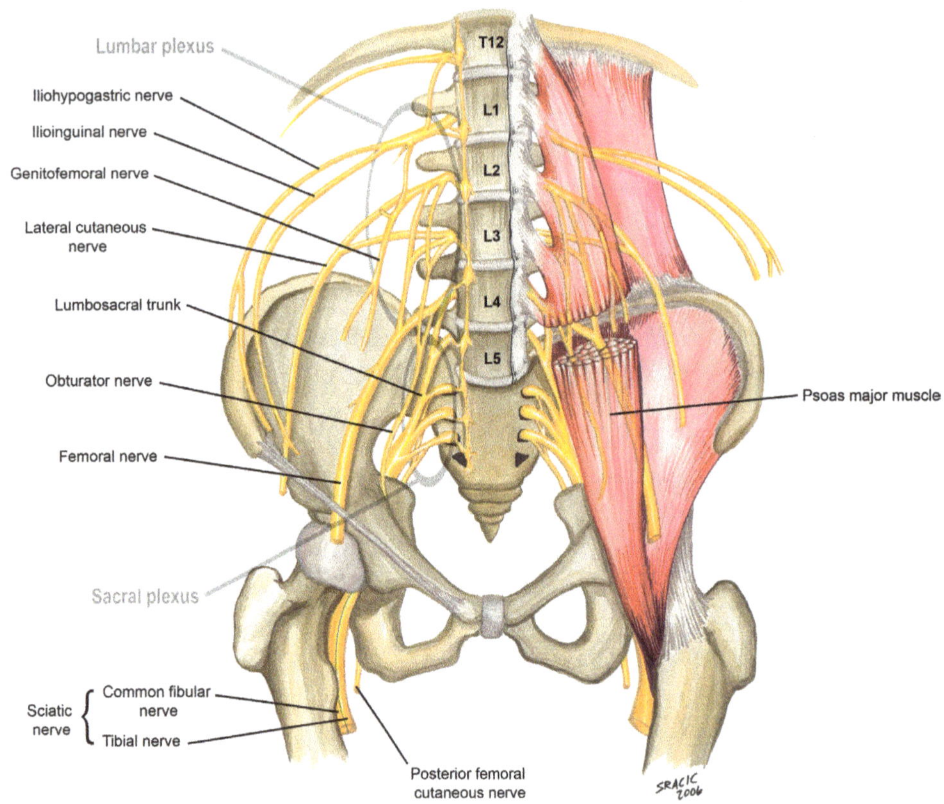

Figure 39.2 Lumbar plexus and sacral plexus.

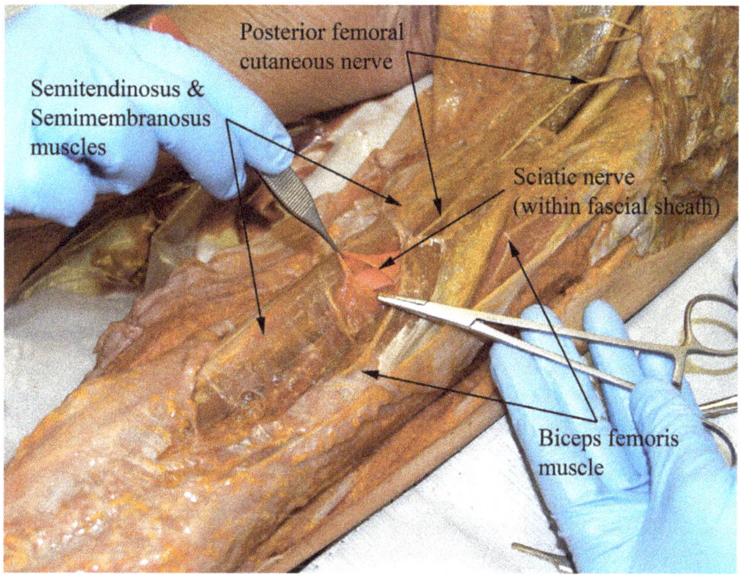

Figure 39.3 Sciatic nerve within the fascial sheath dissected at the posterior midthigh.

of 2 individual nerves, the tibial nerve and common peroneal nerve, traveling together within the same nerve sheath (Figure 39.3).

- Pudendal nerve (S2-S4): Enters the perineum via the lesser sciatic foramen. It is the primary nerve of the perineum, providing sensation to the genitalia as well as motor innervation to the muscles of the perineum.
- Posterior cutaneous nerve of the thigh (also called posterior femoral cutaneous nerve) (S2-S3): Provides cutaneous innervation of the buttocks and proximal medial and proximal posterior surfaces of the thigh (see Figure 39.3).
- Superior gluteal nerve (L4-S1): Leaves the pelvis superior to the piriformis and innervates the gluteal muscles (gluteus medius and gluteus minimus). It also innervates the tensor to the fascia lata.
- Inferior gluteal nerve (L5-S2): Leaves the pelvis inferior to the piriformis and superficial to the sciatic nerve, branching to innervate the gluteus maximus muscle.

Lumbar Plexus Block

40

1. Introduction

The lumbar plexus is composed of 6 nerves supplying the lower abdomen and upper leg. When combined with a sciatic nerve block, the lumbar plexus block can provide complete analgesia to the lower extremity. This serves as an alternative to neuraxial anesthesia, which undesirably also anesthetizes the nonoperative leg and occasionally causes urinary retention. The complete lumbar plexus may be blocked from a posterior approach (aka psoas compartment block); however, the individual nerves of the plexus can be blocked from anterior approaches.

2. Anatomy

The lumbar plexus is formed from the ventral rami of L1-L4 with variable contributions from T12 and L5 (Figure 40.1). The peripheral branches of the lumbar plexus include the iliohypogastric, ilioinguinal, genitofemoral, lateral femoral cutaneous, femoral, and obturator nerves. The plexus forms within the body of the psoas muscle (Figure 40.2). A lumbar plexus block consistently blocks the 3 nerves that supply the lower extremity: femoral nerve, lateral femoral cutaneous nerve, and obturator nerve (Figure 40.3).

The obturator nerve has more variability of location and is separated from the other 2 nerves of the plexus by the psoas muscle. A femoral nerve block ("3-in-1 block") often fails to successfully block the obturator nerve due to the intervening psoas muscle. This is why the lumbar plexus approach is often selected when blockade of all 3 nerves is required.

There are some concerns that the lumbar plexus block may have the potential to cause significant retroperitoneal bleeding due to the relatively deep position of the target structures within the psoas muscle. However, there are only few case reports regarding this complication, whereas a large retrospective analysis of more than 600 lumbar plexus catheters placed for total hip arthroplasty did not find any incidence of significant bleeding or hematoma formation, despite the use of warfarin for deep vein thrombosis prophylaxis in these patients.

While performing a posterior lumbar plexus block, it is recommended to contact the needle with the L4 transverse process before entering the plexus. The bony landmark will serve as a safety measure of needle depth, which should prevent the operator from advancing too deep into the retroperitoneum. Despite variability in distances from skin to the L4 transverse process among patients of varying BMIs, once the transverse process is reached, the distance to the lumbar plexus is no more than 15 to 20 mm. Examination of the spine with ultrasound prior to the block can provide useful information concerning plexus depth from the skin.

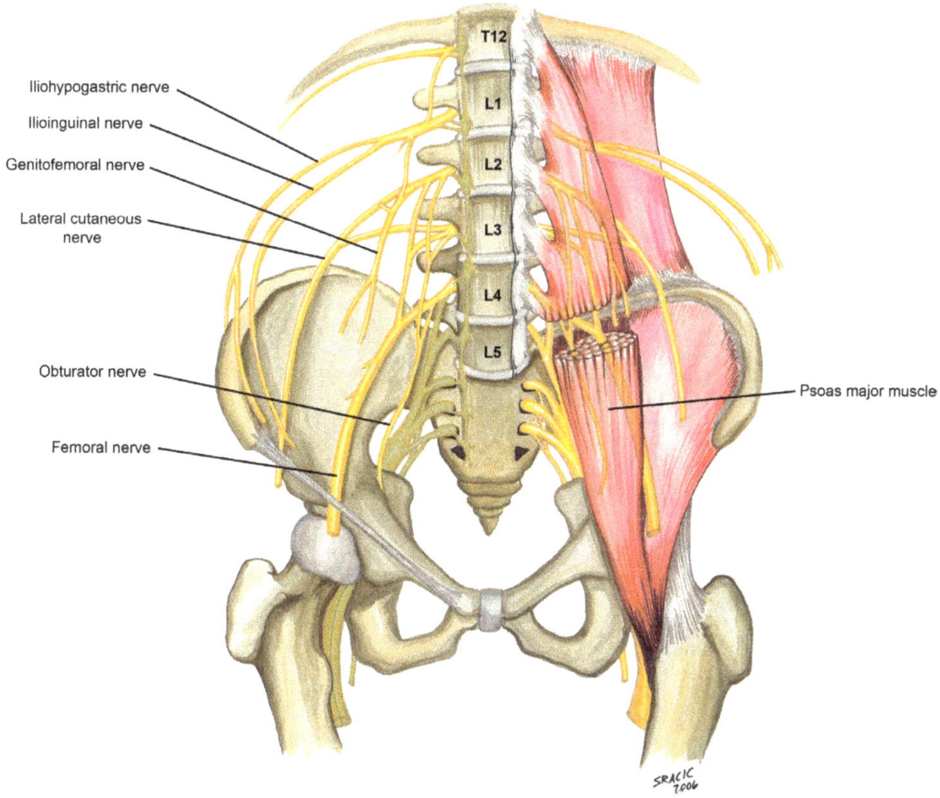

Figure 40.1 Lumbar plexus anatomy.

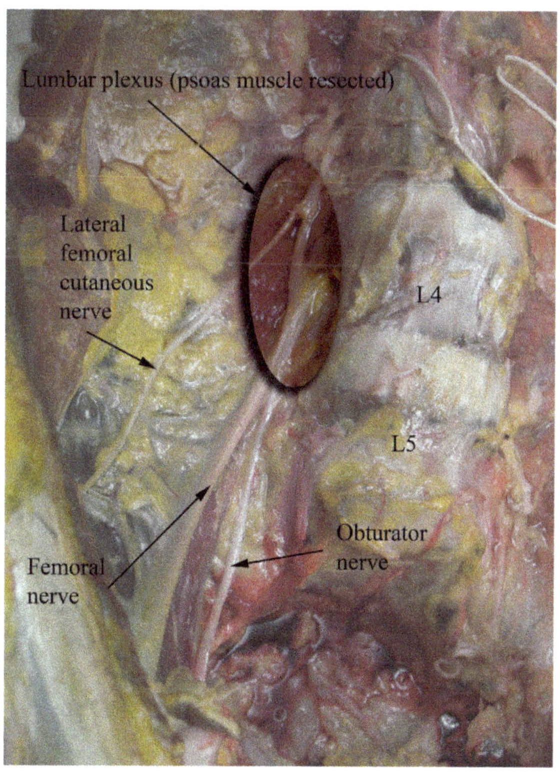

Figure 40.2 Lumbar plexus dissection.

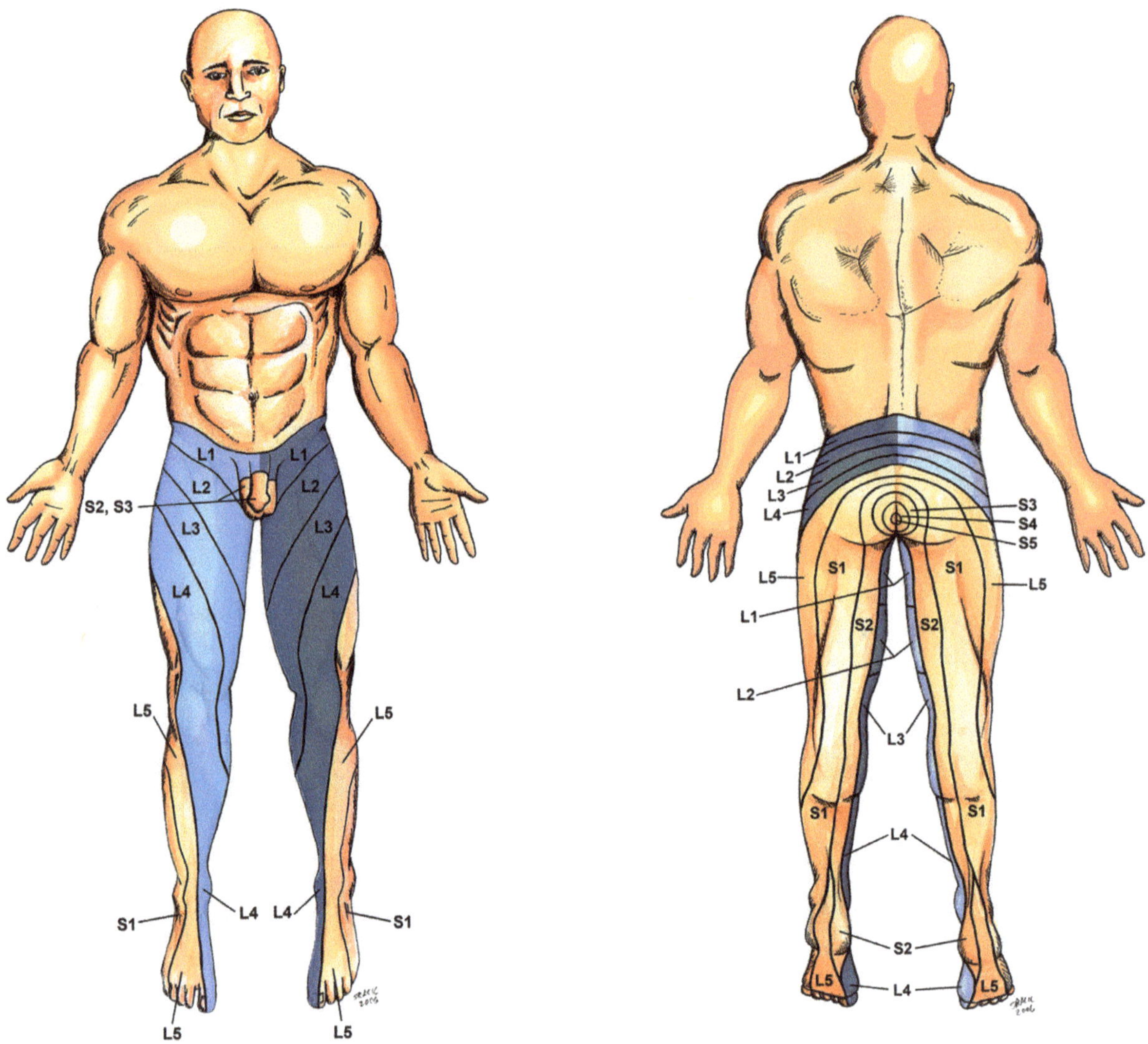

Figure 40.3 Dermatomes anesthetized with the lumbar plexus block.

Posterior lumbar plexus block complications include intrathecal injection, epidural injection or diffusion (the most common complication), intravascular injection, and retroperitoneal bleeding.

3. Procedure

3.1. Landmarks

The patient is placed in the lateral decubitus position with the operative side up. A line is drawn from the top of the posterior iliac crest down to the midline, which is known as the *intercristal line*. This line is positioned over the L4 transverse process in most adults. The intersection of the intercristal line with a line drawn parallel to the spine from the posterior superior iliac spine determines the initial needle insertion point and is 5 cm lateral from the midline in most patients (Figure 40.4).

3.2. Needles

- 21-gauge, 10-cm insulated needle (15-cm needles may be needed for obese patients).
- 18-gauge, 10-cm insulated Tuohy needle for catheter placement. Catheters are introduced 5 cm beyond needle tip.

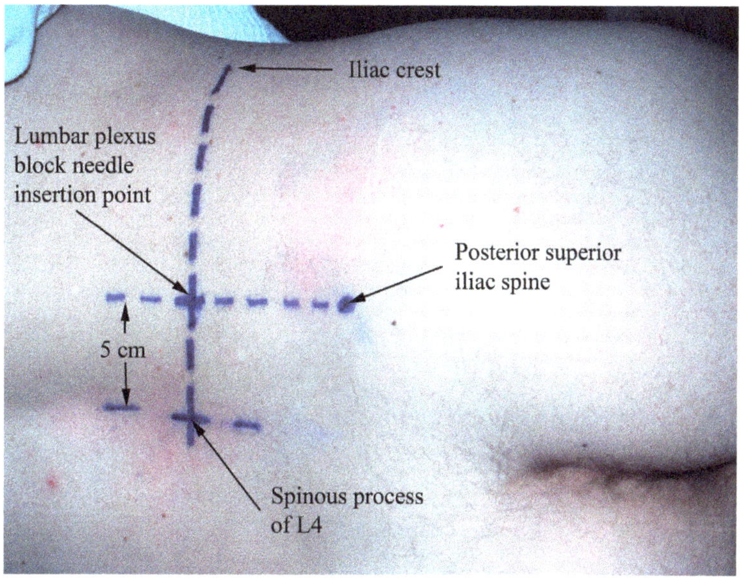

Figure 40.4 Lumbar plexus stimulation block landmarks.

3.3. Stimulation

Initially set the nerve stimulator to 1.0 to 1.2 mA. Insert the needle with a slight medial angulation to the sagittal plane of the patient (Figure 40.5). Watch for a quadriceps muscle twitch (femoral nerve) as evidence of needle proximity to the lumbar plexus, usually 5 to 8 cm from the skin. Make small adjustments of the needle tip in caudal or cephalad directions if there is no contact with the os. Once bone is contacted (usually L4 transverse process), slightly retract the needle and redirect caudally to "walk off" the transverse process. The plexus should be stimulated at a depth of no more than 2 cm beyond the transverse process (penetration beyond 2 cm increases the risk of injury to retroperitoneal structures). Decrease the stimulator current to 0.5 mA. If the twitch remains with this new decreased current, then proceed to inject the local anesthetic.

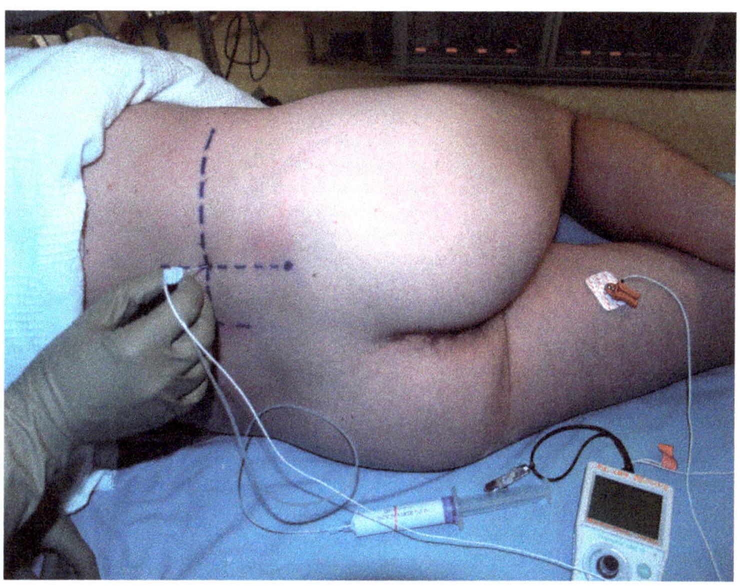

Figure 40.5 Needle placement for the lumbar plexus block.

4. Local Anesthetic

25 to 30 mL of local anesthetic is sufficient.

Teaching Points. Occasionally, stimulation of the hamstring muscles of the posterior thigh will be noted while attempting to perform the lumbar plexus block. This suggests sacral plexus stimulation (sciatic nerve) and indicates the needle tip is too caudal and medial. Injection here may lead to epidural spread or incomplete block of the plexus. Adjustment of the initial needle insertion point 1 cm cephalad and 1 cm lateral compensates for this error.

If os is repeatedly encountered despite "walking off" the transverse process, the needle tip may be too medial and may be hitting the vertebral lamina. Pull the needle back toward the skin and redirect slightly more lateral. The term *os* is specifically used rather than *bone* to remind the physician that lightly sedated patients may become concerned or agitated if they hear the needle described as contacting their bone. The term *os* is less familiar and therefore less alarming to patients, and this term should be used while discussing bony landmarks during regional anesthetic procedures.

5. Ultrasound-Guided Lumbar Plexus Block

In patients with favorable anatomic conditions (normal or below-normal BMI), ultrasound can be utilized for this block. The patient is positioned in the same fashion as for the landmark-based technique. With a curved-linear 2 to 5 MHz transducer positioned to obtain a transverse, paramedian view (Figure 40.6), the vertebral body of L4 and the psoas muscle are visualized (Figure 40.7). A 4-inch needle is introduced in plane until the posterior part of the psoas muscle has been reached. About 25 to 30 mL of local anesthetic is injected. Note that visualization of the lumbar plexus nerves is a rare occurrence. Ultrasound may also be used in combination with the landmark-based nerve stimulation technique to confirm bony anatomic landmarks for this block (L4 transverse process).

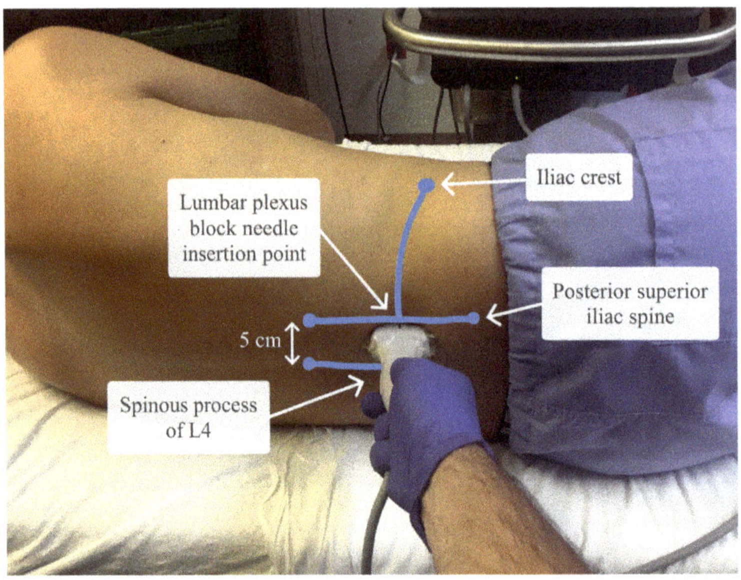

Figure 40.6 Ultrasound: probe positioning for lumbar plexus block (longitudinal scan).

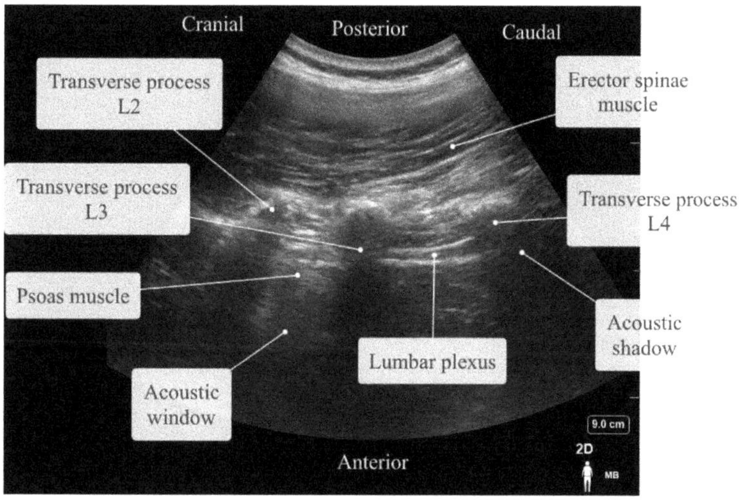

Figure 40.7 Ultrasound: anatomy of the lumbar plexus block.

Teaching Points. In most individuals, current ultrasound equipment does not allow for visualization of the nerves of the lumbar plexus. Consequently, landmark-based nerve stimulation techniques or a combination of ultrasound with nerve stimulation is currently preferred.

41

Femoral Nerve Block

1. Introduction

Femoral nerve block provides analgesia to the anterior thigh, including the flexor muscles of the hip and extensor muscles of the knee. This block has historically been known as the "3-in-1 block," suggesting femoral, lateral femoral cutaneous, and obturator nerves would be blocked from a single injection. However, the obturator nerve is often missed due to variable coursing. To reliably block all 3 aforementioned nerves, refer to the posterior lumbar plexus block in chapter 40.

The femoral nerve block is ideal for surgeries of the hip, knee, or anterior thigh. It is often combined with a sciatic nerve block for near-complete lower extremity analgesia. Complete analgesia of the leg can be achieved without lumbar plexus block by combining a femoral nerve block with parasacral sciatic nerve block (which blocks the obturator more than 90% of the time), or by adding an individual obturator nerve block to the femoral nerve block.

2. Anatomy

The femoral nerve is formed by the dorsal divisions of the anterior rami of L2-L4 and is the largest terminal branch of the lumbar plexus. It travels through the psoas muscle, leaving at the lateral border of the psoas. It then descends caudally into the thigh via a groove formed by the psoas and iliacus muscles, entering the thigh beneath the inguinal ligament (Figure 41.1). The femoral nerve divides into an anterior and posterior branch just after emerging from beneath the inguinal ligament. At this level, it is located lateral and posterior to the femoral artery (Figure 41.2). The anterior branch provides motor innervation to the sartorius and pectineus muscles and sensory innervation to the skin of the anterior and medial thigh. The posterior branch provides motor innervation to the rectus femoris, vastus intermedius, vastus lateralis, and vastus medialis muscles, collectively the "quadriceps muscle." The posterior branch of the femoral nerve also provides sensory innervation to the medial aspect of the lower leg via the saphenous nerve (Figures 41.3 and 41.4). The anatomic location makes this one of the easiest blocks because the landmarks are simply identified (except in cases of the morbidly obese, although the nerve remains in proximity to the femoral artery as in all patients). For the block, the patient should remain supine. The nerve is relatively superficial.

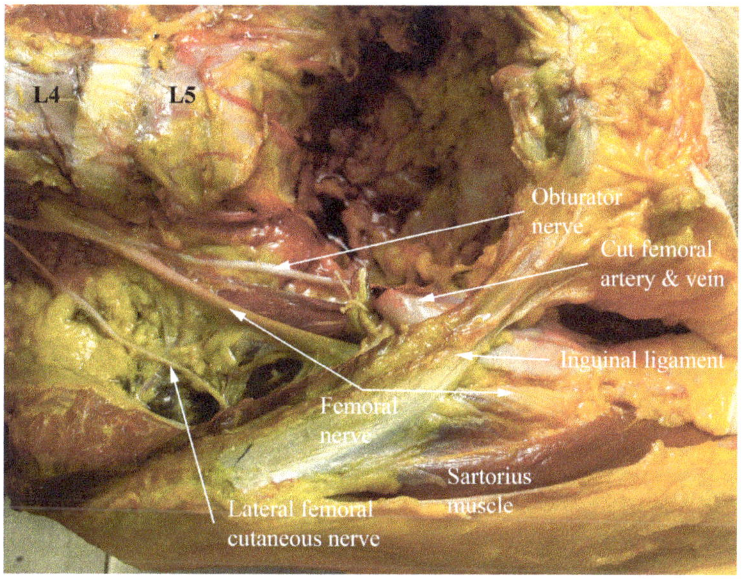

Figure 41.1 Femoral nerve dissection proximal to the inguinal ligament.

3. Procedure

3.1. Landmarks

While the patient is supine, a line (representing the inguinal ligament) is visualized between the anterior superior iliac spine (ASIS) and the pubic symphysis. The femoral nerve passes through the center of the line. This is very useful for positioning the needle in the inguinal crease, particularly in an obese patient. Next, palpate the femoral pulse and mark it at the inguinal crease. The most successful point of needle entry is directly lateral (1–1.5 cm) to the artery in the inguinal

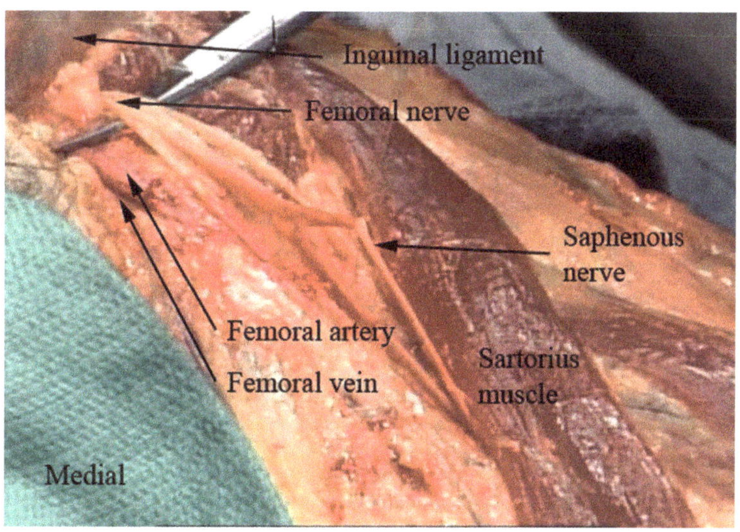

Figure 41.2 Femoral nerve dissection.

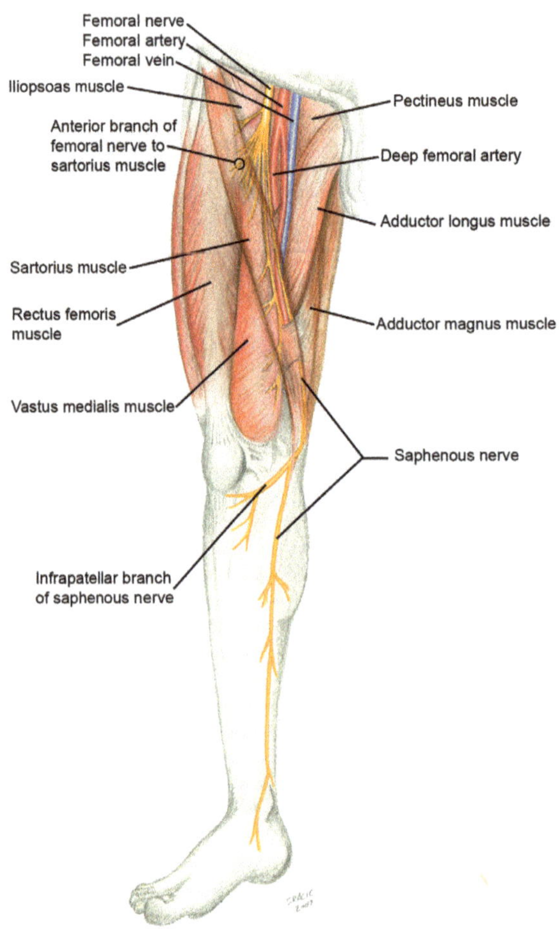

Figure 41.3 Femoral nerve anatomy.

crease. At this location the femoral nerve is wide and superficial, and the needle does not pass through significant muscle mass. Direct the needle cephalad toward the center of the inguinal ligament line (Figure 41.5).

3.2. Needles

- 22-gauge, 5-cm insulated needle.
- 18-gauge, 5-cm insulated Tuohy needle for catheter placement. The catheter is inserted 3 to 5 cm for the femoral block.

3.3. Stimulation

Set the nerve stimulator to 1.0 to 1.2 mA initially. Direct the needle cephalad at approximately a 30° to 45° angle. A brisk "patellar snap" at 0.5 mA or less is indicative of successful localization of the needle near the femoral nerve. The nerve is very commonly superficial, rarely beyond 3 cm deep (Figure 41.6).

3.4. Local Anesthetic

25 to 30 mL of local anesthetic will produce a successful femoral block.

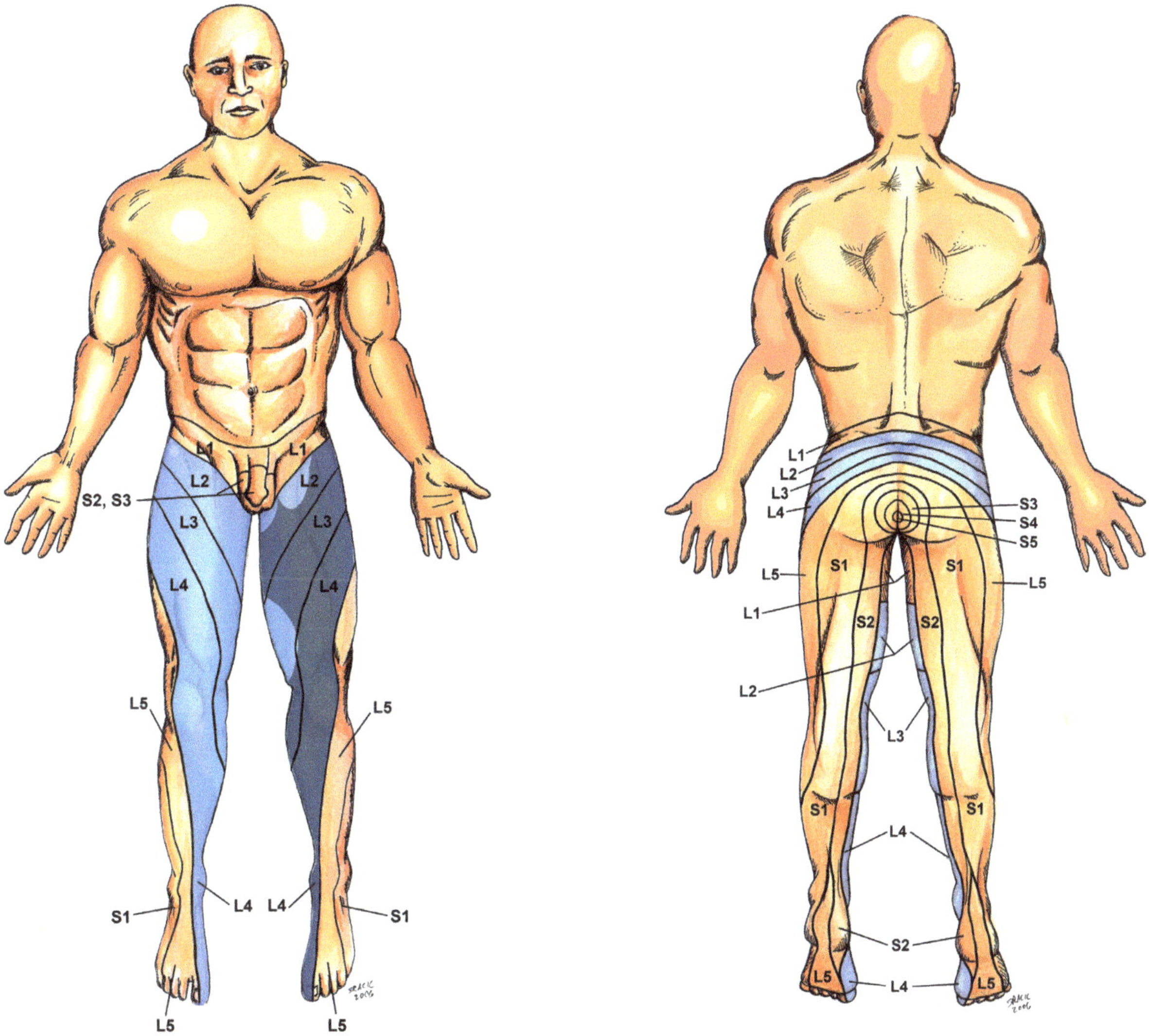

Figure 41.4 Dermatomes anesthetized with the femoral nerve block (dark blue).

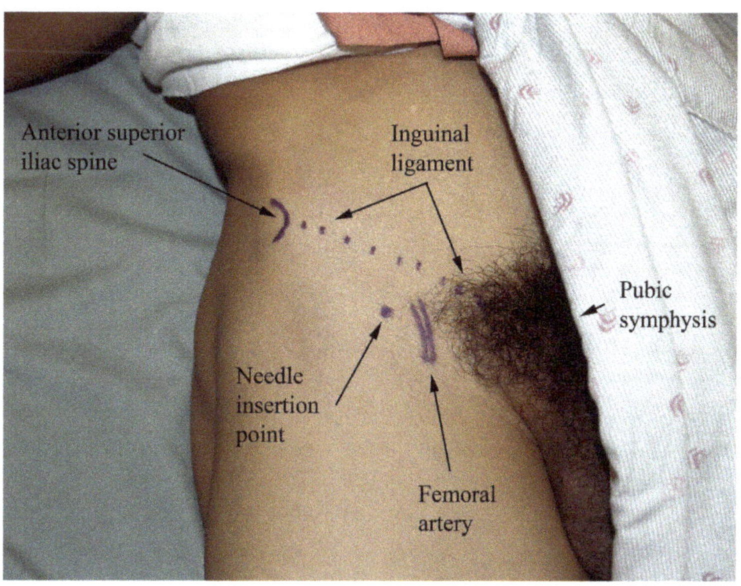

Figure 41.5 External anatomy of the femoral nerve block.

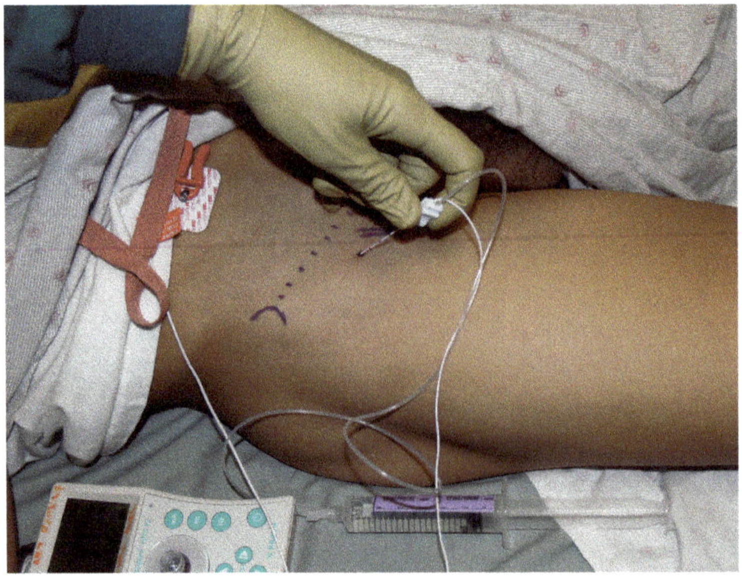

Figure 41.6 Needle position for the femoral nerve block.

Teaching Points. The anterior branch of the femoral nerve is usually encountered with the first needle pass, resulting in stimulation of the sartorius muscle (a contraction of the lower medial thigh). If this occurs, advance the needle tip until either the sartorius twitch is extinguished or a patellar snap is elicited before redirecting the needle. If the sartorious twitch is extinguished without a patellar snap, withdraw the needle toward the skin (without exiting the skin) and redirect it slightly lateral and slightly deeper. The posterior branch of the femoral nerve is typically lateral and deep to the anterior branch. The operator should resist the urge to use the patient's thigh as a hand rest while directing the needle. Stimulation of the femoral nerve can result in brisk vastus muscle twitching that can disrupt needle positioning.

4. Ultrasound-Guided Femoral Nerve Block

4.1. Probe

High frequency (5–12 MHz), linear.

4.2. Probe Position

Place the probe in the inguinal crease, parallel to the inguinal ligament. The femoral nerve will be visualized as a hyperechoic, triangular structure immediately lateral to the femoral artery. The nerve is deep to both the fascia lata and the fascia illiaca at this level.

4.3. Approach and Injection

Insert the needle at the lateral end of the ultrasound probe and advance parallel to the ultrasound beam until it approaches the femoral nerve (Figure 41.7). This allows visualization of the entire needle. Another acceptable approach is to advance the needle to the nerve from a short-axis view (needle seen as a dot) as opposed to the long-axis view. The femoral nerve is easily visualized near the femoral artery in most patients (Figure 41.8). The relatively superficial depth of the femoral nerve at the inguinal crease enhances visualization of the needle under ultrasound. A medial approach to the femoral nerve is typically avoided, since the femoral artery obstructs this approach. Prior to injection, make sure that the needle

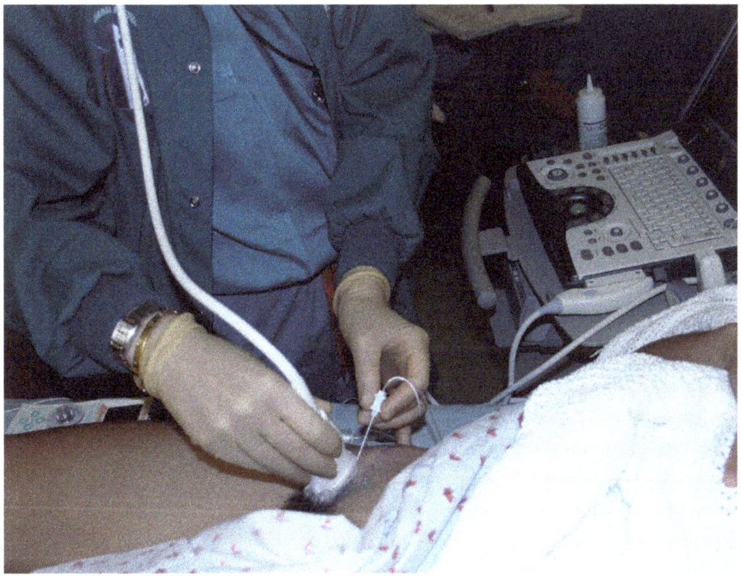

Figure 41.7 Ultrasound probe and needle positioning for the femoral nerve block.

has penetrated the fascia lata (division between subcutaneous tissues of the thigh and underlying muscles and vessels), as well as the fascia iliaca (which surrounds the iliopsoas and femoral nerve). Local anesthetic must surround the entire femoral nerve or surround the medial, lateral, and inferior aspects of the nerve to ensure a successful block (Figure 41.9). If the local anesthetic is distributed only at the superior aspect of the nerve, the needle may not have crossed the fascia iliaca, in which case the block may be delayed or fail.

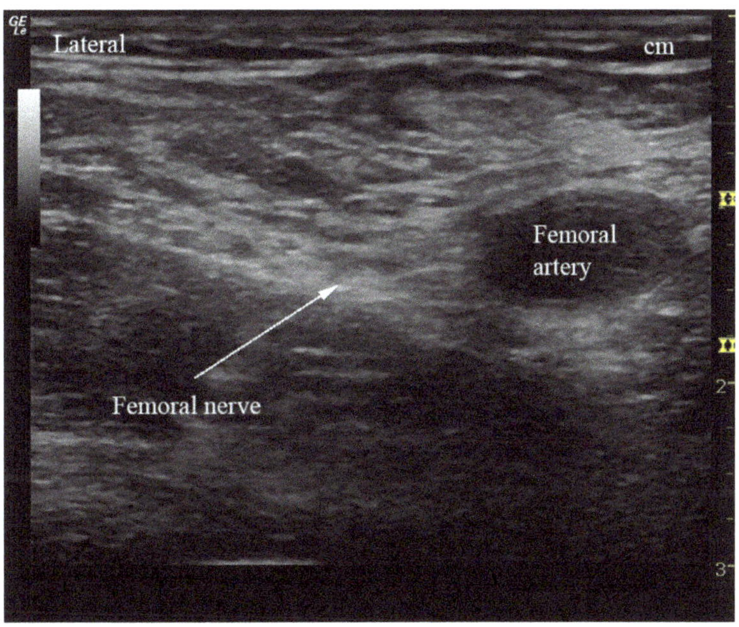

Figure 41.8 Ultrasound anatomy of the femoral nerve.

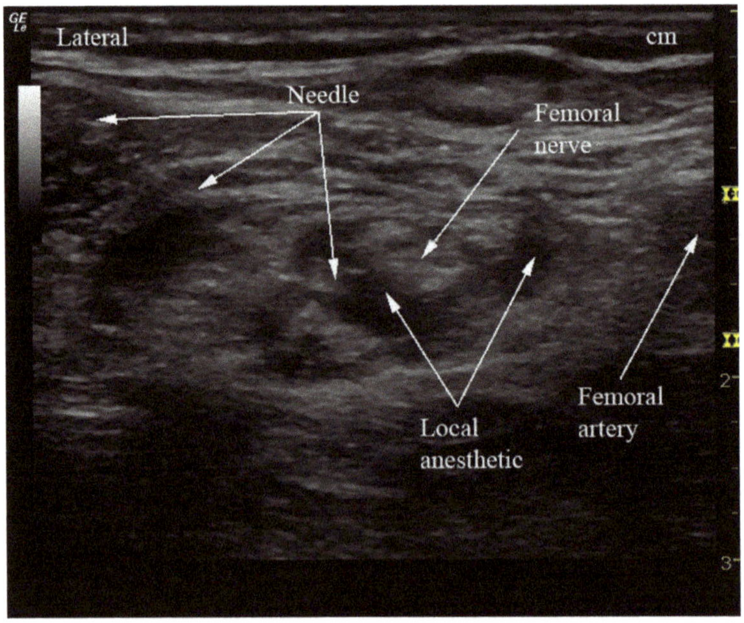

Figure 41.9 Ultrasound image of the femoral nerve post injection.

Teaching Points. Use of the ultrasound can improve the femoral nerve block by:

- Decreasing block latency by as much as 10 minutes
- Improving the sensory component of the block
- Reducing the amount of local anesthetic needed to achieve block success

Individual Nerve Blocks of the Lumbar Plexus

42

1. Fascia Iliaca Block

1.1. Introduction

The fascia iliaca block is a regional anesthetic procedure that takes advantage of both a shared location under the fascia of the iliacus muscle and an anatomic proximity of the femoral and the lateral femoral cutaneous nerve (LFCN). In this procedure, a large volume of local anesthetic can be deposited at various locations inferior to the inguinal ligament and deep to the fascia of the iliacus muscle. With deposition of a large enough volume, local anesthetic can spread to both the femoral and the lateral femoral cutaneous nerves. Cadaver studies suggest that while reliable spread of fluid to the femoral nerve is observed, spread to the LFCN is not so consistent. Clinical studies suggest that selective nerve blocks of the lumbar plexus may be superior to the fascia iliaca block. Injuries or surgeries to the hip or knee are common indications for placement of the fascia iliaca block.

1.2. Anatomy

From the lumbar plexus, the LFCN and the femoral nerve travel anteriorly through the pelvis underneath the fascia of the iliacus muscle. Of note, this is the same fascia as is described during the femoral nerve block procedure. In fact, one of the variations of the fascia iliacus block involves a similar approach as is used for the femoral nerve block.

1.3. Procedure

The fascia iliaca block can be performed using sonography or using superficial anatomic landmarks.

Using anatomic landmarks as a guide, a line is drawn from the anterior superior iliac spine (ASIS) to the pubic tubercle, and this distance is measured. Then, one-third of this distance is approximated from the ASIS medially. The needle is inserted 1 cm inferior to this point until a second "pop" is experienced by the proceduralist (the first "pop" is likely fascia lata, the second "pop" is likely fascia iliaca). Alternatively, the location of the procedure may be identified by measuring 2 cm lateral from the femoral artery and 1 cm inferior to the inguinal ligament.

Using ultrasound, a reliable approach is to identify the "hourglass" outline, formed by the fascia of the internal oblique and sartorius muscles. The iliacus muscle lies deep to this structure and can easily be identified by the following steps:

1. Obtain a sagittal plane view of the ASIS (Figure 42.1) with a high-frequency linear ultrasound probe (10–12 MHz).

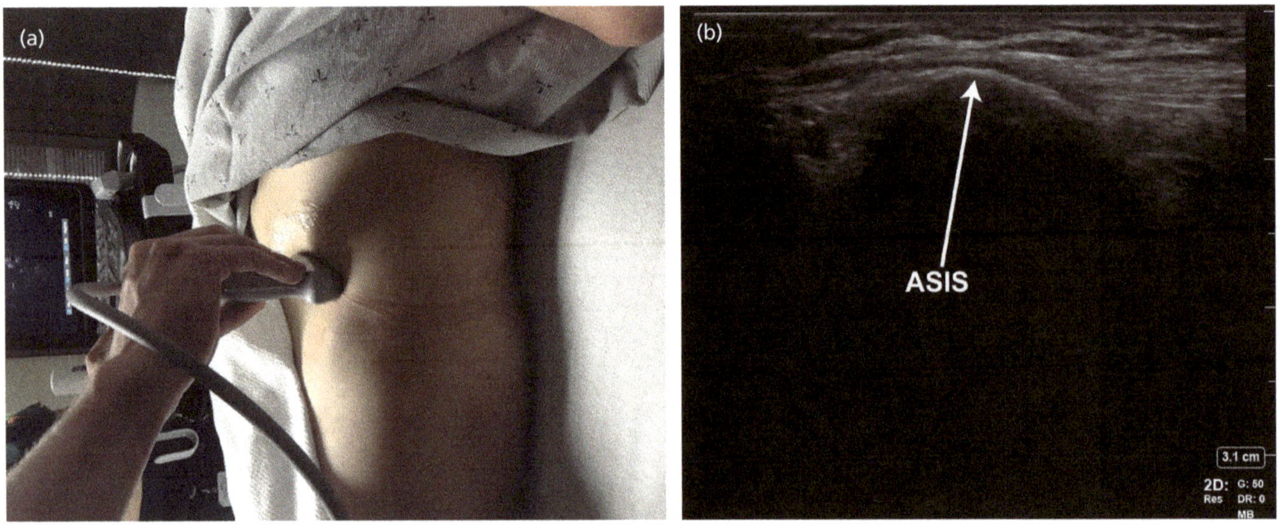

Figure 42.1 A—Ultrasound probe position. B—Ultrasound image of the anterior superior iliac spine (ASIS).

2. Slide medially and inferiorally, maintaining a view of the iliacus muscle (first muscle that is observed during this process)
3. Stop sliding medially once the sartorius and internal oblique muscles are clearly observed, with the iliacus muscle deep to these structures (Figure 42.2).

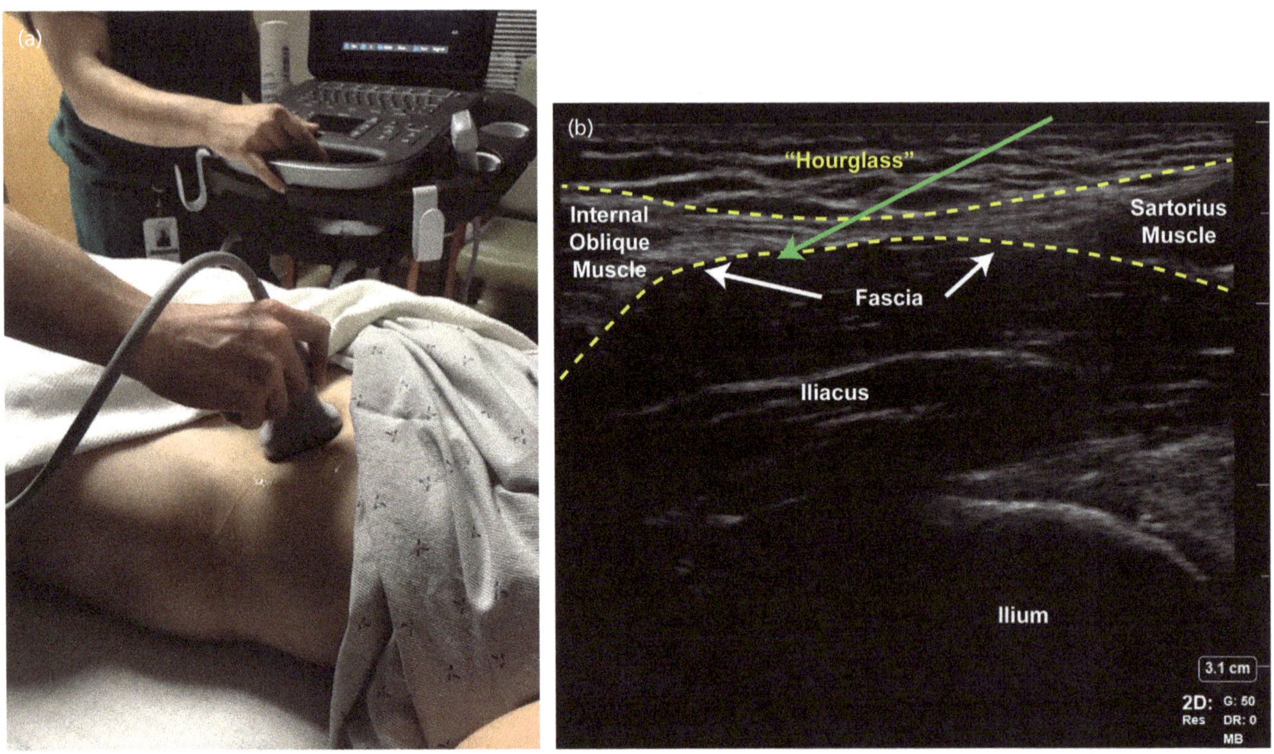

Figure 42.2 A—Ultrasound probe position to view fascia iliaca. B—Ultrasound image of "hourglass" with needle path represented by the blue line.

4. When performing the procedure, the needle is typically advanced in a caudal-to-cephalad approach and local anesthetic is deposited deep to the fascia of the iliacus muscle. Long-acting local anesthetic, 30 to 40 mL, is typically employed for this block.

2. Lateral Femoral Cutaneous Nerve

2.1. Introduction

The LFCN is a purely sensory nerve derived from the L2-L3 nerve roots. It supplies sensory innervation to the lateral aspect of the thigh (Figure 42.3). The LFCN, as part of the lumbar plexus, is included as part of a lumbar plexus block. It can also sometimes be simultaneously anesthetized via a femoral nerve block. Occasionally there arises the need to perform an individual LFCN block for surgeries such as a thigh skin graft harvest or for the diagnosis of meralgia paresthetica (a neuralgia of the LFCN).

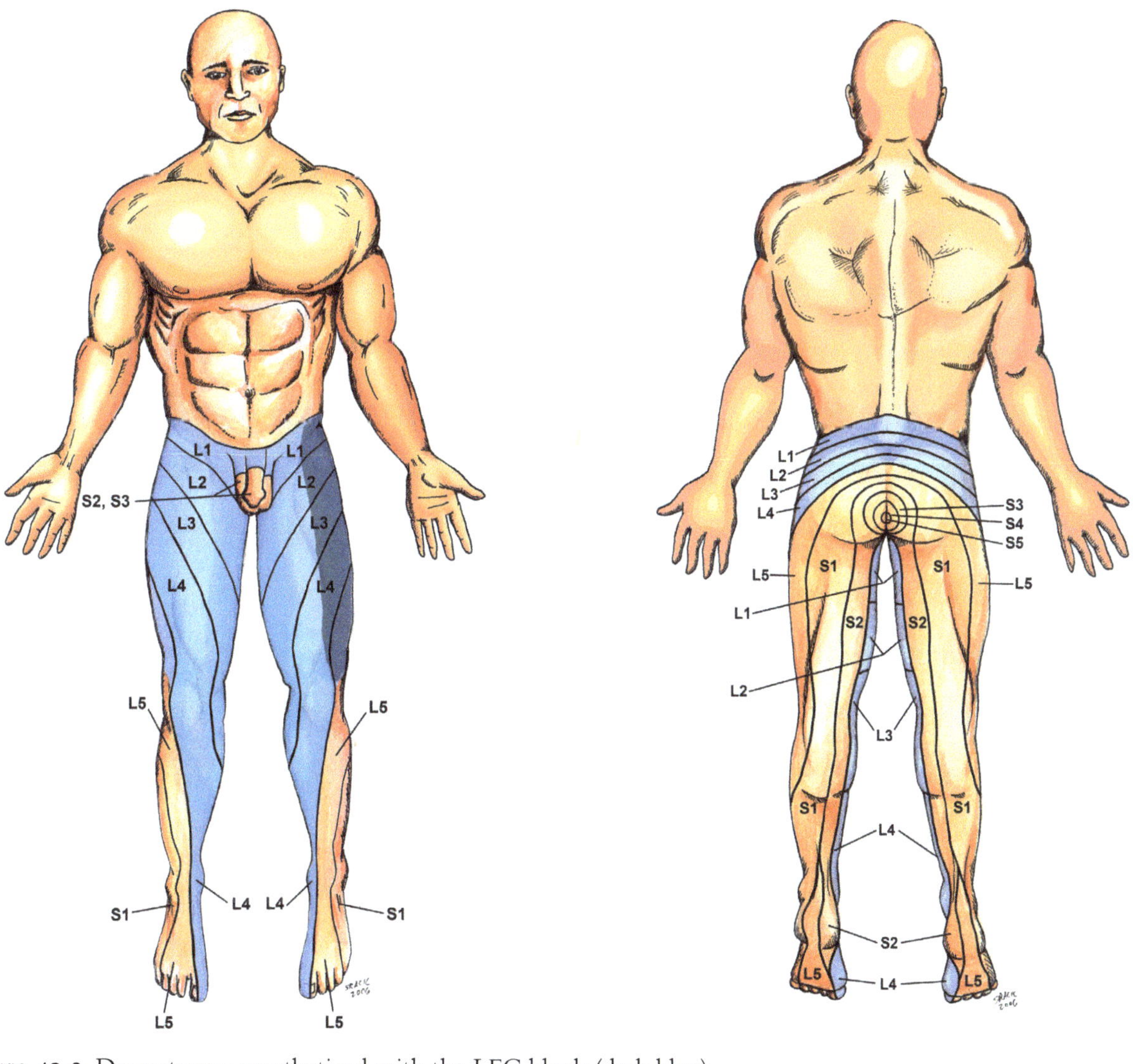

Figure 42.3 Dermatomes anesthetized with the LFC block (dark blue).

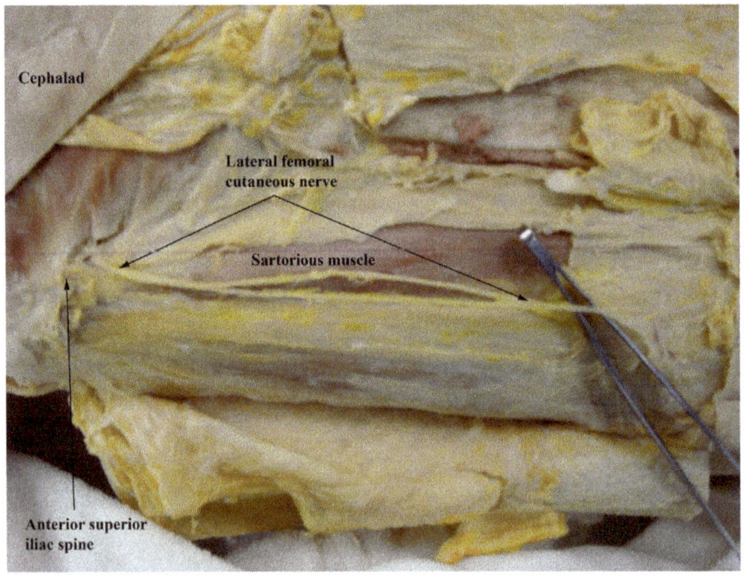

Figure 42.4 Dissection demonstrating the lateral femoral cutaneous nerve.

2.2. Anatomy

The LFCN emerges from the lumbar plexus and travels along the lateral aspect of the psoas muscle. It then crosses diagonally over the iliacus muscle. After passing beneath the inguinal ligament, it enters the thigh and passes medially to the ASIS. The anatomic relationship of the LFCN to the ASIS defines this block (Figure 42.4).

2.3. Procedure

Nerve stimulation is not typically used in this block as the LFCN is purely sensory. Find a point 2 cm caudal and 2 cm medial to the ASIS. Insert the needle perpendicular to all planes and advance needle until a loss of resistance is felt. This signifies the penetration of the fascia lata. Inject 5 mL of local anesthetic and then redirect the needle medially and then laterally, injecting an additional 5 mL at each of these points (Figure 42.5).

3. Block with Ultrasound Probe

3.1. Probe

- High frequency (10–12 MHz), linear.

3.2. Probe position

With the patient in the supine or lateral position, palpate for the ASIS and place the probe along the inguinal ligament. The lateral end of the transducer is placed on the ASIS. Scan medially and inferiorly from the ASIS. Identify the tensor fasciae latae and the sartorius muscle, with the goal to inject between the muscle bodies. The nerve will appear as a small hypoechoic oval structure between the previously mentioned structures in a short-axis view.

3.3. Approach and procedure

Insert the needle in plane, in a lateral to medial orientation, through the subcutaneous tissue and the tensor fasciae latae. A "pop" may be felt as the needle tip enters the plane between the tensor fascia latae and sartorius muscles. Gently

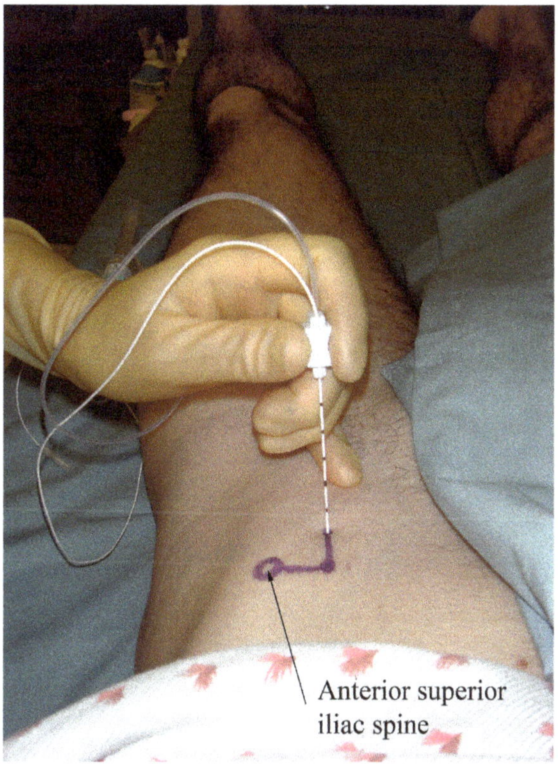

Figure 42.5 Needle position and external landmarks for the lateral femoral cutaneous nerve block.

aspirate, then inject 1 to 2 mL of local anesthetic to verify needle tip position; advance or withdraw and repeat as needed until in the correct plane. Usually 5 to 10 mL of local anesthetic is sufficient for successful block.

> **Teaching Points.** Fascia iliaca block, a variation of the LFCN block, is useful in adults and children. To perform it, draw a line from the ASIS to the pubic tubercle and divide it into thirds. Draw a line where the lateral and middle thirds meet, then insert the needle 1 cm caudally from that point. Two fascial "pops" will be felt, indicating the fascia lata and the fascia iliaca. After the second "pop," drop the needle to a 30° angle and advance it 1 cm. Slowly inject 30 mL of local anesthetic (Figure 42.6). Like the femoral "3-in-1" block, the fascia iliaca block often fails to anesthetize the obturator nerve.

4. Obturator Nerve Block

4.1. Introduction

The obturator nerve is a mixed sensory and motor (mainly motor) nerve originating from the anterior rami of L2-L4. It supplies sensory innervation to the medial aspect of the thigh (Figure 42.7) and motor innervation to the adductor muscles of the medial thigh (adductors longus, brevis, and magnus; gracilis and obturator externus muscles). Rarely is an isolated obturator nerve block performed; more commonly, the obturator nerve is blocked in addition to other anterior approaches to the lumbar plexus nerves.

4.2. Anatomy

The obturator nerve travels as a single nerve from the lumbar region toward the pelvis within the body of the psoas. It crosses the pelvis vertically, exiting from the obturator foramen (immediately below the superior pubic ramus), and

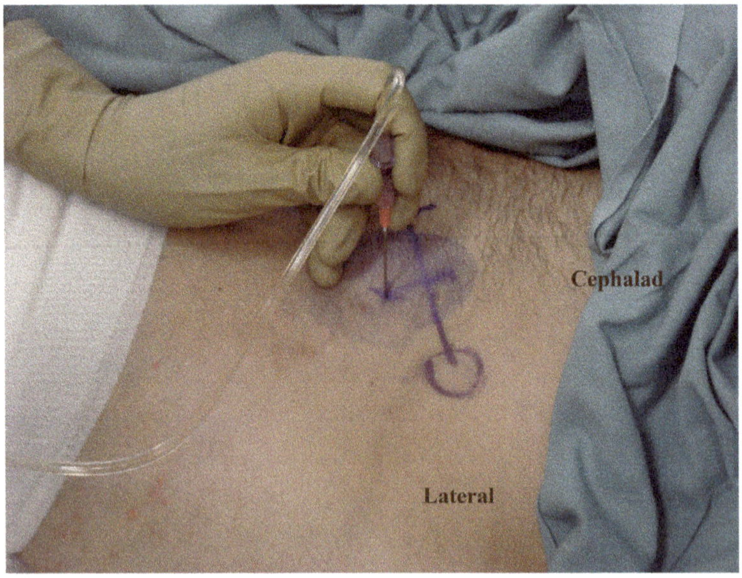

Figure 42.6 Needle position and external landmarks for the fascia iliaca block without ultrasound.

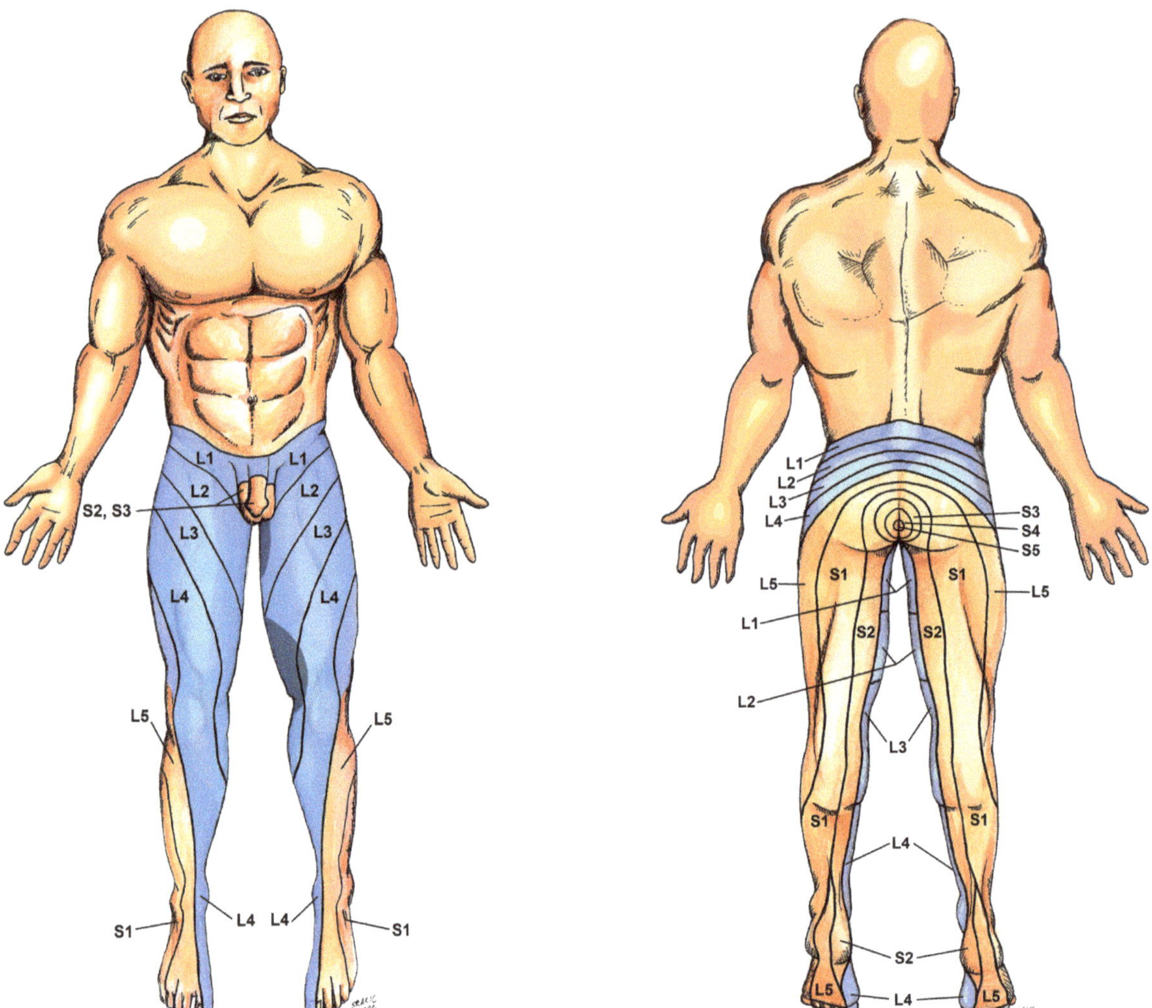

Figure 42.7 Dermatomes anesthetized with the obturator block (dark blue).

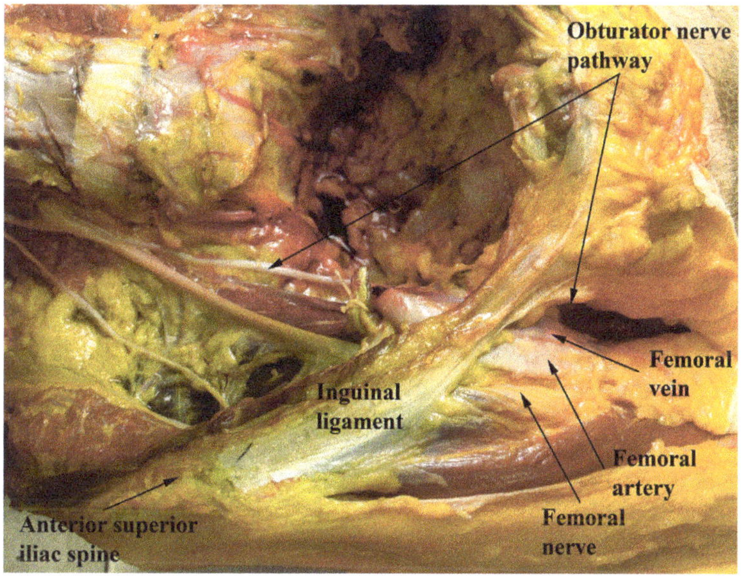

Figure 42.8 Psoas muscle has been removed.

divides into anterior and posterior terminal branches (Figure 42.8). The anterior branch supplies motor fibers to the anterior adductor muscles of the thigh, as well as cutaneous fibers to the medial aspect of the thigh. The posterior branch, which lacks cutaneous fibers, supplies motor fibers to the deep adductor muscles of the thigh, as well as contributing to the innervation of the knee joint.

4.3. Procedure

Set the nerve stimulator to 1.5 mA. With the patient supine with the thigh partially abducted and the knee partially flexed, palpate the pubic tubercle and draw a line 2 cm lateral and 2 cm inferior to the tubercle. At that point, insert a 5- to 10-cm stimulating needle perpendicular to the skin until it contacts the pubic ramus. Then redirect it posteriorly and slightly laterally to "walk off" the pubic ramus and into the obturator foramen. Once the adductor muscles begin to twitch, gradually decrease the stimulator until the twitch is still visible at 0.5 mA or less. At this point it is safe to inject 5 to 10 mL of local anesthetic (Figure 42.9).

5. Block with Ultrasound Probe

5.1. Probe

- High frequency (5–12 MHz), linear.

5.2. Probe position

Place the patient supine with the thigh slightly abducted and externally rotated. The transducer is placed in the femoral crease, and the femoral vessels are identified. The transducer is then swept medially along the crease to identify the adductor muscles and their fasciae. The anterior branch is found between the pectineus and adductor brevis muscles, and the posterior branch is found between the adductor brevis and adductor magnus muscles.

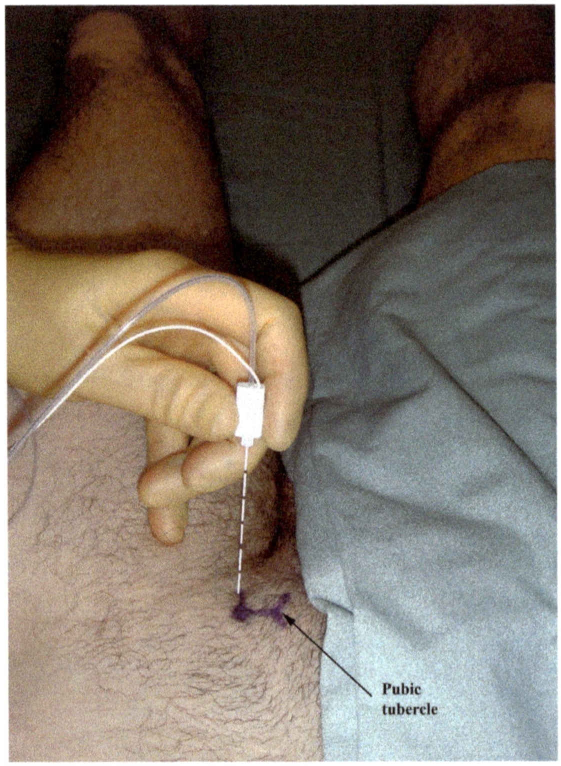

Figure 42.9 Needle position and external landmarks for the obturator nerve block.

5.3. Approach and injection

Advance the needle tip between the pectineus and adductor brevis at the junction of the middle and posterior third of their fascial interface. Inject 5 to 10 mL of local anesthetic. Then advance the needle farther so that it is between the adductor brevis and adductor magnus muscles. Again, inject 5 to 10 mL of local anesthetic. Care must be taken to ensure spread into the interfascial spaces and not into the muscles themselves, which may necessitate needle repositioning.

Teaching Points. The obturator nerve is often not blocked when a femoral or a fascia iliaca block is placed. For less invasive surgeries this may be a nonissue. For more invasive surgeries involving the thigh, it should be included. When it must be blocked, either perform a posterior approach to the lumbar plexus or block it separately, in addition to any other block of the lumbar plexus nerves.

6. Alternative Approach to the Obturator Nerve Block

There is an accessory obturator nerve (L3-L4) that sends a branch to the hip joint and is present in up to a third of patients. When the accessory obturator nerve is not present (71%–92% of cases), the posterior branch of the obturator nerve also sends a branch to the knee joint. The inguinal interadductor obturator nerve block approach landmarks are the inguinal ligament, femoral artery, and long adductor muscle tendon. Directly below the inguinal ligament, draw a line from the medial edge of the femoral pulse to the medial border of the tendon of the long adductor muscle. At the midpoint of this line, insert a 21-gauge, 10-cm insulated needle slightly lateral and posterior, with a superior inclination

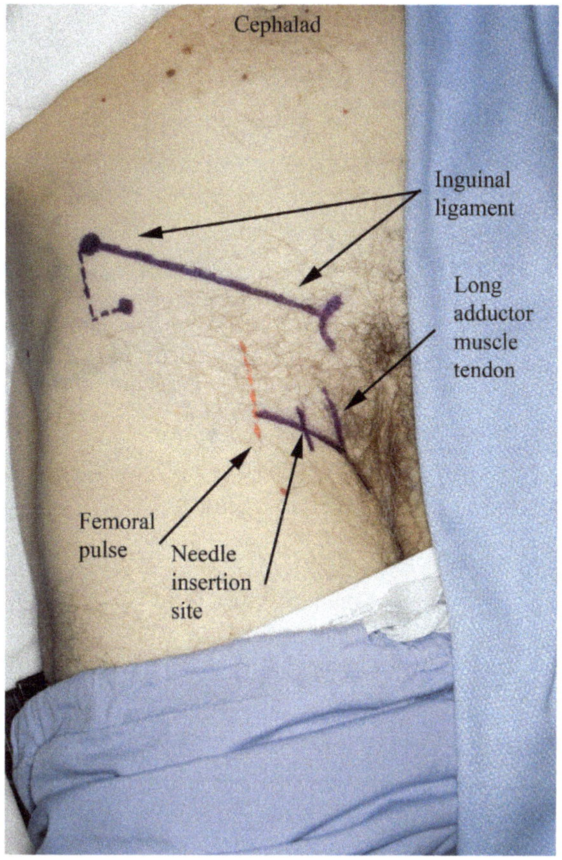

Figure 42.10 External landmarks for the inguinal interadductor obturator nerve block.

(Figures 42.10 and 42.11). Advance until the anterior adductor muscles twitch (anterior obturator branch) and then inject 5 to 7 mL of local anesthetic. Then advance the needle slowly a few millimeters in a slightly lateral direction until the posterior (major) adductor muscles twitch (posterior obturator branch) and inject another 5 to 7 mL of local anesthetic.

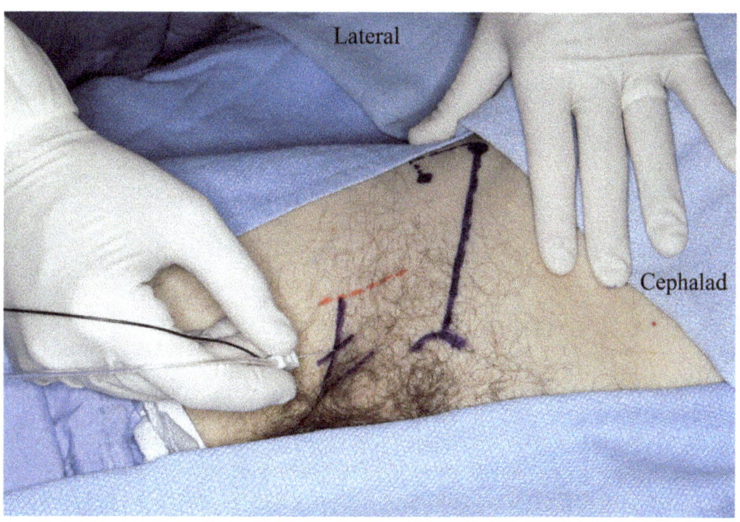

Figure 42.11 Needle position for the interadductor obturator nerve block.

7. Saphenous Nerve Block

7.1. Introduction

The saphenous nerve is the only nerve below the knee not derived from the sciatic nerve. It is a continuation of the femoral nerve. It provides cutaneous innervation over the medial portion of the lower leg. All other innervation, motor and sensory, to the lower leg comes from the sciatic nerve. The saphenous nerve can be blocked with either a lumbar plexus block, a femoral block, or an adductor canal block. It can also be individually blocked directly at the knee or the ankle (see chapter 47, "Ankle Block"). The saphenous nerve block is frequently combined with a sciatic nerve block to anesthetize the entire lower leg.

7.2. Anatomy

Derived from the L3-L4 nerve roots, the saphenous is the largest sensory branch of the femoral nerve. It innervates the medial aspect of the lower leg from just distal to the knee down to the medial malleolus (as far down as the great toe in some patients; Figure 42.12). It travels through the femoral triangle, lateral to the artery and vein, and then becomes more

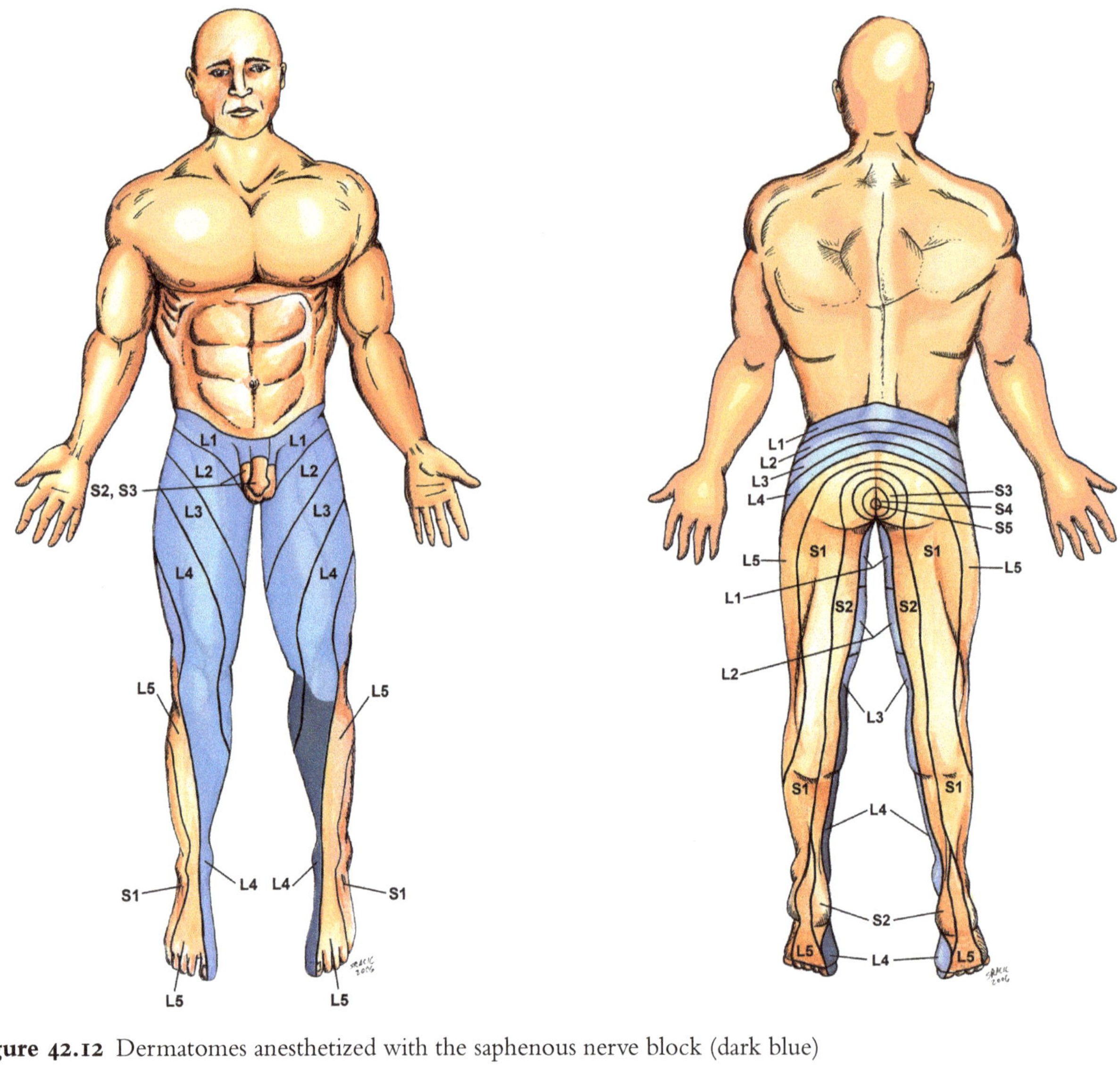

Figure 42.12 Dermatomes anesthetized with the saphenous nerve block (dark blue)

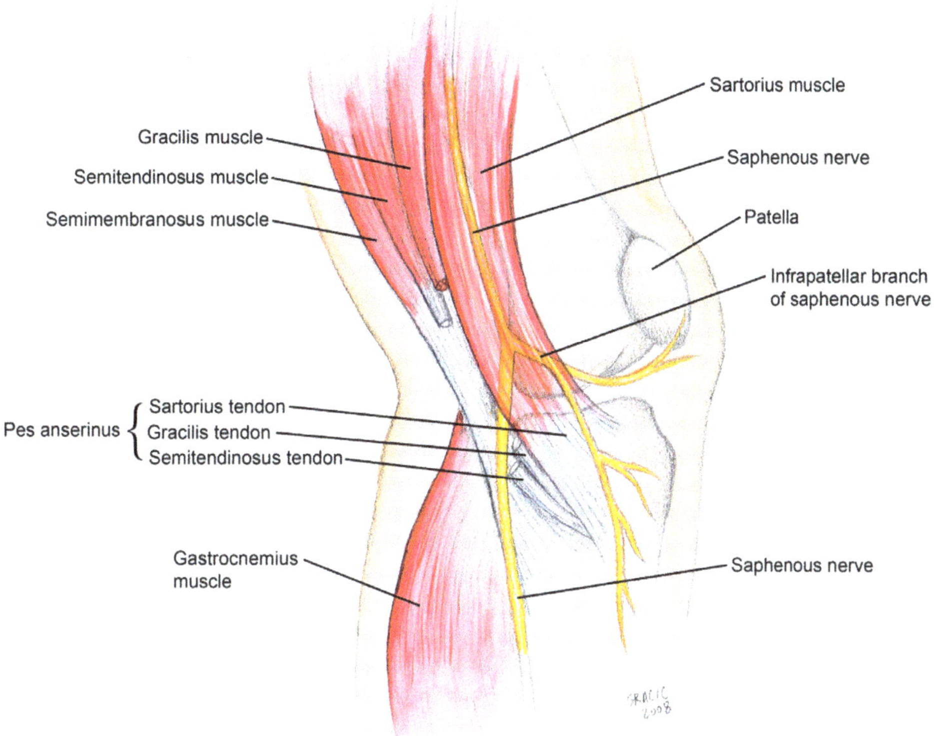

Figure 42.13 Saphenous nerve anatomy at the knee.

superficial as it courses between the sartorius and gracilis muscles (Figure 42.13). Below the knee, it travels with the great saphenous vein. The transsartorial approach is commonly used for a saphenous block (Figure 42.14). Others described later in this chapter include the paravenous, simple field block, and ultrasound-guided approaches.

Teaching Points. For below-knee tourniquet placement, a saphenous nerve block is adequate; otherwise a femoral block would be more appropriate for a thigh tourniquet.

8. Procedure

8.1. Transsartorial approach

The patient should be supine with the leg extended and actively elevated 2 inches. The sartorius muscle is identified medially over the leg just above the knee. Insert a needle 1 to 2 cm above the patella and pass it through the body of the sartorius muscle (Figure 41.3). Look for a loss of resistance indicating subsartorial adipose, aspirate, and then deposit 10 mL of local anesthetic. The distance from skin to loss of resistance is roughly 1.5 to 3.0 cm.

8.2. Paravenous approach

The saphenous nerve lies medial and posterior to the saphenous vein. Place a tourniquet around the leg and hang the leg over the side of the bed for 1 minute so the vein may become identifiable. Once the vein is identified, inject 5 mL of local anesthetic subcutaneously on both sides of the vein below the patella.

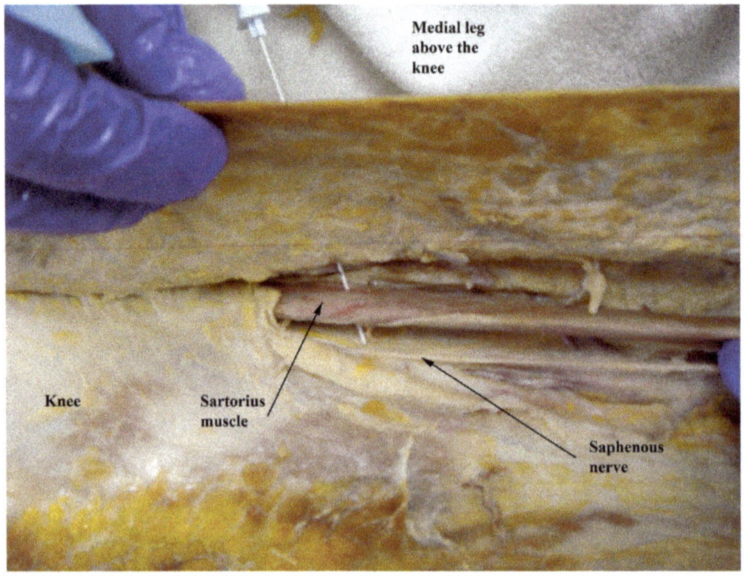

Figure 42.14 Dissection of the saphenous nerve.

8.3. Below-knee field block approach

The patient should be supine. Palpate the tibial tuberosity and inject 5 to 10 mL of local anesthetic into the subcutaneous tissue. Begin at the medial aspect of the tibial tuberosity and inject up to the medial gastrocnemius muscle.

> **Teaching Points.** The saphenous nerve has many smaller branches, and as such a complete block of the entire nerve is very difficult at or below the knee. A femoral nerve block or adductor canal block is recommended if the operative field will include the medial aspect of the lower leg.

9. Ultrasound-Guided Adductor Canal Block

9.1. Introduction

This block is indicated for surgery of the knee, such as total knee arthroplasty or anterior cruciate ligament repair. It provides blockade of the sensory innervation of the knee joint while mostly sparing the motor function of the quadriceps muscle. The adductor canal is also known as Hunter's canal or the subsartorial canal. It is an aponeurotic intermuscular tunnel in the middle third of the thigh.

9.2. Anatomy

The canal is roughly triangular in cross section and bordered by 3 muscles: the vastus medialis anterolaterally, the sartorius medially, and the adductor magnus posteriorly. This muscular tunnel extends from the upper, anterior thigh to the lower, medial thigh. Approximately 12 to 14 cm proximal to the knee, there is a distal opening in the adductor magnus muscle; this opening is known as the adductor hiatus. The adductor canal houses the femoral artery, the femoral vein, the posterior branch of the obturator nerve, and branches of the femoral nerve, specifically the saphenous nerve and nerve to vastus medialis (Figure 42.15)

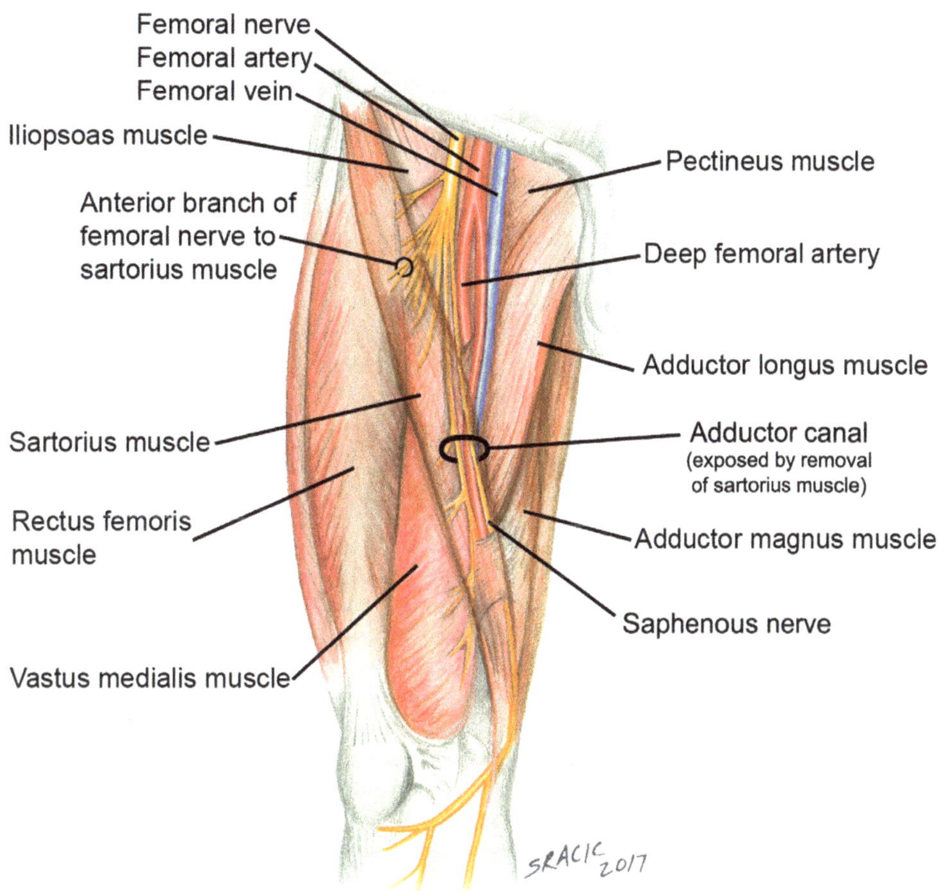

Figure 42.15 Saphenous nerve anatomy.

10. Block with Ultrasound Probe

10.1. Probe

- High frequency (5–12 MHz), linear.

10.2. Probe position

Place the patient supine with the thigh abducted and externally rotated. Place the probe along the medial thigh approximately at the midpoint between the inguinal crease and the medial condyle. Identify the femoral artery, scan cephalad, and track distally if necessary. Identify the sartorius muscle and the canal deep to it. Of note, the saphenous nerve is almost always too small to be reliably imaged; the aim of the technique is to inject local anesthetic under the sartorius and around the femoral artery (within the adductor canal). The probe should be placed just proximal to where the femoral artery dives posteriorly to become the popliteal artery. The probe should be perpendicular to artery (Figure 42.16).

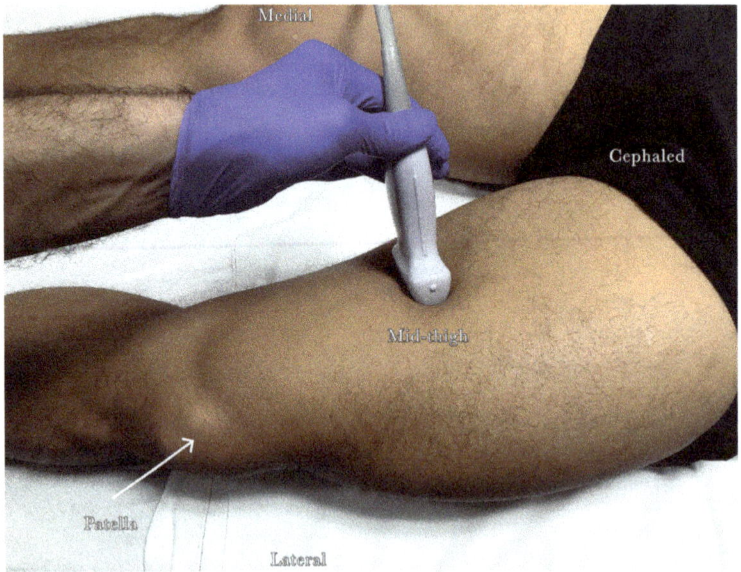

Figure 42.16 Adductor canal surface anatomy.

10.3. Approach and injection

Insert the needle using an in-plane approach from lateral to medial. Advance the needle into the adductor canal. Aspirate prior to injection of the test dose and look for spread of local anesthetic within the adductor canal. If you cannot clearly see the spread, be sure to reposition. Once assured of correct placement within the adductor canal, inject 20 to 25 mL of local anesthetic (Figure 42.17).

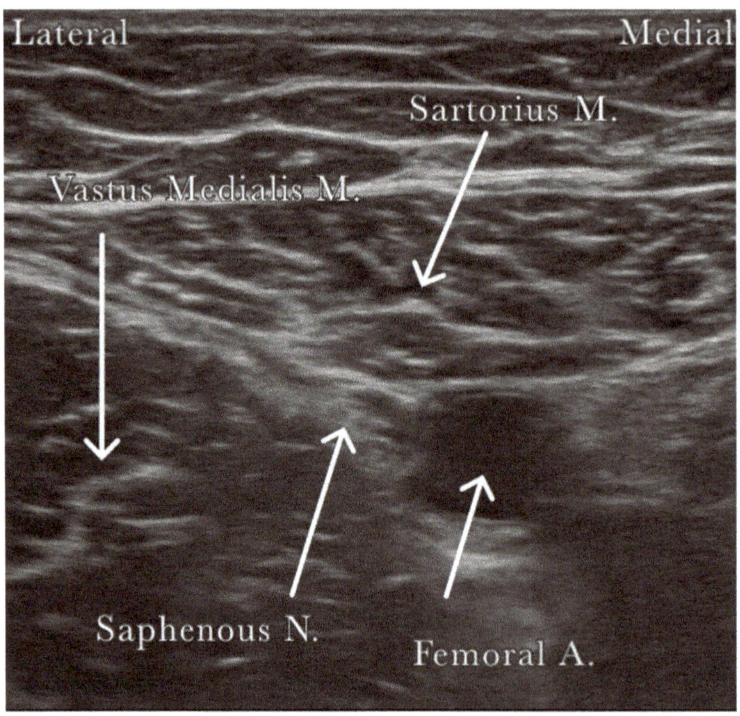

Figure 42.17 Ultrasound image of adductor canal block.

Sciatic Nerve Block: Posterior and Alternative Approaches

43

1. Introduction

The sciatic nerve supplies motor and sensory innervations to the posterior aspect of the thigh as well as to the entire lower leg (except for the medial leg, which is supplied by the saphenous nerve). It is the single largest nerve in the body and can be blocked at several locations along the lower extremity. The classic approach, Labat's, targets the nerve while in the gluteal region. Other sciatic nerve blocks involve different approaches and allow for different positioning; they will be discussed in subsequent sections of the book. Sciatic nerve blocks require adequate setup time because this large nerve resists local anesthetic penetration; this subsequently leads to longer time to block onset. For complete anesthesia of the leg below the knee, the saphenous nerve must also be blocked directly or by an adductor canal block or femoral block.

2. Anatomy

The sciatic nerve arises from the ventral rami of L4-S3 and is actually 2 nerves in close proximity, the tibial and common peroneal (fibular) nerves. They are enclosed in one common preineural sheath and usually do not separate until the level of the midthigh (separation as proximal as the pelvis can occur in up to 12% of the population). The sciatic nerve leaves the pelvis via the greater sciatic foramen and travels under the gluteus maximus (Figure 43.1) and continues distally between the greater trochanter and ischial tuberosity toward the posterior thigh (Figure 43.2). It does not innervate any muscles in the gluteal region, but does give motor innervation to posterior thigh muscles. Its primary function involves motor innervation to all muscles of the lower leg and foot, as well as providing sensory innervations to the skin of most of the leg and foot (Figure 43.3).

Teaching Points. Of the various approaches to the sciatic nerve, Labat's posterior technique (first described in 1924) has the advantage of also blocking the posterior femoral cutaneous nerve (PFCN). PFCN provides sensory innervations to the gluteus and uppermost medial and posterior thigh.

It has been suggested that blocking the PFCN is important when thigh tourniquets are to be used. However, in clinical practice a block of the femoral nerve provides sufficient tourniquet coverage in most cases.

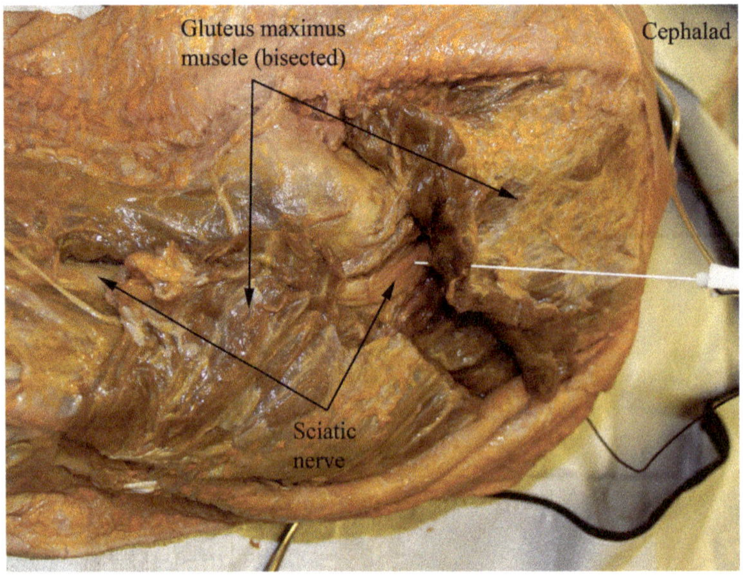

Figure 43.1 Dissected proximal sciatic nerve.

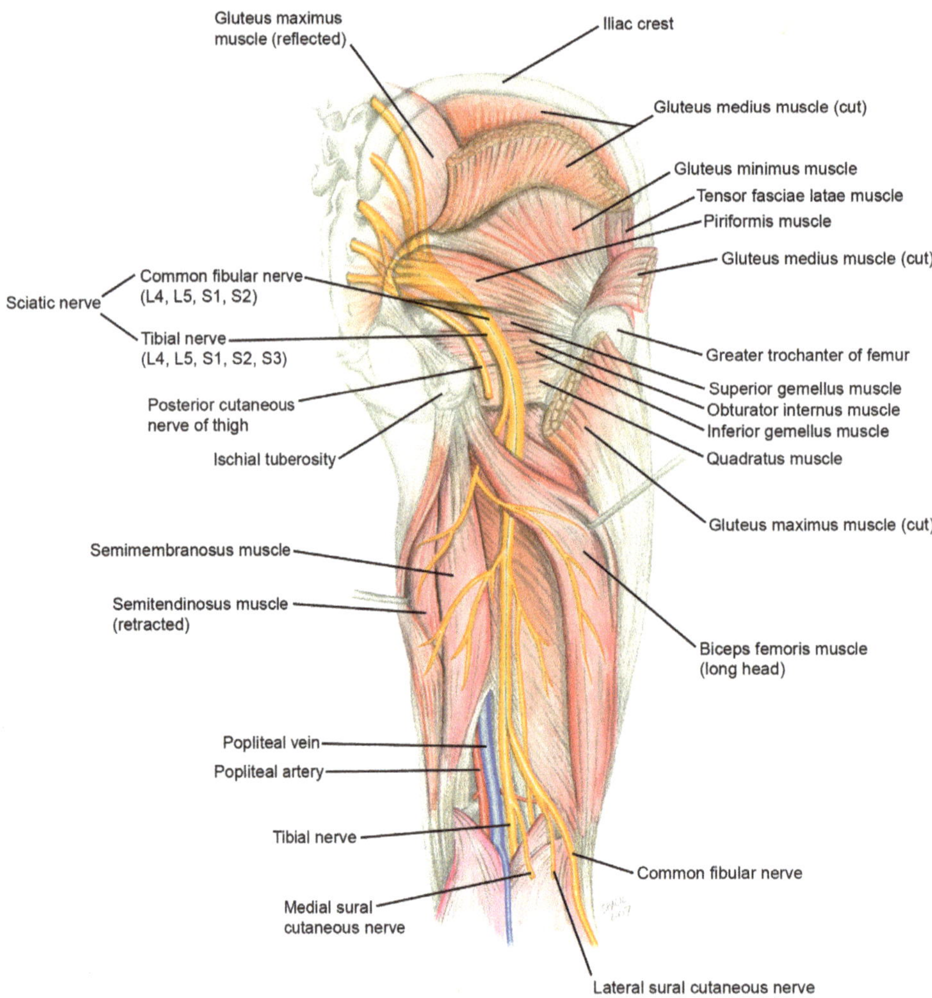

Figure 43.2 Sciatic nerve anatomy.

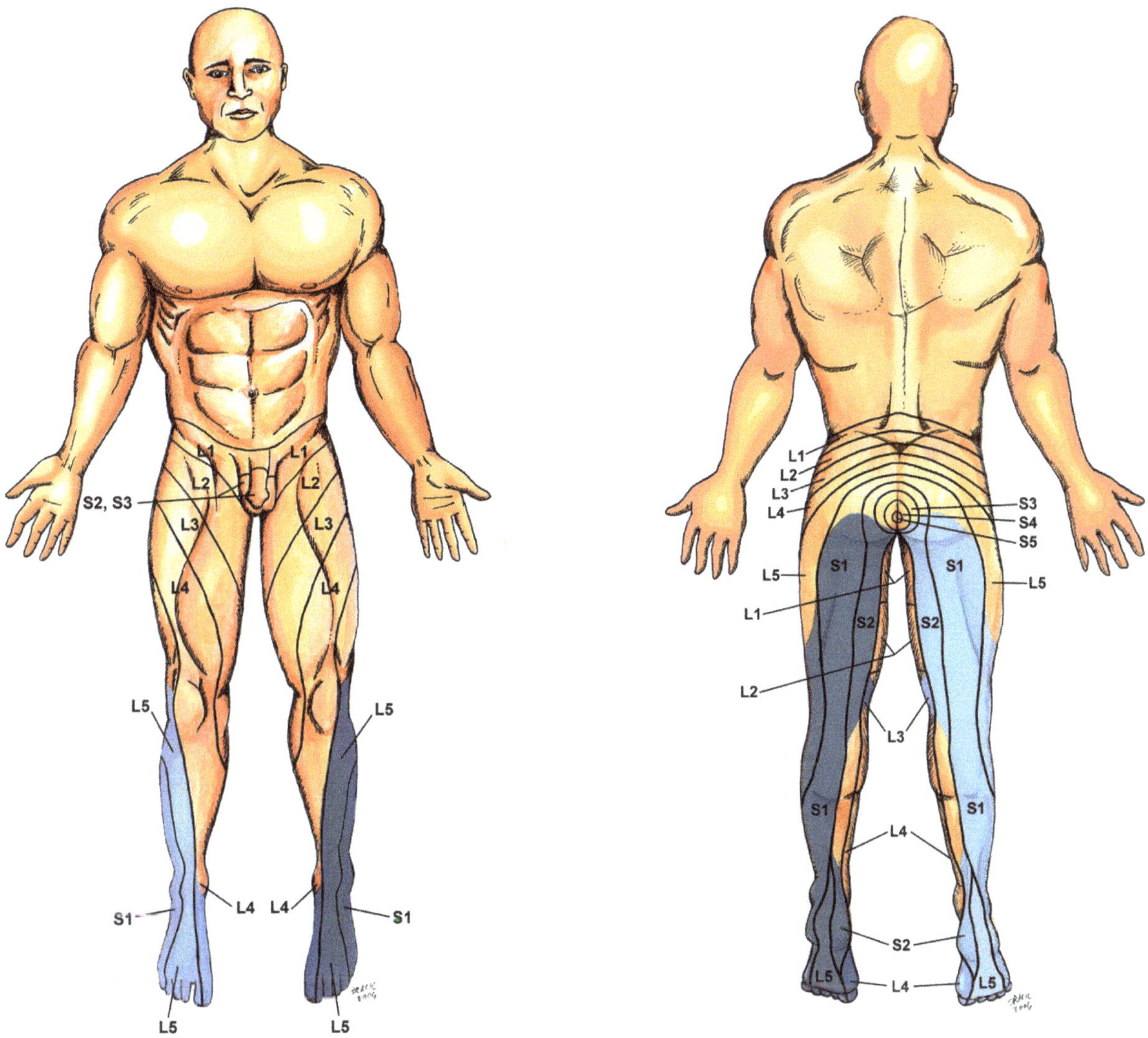

Figure 43.3 Dermatomes anesthetized with a proximal block of the sciatic nerve (dark blue).

3. Procedure

3.1. Landmarks

In the classic Labat's approach, place the patient in the lateral decubitus position with the leg flexed at the knee (if unable to flex the leg, attempt to extend at the hip as far as possible without causing discomfort). Draw a line from the greater trochanter to the posterior superior iliac spine (PSIS). Draw a second line from the greater trochanter to the sacral hiatus (Winnie's modification). Then draw a perpendicular line from the midpoint of the first line to its intersection with the second line; this point will determine the point of needle insertion. A fourth line can be drawn along the "furrow" formed by the medial edge of the gluteus maximus muscle and the long head of the biceps femoris muscle (Figure 43.4). The furrow represents the course of the sciatic nerve as it traverses toward the lower leg. The triangle formed by the first, second, and fourth lines also defines initial needle placement. Adjusting the needle within the triangle can improve success at sciatic nerve stimulation.

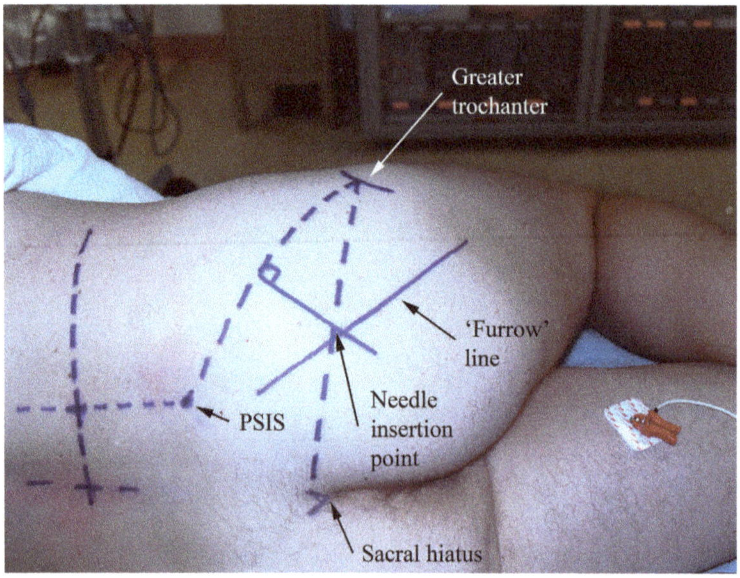

Figure 43.4 Landmarks for posterior approach to the sciatic nerve.

3.2. Needles

- 21-gauge, 10-cm insulated needle (15-cm needle for obese patients may be needed).
- 18-gauge, 10-cm insulated Tuohy needle for catheter placement. Catheter placed 3 to 5 cm beyond needle tip.

3.3. Stimulation

Set the nerve stimulator at 1.0 to 1.5 mA and insert the needle perpendicularly (Figure 43.5). Stimulation of the gluteus maximus muscle is often encountered just before sciatic nerve stimulation; the needle should be advanced through gluteus stimulation without pause as this can be uncomfortable for patients. Plantar flexion/inversion (tibial nerve) or

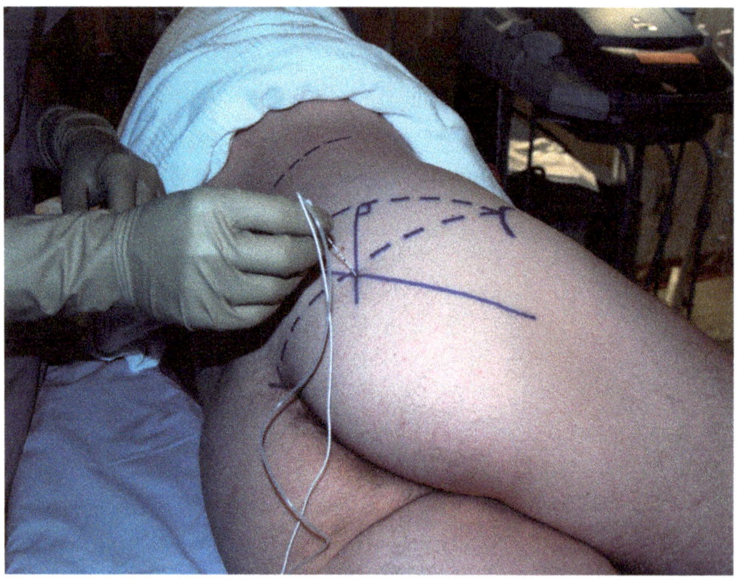

Figure 43.5 Needle position for Labat's approach to the sciatic nerve block.

dorsiflexion/eversion (common peroneal nerve) with 0.5 mA is indicative of successful needle placement in proximity to the sciatic nerve. If hamstring muscle twitch is elicited, the needle has been placed too far medially and can be corrected with a slight lateral adjustment.

3.4. Local Anesthetic

20 to 30 mL of local anesthetic is sufficient.

Teaching Points. Complete anesthesia of the lower extremity can be achieved with a proximal sciatic nerve block and a lumbar plexus block (femoral nerve block often misses the obturator nerve).

Labat's approach is well suited for continuous catheter techniques. Plantar flexion of the foot (tibial nerve stimulation) results in shorter onset times and more frequent success of the block as opposed to dorsiflexion (common peroneal nerve). The addition of the furrow line can be especially useful in obese patients, when palpation of traditional landmarks is difficult.

4. Ultrasound-Guided Posterior Sciatic Nerve Block

4.1. Probe

- Curved low frequency (2–5 MHz) or linear high frequency (5–12 MHz) linear probe used.

4.2. Probe position

Place the patient in the lateral decubitus position (operative side up) and draw a line between the greater trochanter and the ischial tuberosity; the sciatic nerve should bisect the midpoint. The probe should be placed directly on the line perpendicular to the sciatic nerve to allow a transverse view (Figure 43.6). The ischial tuberosity should be seen medially with the greater trochanter laterally as hyperechoic curved structures on the sides of the screen. The sciatic nerve is

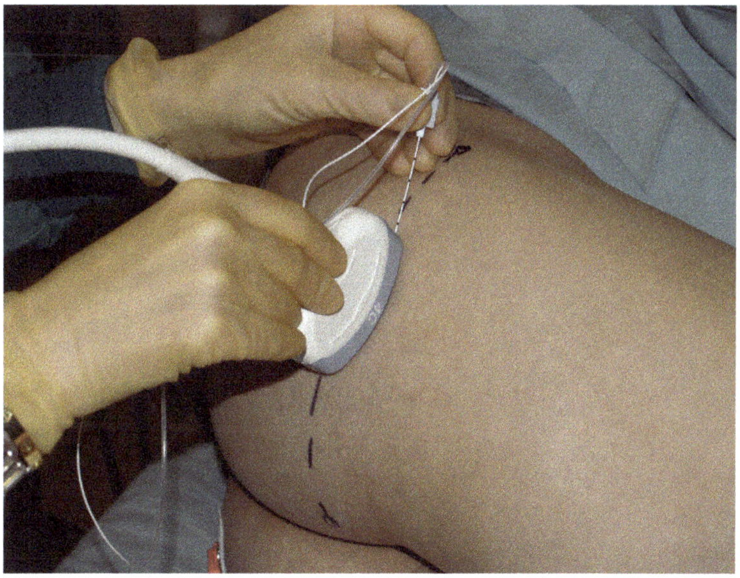

Figure 43.6 Ultrasound probe and needle position for infragluteal sciatic nerve block.

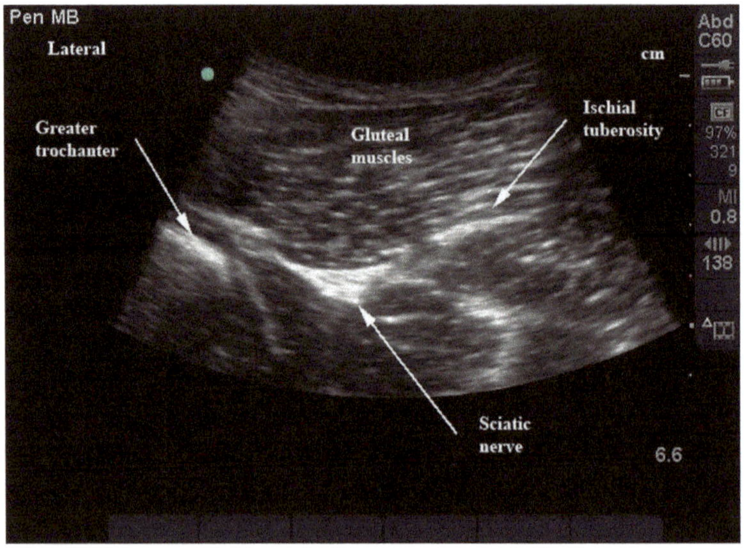

Figure 43.7 Ultrasound image of the sciatic nerve, infragluteal.

located between the 2 landmarks and appears as an elliptical hyperechoic structure (Figure 43.7). The ultrasound probe can be turned 90° to place the nerve in profile, allowing the operator to confirm the nerve as it passes proximal toward the sacrum and distal down the posterior leg.

4.3. Approach and injection

Insert the needle from the lateral aspect of the probe for an "in-plane approach." This approach is preferred because a medial approach will likely have the inferior gluteal artery as an obstacle to the nerve. At this level, the sciatic nerve is located within a discrete subgluteal space located between the anterior surface of the gluteus maximus muscle and the posterior surface of the quadratus femoris muscle. With proper needle placement, 20 to 30 mL of local anesthetic will surround the nerve in an optimal fashion. If this is not achieved, the needle can be adjusted to gain further local spread of local anesthetic around the nerve (Figure 43.8).

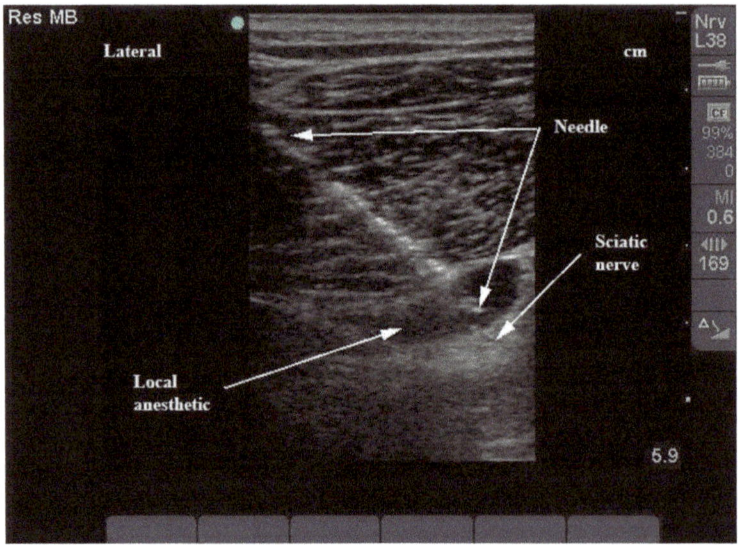

Figure 43.8 Ultrasound image demonstrating local anesthetic injection around the sciatic nerve, infragluteal.

Teaching Points. Use the low-frequency curved probe first to easily identify the sciatic nerve as well as both the greater trochanter and the ischial tuberosity. If only one of the landmarks is visible, increase ultrasound depth to view the other. Once the sciatic nerve is correctly identified, depth can again be decreased to focus only on the nerve. Following nerve identification, a high-frequency linear probe can be used to increase nerve resolution for insertion of the needle and injection of local anesthetic.

5. Alternative Approaches To The Sciatic Nerve Block

5.1. RAJ technique

This posterior approach allows the patient to remain supine. The hip and knee are flexed to a 90° angle (the foot rests on a Mayo stand or is held up by an assistant). This positioning allows for the sciatic nerve to become more superficial as the gluteal muscles are stretched and flattened out. Draw a line connecting the greater trochanter and ischial tuberosity. Insert a 10-cm needle perpendicularly to the midpoint of the line (Figure 43.9).

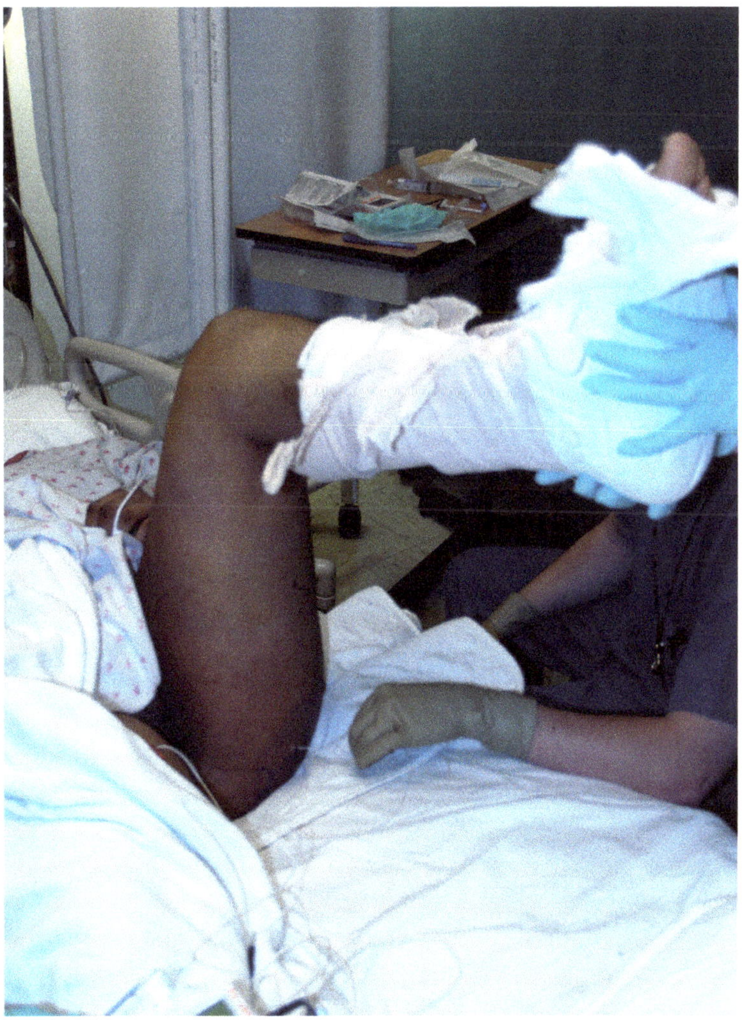

Figure 43.9 Positioning for Raj technique for the sciatic nerve block.

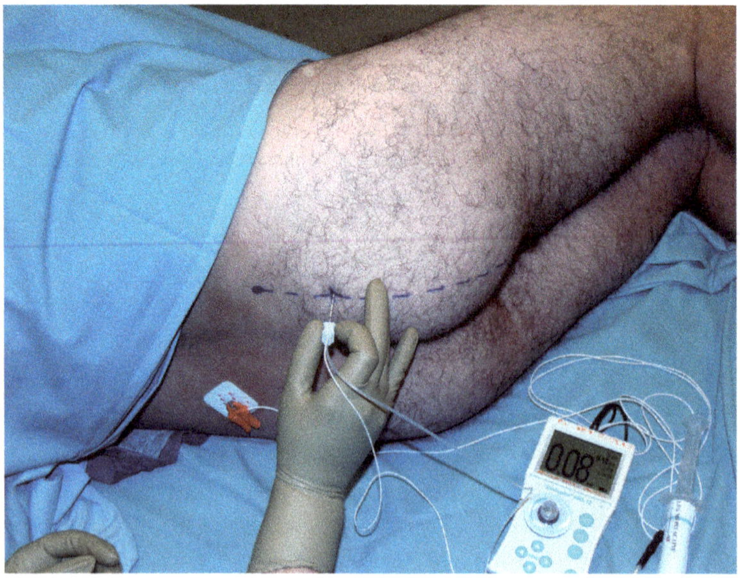

Figure 43.10 Needle position and external landmarks for the parasacral approach to the sciatic nerve block.

> **Teaching Points.** The same landmarks can also be utilized to perform this block in a lateral position.

5.2. Parasacral Technique

This is the most proximal approach to the sciatic nerve, targeting it in the greater sciatic foramen. Place the patient in the lateral decubitus position. This approach will also generally block the obturator nerve, thus enabling the entire lower extremity to be anesthetized with a sciatic and femoral nerve block. Draw a line connecting the PSIS and the ischial tuberosity. Insert a 10-cm needle 6 cm caudal to the PSIS. If bone is contacted, "walk off" the needle caudally until it advances through the sciatic foramen. The nerve is usually found 6 to 7 cm deep (Figure 43.10).

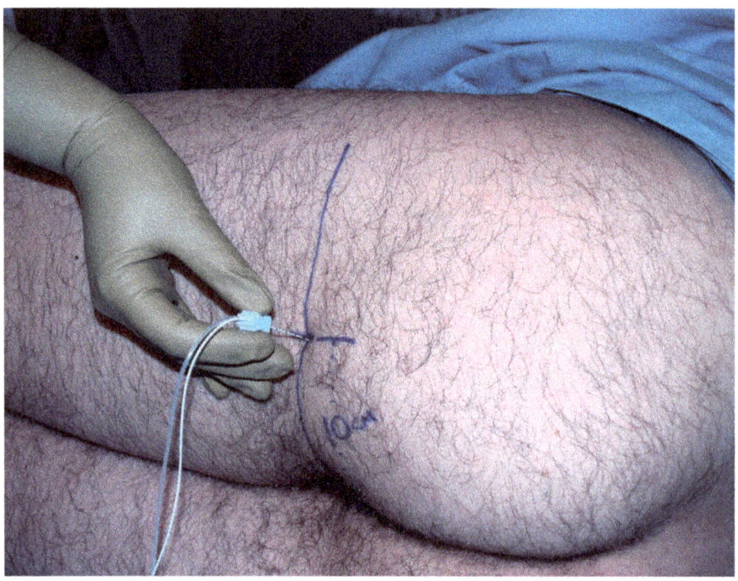

Figure 43.11 Needle position and external landmarks for the subgluteal approach to the sciatic nerve block.

5.3. Midline Technique

There are 2 midline techniques that target the sciatic nerve 10 cm lateral to the midline of the pelvis described by Franco. The first is a midgluteal approach performed with the patient prone. Insert a 10-cm needle at the midpoint of the intergluteal sulcus 10 cm lateral to the midline. Advance the needle parallel to the midline and perpendicular to the bed. If no nerve stimulation response is elicited, adjust the needle slightly medial or lateral. The second technique is a subgluteal approach with the patient in the lateral decubitus position with flexed hips and knees. Insert the needle in the subgluteal fold 10 cm from the intergluteal sulcus, directing it parallel to the bed (Figure 43.11).

44

Sciatic Nerve Block: Anterior Approach

1. Introduction

The anterior approach is useful in patients who are unable to assume a lateral decubitus position (Figure 44.1). It is a deep block that often requires a 15-cm needle and is associated with slightly more discomfort than other approaches. The proximity of the femoral artery anterior to the sciatic nerve in this position increases the risk of inadvertent arterial puncture. Continuous block techniques have been described with this approach, but are somewhat unpopular in the United States.

2. Procedure

2.1. Landmarks

With a supine patient, draw a line from the anterior superior iliac spine to the pubic tubercle, and divide it into thirds. Draw a second line, parallel to the first, medial from the cephalad aspect of the greater trochanter. Then, draw a third line perpendicular from the medial third of the first line until it intersects with the second line. This intersection, located over the lesser trochanter of the femur, will serve as the point of initial needle insertion (Figures 44.2 and 44.3). The lesser trochanter obstructs the route to the sciatic nerve when the leg and foot are in neutral position; internal rotation of the leg by 45° exposes the nerve and allows the needle easy passage to the nerve.

2.2. Needles

- 21-gauge, 15-cm insulated needle.
- 18-gauge, 15-cm insulated Tuohy needle for catheter placement. Catheter placed 5 cm beyond needle tip. Catheters are not recommended.

2.3. Stimulation

Set nerve stimulator at 1.5 mA and advance the needle perpendicularly. If bone is contacted, withdraw and rotate the leg internally. Advance in the same plane as before until a twitch is elicited. If bone is contacted again, the initial insertion site may be distal to the lesser trochanter. In this situation withdraw the needle and externally

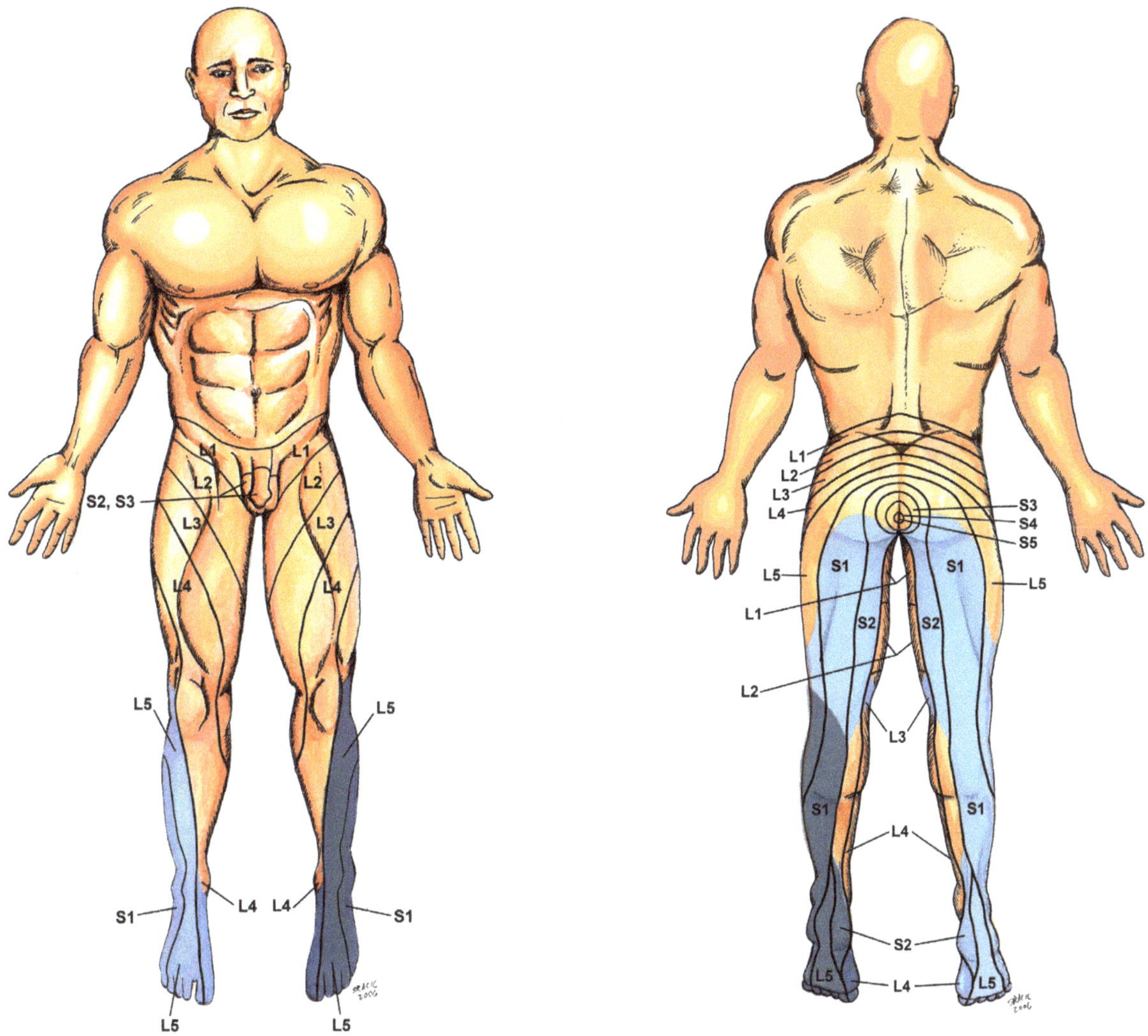

Figure 44.1 Dermatomes anesthetized with the anterior sciatic nerve block (dark blue).

rotate the leg 45° and re-advance the needle. Elicitation of plantar flexion/inversion or dorsiflexion/eversion at 0.5 mA or less are the sought-after endpoints for correct placement. Stimulation of the hamstring suggests the needle is deep to the nerve (Figure 44.4).

2.4. Local anesthetic

25–30 mL of local anesthetic is sufficient.

3. Ultrasound-Guided Anterior Sciatic Nerve Block

3.1. Probe

- Low frequency (2–5 MHz), curvilinear probe.

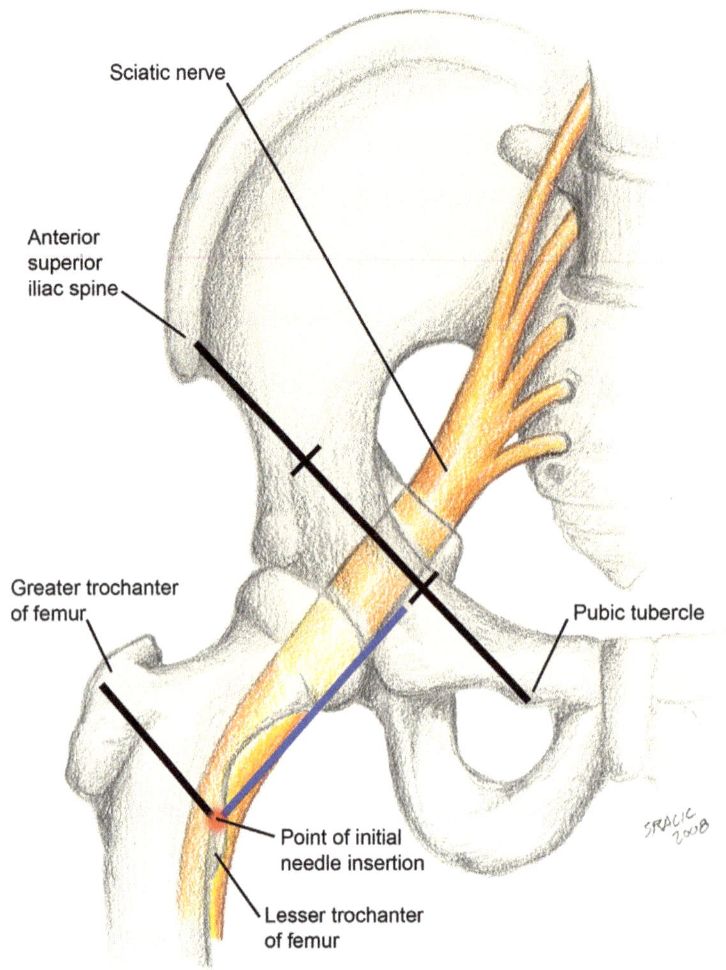

Figure 44.2 Landmarks for anterior sciatic nerve block.

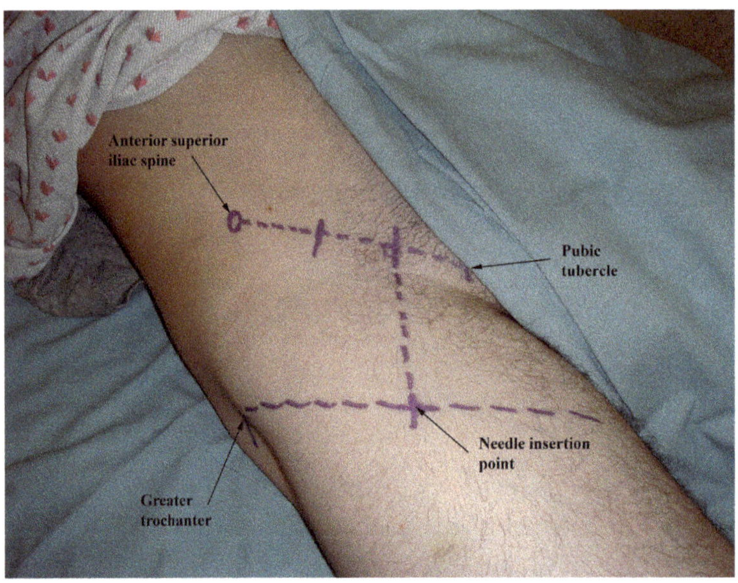

Figure 44.3 External landmarks for anterior sciatic nerve block.

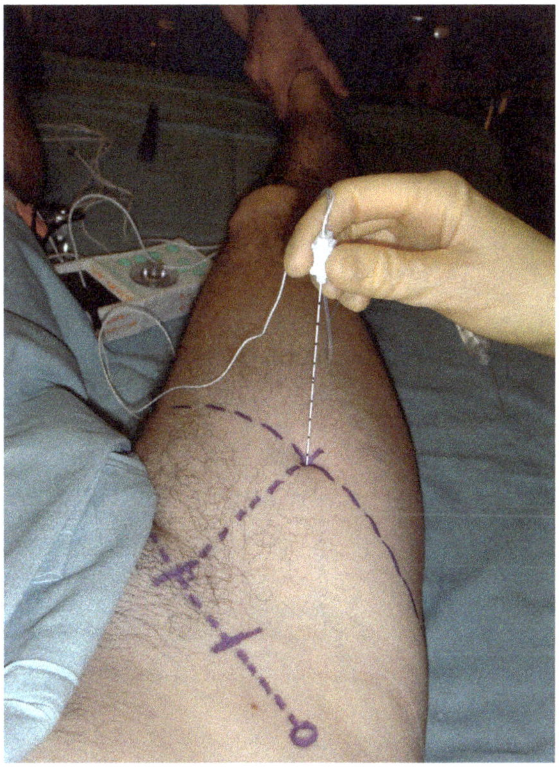

Figure 44.4 Needle position for anterior sciatic nerve block.

3.2. Probe position

The patient is placed supine, with the hip and the knee mildly flexed to facilitate exposure. The transducer is placed approximately 7 cm distal to the inguinal crease in a transverse fashion on the anteromedial aspect of the thigh (Figure 44.5). Obtain a view of the femur and visualize the lesser trochanter. Then slide the probe medially. The sciatic nerve should

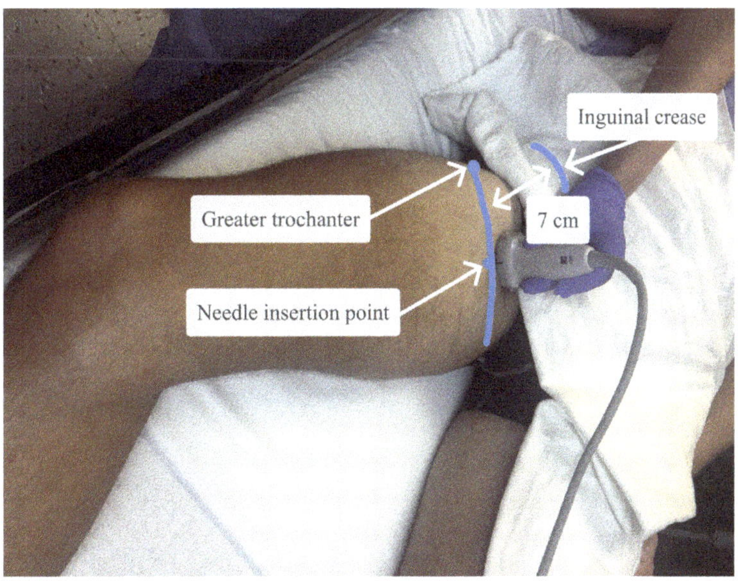

Figure 44.5 Ultrasound probe positioning for anterior sciatic block.

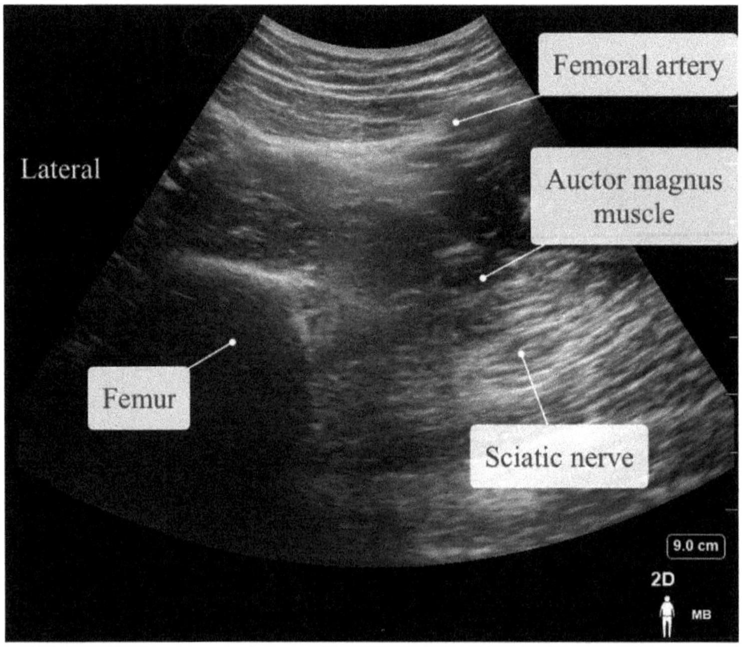

Figure 44.6 Ultrasound anatomy of anterior sciatic block.

appear as an hyperechoic structure between the adductor magnus muscle anteriorly and the gluteus maximus muscle posteriorly (Figure 44.6). If the patient is able to dorsiflex and/or plantar flex the ankle, this maneuver often causes the nerve to rotate or otherwise move within the muscular planes, facilitating identification.

3.3. Approach and injection

With the sciatic nerve identified, insert a 10- to 15-cm needle in plane from the medial aspect of the thigh and advanced toward the sciatic nerve. Once the needle tip is in position near the nerve, inject 1 to 2 mL of local anesthetic to confirm the adequate distribution. The needle position may need to be adjusted some if there is improper spread of local anesthetic or nerve displacement. Twenty milliliters of local anesthetic is usually adequate for successful blockade.

Teaching Points. This approach typically does not reliably block the posterior cutaneous nerve of the thigh.

Sciatic Nerve Block: Lateral Approach

45

1. Introduction

This approach has the advantage of the patient being supine. It may be technically easier than the anterior block and covers the same dermatomes (see Figure 43.3); the needle depth is shallower, thus making it more comfortable. This block of the sciatic nerve is typically performed more distally on the leg, just proximal to the popliteal fossa (Figure 45.1). Due to the more distal approach, care must be taken to ensure adequate anesthesia and analgesia of both the tibial and the common peroneal nerves. Larger volumes of local anesthetic are used to ensure adequate distribution.

2. Procedure

2.1. Landmarks

Palpate the popliteal crease and then palpate approximately 10 cm cephalad in the groove between the vastus lateralis and the biceps femoris muscles (Figure 45.2). If these are difficult to identify, flex the knee.

2.2. Needles

- 21-gauge, 10-cm insulated needle.
- 18-gauge, 10-cm insulated Tuohy needle for catheter placement. Catheter placed 5 cm beyond needle tip.

2.3. Stimulation

Set the nerve stimulator at 1.2 to 1.5 mA. Advance the needle in a horizontal plane until contact is made with the femur (Figure 45.3). Then withdraw the needle back almost to the skin and redirect it roughly 30° posteriorly and advance slowly until stimulation is elicited (Figures 45.4 and 45.5). The nerve is typically 1 to 2 cm beyond the point of initial femur contact. Plantar flexion is a more desirable twitch as it has been shown to result in a more complete sensory block.

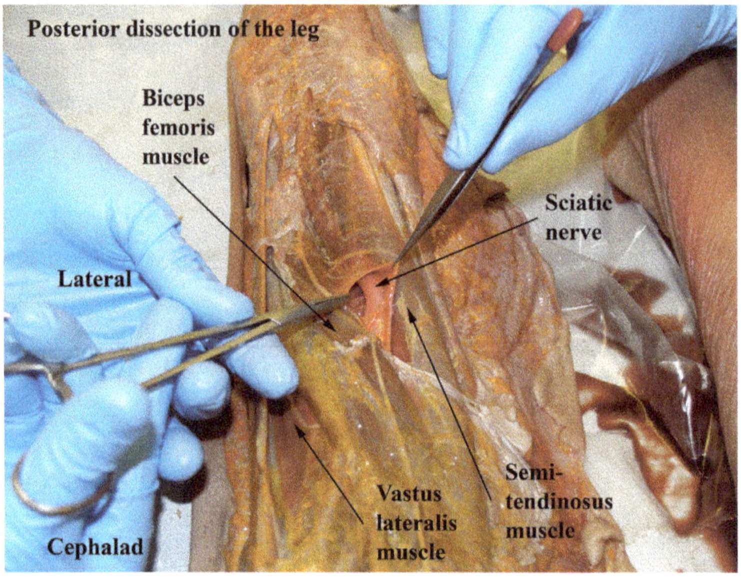

Figure 45.1 Anterior thigh dissection demonstrating the sciatic nerve.

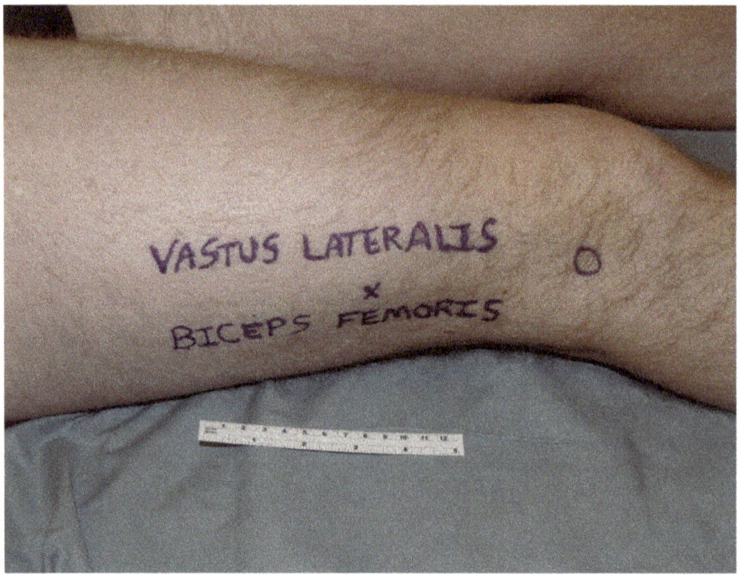

Figure 45.2 External landmarks for lateral sciatic nerve block.

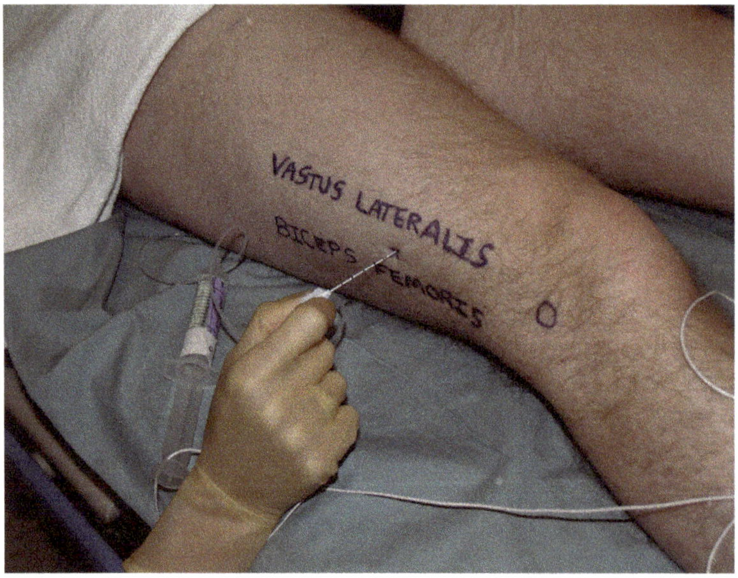

Figure 45.3 Needle position for lateral sciatic nerve block with femur contact.

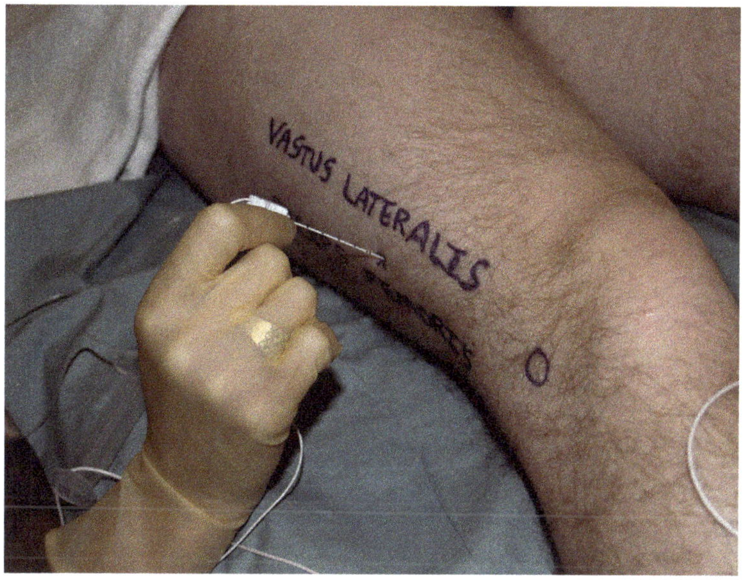

Figure 45.4 Needle redirection 30° for lateral sciatic nerve block.

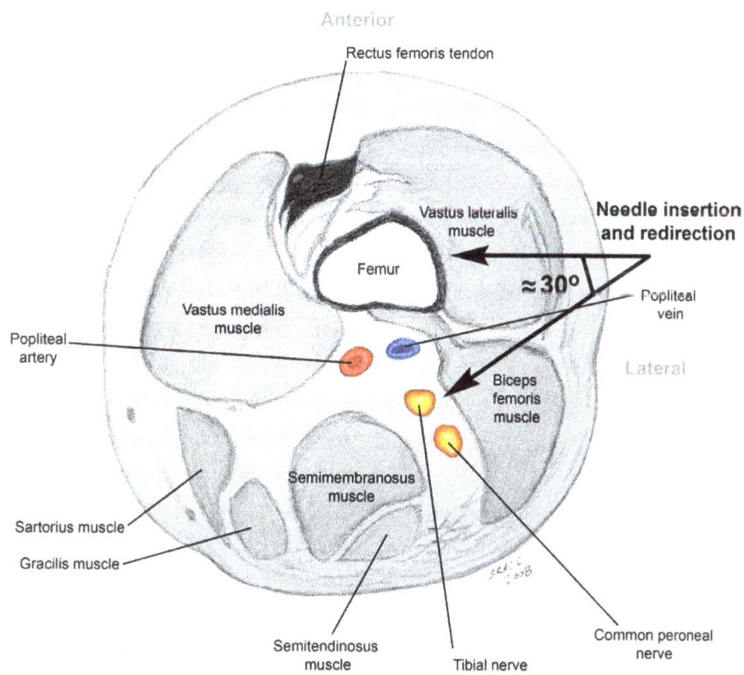

Figure 45.5 Midthigh anatomy.

2.4. Local Anesthetic

30 to 35 mL of local anesthetic is sufficient.

Teaching Points. In the lateral approach, the needle must pass through the biceps femoris muscle. Local stimulation of this muscle is often seen. Advance the needle further to stop twitching. If vastus lateralis stimulation is seen, the needle tip is too anterior and should be repositioned in a more posterior plane.

3. Ultrasound-Guided Lateral Popliteal Sciatic Nerve Block

3.1. Probe

- Midfrequency (5–12 MHz), linear.

3.2. Probe Position

Place the patient supine with the foot and ankle resting on a stack of blankets or a pillow to allow room for the probe beneath the leg. Position the probe approximately 5 cm proximal and parallel to the popliteal crease (transverse view; Figure 45.6). Scan cephalad to caudal until the sciatic nerve is identified. The popliteal artery can be used as a landmark for sciatic nerve identification as the nerve is superficial and lateral to the artery. The sciatic nerve is a round, hyperechoic structure (Figure 45.7). If the probe is moved more distal, the sciatic nerve can be observed to split into the tibial and common peroneal nerves. At this point the probe should be moved more proximally.

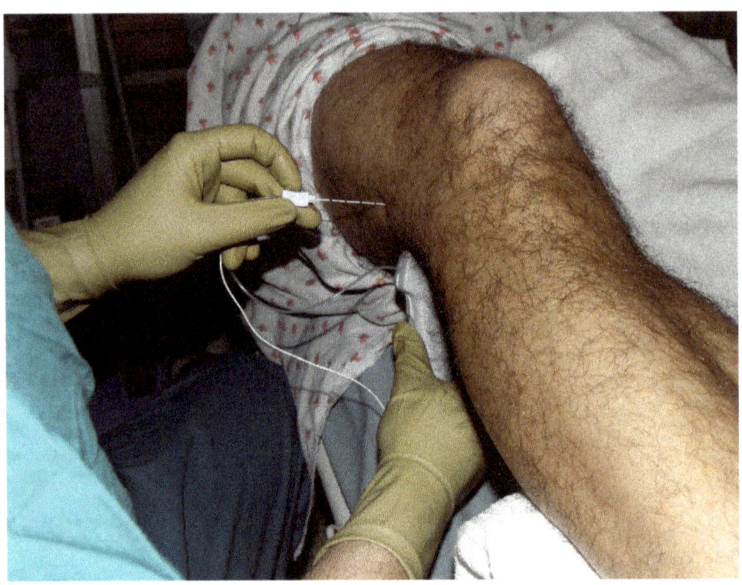

Figure 45.6 Ultrasound probe and needle positioning for lateral sciatic nerve block.

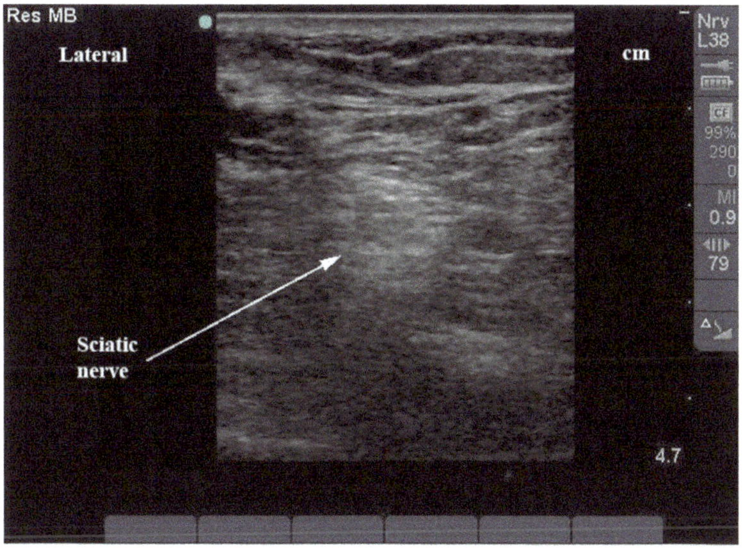

Figure 45.7 Ultrasound image of the sciatic nerve midthigh.

3.3. Approach and Injection

Insert a 21-gauge needle from the lateral side in parallel with the probe; this will allow visualization of the entire needle shaft. Inject 30 to 40 mL of local anesthetic with dynamic repositioning of the needle to completely surround the sciatic nerve with local anesthetic (Figure 45.8).

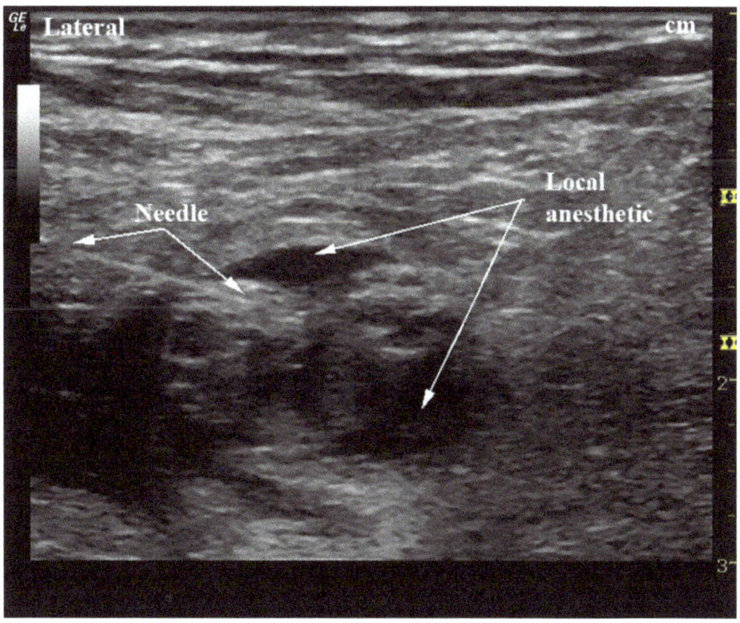

Figure 45.8 Sciatic nerve ultrasound image after local anesthetic injection.

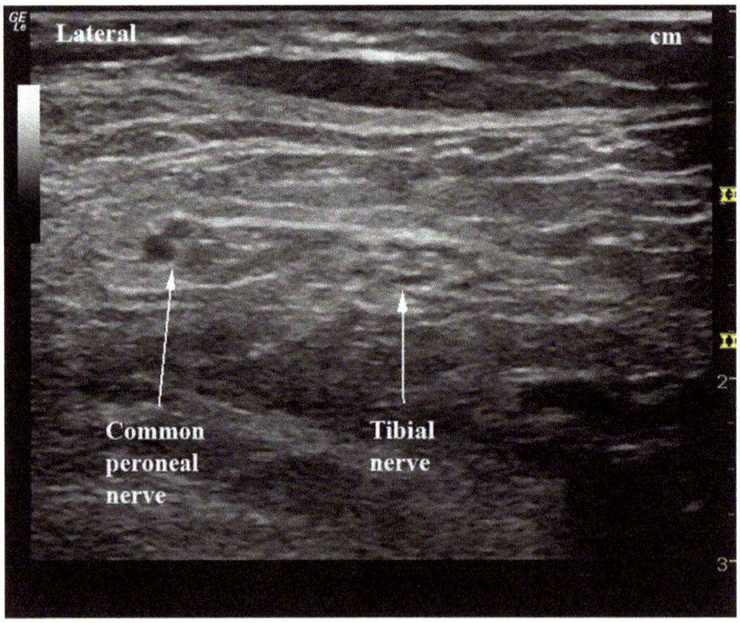

Figure 45.9 Ultrasound image of the common peroneal nerve and tibial nerve distal to the bifurcation of the sciatic nerve.

Teaching Points. Especially in a patient with larger thighs, it can be helpful to begin with the probe positioned just above the popliteal crease. The tibial and common peroneal nerves are seen as 2 hyperechoic round structures (Figure 45.9). Sliding the probe cephalad will result in the 2 structures merging to become the sciatic nerve. This technique ensures block placement proximal to the sciatic splitting. Depositing local anesthetic near the sciatic nerve split is considered optimal for decreasing block latency, since the nerve surface area exposed to local anesthetic is doubled at the split.

Sciatic Nerve Block: Popliteal

46

1. Introduction

The popliteal nerve block is a sciatic nerve block within the popliteal fossa with the patient in the lateral decubitus position or prone. The anatomy of the popliteal fossa allows ultrasound visualization of the sciatic nerve without interference from overlying muscle tissue. It is an ideal block for surgeries of the foot and ankle. It anesthetizes the same dermatomes as the other approachs to the sciatic nerve (Figure 43.3). The popliteal block preserves hamstring function, but all patients should be cautioned to avoid bearing weight on the leg for 24 hours.

2. Anatomy

The popliteal fossa is bordered laterally by the biceps femoris muscle and medially by the semimembranosus muscle. Within the fossa the sciatic nerve typically splits into tibial and common peroneal nerves (Figure 46.1). The needle should be placed just proximal to the splitting of these 2 nerves to avoid an incomplete block (Figure 46.2). Optimal needle placement for simulation blocks is usually 10 cm from the popliteal crease. A larger volume of local anesthetic (30–40 mL) is used to ensure adequate coverage of both nerves in case the nerve has already diverged. The sciatic nerve supplies motor innervation to the entire lower leg via the posterior tibial nerve and the superficial and deep peroneal nerves. The sural nerve is composed of branches from both the tibial and common peroneal nerves, but is sensory only. The sciatic nerve also supplies sensation to the entire lower leg except for the medial lower extremity, which is supplied by the saphenous nerve from the lumbar plexus.

> **Teaching Points.** Vascular puncture and intravascular injection are rare with this block (the nerve is superficial to the popliteal artery and vein). For a complete sensory blockade of the lower extremity, the saphenous nerve must also be blocked.

3. Procedure

3.1. Landmarks

The patient should be prone and the operative leg supported below the knee. The knee should be slightly flexed with the foot resting freely above the bed. If body habitus necessitates, the fossa can be accentuated by having the patient bend the knee against

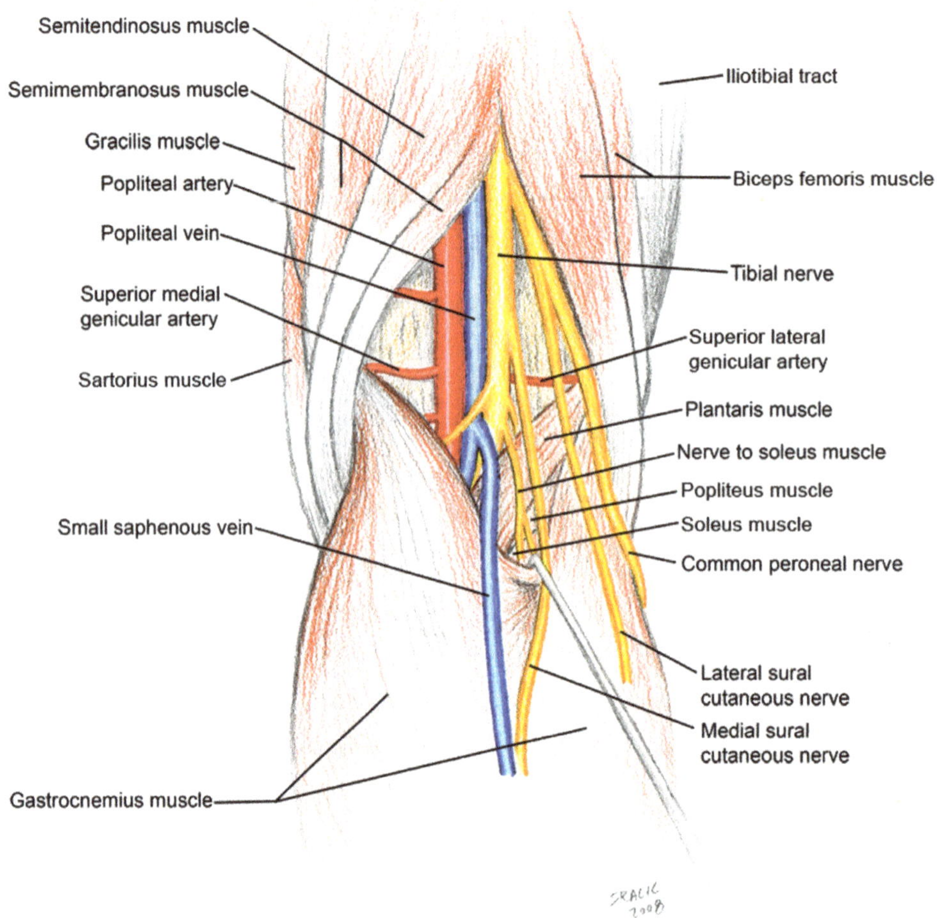

Figure 46.1 Popliteal fossa anatomy.

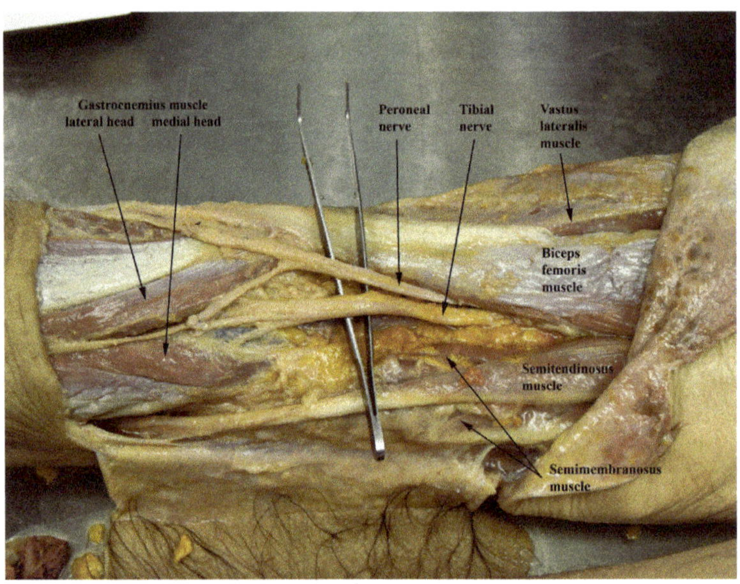

Figure 46.2 Popliteal fossa dissection.

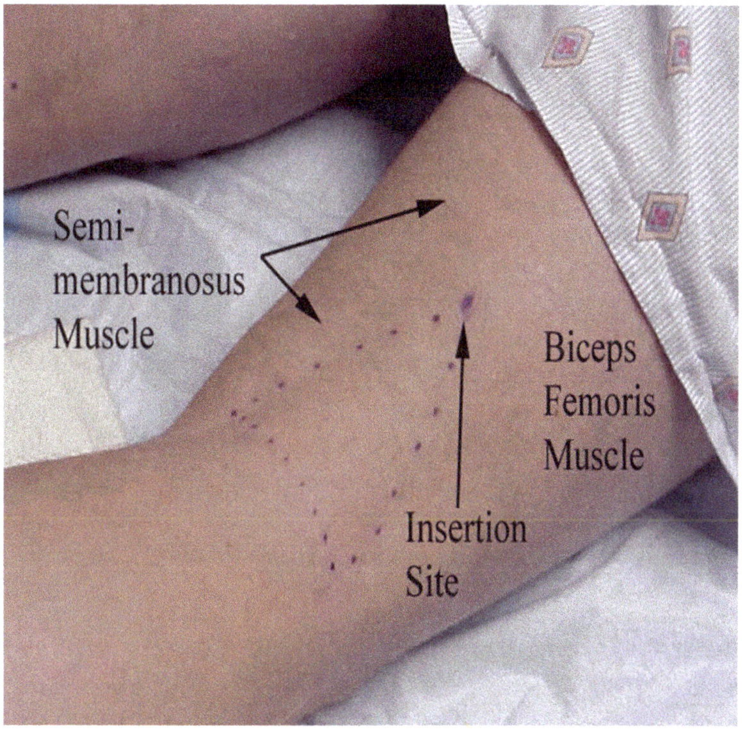

Figure 46.3 External landmarks for popliteal fossa block.

resistance. The borders of the popliteal triangle are as follows: the popliteal crease forms the base, the biceps femoris muscle forms the lateral edge, and the semitendinosus and semimembranosus muscles form the medial border (Figure 46.3). The needle should be inserted at a 45° to 60° angle to the skin in a cephalad direction and at least 7 cm superior to the popliteal crease and approximately 1 cm lateral to the apex of the popliteal triangle (Figure 46.4).

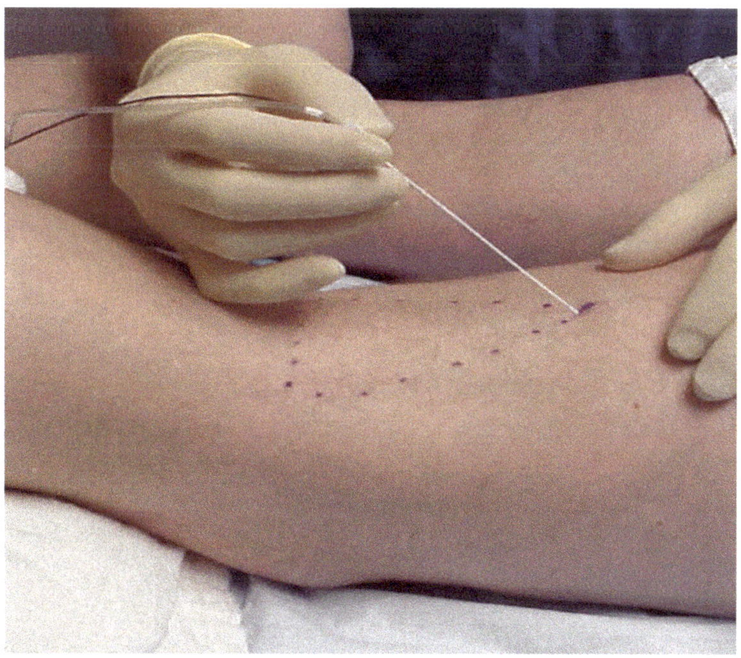

Figure 46.4 Needle orientation for popliteal fossa block.

3.2. Needles

- 21-gauge, 10-cm insulated needle.
- 18-gauge, 10-cm insulated Tuohy needle for catheter placement. Catheter placed 3 to 5 cm beyond needle tip.

3.3. Stimulation

Set the nerve stimulator to 1.0 to 1.2 mA. Stimulation patterns are as follows:

- plantar flexion → posterior tibial nerve
- dorsiflexion → deep peroneal nerve
- eversion of the foot → superficial peroneal nerve
- inversion of the foot → tibial and deep peroneal nerves

Inversion of the foot leads to the best sensory and motor block, with dorsiflexion yielding the second-best block.

If the biceps femoris muscle twitches after needle insertion, the needle should be directed more medially. Conversely, if the semitendinosus and semimembranosus muscles twitch, the needle should be directed more laterally.

3.4. Local anesthetic

In most adults, 30 mL of local anesthetic is sufficient to block the nerves.

Teaching Points. Failure to elicit a motor response with initial stimulation should be corrected with more lateral redirection rather than medial redirection (increase risk of vascular penetration of the medially and deep positioned artery and vein from the nerve). Try to maneuver the stimulating needle as cephalad in the popliteal fossa as possible to attempt to block the nerve before it divides.

4. Ultrasound-Guided Popliteal Sciatic Nerve Block

4.1. Probe

- High frequency (5–12 MHz), linear.

4.2. Probe position

The best image of the sciatic nerve can be obtained in a transverse plane (Figure 46.5), yielding either 1 large or 2 small round, hyperechoic structures depending on the location of the sciatic nerve's divergence. If the popliteal artery is seen, the nerve will be lateral and superficial to the artery (Figure 46.6).

4.3. Approach and injection

The in-plane approach allows for complete visualization of the needle. Place the probe parallel to the popliteal crease at a level proximal to the nerve division. Insert the needle from the lateral side of the probe. Pierce the sciatic sheath and inject 30 to 35 mL of local anesthetic. Needle repositioning may be necessary to surround the nerve structures with local anesthetic.

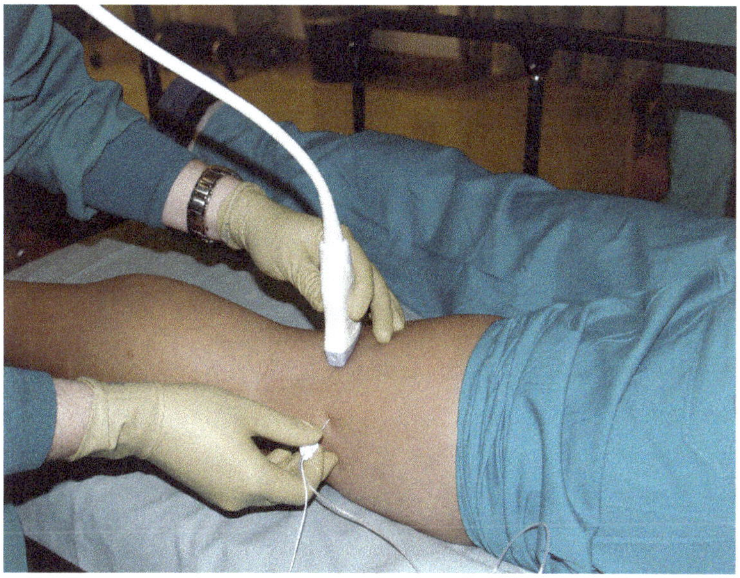

Figure 46.5 Ultrasound and needle positions for popliteal fossa block.

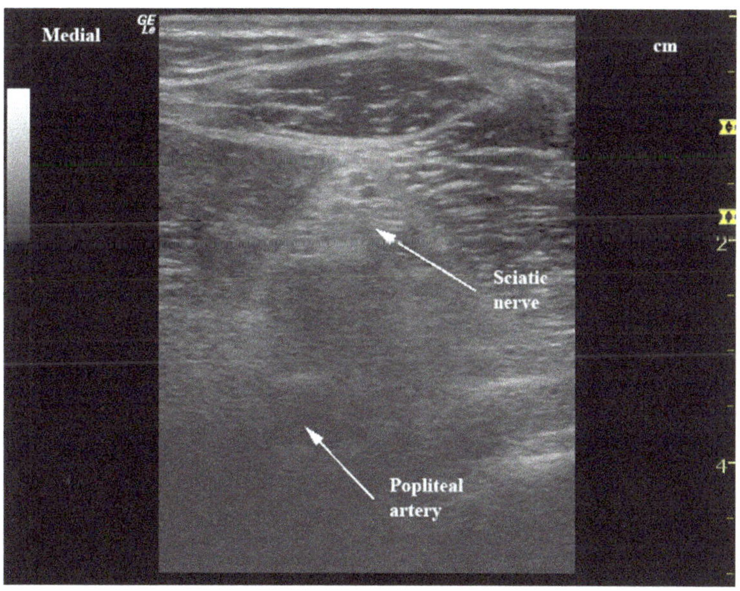

Figure 46.6 Ultrasound anatomy for the popliteal fossa block.

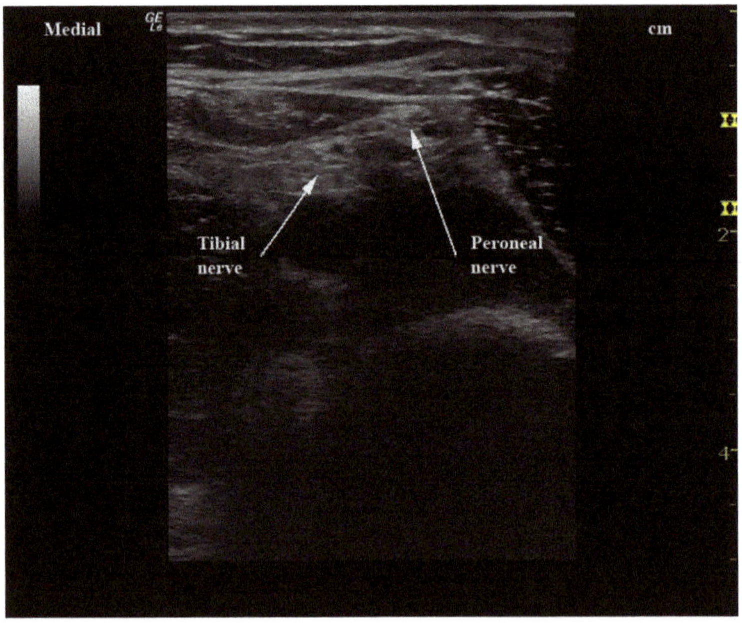

Figure 46.7 Ultrasound anatomy demonstrating the bifurcation of the sciatic nerve.

Teaching Points. Local anesthetic should be injected just proximal to nerve divergence. Scan the leg in the cephalad direction and look for the tibial and peroneal nerves to coalesce to form the sciatic nerve (Figure 46.7.). The popliteal block is performed in the same area as the lateral sciatic block but with the patient prone instead of supine. The common peroneal and tibial nerves can be separately blocked more distally; 2 separate injections are required however.

Ankle Block

47

1. Introduction and Anatomy

Five peripheral nerves supply the foot: the tibial nerve, the deep peroneal nerve, the superficial peroneal nerve, the sural nerve, and the saphenous nerve. All cross the ankle and are derived from the sciatic nerve except for the saphenous nerve, which is derived from the femoral nerve. The tibial and deep peroneal nerves supply deep structures of the foot and therefore must be blocked beneath the deep fascia of the ankle. The remaining nerves supply sensory innervation to the skin and can be blocked superficially (Figure 47.1). The ankle block works very well for foot and toe surgery, and facilitates early ambulation.

2. Procedure

Tibial Nerve. This nerve is located posterior to the posterior tibial artery at the level of the medial malleolus. Palpate the artery and insert the needle, passing posterior to the artery. A nerve stimulator can be used to help localize the nerve. The needle will typically contact the medial malleolus; after this contact occurs, slightly withdraw the needle. Inject 3 to 5 mL of local anesthetic (Figure 47.2).

Deep Peroneal Nerve. This nerve runs lateral to the dorsalis pedis artery at the level of the foot. Palpate the artery and insert the needle lateral to the artery. If bone is contacted, withdraw the needle slightly before injecting 2 to 4 mL of local anesthetic (Figure 47.3).

Superficial Peroneal Nerve. Inject a subcutaneous wheal of local anesthetic (5 mL) from the anterior border of the tibia to the lateral malleolus (Figure 47.4).

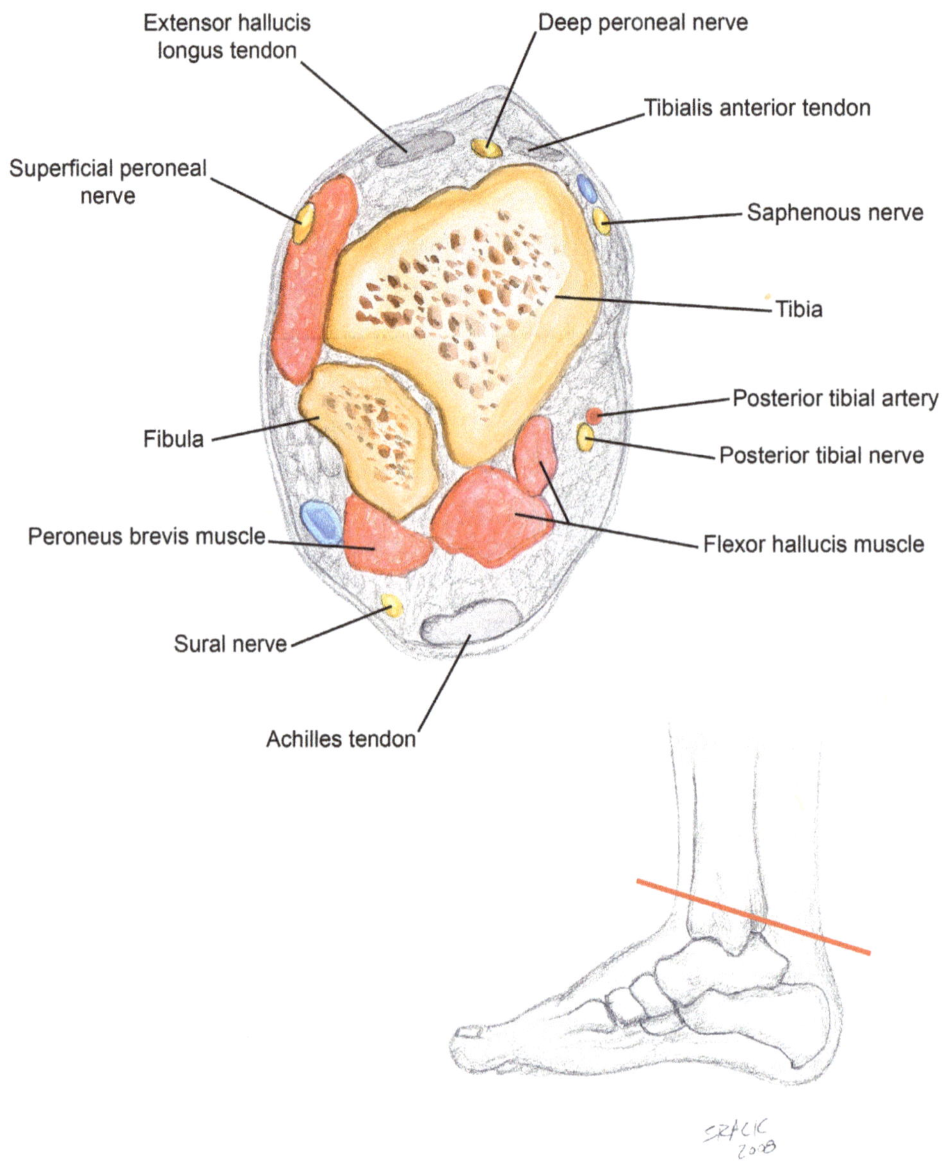

Figure 47.1 Ankle anatomy.

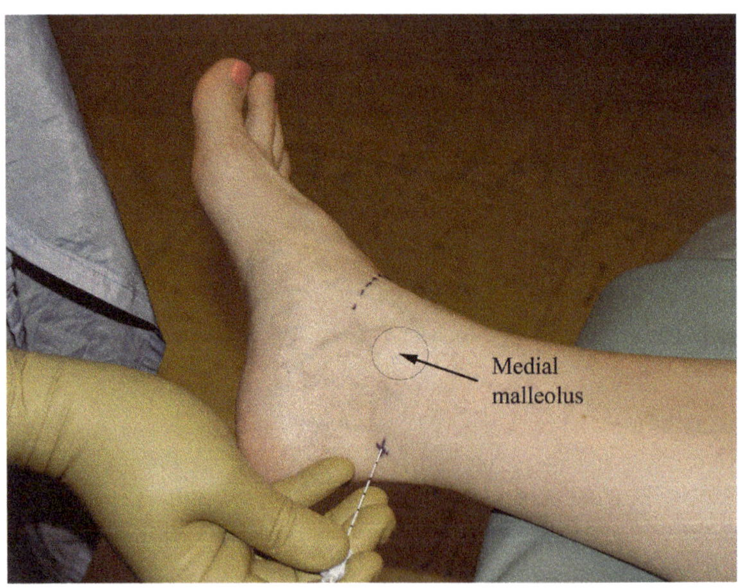

Figure 47.2 Needle position for tibial nerve block.

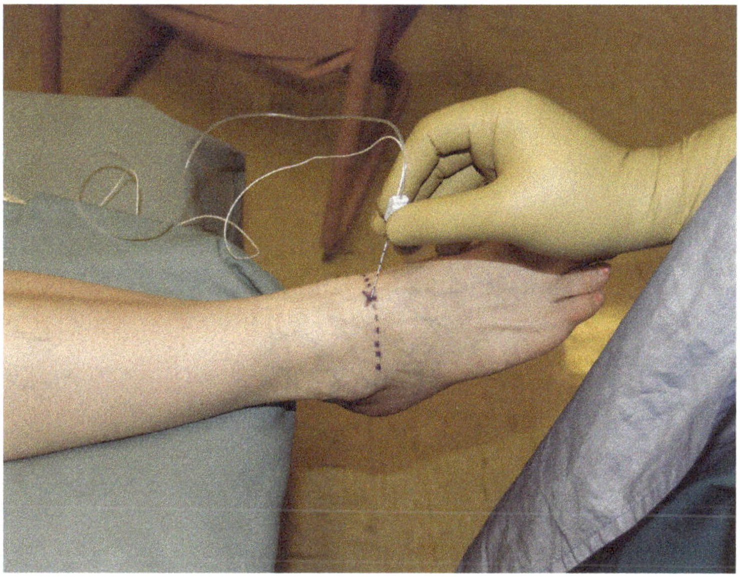

Figure 47.3 Needle position for deep peroneal nerve block.

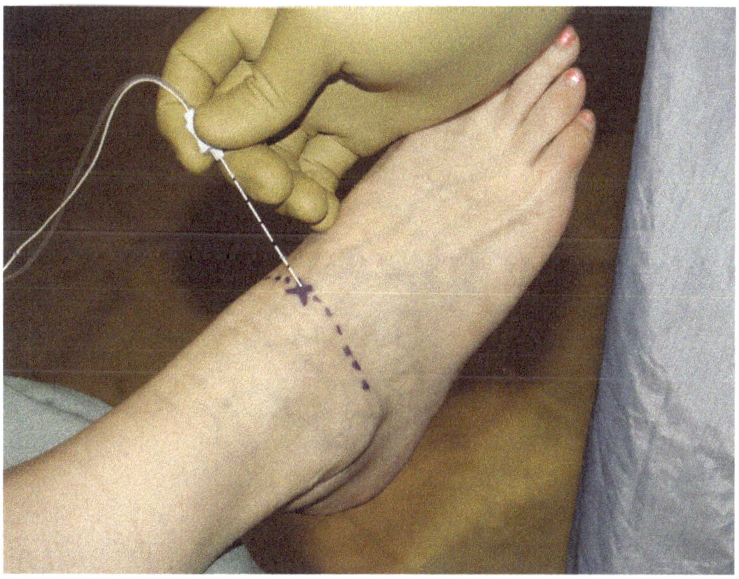

Figure 47.4 Needle position for superficial peroneal nerve block: subcutaneous injection along dotted line toward lateral malleolus.

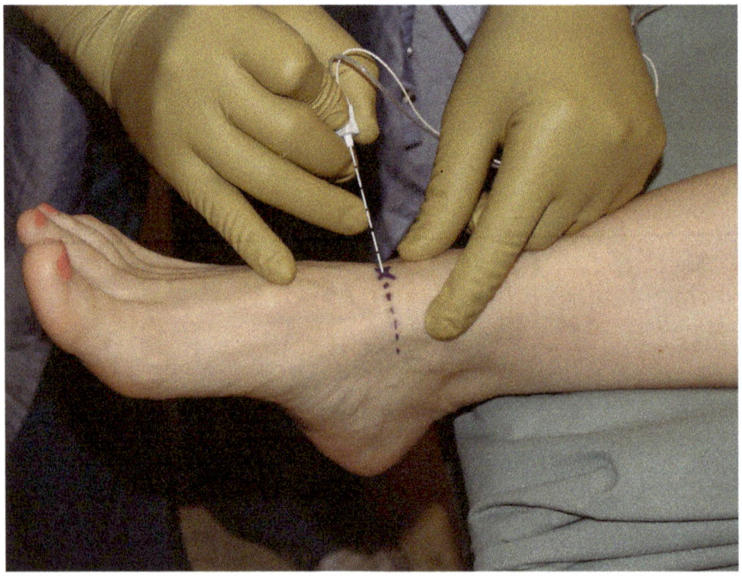

Figure 47.5 Saphenous nerve block needle position with injection directed toward medial malleolus.

Saphenous Nerve. Inject a subcutaneous wheal of local anesthetic (5 mL), directing it posteriorly from the tibial ridge to the medial malleolus (Figure 47.5).

Sural Nerve. Insert the needle between the Achilles tendon and the lateral malleolus, and subcutaneously infiltrate 5 mL of local anesthetic along this course (Figure 47.6).

Needle. 22-gauge, 5-cm, b-bevel needle.

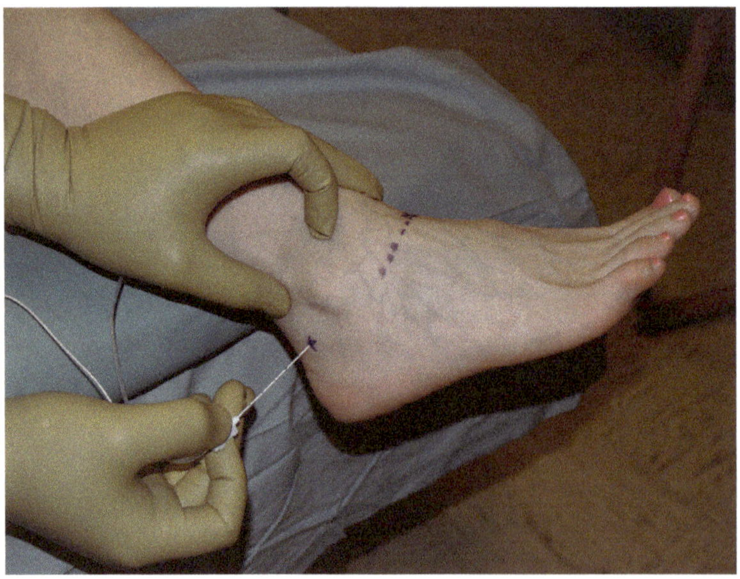

Figure 47.6 Needle position for sural nerve block.

Teaching Points. Do not use epinephrine-containing local anesthetic for this block. If a paresthesia is elicited, the needle should be redirected prior to injection because intraneural injection can cause significant damage in these small nerves. Injection around the ankle can be uncomfortable; preemptive analgesia can be very helpful.

48

Paravertebral Nerve Block

1. Introduction

Paravertebral nerve blocks (PVBs) have been an established technique for providing analgesia to the chest and abdomen for many years. PVBs are highly versatile and may serve as an anesthetic for chest trauma, chest tubes, thoracotomy, thoracoscopy, cardiac surgery, breast surgery, herniorrhaphy, laparoscopic surgery, cholecystectomy, nephrectomy, and other abdominal surgeries. In addition, PVBs are a valuable tool in treating acute and chronic pain conditions of the chest and abdomen (Table 48.1).

2. Anatomy

The paravertebral space is a wedge-shaped anatomic compartment adjacent to the vertebral bodies that is contiguous between vertebral levels and contains the intercostal nerves, arteries and veins, adipose tissue, and sympathetic trunk. Its boundaries are defined anterior-laterally by the parietal pleura; posteriorly by the superior costotransverse ligament (SCTL) (thoracic levels), transverse process, and ribs; medially by the vertebrae, vertebral disk, and intervertebral foramina; and superiorly and inferiorly by the ribs and transverse processes (Figure 48.1). The space is further divided into an anterior (ventral) and posterior (dorsal) compartment by the endothoracic fascia. Studies have suggested that to inject as close to the spinal nerves as possible, this fascial layer should be crossed and local anesthetic deposited into the ventral compartment. Within the paravertebral space, the spinal nerves are essentially "rootlets," and are not as tightly bundled with investing fascia as they are more distal. This anatomy enhances local anesthetic contact; the nerve roots facilitate dense nerve blockade when a small volume of local anesthetic is introduced into the space. Additionally, the sympathetic chain is located deep to the endothoracic fascia. Injection of local anesthetic results in ipsilateral motor, sensory, and sympathetic blockade. The use of the peripheral nerve stimulator or ultrasound to more accurately place the needle in the ventral compartment can reduce the number of paravertebral injections needed. However, many providers are disinclined to rely on the multisegmental spread of local anesthetic but instead prefer the multiple-injection technique, injecting each individual level required. This places less emphasis on needle position within the paravertebral space. Both techniques are acceptable.

The average depth of needle tip to transverse process contact is 5 to 6 cm in the thoracic spine, with the depth being greater at the upper (T1-T3) and lower (T9-T12)

Table 48.1:
Paravertebral injection location by type of surgery

Surgery	Dermatomes
Mastectomy with axillary dissection	T1-T6
Mastectomy	T2-T6
Breast biopsy	Level of biopsy with 1 level above and below
Cardiac surgery	T2-T6
Thoracic surgery	T4-T9
Rib fractures	Level of fracture with 1 level above and below
Inguinal hernia	T9-L1
Umbilical hernia	T9-T11 bilaterally
Nephrectomy	T8-T12
Cholecystectomy	T6-T10
Appendectomy	T10-T12

thoracic levels, and 6 to 7 cm in the lumbar spine. The average width of the thoracic transverse processes is 10 mm, whereas it is 5 to 7 mm in the lumbar region. However, body mass index has been shown to significantly influence the skin-to-paravertebral depth at these levels.

Complications from paravertebral blocks include inadvertent vascular puncture, hypotension, hematoma, epidural spread (via the intervertebral foramina), intrathecal spread (via the dural cuff), pleural puncture, local anesthetic toxicity, and pneumothorax.

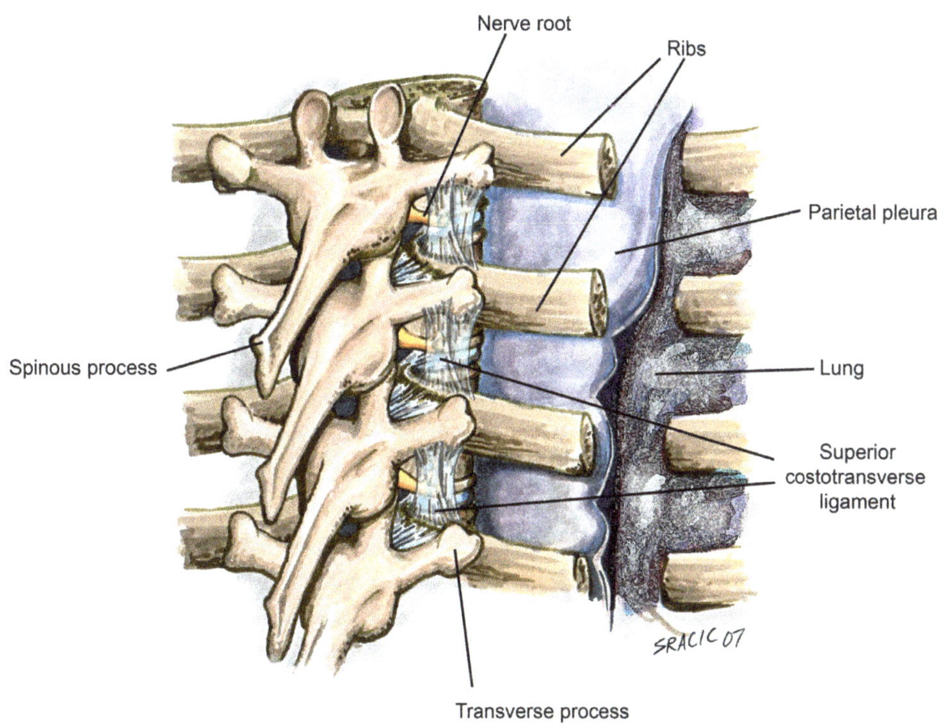

Figure 48.1 Paravertebral anatomy.

Since hemorrhage is not controllable at this site, this is considered a "deep" block by the American Society of Regional Anesthesia and Pain Medicine (ASRA), and thus it is recommended that the same anticoagulation guidelines as for neuraxial techniques apply.

3. Procedure

3.1. Transducer and needles

- 5–15 MHz linear array or 4-8 MHz curvilinear ultrasound transducer probe, depending on body habitus
- 21-gauge, 10-cm Tuohy needle
- 10-cm insulated needle for stimulation technique
- 18-gauge, 10-cm Tuohy needle for continuous catheters

3.2. Landmarks

The patient is placed with the neck and back flexed and the shoulders relaxed forward. The spinous process of each level planned for the block is palpated and marked at its superior aspect. The T7 or T8 spinous process can be identified by palpation and in concordance with the inferior angle of the scapula. In thoracic paravertebral blocks, the numbered spinous process corresponds to the next numbered nerve root caudally because of the cephalad angulation of the thoracic transverse processes.

For example, a paravertebral block performed at the C7 spinous process blocks the T1 nerve root if the needle is passed caudally (Figure 48.2). From the midpoint of each spinous process, the needle entry site is marked 2.5 cm laterally (Figure 48.3). In the thoracic area, these marks will overlie the transverse process of the next vertebral body, as noted earlier. In the lumbar area, the transverse process is usually at the same level as the spinous process.

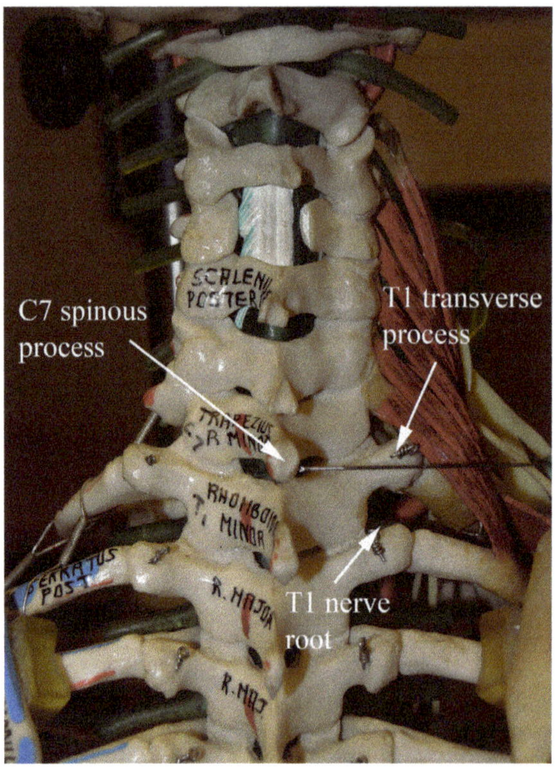

Figure 48.2 Relationship between cervical vertebrae spinous processes and cervical vertebrae transverse processes.

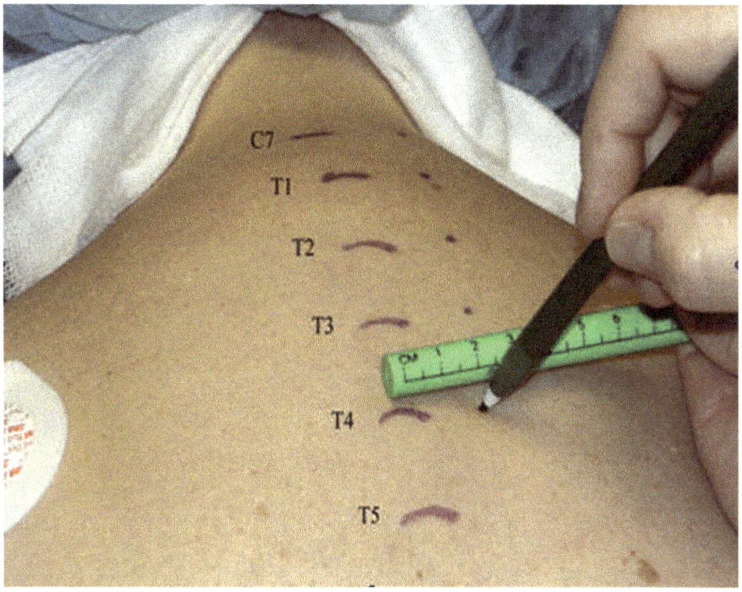

Figure 48.3 Measuring from spine midpoint 2.5 cm laterally.

3.3. Block without stimulation

Place a skin wheal of lidocaine local anesthetic at each level to be blocked. The Tuohy needle is attached via extension tubing to a syringe of local anesthetic. Grasp the shaft of the needle in your dominant hand and advance it anteriorly in the parasagittal plane (perpendicular to the back) until it contacts the transverse process (2–5 cm deep, depending on the body habitus of the patient). If you cannot identify the transverse process at an appropriate depth, assume that the needle tip lies between adjacent transverse processes, and redirect the needle cephalad and then caudad until the transverse process is successfully contacted (Figure 48.4). An optional technique employs a spinal needle for this initial localization. Ultrasound can also be used to determine transverse process depths prior to the procedure. This depth should be noted as the estimated distance to subsequent transverse processes. With the needle contacting the transverse process, grasp the

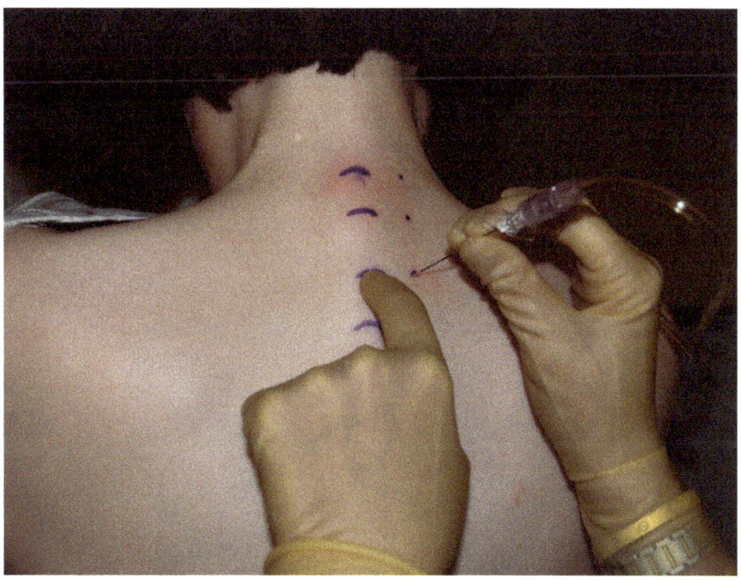

Figure 48.4 Finding the transverse process

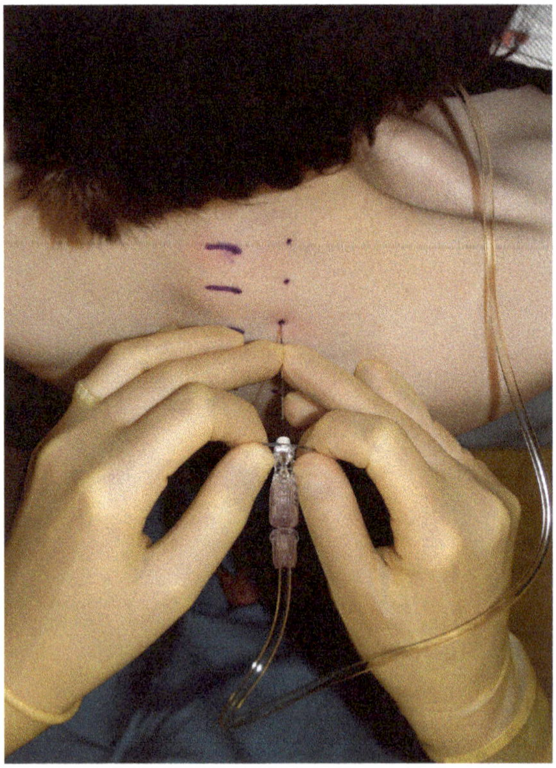

Figure 48.5 Finger Backstop

needle shaft with your fingers 1 cm from the skin surface (Figure 48.5). The fingers now serve as a "backstop" to prevent the needle passing beyond 1 cm into the paravertebral space and possibly into the pleura of the lung. Then withdraw the needle tip to the subcutaneous tissue and angle it to "walk off" the caudad edge of the transverse process, advancing no more than 1 cm into the space. Often, a loss of resistance or "pop" is appreciated, indicating that the needle tip has penetrated the SCTL; however, resistance loss may not be encountered, since the SCTL is less dense than the ligamentum flavum and may have gaps. A loss of resistance syringe may aid in detecting this subtle finding. Additionally, a hanging drop technique can be employed to rule out intrapleural placement.

After gentle aspiration for blood and air, inject local anesthetic into the space. Resistance to local anesthetic injection indicates that the needle tip is not in the paravertebral space or has not penetrated the ligament. If this occurs, advance the needle no more than 0.5 cm until the resistance lessens (the tip has passed beyond the ligament) or bone is contacted (necessitating reposition of the needle). The reason for the caudal direction of needle placement is that if initial bone contact is inadvertently with the rib (too deep to the paravertebral space), "walking off" caudally will lead to needle contact with the transverse process at a more superficial point ("stepping up"), thus minimizing unintended deep needle insertion and pneumothorax (Figure 48.6). Catheters should be placed a maximum of 2 to 3 cm beyond the needle tip, since more distal placement is associated with intraforaminal passage, epidural placement, and pleural puncture.

3.4. Block with stimulation

After identifying landmarks and prepping the area, attach a 21-gauge insulated needle to a nerve stimulator and turn the current to 2.5 mA. Advance the needle through the skin, perpendicular in all planes. Occasionally, contractions of the paraspinal muscles are seen at this point. Place the needle into the paravertebral space as described previously for nonstimulating paravertebral blocks.

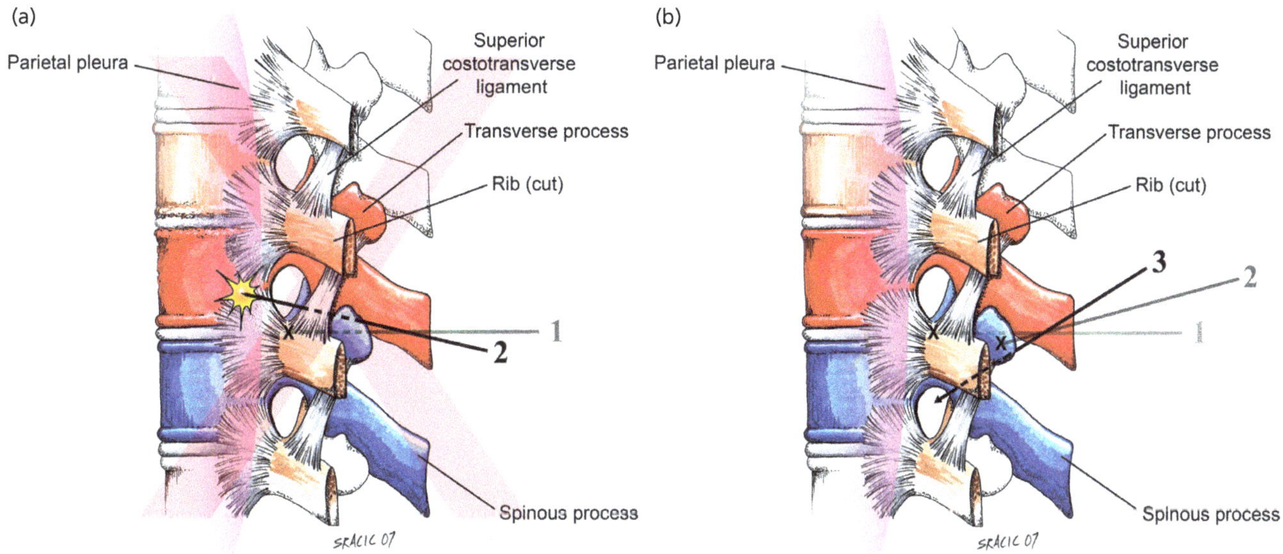

Figure 48.6 Cephalad versus caudal needle redirection for thoracic paravertebral blocks with erroneous initial needle contact with the rib. (a) In this figure the needle inadvertently contacts the rib (a-1) rather than the desired transverse process. If the provider directs the needle cephalad as depicted (a-2), inadvertent needle penetration of the pleura is possible. Therefore, cephalad needle redirection is *not* recommended. (b) In this figure the needle again incorrectly contacts the rib (b-1); however, with caudad redirection (recommended), this error is detected when the needle "steps up" onto the transverse process (b-2). With correct contact of the needle with the transverse process, the needle can be directed caudad into the paravertebral space with confidence using the 1-cm finger "backstop" (b-3).

Once the needle has advanced through the SCTL, any paraspinal contractions will stop, and an intercostal muscle twitch will typically be observed. The patient can often confirm the contraction of his or her chest wall. Gently manipulate the needle tip to continue to view this twitch as you decrease the stimulator current to approximately 0.8 mA. The needle tip should now be within the ventral compartment of the paravertebral space and beyond the endothoracic fascia. Inject local anesthetic as specified earlier. The stimulation technique provides a more objective indication of correct needle placement within the space.

3.5. Ultrasound-guided, parasagittal or longitudinal, in plane

Position the probe in the parasagittal plane over the appropriate ribs (Figure 48.7a). Move the probe medially until the adjacent 2 transverse processes are seen along with the hyperechoic pleural boundary. The transverse processes are flatter, more shallow, and medial in comparison to the ribs. Infiltrate the skin entry point with local anesthetic as above. Advance the needle from the superior aspect of the probe into the paravertebral space. Similar to the landmark technique, loss of resistance may be felt when passing through the SCTL. The visceroparietal pleural interface may be visualized with the use of M-mode sonography to rule out pneumothorax. Anterior pleural depression indicates the confirmation endpoint for injection volume. In addition, local anesthetic will also spread longitudinally in both craniocaudad directions beneath the superior costotransverse ligament and above adjacent transverse processes (Figure 48.7b).

3.6. Ultrasound-guided, transverse, in plane

Position the probe in the transverse plane between adjacent transverse processes (Figure 48.8a). Adjust the probe in the cephalocaudal plane to locate the intercostal space and eliminate shadowing from adjacent ribs. Identify the internal

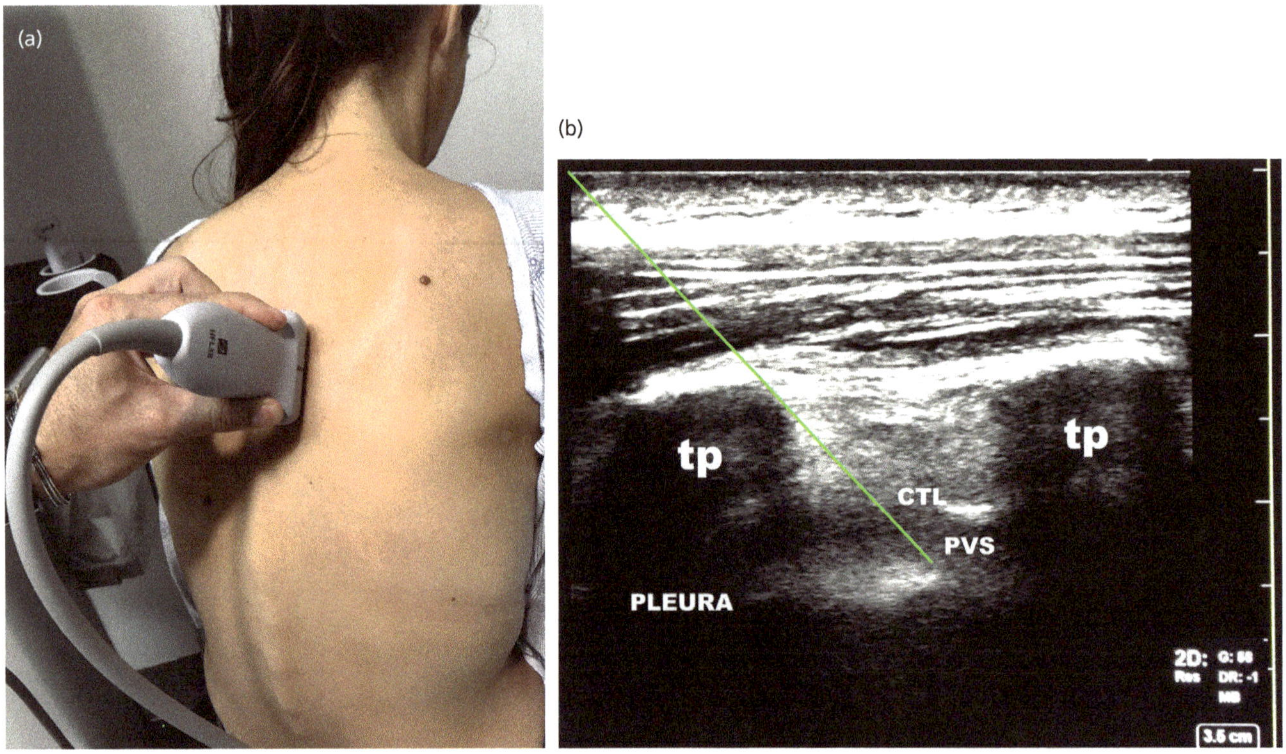

Figure 48.7 (a) Parasagittal probe position; (b) parasagittal ultrasound scan.

Legend: tp: transverse process; CTL: superior costotransverse ligament; PVS: paravertebral space. The green line represents the needle trajectory.

intercostal membrane, pleura, transverse process (medially), and the apex of the thoracic paravertebral space. Infiltrate the skin entry point with local anesthetic as above. Advance the needle in plane from the lateral aspect of the probe through the internal intercostal membrane (Figure 48.8b).

3.7. Local anesthetic

For multiple injection techniques, 3 to 5 mL of local anesthetic (usually 0.5% ropivacaine) is injected at each level. Smaller volumes are injected when bilateral paravertebral blocks (more than 6 injections) are required. Larger volumes of 10 to 20 mL can be injected at a single thoracic level with typical spread of the local anesthetic 1 to 2 paravertebral levels above and below the injection level, particularly when ultrasound or stimulation is used. Each syringe of local anesthetic can contain epinephrine 1:400,000 as a marker of intravascular injection. Rate of catheter infusion for postoperative pain is 8 to 12 mL/h (0.2% ropivacaine).

3.8. Continuous paravertebral nerve block

Landmarks. These are the same as a single injection block

Needles. 18-gauge, 10-cm Tuohy needle and a 20-gauge flexible catheter.

Position. The sitting position is preferable for catheter placement because of ease of landmark identification. When placing the catheter in an intubated or heavily sedated patient, lateral decubitus position with the block side up is usually preferred.

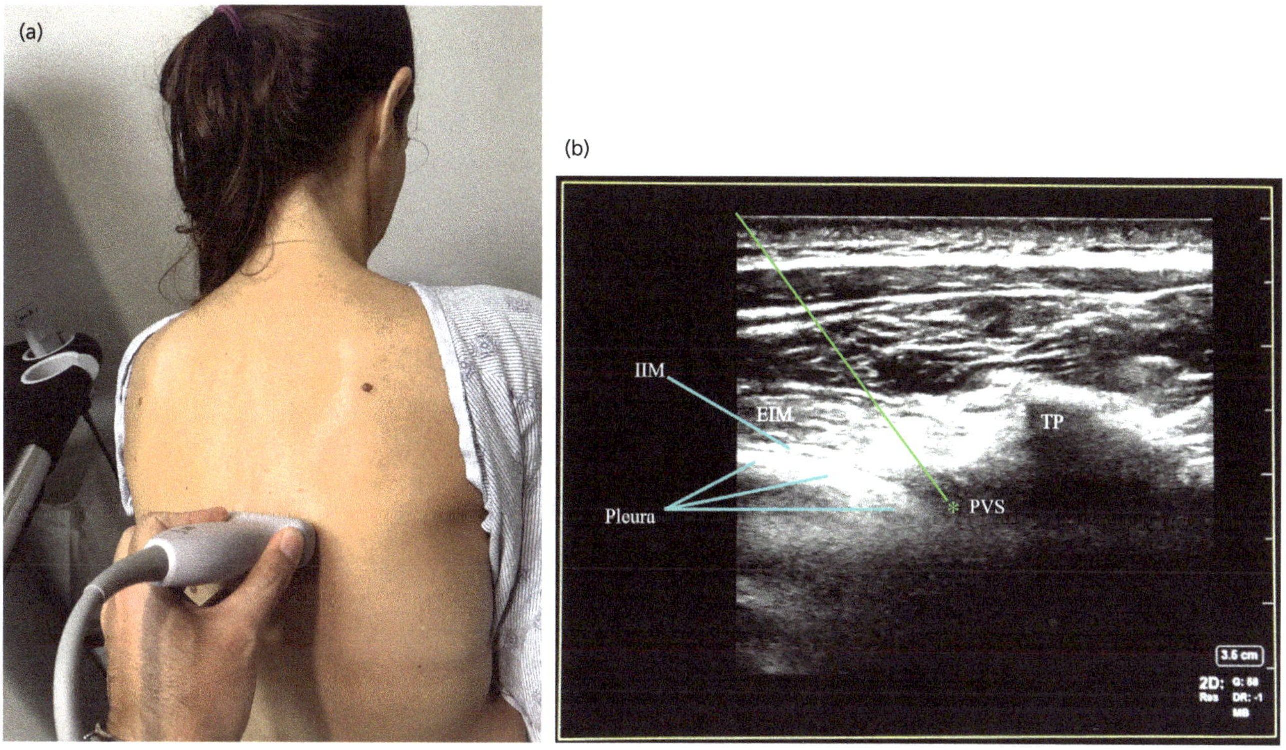

Figure 48.8 (a) Transverse probe position; (b) Transverse ultrasound scan.

Legend: IIM: internal intercostal membrane; TP: transverse process; EIM: external intercostal muscle; PVS: paravertebral space. The green line represents the needle trajectory.

Placement. Similar to the single-injection paravertebral block, lidocaine is used to anesthetize the needle entry site on the skin. Advance the needle anteriorly in the parasagittal plane until it contacts the transverse process, about 2 to 5 cm deep depending on the patient's body habitus. Withdraw your needle, angle it 10° to 15° to "walk off" the caudal edge of the transverse process into the paravertebral space. The needle depth should be about 1 cm beyond where it made contact with the transverse process. There may be a slight "pop" or loss of resistance once the needle pierces the SCTL and enters the paravertebral space. Inject 5 mL of local anesthetic to hydro-dissect and open up the space.

Before attaching your catheter to thread into the PVB space, a hanging drop technique may be utilized to confirm that the needle is not in the intrapleural space. Have the patient take a deep breath. If the needle is in the intrapleural space, the local anesthetic is pulled into the pleura during inspiration. If the needle is in the PVB space, you will notice a slight movement of the drop inward with each inspiration. This respiratory variation is indicative that the needle is in the correct location. Place the catheter through the Tuohy needle and advance it 2 to 3 cm beyond the needle tip. If it is difficult thread, withdraw the catheter, rotate the needle 90°, and reinsert the catheter into needle. Once the catheter has advanced easily, withdraw the needle and secure the catheter to the patient skin. Aspirate to make sure the catheter is negative for blood and cerebrospinal fluid before initiating the infusion. Inject some local anesthetic to make sure the catheter is functional and is not kinked distally prior to taping. Use of liquid skin adhesive at the point where the catheter enters the skin will reduce dislodgement and leaking. Catheters should be placed a maximum of 2 to 3 cm beyond the needle tip, since more distal placement is associated with intraforminal passage, epidural placement, and pleural puncture. Continuous paravertebral catheters can also be placed with ultrasound guidance as discussed in this chapter.

Teaching Points. At the thoracic levels it is common to appreciate a loss of resistance or a subtle "pop" as the needle passes through the SCTL. In the lumbar region, there is no SCTL. If a distinct "pop" is sensed here, the needle has likely punctured the psoas fascia and should be withdrawn to a more shallow depth, still remaining anterior to the transverse process. In addition, it is important to note that in the lumbar region, the transverse process is very thin, so the needle should be inserted only 0.5 cm past the transverse process. If using the ultrasound or nerve stimulator technique for thoracic paravertebral blocks, be aware that a blunt-tip Tuohy needle is not being used, which may increase the risk of pleural puncture.

Transversus Abdominis Plane Block

49

1. Introduction

Tranversus abdominis plane (TAP) infiltration is a field block that has demonstrated efficacy in the treatment of postsurgical abdominal pain. The cutaneous sensory analgesic coverage of the block does not have dermatomal distribution, which is due to the significant variability of innervation supplying the anterolateral abdominal wall. Visceral analgesia is not a component of this nerve block; only somatic analgesia and muscular relaxation of the abdominal wall are achieved. TAP blocks have been found to be amenable for numerous abdominal surgeries, including hysterectomy, cesarean delivery, gynecologic laparoscopy, laparoscopic cholecystectomy, laparoscopic gastric bypass surgery, laparoscopic donor nephrectomy, inguinal hernia repair, appendectomy, gastrectomy, and prostatectomy. TAP blocks can be particularly useful to provide analgesia following laparotomy for trauma when epidural analgesia is contraindicated.

2. Anatomy

The TAP is identified as the anatomic space located between the transversus abdominis and internal oblique muscles (Figure 49.1). Somatic afferents that supply the anterior and lateral abdominal wall travel through this space from the anterior rami of the T7-L1 spinal nerves. As the nerves course medially, the spinal nerve branches continually exit the plane anteriorly prior to termination of the plane at the rectus abdominis. Since cadaveric dissection has revealed that the nerves are bound to the transversus abdominis muscle by a layer of fascia, local anesthetic should be deposited beneath this layer. Although it is possible to have variable involvement of T6-T8 more posteriorly in the TAP, nerves identified between the inguinal ligament and costal margin at the anterior axillary line are typically derived from T9-L1, although this is variable. The T9-L1 nerves can be blocked prior to their branching by depositing local anesthetic further posteriorly beyond the midaxillary line with a TAP block.

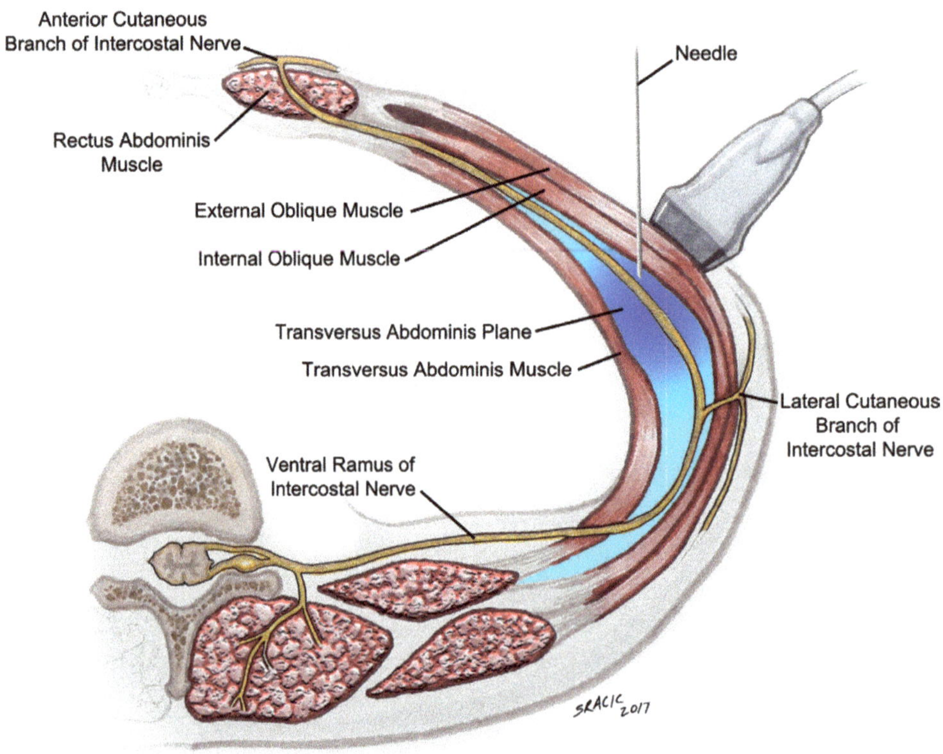

Figure 49.1 Transversus abdominis plane.

There are no unique contraindications to the TAP block, and standard contraindications for any regional techniques apply. Since the block is placed peripherally, it may be considered as an analgesic option when the coagulation status prohibits the use of epidural or other deep techniques as described by the American Society of Regional Anesthesia and Pain Medicine (ASRA) guideline "Regional Anesthesia in the Patient Receiving Antithrombotic or Thrombolytic Therapy." Local anesthetic systemic toxicity (LAST) may be more likely with this technique, since high doses and volumes of local anesthetic are injected, particularly with bilateral procedures. An increased risk of LAST in parturients has also been suggested, and decreased dosing is advised in this patient population. Puncture of peritoneal structures has been reported in case reports involving injury to the liver, small bowel, and colon. Intraperitoneal needle placement is less likely to occur with the use of ultrasound guidance.

3. Procedure

3.1. Transducer and needles

- Probe. High frequency (5–12 MHz), linear
- 21-gauge, 10-cm Tuohy needle

3.2. Landmarks

The abdominal wall is approached along the midaxillary line by palpation of the costal margin cephalad and the iliac crest caudal. The lumbar triangle of Petit was an initial anatomic description for a landmark-based approach that has lost favor to the more reliable ultrasound-guided techniques. The posterior location of this triangle makes it less accessible in the supine positioning of most patients after abdominal surgery (Figure 49.2).

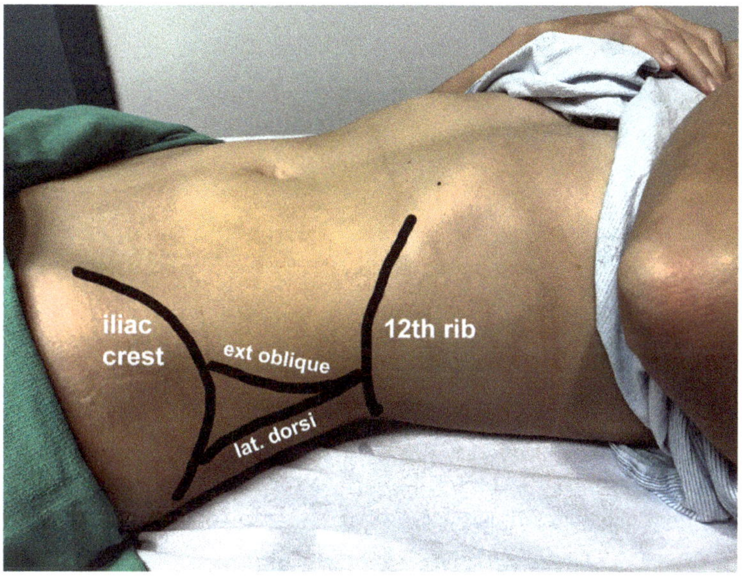

Figure 49.2 TAP block external anatomy.

A landmark technique at this triangle described a "fascial click" once the needle had passed through the internal oblique muscle into the TAP space. A later technique described a more medial approach, with a "double click" indicating advancement through the external and internal oblique muscles. Nevertheless, when verifying with ultrasound after needle placement, one study found that landmark-based techniques resulted in correct placement less than 25% of the time. With the advent of ultrasound technology, this approach has been largely abandoned.

3.3. Ultrasound-guided technique, transverse in plane

Depending on the location of the incision, the following approaches should be used:

1. For incisions *above* the umbilicus: Use the subcostal TAP approach (Figure 49.3).
2. For incisions *below* the umbilicus: Use an abdominal TAP approach (Figure 49.4).
3. For midline incisions: Bilateral TAP blocks are required.
4. Midline incisions above and below the umbilicus: Bilateral subcostal and abdominal TAP blocks should be considered. Place the ultrasound probe in the transverse orientation along the anterolateral abdominal wall between the costal margin and the iliac crest.

An initial imaging depth of 4 to 6 cm is typically appropriate to visualize the external oblique, internal oblique, and transversus abdominis muscles. After identifying these muscles, slide the probe posterolaterally to the midaxillary line and attempt to demarcate the tapering of the transversus abdominis and internal oblique muscles into the thoracolumbar fascia. The target for the needle tip is below the transversus abdominis fascia, 1 cm anterior to the muscle tapering laterally (Figure 49.5). Another method is targeting the TAP just posterior to the midaxillary line. While in plane, advance the needle from the anterior aspect of the probe. An endpoint to injection of local anesthetic at this location will depict a hypoechoic oval shape if in the correct plane and indentation of the transversus abdominis muscle into the peritoneum.

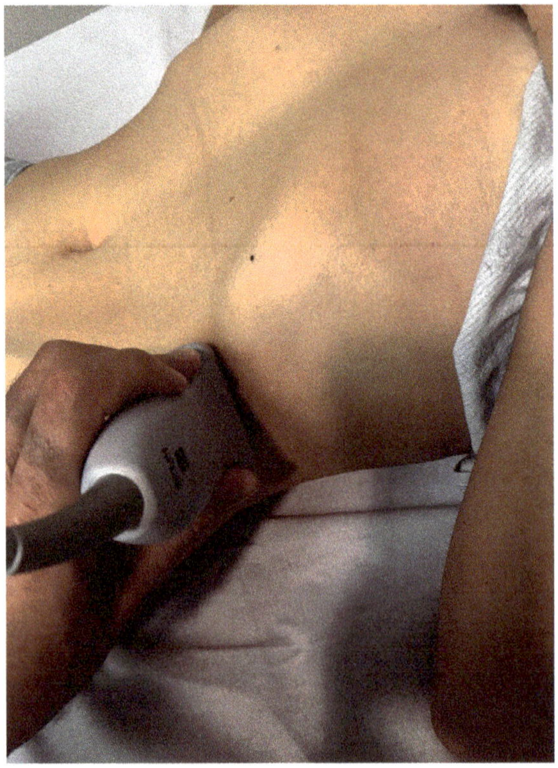

Figure 49.3 A subcostal TAP is performed immediately caudad to the 12th rib.

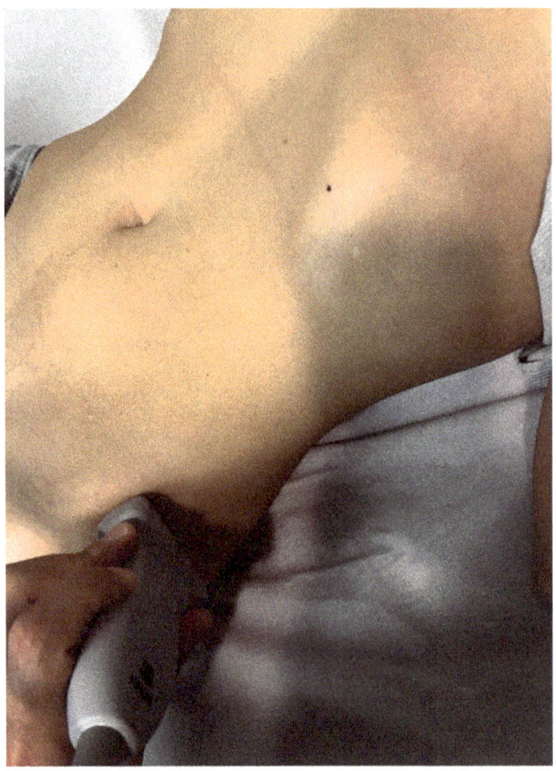

Figure 49.4 An abdominal TAP is performed immediately cranial to the iliac crest.

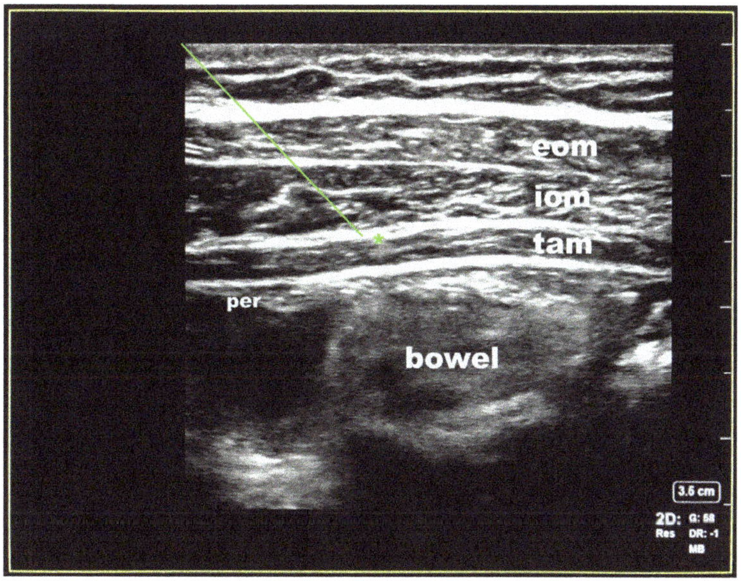

Figure 49.5 TAP ultrasound anatomy

Legend: eom: external oblique muscle; iom: internal oblique muscle; tam: transversus abdominis muscle; per: peritoneum.

4. Local Anesthetic

The volume for injectate is typically 15 to 20 mL per side (0.25%–0.75% ropivacaine or bupivacaine). While the duration of analgesia after TAP infiltration with nonliposomal local anesthetic ranges from 12 to 48 hours, liposomal bupivacaine formulations may extend analgesia up to 72 hours.

> **Teaching Points.** Variation in anatomy makes location of the triangle of Petit inaccurate. Increased failure rate and chance of complications should discourage the use of the landmark-based technique if possible. A posterior target in the TAP near the thoracolumbar fascia is more likely to capture a greater portion of the spinal nerve branches supplying the abdominal wall. An endpoint for injectate is an ovoid dissection of the plane between the transversus abdominis and internal oblique muscles, deep to the fascia that envelops the transversus abdominis muscle.

50

Quadratus Lumborum Block

1. Introduction

The quadratus lumborum (QL) blocks were initially developed as variants of the ultrasound-guided posterior transversus abdominis plane (TAP) block by Rafael Blanco. These blocks have greater dermatomal coverage of the abdominal trunk due to their more posterior approach. The QL block consists of 3 different approaches based on injection location relative to the psoas muscle: lateral (QL1), posterior (QL2), or anterior/transmuscular (QL3). The QL blocks can provide anesthesia and analgesia for abdominal and flank surgeries (Table 50.1). One particular benefit of this plane block is that it not only offers the potential to decrease somatic pain, but also may reduce visceral pain. This is likely accomplished by spread of the injected local anesthetic to the paravertebral space or to the sympathetic fibers of the thoracolumbar fascia. Spread of local anesthetic to the paravertebral space from this procedure is most likely accomplished when the solution is injected anterior or posterior to the QL muscle.

2. Anatomy

The 3 muscles of the lateral abdominal wall consist of the external oblique muscle superficially, the transversus abdominis muscle posteriorly, and the internal oblique muscle between them. The internal oblique and transversus abdominis muscles converge posteriorly into an aponeurosis of thoracolumbar fascia. The thoracolumbar fascia is a sheet of fused fascial aponeuroses that envelops the posterior muscles of the thoracolumbar trunk. It divides into 3 layers: (1) the anterior layer, which covers the anterior surface of the QL and merges medially with the fascia of the psoas major and laterally with the transversalis fascia; (2) the middle layer, which is sandwiched between the erector spinae muscles and the QL muscle; and (3) the posterior layer, which covers the posterior surface of the erector spinae muscles.

At the lateral border of the erector spinae muscle, the middle thoracolumbar fascia fuses with the deep lamina of the posterior thoracolumbar fascia to form a triangular structure called the lumbar interfascial triangle, which is the hypothetical site of action of the QL block. The thoracolumbar fascia contains mechanoreceptors, nociceptors, and sympathetic fibers. Furthermore, the confluence of fascial layers at this level provides potential planes of local anesthetic spread, primarily in a craniocaudad direction. A layer of transversalis fascia covers the thoracolumbar fascia, the anterior surface of the QL muscle, and the anterolateral surface of the psoas major. The transversalis fascia divides into 2 layers at the diaphragm: the inferior diaphragmatic fascia, and the endothoracic

Table 50.1:
Quadratus lumborum (QL) blocks

Type of Block	Benefits	Risks	Dermatomal Coverage
Lateral (QL1)	Greater extent of dermatomal coverage compared with the conventional TAP block	Intraperitoneal injection and possible bowel injury	T7-L1
Posterior (QL2)	Decreased risk of peritoneal puncture compared with QL1, since the needle is directed more posteriorly	Vascular injury in the paravertebral space	T7-T12
Anterior (QL3)	Decreased risk of peritoneal puncture, as the psoas muscle acts as a posterior barrier along the needle path	Inadvertent psoas compartment block, with the attendant risk of bleeding in anticoagulated patients	T11-L4
Subcostal (QL4)	Greater extent of dermatomal coverage over the lower thorax and complete abdomen	Intraperitoneal injection, possible bowel injury, possible diaphragmatic injury, and renal puncture	T6-L1

fascia (passing behind the lateral and medial arcuate ligaments), the latter of which may provide a point of access into the thoracic paravertebral space.

The lateral (QL1) block anesthetizes the lateral and anterior cutaneous branches of intercostal nerves from T7 to L1, with extension to the paravertebral space at these levels. The posterior (QL2) block covers the same dermatomes, but it also produces relief of visceral pain, suggesting its site of action at the sympathetic nerves in the paravertebral space. The anterior (QL3) block has been reported to cover the T11-L4 dermatomes, with analgesia achieved in the distribution of both the lumbar plexus and TAP blocks (Figure 50.1).

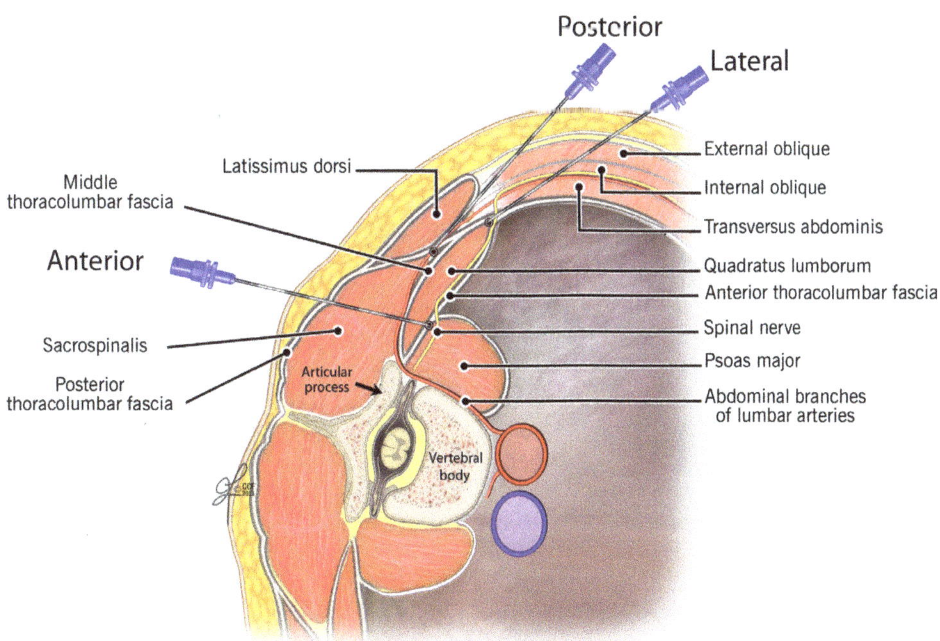

Figure 50.1 Quadratus lumborum block approaches and relevant anatomy.

3. Procedure

3.1. Equipment

- Lateral (QL1) and posterior (QL2) approaches: High frequency (6–15 MHz) linear ultrasound probe transducer
- Anterior (QL3) approach: Lower frequency (2–6 MHz) curvilinear ultrasound transducer
- 21- or 22-gauge, 9- to 10-cm echogenic needle

Lateral (QL1) Block. The patient can be positioned in either the supine position or the lateral position. The arm on the side to be blocked should be slightly abducted to provide access to the ipsilateral flank. The ultrasound probe is placed on the flank, slightly cephalad to the iliac crest, in a transverse orientation. The 3 muscle layers of the lateral abdominal wall (external oblique, internal oblique, transversus abdominis) and the QL muscle are visualized (Figure 50.2). Sliding the probe posteriorly will allow visualization of the latissimus dorsi superficially, the erector spinae muscles medially, and the QL deep to both (situated anterolateral to the apex of the L3 and L4 transverse processes). The psoas muscle is located deep to the QL muscle and paramedian, adjacent to the vertebral body.

The needle is inserted in plane to the probe in an anterolateral to posteromedial direction, through the external oblique, internal oblique, and transversus abdominis muscles, to reach the anterolateral edge of the QL muscle. Once it is properly positioned, inject local anesthetic at the anterolateral aspect of the QL muscle, superficial to the transversalis fascia, leading to spread similar to a TAP block in the abdominal wall with extension into the thoracic paravertebral space via the endothoracic fascia in the thoracic wall. Local anesthetic spread between the QL and the medial layer of the thoracolumbar fascia is desirable.

Posterior (QL2) Block. The patient can be positioned similarly to the lateral (QL1) block. The ultrasound probe is placed on the flank, slightly cephalad to the iliac crest, in a transverse orientation. Sliding the ultrasound probe posterolaterally will bring into view the posterior border of the external oblique muscle (the "hook" sign), creating a roof over the QL muscle. The latissimus dorsi is located superficially, the erector spinae muscles medial, and the QL deep to

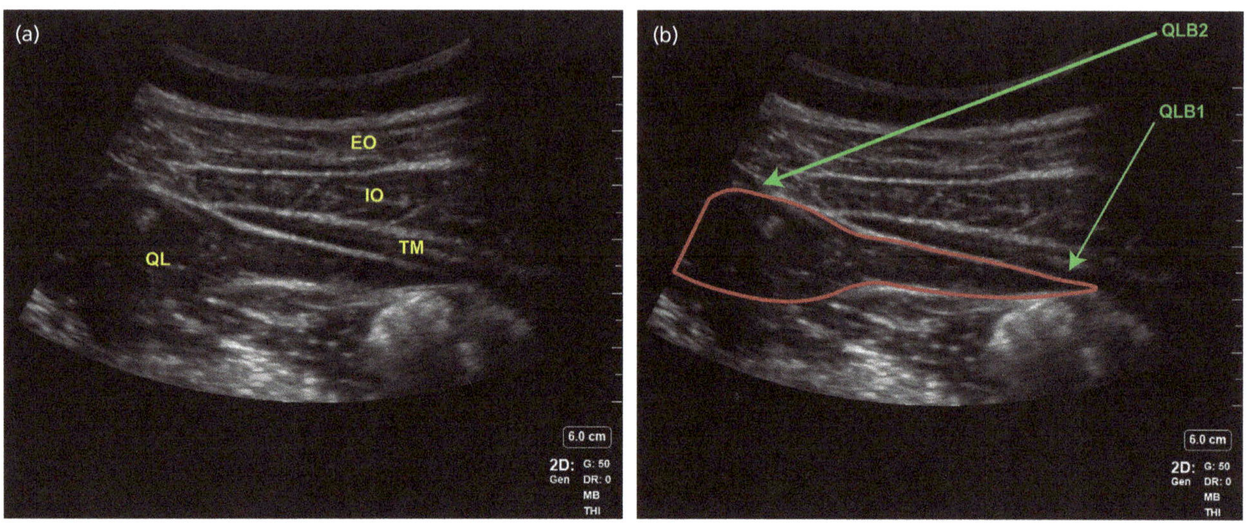

Figure 50.2 50.2a (left) and 50.2b (right). Lateral view of quadratus lumborum muscle. Labeled anatomic structures include (yellow) in Figure 50.2a: EO: external oblique muscle; IO: internal oblique muscle; TM: transversus abdominus muscle; QL: quadratus lumborum muscle. The outline of the QL muscle is in red, found in figure 50.2b. The green arrows signify the path of the needle, with the arrowhead representing the tip of the needle, where local anesthetic should be injected for the indicated block. This lateral sonographic view typically allows for the patient to be lying in the supine position and is most optimal for placement of the QL 1 and 2.

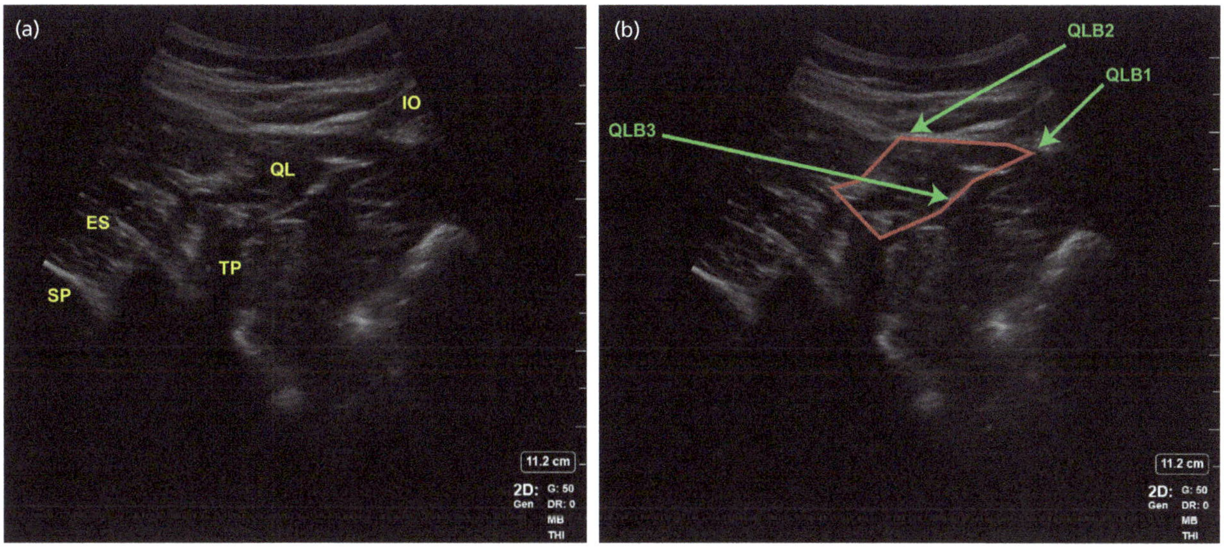

Figure 50.3 50.3a (left) and 50.3b (right). Posterior view of quadratus lumborum muscle. Labeled anatomic structures included (yellow) in Figure 50.3a: SP: spinous process of thoracic vertebrae; ES: erector spinae muscles; QL: quadratus lumborum muscle; PM: psoas muscle; IO: internal oblique muscle. The outline of the QL muscle is in red, found in figure 50.3b. The green arrows signify the path of the needle, with the arrowhead representing the tip of the needle, where local anesthetic should be injected for the indicated block. This posterior sonographic view typically requires the patient to be lying in the lateral decubitus position and is most optimal for placement of the QLB3.

both (situated anterolateral to the apex of the L3 and L4 transverse processes). The psoas muscle is located deep to the QL muscle and paramedian, adjacent to the vertebral body (Figure 50.3).

Tilting the probe caudally will reveal a bright hyperechoic line corresponding to the intermediate layer of the thoracolumbar fascia and the lumbar interfascial triangle.

Insert the needle in plane to the probe in a lateral to medial direction, through the external oblique, internal oblique, and transversus abdominis muscles, to reach the anterolateral edge of the sacrospinalis muscle, at the posterior border of the QL muscle. Once the needle tip is properly positioned, inject local anesthetic, noting spread extending past the middle layer of the thoracolumbar fascia into the lumbar interfascial triangle.

Anterior (QL3) Block. The patient is positioned in the lateral position, with the operative side up. The ultrasound probe is placed cephalad to the iliac crest in the midaxillary line, in a transverse orientation. Slide the probe posteriorly to insonate the QL muscle, its attachment to the lateral edge of the L4 transverse process, the psoas major anteriorly, and the erector spinae muscle posteriorly, forming a "shamrock sign" with 3 leaves.

Insert the needle in plane to the probe in a slight posteromedial to anterolateral direction, through the erector spinae (sacrospinalis) and QL muscles and anterior thoracolumbar fascia, to place the needle tip in the interfascial plane between the QL and the psoas muscles. The goal is for the local anesthetic to spread cranially between the QL and psoas muscles to reach the thoracic paravertebral space.

3.2. The subcostal approach (paramedian oblique sagittal)

To obtain an oblique sagittal view of QL muscle, the transducer is positioned 6 to 8 cm lateral to the lumbar spinous process at the L1-L2 level just above the crossover point of the erector spinae and the QL. Using a curvilinear transducer with the orientation marker of the ultrasound, it is directed cranially, and the probe is slightly tilted medially. In addition, the cranial part of the ultrasound probe is slightly tilted medially and the caudal part of the probe laterally. The needle

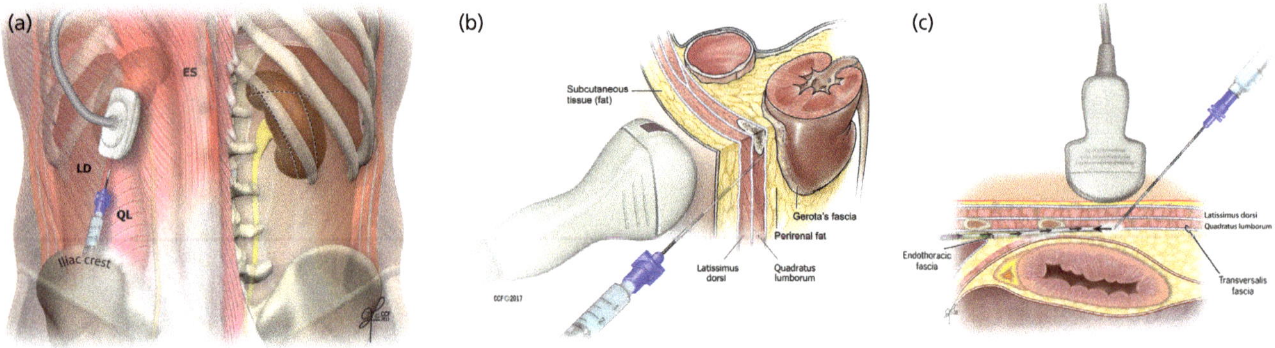

Figure 50.4 Subcostal QL approach and the relevant anatomy.

is advanced in plane in a caudal to cephalad direction, through the latissimus dorsi and QL muscles; local anesthetic is deposited anterior to the QL muscle, between the QL muscle and the anterior layer of the thoracolumbar fascia (ATLF).

The needle tip is then advanced farther cephalad, and local anesthetic is deposited incrementally, observing spread in a cephalad direction close to the 12th rib, creating a lunar-shaped distribution with anterior displacement of the ATLF (Figure 50.4).

Local Anesthetic. Fifteen to 25 mL of local anesthetic is sufficient for most adult patients.

Teaching Points. The lateral (QL1) block risks intraperitoneal injection and possible bowel injury, since the peritoneum lies beyond the needle tip along the needle path. Blanco has since abandoned this approach in favor of the posterior (QL2) approach for this reason.

The posterior (QL2) approach is believed to be safer than the lateral (QL1) approach, since the needle path is directed more posteriorly and thus avoids the risk of breaching the peritoneum. The psoas muscle also acts as a protective barrier over the peritoneum. Blanco suggests it may be safer than a TAP block due to the superficial plane of injection. Blanco warns that the interfascial plane of injection of the posterior (QL2) block contains vessels exiting from the paravertebral space, which could be a risk factor for hematoma in anticoagulated patients.

The anterior/transmuscular (QL3) approach is theoretically safer than the posterior and lateral approaches because it directs the needle path away from the peritoneal cavity. Additionally, there is a risk of injection within the psoas muscle, which would result in a psoas compartment block. Thus it is reasonable to categorize the anterior (QL3) approach within the same risk profile as the lumbar plexus block, with its associated risk of bleeding in anticoagulated patients.

Neuraxial Anesthesia/Analgesia

51

1. Introduction

Neuraxial anesthesia encompasses epidural anesthesia, spinal anesthesia, and combined spinal and epidural anesthesia (CSE). Neuraxial anesthesia has been used for more than 50 years to provide adequate surgical anesthesia and/or analgesia to different regions of the human body depending on the level of blockade. These procedures can be used as the sole intraoperative anesthetic or in combination with general anesthesia for numerous surgeries, which include thoracic, abdominal, vascular, urologic, and orthopedic surgery for lower extremities. In addition, epidurals are commonly used for labor analgesia and chronic pain relief.

Spinal and epidural infusions are highly varied based on local anesthetic availability and regional practice standards. The recommendations provided here are examples only and certainly are not representative of the full breadth of neuraxial injection possibilities.

2. Anatomy

To perform adequate neuraxial anesthesia, one must understand the anatomy of the vertebral column, ligaments, meninges, and spinal cord.

The vertebral column is composed of 7 cervical vertebrae, 12 thoracic vertebrae, 5 lumbar vertebrae, and 9 fused sacral and coccygeal vertebrae. The cervical and lumbar columns are curved in a convex manner, while thoracic and sacral columns are concave (Figure 51.1). The stability of the vertebral column is maintained by several ligaments (from posterior to anterior): supraspinous ligament, interspinous ligament, and ligamentum flavum. Additionally, anterior and posterior longitudinal ligaments bind the vertebral column to provide further stability.

The epidural space overlies the spinal meninges and encompasses nerve roots, arteries, veins, and adipose tissue. The epidural space is defined anteriorly by posterior longitudinal ligament, laterally by intervertebral foramina, and posteriorly by ligamentum flavum.

The meninges consist of 3 separate membranes, which include the dura mater (outermost layer), arachnoid mater (middle layer), and pia mater. The area between the arachnoid mater and pia matter is classified as the subarachnoid space that contains cerebral spinal fluid (CSF). Injection of local anesthetic into the subarachnoid space results in bilateral sensory, motor, and sympathetic blockade (Figure 51.2).

The spinal cord starts at the foramen magnum and extends distally to L1 in adults or L3 in children from newborns to 1 year of age. The end of the spinal cord is termed *conus medullaris*.

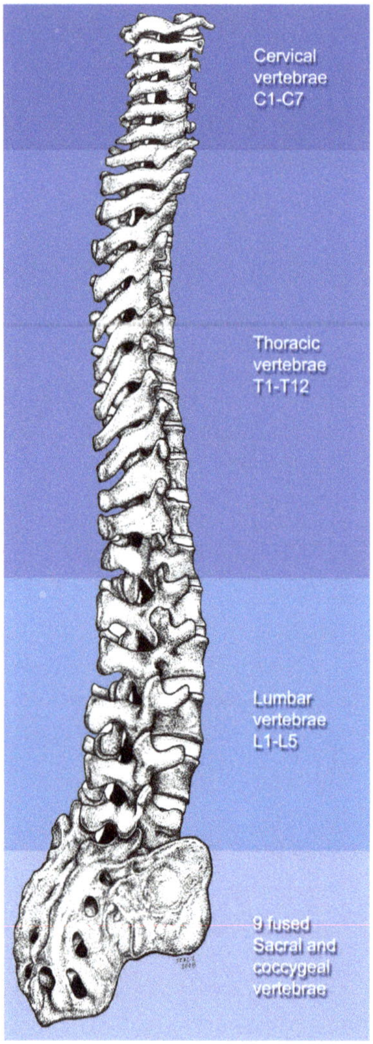

Figure 51.1 Human spine.

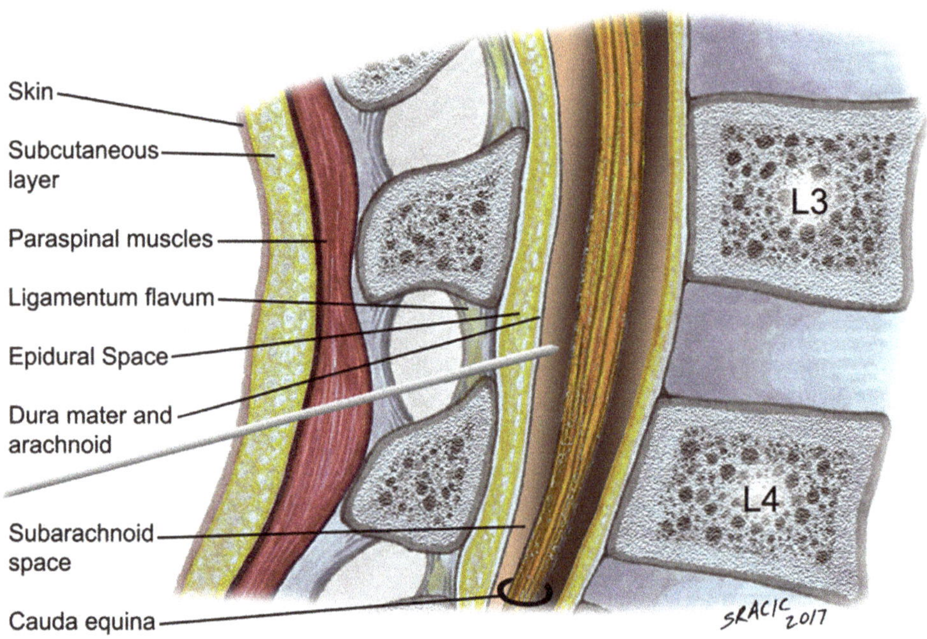

Figure 51.2 Neuraxial block anatomy.

Complications from neuraxial anesthesia include postural puncture headache, hypotension, bradycardia, hematoma formation, abscess, total spinal anesthesia, and nerve injury.

3. Procedure

3.1. Single-injection spinal anesthesia

The patient is placed sitting upright, with the neck and back flexed and lower back pushed out to optimize the space between the lumbar vertebrae (Figure 51.3a). A footstool under the patient's feet and a pillow for the patient to hold can help the patient maintain this position comfortably. Palpate the midline to feel for spinous processes. Depending on the level of blockade, additional anatomic landmarks or ultrasound can be used to determine specific vertebral bodies that correspond to a dermatomal level. For example, the iliac crests can be palpated as a landmark to the L4-L5 dermatome level. Ultrasound identification of vertebral levels is more objectively accurate.

The skin at the needle entry point is cleaned with aseptic cleaning solution and the surrounding area covered with sterile drapes. Lidocaine is often used to anesthetize the skin prior to needle insertion (Figure 51.3b). An introducer needle is then inserted perpendicular to the skin. Next, the spinal needle is inserted through the introducer. Once the spinal needle advances through the dura mater, a slight "pop" is felt. The stylet is then removed from the spinal needle and CSF flow should be appreciated within the next 5 to 10 seconds (Figure 51.3c). If no CSF flow is present, reinsert the stylet and advance the spinal needle until a slight "pop" can be appreciated. After free flow of CSF is confirmed, the desired local anesthetic solution is injected slowly (Figure 51.3d). After completion of injection, the spinal needle and introducer are removed and the patient is placed into surgical position. Standard American Society of Anesthesiologists (ASA) monitors should be in place and monitored every 3 to 5 minutes. Vital sign monitoring should continue until the spinal block resolves.

3.2. Epidural anesthesia

Epidural anesthesia requires the same patient positioning and preparation as for spinals. A larger-gauge Tuohy needle (usually 17 gauge or 18 gauge) is advanced through the skin. The needle travels through an area of high resistance (supraspinous ligament, interspinous ligament, and ligamentum flavum) into an area of low resistance (epidural space). Typically a glass syringe filled with saline and a small air bubble (air-only techniques should be avoided) is attached to the Tuohy needle as it is advanced toward the ligamentum flavum. The plunger of the syringe should not inject if positioned properly into ligamentum flavum, As the Tuohy needle is slowly advanced, a sudden "loss of resistance" on the plunger will be appreciated, and fluid will be easily injected into the epidural space. A flexible (20-gauge) catheter is

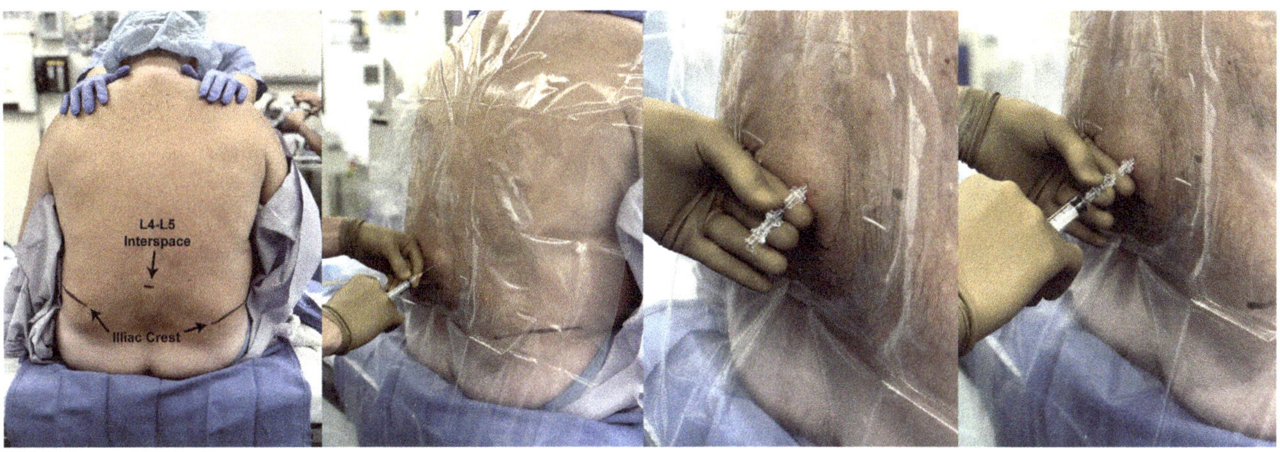

Figure 51.3 Single injection spinal anesthesia.

then advanced 3 to 4 cm into the epidural space and the Tuohy needle is removed over the catheter that is left in place. A 3-mL test dose of local anesthetic (typically lidocaine with epinephrine) is injected into the epidural catheter, and the patient is observed for signs of intravascular or subarachnoid injection. Systolic blood pressure greater than 15 mmHg or heart rate increase of 10 beats per minute can signify intravascular test dose. Immediate sensory blockade can signify subarachnoid injection. If test dose is positive, the epidural catheter should be removed and the procedure repeated for proper epidural placement.

3.3. Ultrasound guidance for neuraxial blockade

By landmark identification alone, practitioners can still be misled in regard to the estimated level of vertebral interspace for needle insertion. Ultrasound guidance can improve the accuracy of desired needle placement. The anatomy of neuraxial structures, such as the transverse process, vertebral bodies, and intrathecal space, can be identified with a curved low-frequency ultrasound probe (4–7 MHz). In the axial plane, the transverse processes can be identified as linear, hyperechoic structures. At midline, the intrathecal space can be identified as a hypoechoic region deep to the transverse process (Figure 51.4). Information provided through ultrasound scanning allows for needle placement at the exact desired level of vertebral process. In addition, one can also estimate the depth to intrathecal space by using the ultrasound probe prior to needle insertion. Occasionally, initial ultrasound scanning can result in other anatomic findings that may modify the anesthetic plan, and therefore it is highly recommended in all cases when the technology is available.

3.4. Needles/catheter

- For spinal anesthesia: 20-gauge introducer needle, 3.5 to 5 inch × 24- to 27-gauge pencil point (Whitacre or Pencan) spinal needle
- For epidural anesthesia: 17- or 18-gauge Tuohy needle with a 20-gauge flexible catheter

3.5. Local anesthetic

For single-injection spinals, 2 to 3 mL of local anesthetic is injected into the lumbar subarachnoid space for procedures of the abdomen, lower extremity, and perineum. Isobaric bupivacaine 0.5%, tetracaine 0.5%, or ropivacaine 0.5% is utilized for procedures with an expected the duration of 3 to 6 hours depending on several factors. The dose of local anesthetic and addition of a vasoconstrictor such as epinephrine are the main determinants of spinal duration. Pregnancy and patient height may also affect spinal duration to a certain degree. For shorter procedures, 2 hours or less, 2% lidocaine, 1.5%

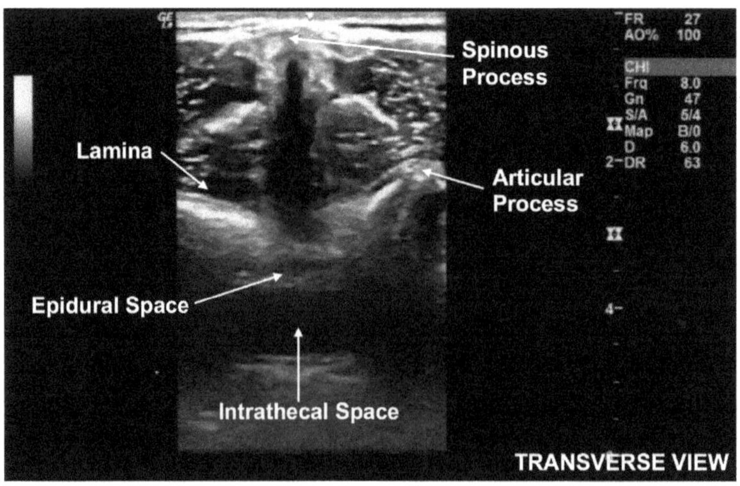

Figure 51.4 Neuraxial structures via ultrasound.

mepivacaine, and 3% 2-chloroprocaine may be used. The risk of transient neurologic symptoms has been reported to be between 10% and 40% with lidocaine and mepivacaine, and chloroprocaine is preferred for shorter procedures.

For abdominal procedures, mostly cesarean sections, a higher-level spinal is achieved by using a hyperbaric solution of local anesthetic, typically 0.75% bupivacaine with dextrose. After the injection of a hyperbaric solution, the patient is placed from a sitting to supine position and immediately in slight Trendelenburg position to encourage a higher spinal block level. For cases of the perineal area such as hemorrhoidectomy or anal fistula repair, a hypobaric spinal solution may be placed with the patient in the prone jackknife position.

Single injection spinals are typically not used in the thoracic spine due to concern for a "total spinal" and blockade of the cardiac accelerator fibers from the T1-T4 nerve roots.

For epidural blockade, generally 1 to 2 mL of local anesthetic will be required for each dermatome level to be blocked. For instance, at the level of L4, up to 20 mL of local anesthetic solution can be administered to achieve a sensory blockade at T7.

- For short procedures, 3% 2-chloroprocaine can be used with an onset time of 10 to 15 minutes and an expected duration of 45 to 60 minutes.
- For procedures lasting less than 2 hours, 2% lidocaine or 1.5% mepivacaine can be used with an onset time of 15 minutes and an expected duration of 80 to 160 minutes; 1:200,000 epinephrine can be added to these local anesthetics to prolong the duration of action by about 50%.
- For procedures lasting longer than 2 hours, 0.5% bupivacaine or 0.5% ropivacaine can be used with an onset time of 15 to 20 minutes and an expected duration of 140 to 200 minutes.

3.6. Adjuvants

For continuous epidural analgesia, opioids (frequently fentanyl) can be added to the local anesthetic solutions to provide multimodal analgesia. For instance, an epidural solution may contain 0.125% bupivacaine plus fentanyl 5 mcg/mL at a rate of 6 to 10 mL/h. Epidural rates can be adjusted based on pain score, motor blockade, hemodynamics, respiratory depression, nausea, or itching.

Additionally, other adjuvants such as clonidine, neostigmine, ketamine, and midazolam have been studied to various degrees. Side effects of clonidine must be monitored. They include hypotension (most common), bradycardia, and dry mouth.

Regional Anesthesia Complications

52

1. Introduction

Regional anesthesia offers numerous opportunities for improved pain control and increased patient satisfaction compared with general anesthesia. As regional anesthesia techniques and utilization expand, the ability to evaluate, diagnose, and treat possible complications becomes exceedingly important. This chapter reviews neural anatomy, the effects of local anesthetics, and common perineural additives and then discusses the etiology, evaluation, and treatment of peripheral nerve block complications.

2. Peripheral Nerve Anatomy

The multiple tissue layers of peripheral nerve microanatomy offer protection to nerve cell bodies and axons and barriers to local anesthetics. Peripheral nerves are bundled into fascicles composed of both afferent and efferent nerve fibers with variable sympathetic fiber input. Each fiber, termed an *axon*, is encircled by endonerium, a connective tissue containing glial cells (Figure 52.1).

Clusters of axons, bundled with capillaries and fibroblasts, are surrounded by a dense connective tissue layer called perineurium to create a fascicle. Epineurium, another dense connective tissue layer, then encases groups of fascicles. Neural health requires regulation of the endoneurium environment by perineurium and the endoneurial capillaries. Tight endothelial junctions create the blood-nerve barrier with blood flow regulated by the sympathetic nervous system. Given the high metabolic activity of nerves, blood flow may reach 40 mL/100 g/min.

Nerve fibers are classified by function, size, and presence or absence of myelin (Table 52.1). Both increased diameter and myelin are associated with increased conduction velocity. Concomitantly, myelinated nerve fibers frequently have a diameter exceeding 1 micron. Motor and sensory functions requiring critical speeds are typically associated with large-diameter, myelinated fibers (A-fibers), while autonomic functions are usually controlled by small-diameter fibers.

2.1. Nerve Cell Ion Gradient

Impulse propagation also requires changes in the nerve membrane charge through the movement of ions. At rest, ion channels establish electrical and chemical gradients across the resting nerve axon membrane through a cellular energy- requiring process. Sodium (Na^+) ions are moved out of the cell and potassium (K^+) ions into the cell, by an active Na^+/K^+ adenosine triphosphatase (ATPase) pump, with a 3:2 ratio, respectively. This

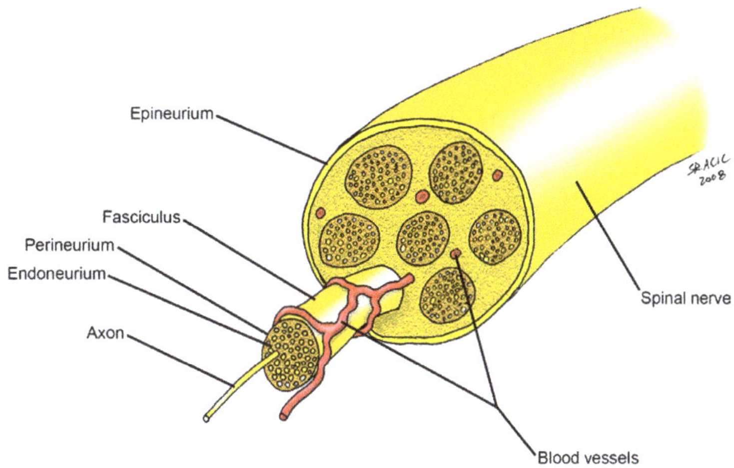

Figure 52.1 Histological representation of a peripheral nerve.

produces high intracellular K^+ and high extracellular Na^+ concentrations, generating potential energy through a chemical gradient. By this concentration gradient, K^+ flows out of the cell through passive ion channels. The combination of the active pumping (Na^+) and passive leakage (K^+) of positive ions out of the axon creates an electrical gradient and a negative intracellular charge (–70 to –90 mV) compared with the outside, resulting in a resting electrical potential difference.

Action potentials are momentary, localized episodes of depolarization in which a positive charge is conducted along nerves by the movement of Na^+ ions down both electrical and chemical gradients. Sufficient nerve stimulation opens voltage-gated Na^+ channels, resulting in a rapid influx of Na^+ ions. If the stimulus is sufficient to raise the membrane potential (termed *threshold potential*) greater than –60 mV, a widespread opening of Na^+ channels is triggered, generating a further rapid influx of Na^+ ions. Membrane depolarization results in a potential difference, compared with adjacent areas, producing an electrical current. This raises the membrane potentials of contiguous areas and creates a wave of depolarization of the adjacent nerve membranes (unmyelinated nerves) or adjoining nodes of Ranvier (myelinated nerves). This action potential is then propagated down the nerve axon. The increased intracellular Na^+ concentration causes the membrane potential to bypass neutral and depolarization peaks (+50 mV), stimulating a stop in Na^+ influx. This triggers voltage-dependent K^+ channels to open, and extracellular K^+ movement reverses the membrane potential (repolarization). The Na^+/K^+ ATPase pump, activated by increased intracellular Na^+, reestablishes the resting membrane potential in preparation for another action potential.

Myelin, produced by Schwann cells, surrounds most peripheral axons, augments nerve electrical insulation, and amplifies impulse propagation. In a process called *saltatory conduction*, impulses skip between gaps (nodes of Ranvier) in the nerve myelin sheath to travel 60–100 m/s by jumping 3 to 5 nodes of Ranvier (60–100 mm).

Table 52.1:
Properties of different nerve fibers

Nerve Fiber	Myelination	Size	Function	Conduction Speed
A-alpha/A-beta	Myelinated	2–33 μm	Motor, proprioception	30–120 m/s
A-gamma	Myelinated	3–6 μm	Muscle tone	15–35 m/s
A-delta	Myelinated	1–4 μm	Pain, touch, temperature	5–25 m/s
B-fiber	Myelinated	<3 μm	Autonomic function	3–15 m/s
C-fiber	Unmyelinated	0.3–1.3 μm	Sympathetic innervation	2 m/s

3. Effects of Local Anesthetics

3.1. Sodium Channel Blockade

Local anesthetics block nerve conduction by reversibly binding with intracellular voltage-gated Na^+ channels. Local anesthetic binding affinity is highest when the sodium channel is open and least when the channel is closed; consequently, a stimulated nerve is more sensitive to local anesthetic than a resting nerve. Furthermore, as local anesthetics are water-soluble salts in an acidic solution, they must be converted into a lipid-soluble (nonionized) form to diffuse across the cell membrane. The proportion of drug transformed to the nonionized form is correlated with tissue pH and drug pKa. After moving intracellularly, a decreased intracellular pH regenerates the ionized form, which is then available to bind the sodium channel. Threshold potentials are not achieved and nerve impulse conduction obstructed when enough sodium channels are interrupted. The patient experiences neural blockade first with decreased pain and temperature sensation, followed by touch, deep pressure, and finally motor function. Large fibers (touch, pressure, and motor) require higher local anesthetic concentrations to produce adequate blockade compared with small myelinated fibers (pain). Dissociation of the local anesthetic from the Na^+ channels is related to the drug's affinity for the receptor (e.g., lidocaine dissociates rapidly and is short-acting while bupivacaine dissociates slower, lasting far longer).

3.2. Toxicity

Local anesthetics are neurotoxins. Although the exact mechanism is unknown, toxicity is likely a combination of inhibition of rapid axon transport, disruption of the axon microskeleton, axonal degeneration, and ischemia. Small, unmyelinated fibers are more vulnerable to damage. With increased local anesthetic dose, the epineurium becomes disrupted and permeable to granulocytes, which infiltrate the subjacent endoneurium and cause endoneurial edema. Damage to supporting Schwann cells may appear as lipid droplet accumulation in the cell; however, Schwann cell injury may be temporary as these cells replicate quickly. Additionally, local anesthetics can cause ischemia by reducing blood flow within endoneurial capillaries. This may be caused by decreasing the production of natural vasodilating substances such as nitric oxide or prostaglandins. Growing nerves also produce growth cones at the terminal ends of the axon, which interact with nerve growth factor and Schwann cells to direct growth direction and rates. Local anesthetics induce growth cone collapse when applied at increasing concentrations. Local anesthetics also delay nerve growth by retraction of the filopodia (cytoplasmic projections) of the growth cones. Even at very low concentrations of local anesthetics, nerve axonal growth is delayed and axon transport is inhibited. The clinical significance of this growth inhibition by local anesthetics is unclear.

4. Other Regional Anesthesia–Related Complications

4.1. Local anesthetic systemic toxicity

The classic description of local anesthetic systemic toxicity (LAST) begins with perioral numbness and tinnitus progressing to neurologic excitation, seizure, and cardiac arrest. However, LAST can present at any point along this continuum, and treatment depends on the presentation. Tinnitus, metallic taste, and other mild manifestations are often self-limited and are managed with patient monitoring. LAST-induced seizures are treated with benzodiazepines to end seizure activity, while avoiding propofol with its cardiac depressant effects. Normal oxygenation and ventilation status must also be monitored and maintained. If cardiac manifestations occur, Advanced Cardiac Life Support (ACLS) protocols are activated and 20% lipid emulsion infused (1.5-mL/kg bolus followed by 0.25-mL/kg/min infusion). The infusion can be increased with refractory symptoms (0.5 mL/kg/min) and the bolus repeated an additional 2 times for persistent cardiovascular collapse. Distinctive from current ACLS guidelines, vasopressin, calcium channel blockers, beta blockers, and additional local anesthetics are avoided in the treatment of LAST-associated arrhythmias as evidence suggests this may lead to refractory arrest. Similarly, epinephrine dosing is reduced to 1-mcg/kg boluses during resuscitation. While the current recommendations for the use of lipid emulsion are only for cardiac symptoms, earlier administration has been proposed with significant or unclear neurologic manifestations.

4.2. Falls

Nerve blocks of the lower extremity have proven effective at providing analgesia; however, their association with increasing fall risk is concerning. In hospitalized patients, independent of nerve blockade, the risk of fall has been found to be approximately 1.7%. Reviews of lower extremity blockade suggest the highest fall risk occurs in continuous lumbar plexus blocks (fall incidence 2.2%). This rate is similar to patients undergoing total knee replacement without nerve blockade (fall incidence 2%), suggesting that nerve blockade alone is not singularly responsible for all patient falls. In recent years, more distal blocks, such as the adductor canal block, have gained support in an effort to decrease motor weakness, while improving early physical therapy following lower extremity surgery. Unfortunately, the loss of extremity proprioception is still present with any block; therefore, distal blocks should not erroneously be suggested as improving fall safety, and all patients should be counseled for this risk.

4.3. Respiratory Side Effects

Phrenic Nerve Block. Brachial plexus blockade is known to be associated with transient phrenic nerve paralysis. In general, it is assumed that when performing an interscalene block the incidence of phrenic nerve blockade will approach 100%. This incidence can be decreased by using smaller injectate volumes or a more caudal approach, although not reliably eliminated. At the C5 level, the phrenic nerve lies approximately 1.8 mm from the brachial plexus, but 3 cm caudally they are nearly 11 mm apart. Therefore, a more caudal approach can decrease the chance of phrenic blockade. Notably, supraclavicular blocks are also associated with phrenic nerve blockade (incidence approaching 50%) while infraclavicular blocks are less likely (3% incidence).

Pneumothorax. Iatrogenic pneumothorax is another potential risk with brachial plexus blocks. This is most often associated with the supraclavicular landmark-based approach (incidence of 6.1%) with 18-gauge cutting needles. Ultrasound guidance has greatly decreased, but not eliminated, this complication. In 2014, Gauss et al. evaluated more than 6300 ultrasound-guided supra- and infraclavicular nerve blocks and reported a 0.06% and 0.07% pneumothorax incidence, respectively.

4.4. Neuraxial and Deep-Tissue Hematoma

Neuraxial and deep-tissue hematomas are rare but potentially devastating complications of neuraxial anesthesia, analgesia, and/or deep-tissue regional nerve blockade. To better understand the risk of causing a neuraxial or deep-tissue hematoma in the periprocedural period when using central neuraxial or deep-tissue nerve blockade in the presence of antithrombotic therapy, one needs an understanding of the pharmacokinetics and pharmacodynamics of the antithrombotic agents that may be used. Each agent has unique properties that affect how the anesthetic may be more safely managed. In recent years, newer and more potent or longer-lasting agents have been introduced to the pharmaceutical market, which has resulted in greater confusion among providers who perform neuraxial anesthesia and deep-tissue regional nerve blocks.

Table 52.2 presents recommendations for neuraxial and deep-tissue regional nerve blocks that are compiled, reviewed, and updated on an annual basis by the Massachusetts General Hospital (MGH) Medical Education and Safety Advisory Committee (MESAC). This committee is composed of a multidisciplinary team of experts who compile a succinct list of recommendations for placement of neuraxial and deep-tissue regional nerve blocks in the setting of anticoagulant/antithrombotic medications. These recommendations are mainly derived from the fourth edition of the American Society of Regional Anesthesia and Pain Medicine (ASRA guidelines), but they also use the European Society of Regional Anesthesia guidelines (for some of the drugs that were not included in ASRA guidelines), drug package insert material, and expert consensus from multiple departments at MGH (e.g., Anesthesiology, Critical Care, and Pain Medicine; Cardiology; Hematology; Pathology; Pharmacy). These guidelines apply to patients of normal body weight and organ function, unless otherwise noted. Clinical judgment should be used in treating children and patients of advanced age, patients with decreased renal function (CrCl <50), or patients with high or low body mass index. Clinical judgment

Table 52.2:
Suggested guidelines for use of anticoagulation with neuraxial interventions and deep-tissue regional anesthesia procedures

Massachusetts General Hospital, Department of Anesthesia, Critical Care and Pain Medicine
SUGGESTED GUIDELINES FOR ANTICOAGULATION AND NEURAXIAL INTERVENTIONS 2018

Drug (Generic)	Common Trade Names	Interval for Catheter Placement or Neuraxial Procedure After Last Dose	Interval for Catheter Removal After Most Recent Dose	Recommended Interval to Restart Med After Neuraxial Procedure or Removal of Epidural Catheter
ASPIRIN	ECOTRIN, BUFFERIN	No Significant Risk when taken alone. Precaution should be taken if used in conjunction with other antiplatelet medications		
ABCIXIMAB	REOPRO	48 Hours	48 Hours	24 Hours
ALTEPLASE	ACTIVASE	Minimum of 48 hours, PLUS normalization of clotting studies including fibrinogen	if t-PA has been given, check fibrinogen and remove catheter if level >100	10 Days
APIXABAN (Therapeutic)	ELIQUIS (5 -10 mg BID)	3 days (SCr < 1.5) 4 days (SCr ≥ 1.5, ≥ 80 years, ≤ 60 kg)	48-72 Hours	6 Hours; If traumatic placement occurs, delay administration by 48 hours
APIXABAN (Prophylactic)	ELIQUIS (2.5 mg BID)	26-30 Hours	26-30 Hours	6 Hours
BETRIXABAN (Prophylactic)	BEVYXXA	5 Days (CrCl ≥ 30) 6 Days (CrCl 15-29, concomitant P-gp inhibitors)	72 Hours	5 Hours; If traumatic placement occurs delay administration by 72 hours
ARGATROBAN	ACOVA	At least 6 Hours Check for normal PTT or ACT	Check for normal PTT or ACT	2 Hours
BIVALIRUDIN	ANGIOMAX	At least 6 Hours Check for normal PTT or ACT	Check for normal PTT or ACT	2 Hours
CANGRELOR	KENGREAL	3 Hours	3 Hours	8 Hours
CILOSTAZOL (alone or with aspirin)	PLETAL	42 Hours	42 Hours	5 Hours
CLOPIDOGREL	PLAVIX	7 Days	7 days (If single 75 mg dose given, Urgent Anesthesia consult and hold further dosing)	6 Hours
DABIGATRAN (Therapeutic)	PRADAXA	4 days (CrCL >50) 5 days (CrCl ≤ 50)	4 days (CrCL >50) 5 days (CrCl ≤ 50)	6 Hours

Table 52.2:
Continued

Massachusetts General Hospital, Department of Anesthesia, Critical Care and Pain Medicine
SUGGESTED GUIDELINES FOR ANTICOAGULATION AND NEURAXIAL INTERVENTIONS 2018

Drug (Generic)	Common Trade Names	Interval for Catheter Placement or Neuraxial Procedure After Last Dose	Interval for Catheter Removal After Most Recent Dose	Recommended Interval to Restart Med After Neuraxial Procedure or Removal of Epidural Catheter
DABIGATRAN (Prophylactic)	PRADAXA (≤220 mg per day)	3 Days	48 Hours	6 Hours
DALTEPARIN (Therapeutic)	FRAGMIN	24 Hours	24 Hours	4 Hours
DALTEPARIN (Prophylactic)	FRAGMIN (≤ 5000 units QD)	12 Hours	12 Hours	4 Hours
DIPYRIDAMOLE	PERSANTINE	24 Hours	24 Hours	6 Hours
DIPYRIDAMOLE + ASPIRIN	AGGRENOX	24 Hours	24 Hours	6 Hours
EDOXABAN (Therapeutic)	SAVAYSA	3 days (CrCl >50) 5 days (CrCl ≤ 50, ≤60 kg, concomitant P-gp inhibitor drug use) Consult Cardiology before discontinuing	48-72 Hours	6 Hours
ENOXAPARIN (Therapeutic)	LOVENOX (> 60 mg total daily dose OR 1mg/kg BID OR 1.5 mg/kg QD)	24 Hours	24 Hours	4 Hours
ENOXAPARIN (Prophylactic)	LOVENOX (≤ 60 mg total daily dose)	12 Hours	12 Hours	4 Hours
Note: LOW MOLECULAR WEIGHT HEPARIN: Prophylactic dosing may be started 6-8 hours postoperatively. Therapeutic dosing or BID dosing should be started at least 24 hours postoperatively. Epidural catheters should be removed prior to initiation of therapy.				
EPTIFIBATIDE	INTEGRILIN	8 Hours	8 Hours	24 Hours
FONDAPARINUX *(See Note)*	ARIXTRA (5 mg, 7.5 mg, 10 mg)	7 Days	>4 Days/monitor	6 Hours
FONDAPARINUX *(See Note)*	ARIXTRA (2.5 mg)	36-42 Hours	36-42 Hours	6 Hours
Note: FONDAPARINUX should not be given if regional anesthesia is anticipated or has been used. If, however, FONDAPARINUX is given, the above guidelines are suggested.				

(continued)

Table 52.2: Continued

Massachusetts General Hospital, Department of Anesthesia, Critical Care and Pain Medicine
SUGGESTED GUIDELINES FOR ANTICOAGULATION AND NEURAXIAL INTERVENTIONS 2018

Drug (Generic)	Common Trade Names	Interval for Catheter Placement or Neuraxial Procedure After Last Dose	Interval for Catheter Removal After Most Recent Dose	Recommended Interval to Restart Med After Neuraxial Procedure or Removal of Epidural Catheter
HEPARIN IV/SC (Therapeutic)	HEPARIN (treatment dosing)	IV: 4-6 Hours, PTT < 35 SC: 8-12 Hours, PTT <35	IV: 4-6 Hours, PTT < 35 SC: 8-12 Hours, PTT <35	1 Hour
HEPARIN SC (Prophylactic)	HEPARIN, prophylaxis dosing (≤ 15,000 units/day)	4-6 Hours; or PTT<35	4-6 Hours; or PTT<35	1 Hour
NSAID	CELEBREX, MOTRIN, NAPROSYN, etc.		No Significant Risk	
RIVAROXABAN (Therapeutic)	XARELTO (>10 mg total daily dose)	3 days (CrCl > 50) 4-5 days (CrCl ≤ 50)	48-72 Hours	6 hours; If traumatic placement occurs delay administration by 24 hours
RIVAROXABAN (Prophylactic)	XARELTO (10 mg daily)	24 Hours	24 Hours	6 Hours
PRASUGREL	EFFIENT	7-10 days	7-10 Days	6 hours
TICAGRELOR	BRILINTA	5 days	5 days	6 hours
TIROFIBAN	AGGRASTAT	8 Hours	8 Hours	24 Hours
VORAXAPAR	ZONTIVITY	30 days	Voraxapar should not be given if regional anticipated/has been used	24 Hours
WARFARIN	COUMADIN	3-5 Days, INR <1.5	If > 24 Hours, check INR < 1.5	Same Day

These guidelines apply to patients of normal body weight and organ function unless otherwise noted. Clinical judgment should be used in treating children and patients of advanced age, patients with decreased renal function (CrCl < 50), or patients with high or low BMI. Clinical judgment should be considered in the obstetric population on prophylactic doses of anticoagulants- in some instances, the risk of post-procedural spinal epidural hematoma may be lower than the risk of general anesthesia . It may, therefore, be appropriate to proceed with neuraxial procedures in these parturients without delay. Caution if patient on more than one anticoagulant or if taking SSRIs. Consider increasing interval to restart anticoagulants after multiple attempts or traumatic procedure. Close neuro monitoring is recommended in the period after restarting meds post-procedure.

should be considered in the obstetric population on prophylactic doses of anticoagulants—in some instances, the risk of postprocedural spinal epidural hematoma may be lower than the risk of general anesthesia. It may, therefore, be appropriate to proceed with neuraxial procedures in these parturients without delay. Caution should be exercised if a patient is on more than one anticoagulant or is taking selective serotonin reuptake inhibitors. Consider increasing the time interval before restarting anticoagulants after multiple attempts or traumatic procedure. Close neuromonitoring is recommended in the period after restarting anticoagulation medications postprocedure.

5. Block Additives

Nonlocal anesthetic perineural adjuncts have been described as increasing anesthetic or analgesic duration. While epinephrine is the most common perineural additive, it only prolongs the duration of short-acting local anesthetics (e.g., lidocaine). Additionally, pathologic examination of nerves subjected to high local anesthetic concentrations reveals dose-dependent axonal degeneration, which is more severe if epinephrine is added. This is thought to be due to decreased nerve blood flow. Epinephrine does serve a valuable role as a marker for intravascular injection to avoid LAST, but it should be dosed sparingly and at dilute concentrations (1:400,000). While other additives, including clonidine, dexmedetomidine, dexamethasone, and buprenorphine, have shown variable success with prolonging peripheral block duration, toxicity has remained a concern. However, basic science work has indicated that the local anesthetic is the most neurotoxic agent. Many of these additives also can be associated with side effects, such as clonidine or dexmedetomidine contributing to sedation and hypotension and buprenorphine increasing nausea.

6. Peripheral Nerve Damage After Nerve Block

6.1. Etiology of Nerve Injury

In addition to direct local anesthetic toxicity, peripheral nerves can be damaged by needle injury, compression, stretch, ischemia, complete transection, and surgical insult. Direct needle trauma can be associated with significant nerve injury, especially if the needle penetrates the perineurium and enters the fascicle. Fortunately, the perineurium is very strong and pressures up to 1000 mmHg have been reported without rupture. The use of a blunt-tip needle may decrease neural penetration and minimize fascicular injury. Local anesthetic injection into the fascicle causes direct axonal damage from the needle and local anesthetic toxicity, and it increases fascicular pressure, compromising endoneurial blood flow. Studies in rat tibial nerves demonstrate that nerves can tolerate ischemia for up to 6 hours without permanent sequelae; however, this decreases to 4 hours if ischemia is combined with nerve compression.

6.2. Incidence of Nerve Injury

Barrington and Snyder, in a 2011 publication, suggested that the total number of neurologic complications may be increasing with the growth of regional anesthesia; however, the incidence likely remains unchanged. Brull et al. (2007) reviewed 32 studies published over 10 years and concluded that the rate of neuropathy after a peripheral nerve block was 3%. However, permanent neurologic injury after regional anesthesia was rare. More recently, Barrington et al., in a review of more than 7100 peripheral nerve blocks from the Australasian Regional Anesthesia Collaboration database, published an incidence of 0.4 per 1000 blocks for late neurologic complications related to peripheral nerve blockade. Thirty patients were noted to have postoperative nerve injury and only 3 of these were determined to be related to regional anesthesia, after extensive neurologic evaluation. Interestingly, they also reported a rate of LAST as 0.98 per 1000 blocks.

While peripheral nerve injury may be thought to be associated with regional anesthesia, Ben-David et al. (2002), in a closed-claims analysis of upper extremity nerve injuries associated with anesthesia, found nerve injury to be associated more frequently with general anesthesia (61%) versus regional anesthesia (36%). Whether peripheral nerve blocks are associated with an increased rate of iatrogenic nerve injury has been examined by several studies. A retrospective review by Welch et al. (2009) of more than 380,000 perioperative peripheral nerve injury patients over 10 years noted nerve iatrogenic injuries at a rate of 0.03%. Iatrogenic injuries were associated with general anesthesia, epidural anesthesia, and certain types of surgery; however, they were not associated with peripheral nerve blocks. In a prospective study of 521 patients who received interscalene block for shoulder surgery, Borgeat et al. (2001) found paresthesias or dysesthesias in 14% of patients 10 days after surgery. Symptoms persisted in 7.9% of patients at 1 month; 3.9% at 3 months; 0.9% at 6 months; and 0.2% at 9 months. Notably, no patients had motor weakness. Candido et al. (2005), in a similar study, noted a 3.3% incidence at 1 month postoperative. In both of these studies, most of the neurologic dysfunction was thought to be unrelated to the block. In addition, a retrospective analysis of 12,000 total knee arthroplastics over 20 years found an incidence of peripheral nerve injury of 0.79% that has remained unchanged despite the rapid growth of peripheral nerve block utilization.

Certain surgeries have been associated with a higher risk of nerve injury in multiple retrospective studies. The ASRA, in a practice advisory on the neurologic complications associated with regional anesthesia, noted that these risk factors included surgeries with prolonged tourniquet time, trauma, inflammation, ischemia, or excessive neural stretch. Entry points for multiple orthopedic surgeries run close to multiple neural structures and may contribute to postoperative neural injury. Two examples of surgeries with an increased incidence of nerve injury related to surgical insult and independent of regional anesthesia are lateral femoral cutaneous nerve injury with anterior hip procedures (14%–88%) and variable nerve injury with shoulder arthroscopy (0%–10%). Regardless of the complication rate quoted to the patient, many neurologic symptoms arising from the surgical procedure may be initially attributed to a regional anesthetic block–induced neuropathy. Consequently, the regional anesthesiologist will be called to evaluate these patients.

7. Evaluation of Nerve Injury After Regional Anesthesia

Evaluation begins by localizing the region of pathology and the nerves involved. This starts with a careful history and physical examination and continues with electrophysiological tests and neuroimaging if needed (Figure 52.2).

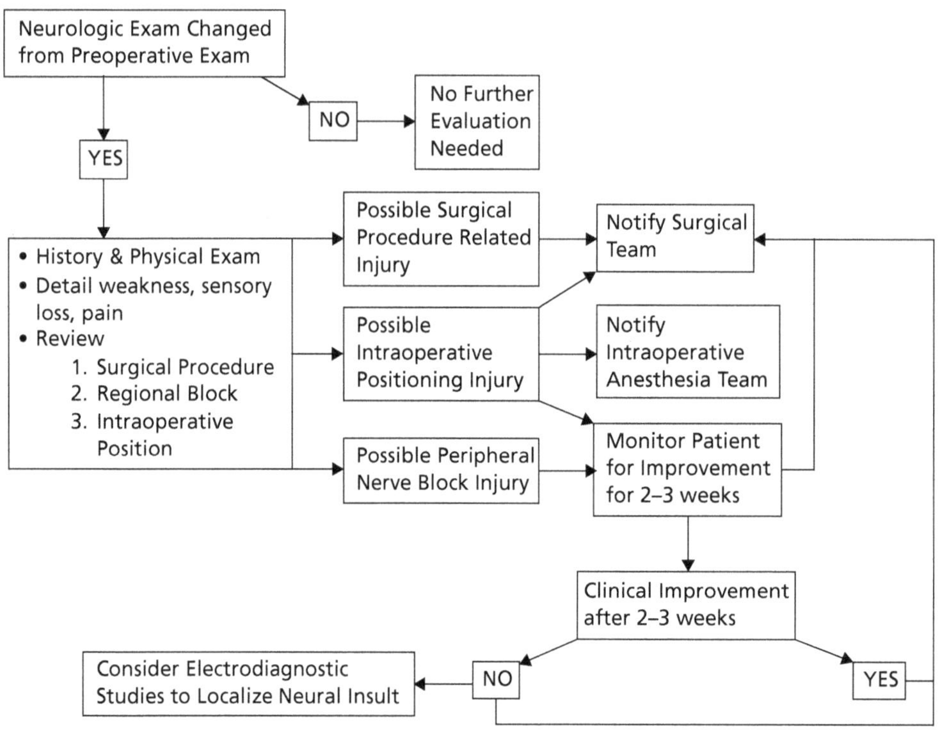

Figure 52.2 Evaluation of a patient with a possible neurologic injury.

7.1. History

In order to evaluate for preexisting neurologic deficits, a normal or abnormal neurologic examination should routinely be documented prior to regional procedures. Preexisting peripheral neuropathy (e.g., diabetes) may predispose patients to postoperative nerve injury with or without a peripheral nerve block, and they should be counseled prior to regional anesthesia regarding this risk. Once neurologic injury is a concern, new neurologic deficits should be described in detail. Symptoms of a nerve injury may not become apparent for 2 to 3 weeks after initial injury due to distracters, including casts, splints, and pain. Surgical, block, and positioning details should be reviewed, as the neurologic complaint is sometimes not on the blocked side or extremity. Weakness, sensory loss, and pain sources should all be clarified and documented.

7.2. Physical Examination

Strength, pinprick, fine touch, position sense, and reflexes must be examined and documented. Notably, muscle atrophy on the first postoperative day usually indicates a preexisting condition. Evaluate thoracic or abdominal sensation if neuraxial involvement is possible. Herniated discs may occur postoperatively, and patients should be evaluated for clinical manifestations of common radiculopathies.

7.3. Electrophysiologic Studies

Nerve conduction studies and electromyography (EMG) assist in determining the location and type of nerve injury; however, they do not reveal the cause of the injury. For both, a nerve is stimulated and a response recorded either in the innervated muscle (motor conduction studies) or over another portion of the stimulated nerve (sensory nerve conduction studies). The latencies, amplitudes, conduction velocities, and direct evoked responses are recorded. Sensory nerves are more susceptible to injury, and sensory studies may assist in diagnosing radicular nerve injury from a herniated disc versus another cause. The pathology, electrodynamics, and anticipated recovery after nerve injury are summarized in Table 52.3. The majority of nerve injuries are related to compression or neurapraxia (transient dysfunction of myelin in a focal area). These are recognized acutely with conduction block or focal slowing on nerve conduction studies, suggestive of a localized nerve injury (e.g., demyelination from a compression injury). Patients with predominantly sensory symptoms and/or findings of conduction block or focal slowing have an excellent prognosis (i.e., expected complete recovery ≤3 months). Both axonal loss and demyelination also cause reduced amplitudes of evoked responses; however, with axonal injury, the latency has minimal change. In cases of axonal injury, electrodiagnostic studies cannot acutely differentiate between axonotmesis (injury only to axon) or neurotmesis (injury to neural tube). As peripheral nerve axons will regenerate if the neural tube is intact (axonotmesis), serial studies (every 2 to 3 months) will demonstrate axonal regeneration and reinnervation starting with muscles contiguous to the injured area with distal improvement over time. Notably, axonal recovery is noted on electrodiagnostic studies prior to clinical motor improvement. However, with more severe injury (neurotmesis), recovery is not observed on serial studies. If an injury is judged to be unlikely to result in spontaneous recovery, surgical options should then be explored. Functional neurologic outcomes are improved if surgical intervention occurs no greater than 6 to 9 months after injury as axonal damage is not definitively evident until Wallerian degeneration has occurred with muscle denervation (up to 3 weeks after injury). In the acute perioperative period, electrodiagnostics are limited to confirming neurapraxia at a site of compression and defining preexisting neurologic disease. Consequently, electrodiagnostic studies are performed 14 to 21 days after injury to localize the neurologic insult and define severity and prognosis.

Limitations to electrophysiologic studies include inaccessible nerve locations for practical testing (e.g., lumbar plexus block) and the aforementioned normal studies for up to 2 weeks after a nerve lesion; however, this can be helpful in determining a preexisting or new-onset injury.

Table 52.3:
Pathology, electrodynamics, and recovery after nerve injury

Injury Type	Pathology	Electrodynamic Changes		Prognosis and Recovery
		Acute	Chronic	
Neuropraxia	• Interruption of nerve conduction within an axon; no anatomic disruption.	• Conduction block • Focal slowing • Decreased amplitude	Acute findings improve	Mildest injury Complete recovery (≤3 months)
Axonal loss or interruption				(Both) • Neurosurgical consultation if no improvement in 3–4 months
Axonotmesis	• Partial or no interruption of connective tissue framework	• Decreased amplitude	• Improvement (axonal regeneration)	
Neurotmesis	• Disruption of axon and connective tissue	• Decreased amplitude	• No improvement	

7.4. Radiographic Studies

Neuroimaging, including Magentic Resonance Imaging (MRI), Computerized Tomography, bone scans, angiography, and magnetic resonance neurography (MRN), may aid in localizing a peripheral nerve injury. Peripheral nerve ultrasound recently has been found to be highly sensitive in identifying peripheral nerve pathology, specifically in mononeuropathies and brachial plexopathies when compared with MRI evaluation.

8. Treatment Options

Treatments for neuropathies are either conservative or surgical. If severe nerve dysfunction occurs after peripheral nerve block and the lesion has been localized by physical examination, neuroimaging, and electrophysiologic tests, neurosurgery should be consulted to evaluate for surgical correction. A retrospective series by Kim et al. (2004) of 119 surgically treated femoral nerve lesions recommended operative exploration for patients without EMG improvement after 3 to 4 months. Operative exploration includes operative nerve examination by direct visualization and electrodiagnostic studies. Neurolysis, including resection of the neuroma and reapproximation of the nerve and its fascicles, may be indicated if a conduction block is noted to enable healthy axons to grow slowly down the nerve within each fascicle. If a reversible etiology is not found, physical therapy should be instituted with strength training and range-of-motion exercises to minimize contracture and muscle atrophy. Electrodiagnostics continue to be repeated at 6 weeks, 3 months, and 6 months after the event. In addition to surgical and conservative measures, the use of stem cells has been described in the animal model and may prove helpful in the future. At this time it remains experimental. Several medications that alter the production of interleukins and growth factors have shown promise in attenuating injury responses in animal models.

9. Conclusion

With the escalating use of regional anesthetic techniques, anesthesiologists are likely to encounter more consultations regarding potential injuries. In this regard, it is imperative that patients have access to the acute pain team until complete block resolution has occurred and that providers know how to evaluate patients both pre- and postoperatively for possible neurologic deficits. Furthermore, providers must be prepared to respond to LAST emergencies and other complications associated with regional anesthesia throughout the body.

Continuous Peripheral Nerve Blocks

53

1. Introduction

The continuous peripheral nerve block (CPNB) catheter allows the benefits of regional anesthesia to be extended beyond the 8 to 20 hours achieved with single-injection, long-acting local anesthetics. A CPNB is typically used to provide the following:

- anesthesia for surgery and prolonged analgesia postoperatively (e.g., shoulder, hip, or knee arthroplasty);
- prolonged analgesia and anesthesia for patients with significant trauma who require multiple surgeries;
- diagnostic or therapeutic treatment for chronic pain syndromes; or
- pain control for patients during aggressive postoperative physical therapy and rehabilitation (e.g., with use of a continuous passive motion device).

Only those with previous experience and competence in single-injection blocks should consider performing CPNB. Please see the chapters on single-injection blocks for the appropriate approaches and indications. Follow these chapters for anatomy, patient positioning, landmarks, needle advancement, and stimulation. *Note: The medical materials are displayed in this chapter for illustration purposes only and should not be considered an endorsement of any product.*

2. Procedure

2.1. Equipment

- 18-gauge continuous-block needle system (e.g., the Contiplex Tuohy needle system [Figure 53.1] [B Braun Melsungen AG, Melsungen, Germany]) needles in 5-cm, 10-cm, and 15-cm lengths (Figure 53.2). This is an insulated Tuohy design with an uninsulated tip; the system includes the needle and an integrated stimulating wire and extension tubing with a diaphragm allowing for catheter insertion.
- Multiorifice catheter (comes with the Contiplex Tuohy)
- Ultrasound with appropriate transducer, sterile ultrasound transducer cover, and sterile ultrasound gel or nerve stimulator (Figures 53.3 and 53.4)
- Chlorhexidine preparation
- Surgical marking pen
- Sterile drape
- Local anesthetic for skin anesthesia
- 3-mL syringe and 25-gauge needle for local anesthetic infiltration

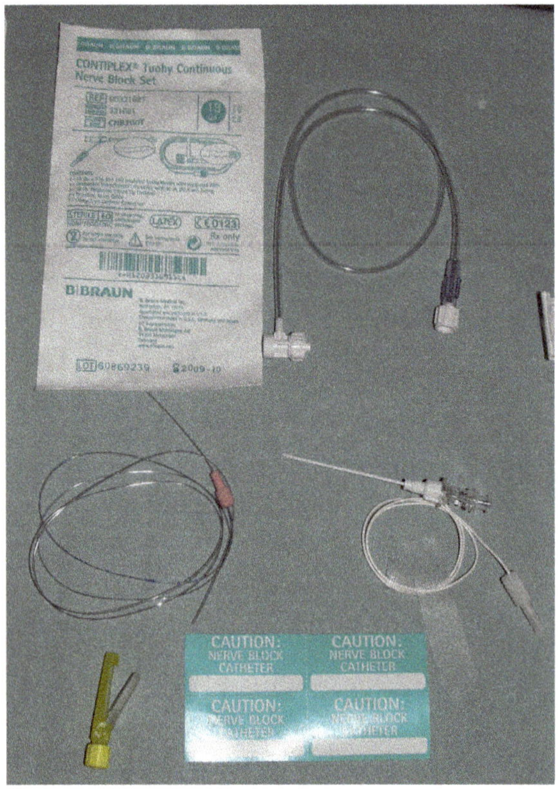

Figure 53.1 Contents of Contiplex Tuohy package (B Braun Melsungen AG, Melsungen, Germany; used with permission).

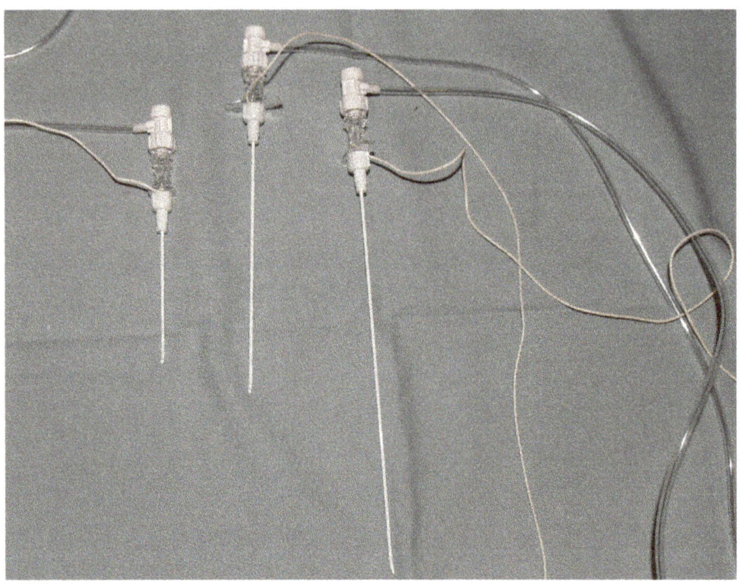

Figure 53.2 Contiplex needles, left to right: 5 cm, 10 cm, and 15 cm (B Braun Melsungen AG, Melsungen, Germany; used with permission).

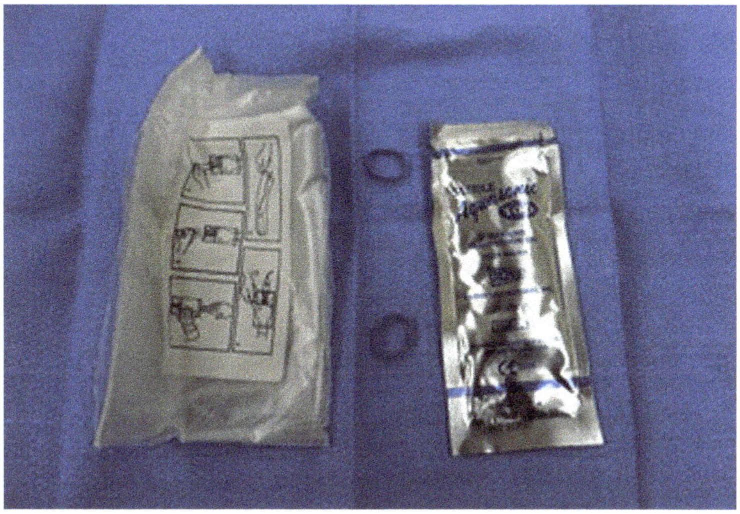

Figure 53.3 Ultrasound sterile probe cover and sterile gel.

- No. 11 scalpel blade—if tunneling is planned
- Skin adhesive (e.g., Dermabond [Ethicon Inc., Somerville, NJ])
- Surgical skin adhesive strips (e.g., Steri-Strips [3M, Saint Paul, Minn])
- Adhesive spray (e.g., Hollister Medical Adhesive [Hollister Inc., Libertyville, Ill])
- Transparent dressing (e.g., Tegaderm [3M])
- AmbIT (Sorenson Medical Inc., West Jordan, Utah) CPNB infusion pump and tubing (Figure 53.5)
- 16-gauge Angiocath needle (BD Medical, Sandy, Utah)

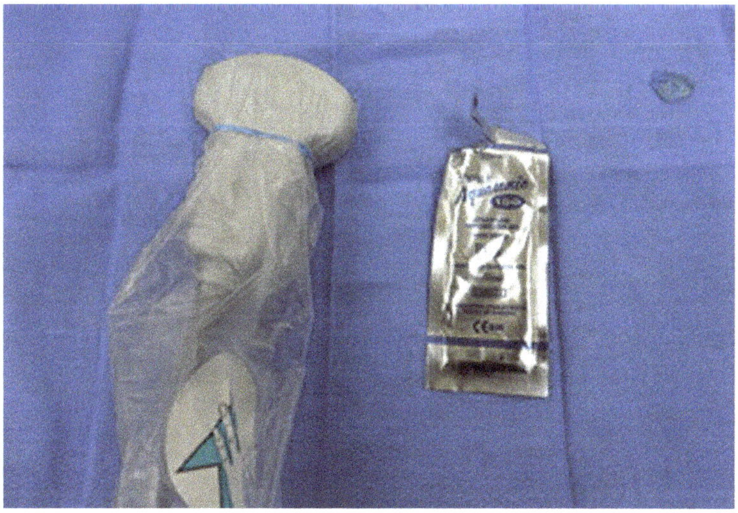

Figure 53.4 Ultrasound probe in sterile cover.

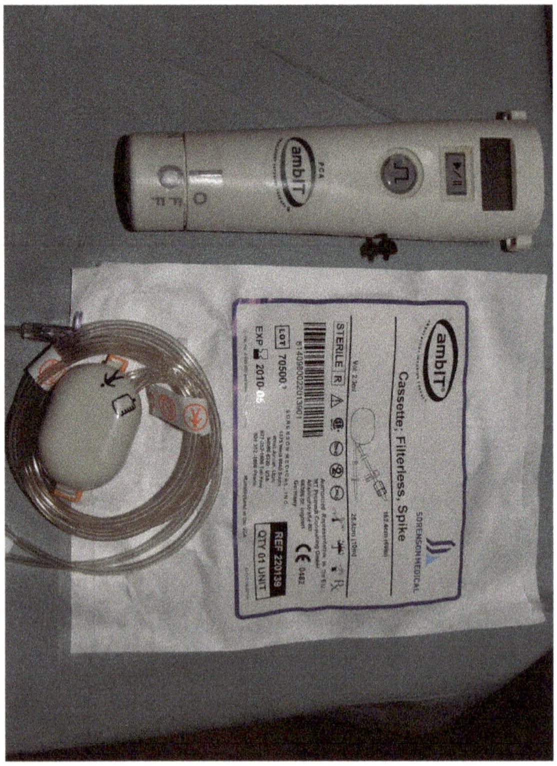

Figure 53.5 AmbiT (Sorenson Medical Inc, West Jordan, Utah; used with permission) pump and tubing.

2.2. Infection control

Regional blocks are placed under sterile conditions. Medical personnel should wear a mask, hat, and sterile gloves. A surgical gown can also be considered. Finally, an antimicrobial dressing (e.g., BioPatch [Johnson & Johnson Wound Management, Ethicon Inc.]) may be placed around the catheter site, if available.

2.3. Steps for catheter placement

- Position the patient as for a single-injection block, ensuring that the patient is on standard monitors and has intravenous access for medications.
- Landmarks for catheter placement are identical to those used for single-injection nerve blocks.
- After identifying skin landmarks, use a chlorhexidine sponge for skin disinfection (povidone-iodine solution is an alternative, although less effective, skin disinfectant) and repeat the preparation before draping the patient.
- Connect the venous valve side port to the Contiplex Tuohy needle. Flush the needle with local anesthetic solution or normal saline, and attach the stimulating wire to the nerve stimulator if using the nerve stimulator.
- Remove the CPNB catheter from its package and place the catheter in a sterile and easily accessible position. Place the ultrasound transducer in the sterile probe cover, use sterile sonographic gel on the patient's skin, and obtain a good ultrasound image.
- Inject a local anesthetic skin wheal at the needle insertion site.
- Orient the block needle so that the bevel is toward the ultrasound probe. Note that the white wire coming from the needle hub is located 180° opposite the needle bevel. Thus, the wire provides a visual guide to bevel orientation at all times. Proper orientation can facilitate needle visualization.

- Advance the needle using the same techniques as in a single-injection block, maintaining appropriate bevel orientation.
- If using stimulation, inject local anesthetic when successful stimulation is achieved, using the same procedure as for single-injection blocks. Care should be taken not to inject the anesthetic too quickly.

If using ultrasound, when the needle is in the appropriate position, inject normal saline through the needle to confirm spread around the target nerve. After confirmation, inject the local anesthetic solution.

2.4. Threading the catheter

- Set your ultrasound probe down on a sterile surface.
- Stabilize the Tuohy needle with one hand (it may be helpful to hold the needle with part of the hand braced against the patient [Figure 53.6]).
- Hold the catheter at the distal tip and advance it through the center of the diaphragm (see Figure 53.6). Continue to thread the catheter until it reaches the end of the needle. Advance the catheter in small increments until it reaches the desired distance, usually 1 to 2 cm beyond the tip of the needle.

After threading the catheter, confirm its location with ultrasound (Figure 53.7) and have an assistant inject normal saline through the catheter injection hub. Adjust the catheter position as needed to optimize position. Set the ultrasound down and remove the injection port from the catheter and carefully remove the needle while maintaining the catheter in the same position. After the needle is out, hold the catheter at the skin and reconfirm its position by ultrasound and injection of normal saline if necessary.

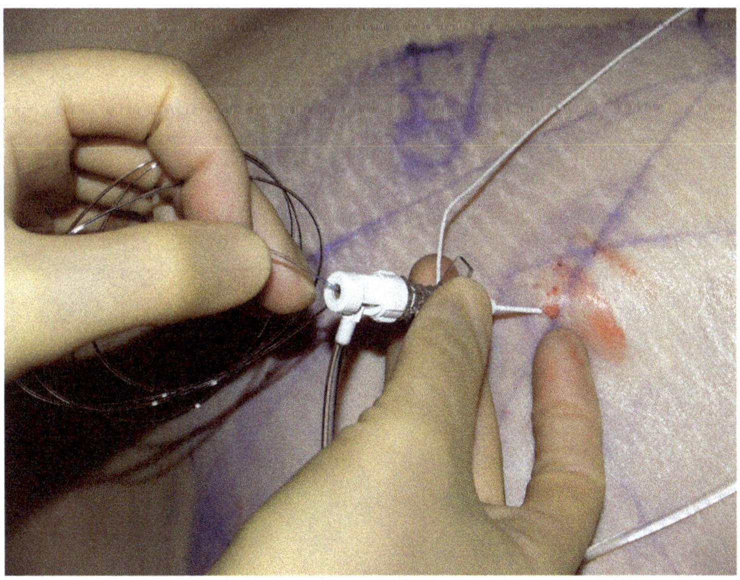

Figure 53.6 Stabilize the Tuohy needle with one hand. It is helpful to have one part of the hand braced against the patient and the other holding the proximal end of the needle near the diaphragm. Hold the catheter at the distal tip and push it through the center of the diaphragm.

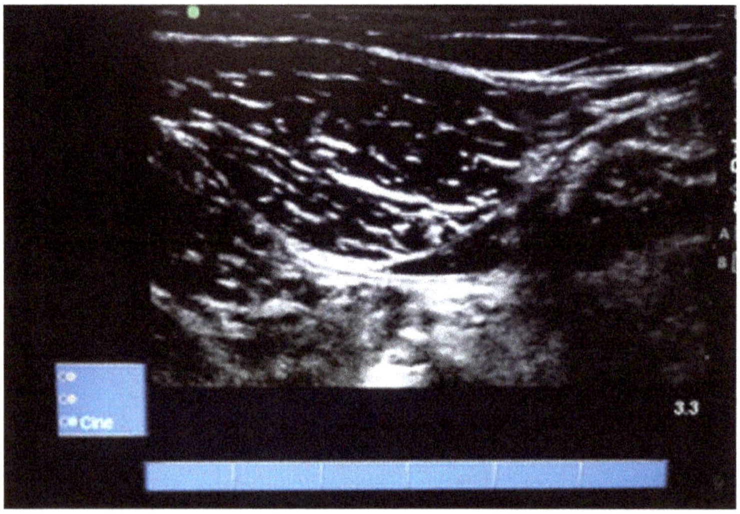

Figure 53.7 Ultrasound image of catheter in pool of local anesthesia.

Teaching Points

- Use the nondominant hand to hold the needle. The hand is braced against the patient with the needle held at the most proximal end (see Figure 53.6).
- Use the dominant hand to thread the catheter.
- Increased resistance to catheter threading at the needle tip is common, and increased force is often needed to pass the catheter beyond the needle tip.
- If the catheter will not advance, try the following techniques:
  - Have an assistant hold the ultrasound while you thread the catheter under direct ultrasound vision.
  - Relax the hand on the needle, allowing it to assume a natural position, and then grip the needle and attempt to thread the catheter again.
  - Rotate the needle 45° and retry.
  - Put a slight backward tension on the needle and retry.
  - Finally, attempt to thread the catheter while simultaneously infusing a small amount of local anesthetic or normal saline through the needle extension tubing.

2.5. Securing the catheter

- If the catheter is not to be tunneled, hold it steady while removing the needle (similar to an epidural catheter placement).
- If the catheter was placed without ultrasound guidance, place the syringe connector on the end of the catheter, aspirate, and test dose the catheter with 5 mL of either 1.5% mepivacaine or 0.5% ropivacaine with 1:400,000 epinephrine.
- After a negative test dose (no increase in heart rate or aspiration of blood), ensure that the site is clean and dry. Use skin adhesive (Dermabond) to seal the area where the catheter exits the skin. Allow the adhesive to dry.
- Spray a light coating of spray adhesive around the catheter. Ensure that the area sprayed is larger than the area of the transparent dressing (Tegaderm) that will be used to cover the site. Allow time for the spray adhesive to become sticky.
- Loop the catheter on the skin and apply 3 skin adhesive strips (Steri-Strips) to hold the catheter in place.

- Apply the transparent dressing over the catheter and skin strips, ensuring that all the edges of the dressing are completely adherent to the skin. Do not place tape over or around the transparent dressing; this can result in tape burns from skin traction and loss of dressing adherence because of trapped moisture.
- Label the catheter with side and type of CPNB infusion (e.g., right femoral block) and date placed.

2.6. Tunneling the catheter

CPNB catheters expected to remain in place for more than 5 days can be tunneled. Tunneling makes the catheter less likely to fall out and may decrease the risk of infection.

- After successfully threading the catheter, maintain a neutral catheter position and withdraw the needle 0.5 to 1 cm.
- Anesthetize the skin with local anesthetic along a track 2 to 4 cm lateral to the needle insertion site (Figure 53.8).
- Make a small skin nick with the no. 11 scalpel blade at the needle insertion site (Figure 53.9).
- Insert a 16-gauge Angiocath needle starting at the lateral aspect of the localized skin. The tip of the Angiocath should exit the skin incision made by the scalpel blade immediately adjacent to the Tuohy needle. Try to avoid leaving a skin bridge between the Angiocath and the Tuohy needle. Note that the CPNB needle is protecting the catheter during this procedure (Figure 53.10).
- Remove the Angiocath needle and leave the Angiocath in place.
- Remove the Tuohy needle and leave the catheter in place.
- Thread the CPNB catheter through the tip of the Angiocath and pull the CPNB catheter through (Figure 53.11).
- Pull the regional anesthesia catheter until it seats within the skin nick. Do not allow the catheter to kink at this point (Figure 53.12a).
- Carefully remove the Angiocath without displacing the CPNB catheter (Figure 53.12b).
- Test dose the catheter or reimage it with ultrasound.

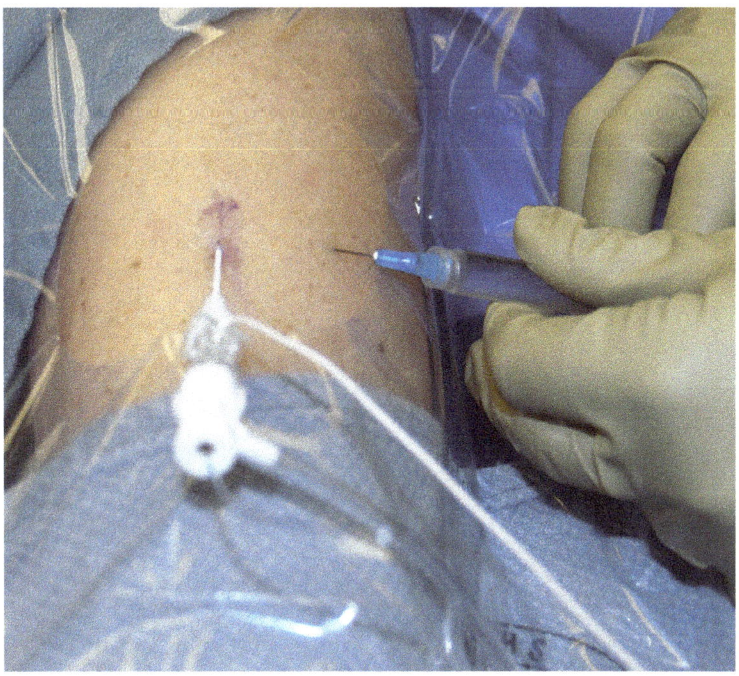

Figure 53.8 Create a local anesthetic skin wheal, starting 2 to 4 cm lateral to the needle position and moving in a straight line toward the needle insertion site.

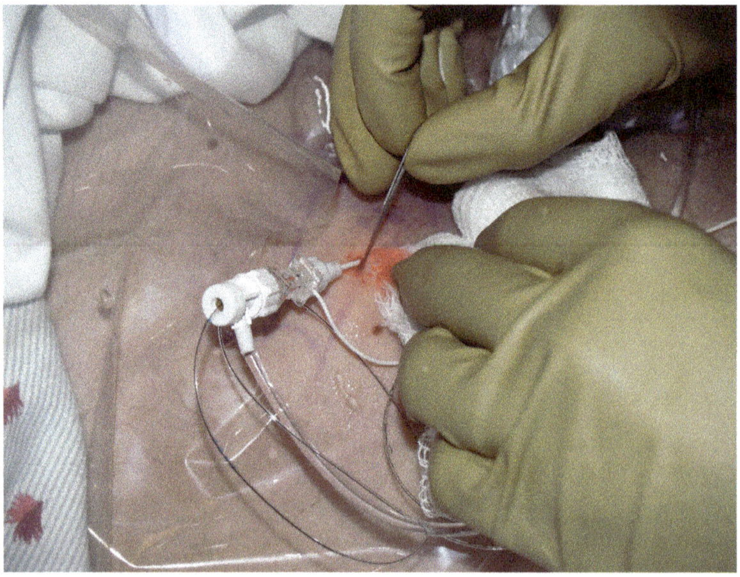

Figure 53.9 Make a skin nick with the no. 11 scalpel blade at the needle insertion site.

- Clean and dry the CPNB catheter site. Glue both sites closed with skin adhesive glue (Figure 53.13).
- Secure the catheter as previously described (Figures 53.13b through 53.16).

2.7. Continuous paravertebral catheters

Some different equipment and techniques are required to place thoracic paravertebral catheters; for instance, a single-orifice (open-tip) epidural catheter may be used rather than a multiorifice catheter. Using a single-orifice catheter may decrease some of the leaking problems that are common with paravertebral catheters.

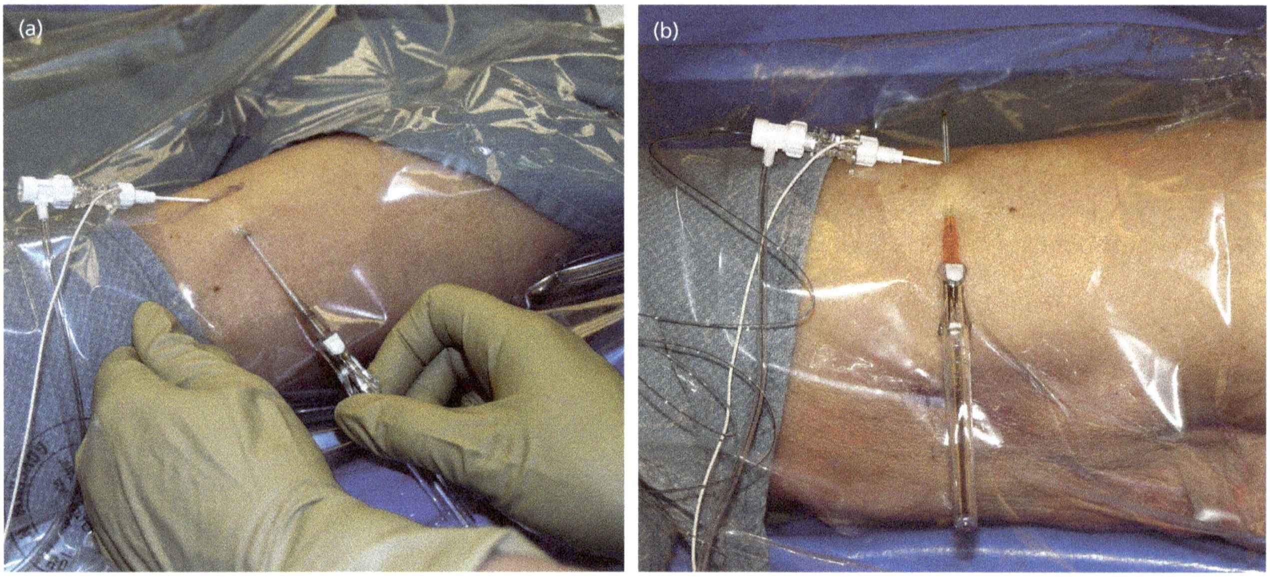

Figure 53.10 (a) Insert a 16-gauge Angiocath (BD Medical, Sandy, Utah; used with permission) needle starting at the lateral aspect of the localized skin wheal. (b) The tip of the Angiocath should exit the skin incision made by the scalpel blade immediately adjacent to the Tuohy needle.

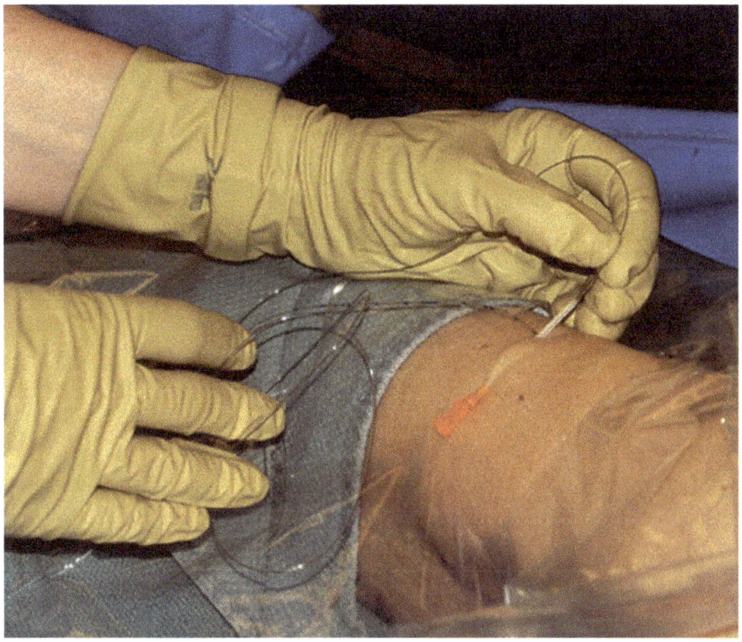

Figure 53.11 Thread the distal end of the CPNB catheter through the Angiocath and pull the CPNB catheter through.

2.8. Equipment for paravertebral catheters

- 18-gauge Tuohy epidural needle (this has centimeter markings on the needle)
- Side port and diaphragm from the 18-gauge Contiplex Tuohy needle
- Epidural catheter
- 22-gauge Tuohy needle used for single-injection paravertebral blocks

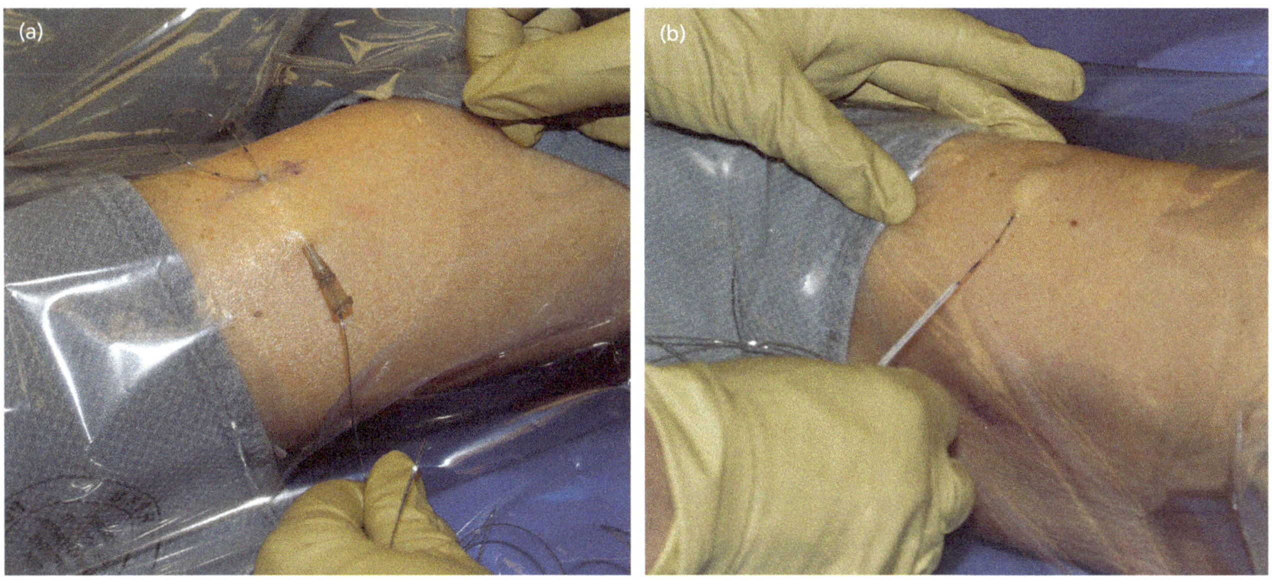

Figure 53.12 (a) Pull the regional anesthesia catheter until it seats within the skin nick and (b) remove the Angiocath.

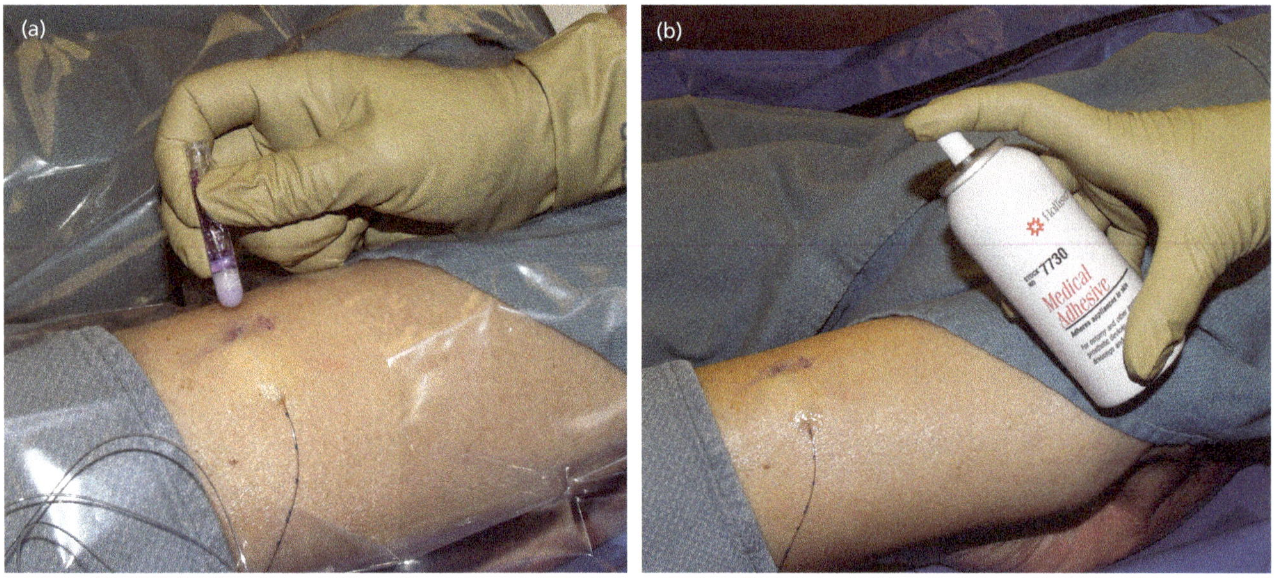

Figure 53.13 Clean and dry the CPNB catheter site. (a) Glue both sites closed with skin adhesive glue, and (b) spray a light coating of adhesive spray around the catheter.

Landmarks for Paravertebral Catheters. Landmarks are the same as for a single-injection paravertebral block. In our practice we have found it helpful to use ultrasound guidance to locate paravertebral landmarks; however, we do not use live ultrasound to place paravertebral catheters.

2.9. Procedure for paravertebral catheters

- Attach the side port of the Contiplex Tuohy needle to the 18-gauge epidural Tuohy needle.
- Use the 22-gauge single-injection Tuohy needle as a finder needle to locate the transverse process at the level where the catheter will be placed (Figure 53.17).

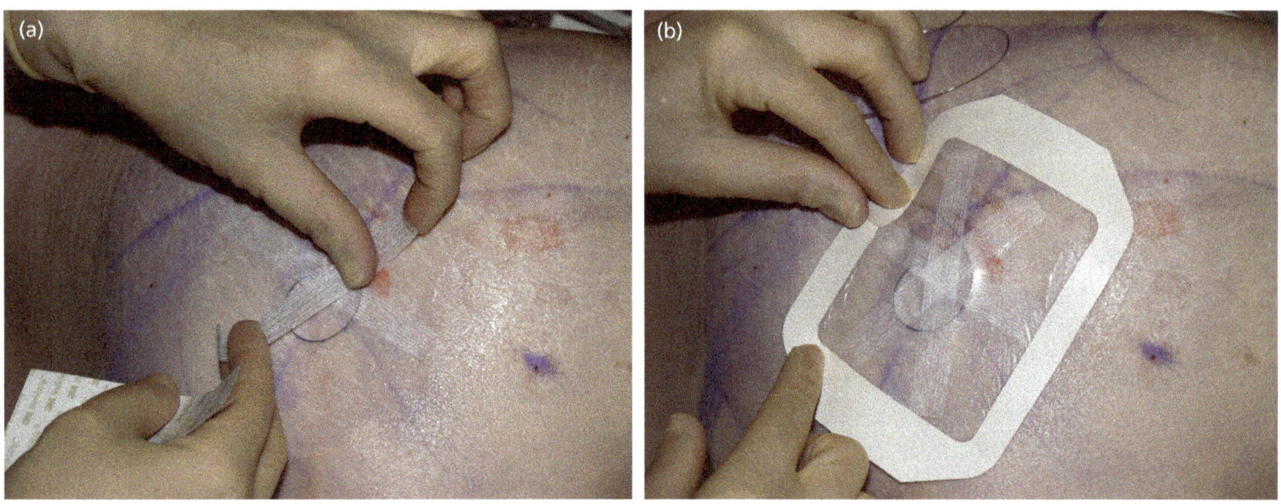

Figure 53.14 (a) Loop the catheter on the skin and apply three skin adhesive strips to hold the catheter in place. (b) Apply a transparent skin dressing over the area. Ensure that all edges of the skin dressing are completely adherent to the skin. The catheter dressing should not prevent visual inspection of the catheter site.

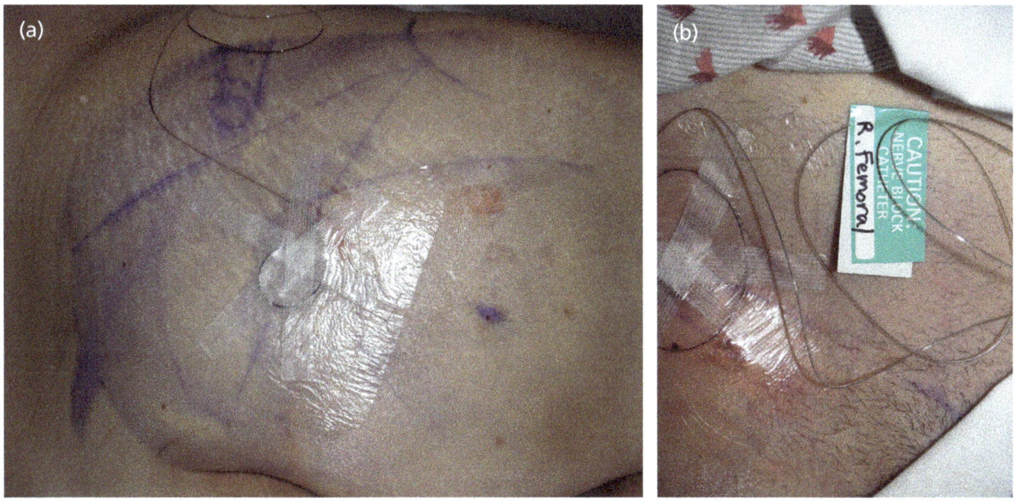

Figure 53.15 (a) Do not place tape around the clear skin dressing. (b) Label the CPNB catheter.

- Replace the finder needle with the 18-gauge epidural Tuohy needle.
- Enter the paravertebral space with the 18-gauge Tuohy needle in the same manner as for single-injection paravertebral block (Figure 53.18).
- Slowly bolus 10 to 15 mL of an appropriate local anesthetic solution containing epinephrine through the 18-gauge Tuohy needle.
- Attempt to thread the epidural catheter through the diaphragm and needle 2 to 4 cm past the end of the Tuohy needle into the paravertebral space. The paravertebral space is small, and these catheters are frequently difficult to thread. Directing the needle bevel caudal may make it easier to thread the catheter

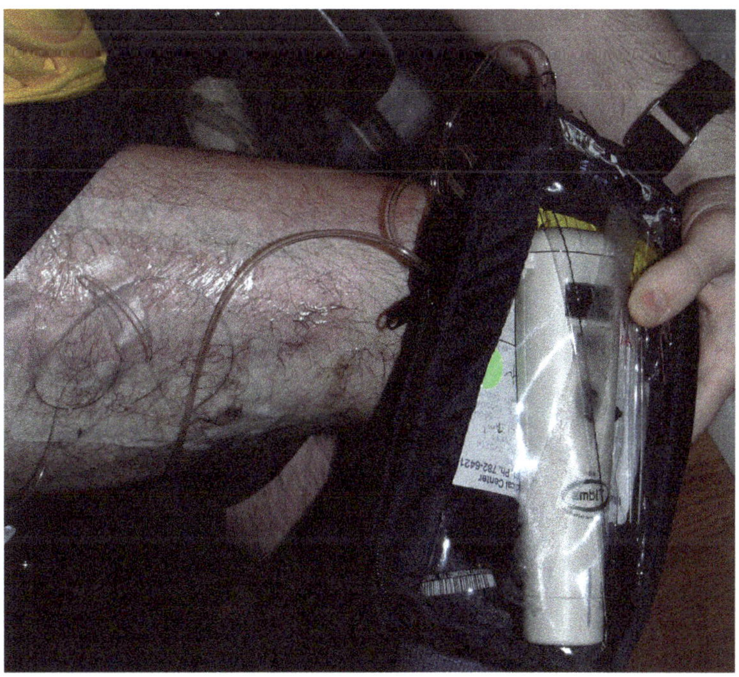

Figure 53.16 Start the local anesthetic infusion.

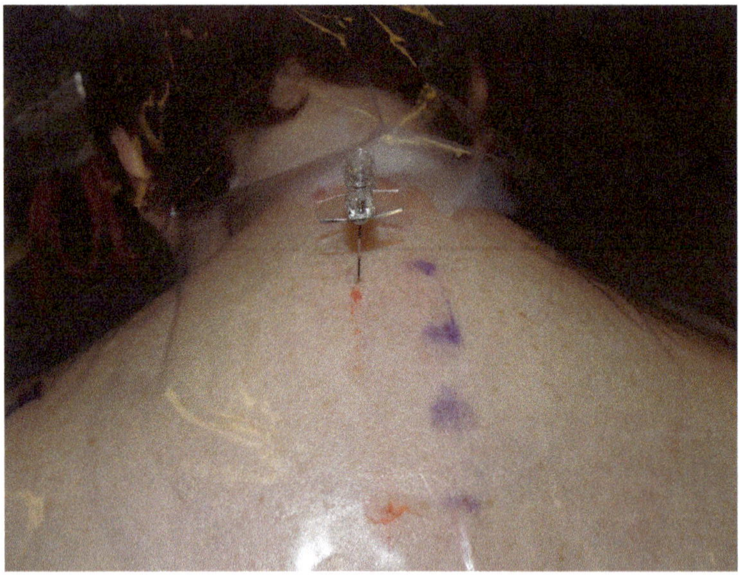

Figure 53.17 22-gauge Tuohy needle used as a finder of the transverse process.

- If you are unable to thread the catheter, rotate the needle 90° laterally or angle the needle tip either cephalad or caudad. All 3 maneuvers are often required.
- After threading the catheter, remove the Tuohy needle, taking care not to withdraw the catheter as well.
- Attach the syringe connector to the catheter. Ensure that you can inject through the catheter by using normal saline. If you cannot inject anesthetic through the catheter, first remove the syringe connector and reapply it (these often do not seat properly on the catheter if they have been removed and reapplied multiple times); if that does not work, then pull the catheter back 0.25 cm and reattempt to inject. Test dose the catheter with 5 mL of local anesthetic containing 1:400,000 epinephrine.
- Secure the catheter in the same manner as for a nontunneled CPNB catheter. Pay particular attention to sealing the catheter exit site with skin adhesive glue. A watertight seal is necessary to prevent leakage of local anesthetic solution around the catheter.

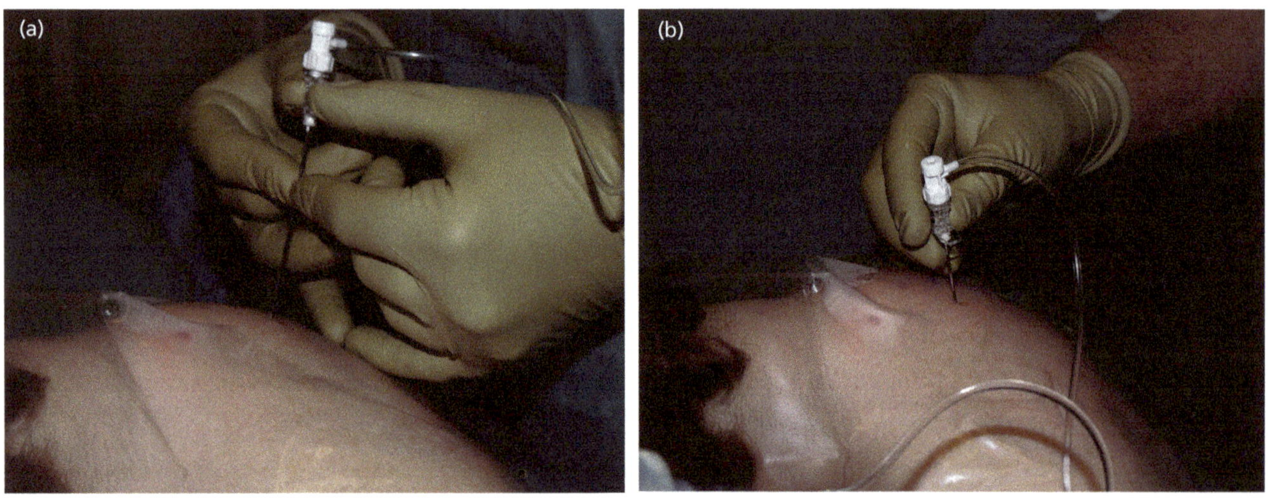

Figure 53.18 (a) 18-gauge epidural Tuohy needle with the side port of the Contiplex Tuohy needle attached. (b) Push the needle tip caudad to facilitate catheter threading.

3. Infusions

The maximum number of catheters is usually 2 (on rare occasions 3). Total infusion amounts (continuous plus bolus) greater than 20 mL/h are usually avoided. However, based on patient condition and the judgment of the provider, certain patients may receive more than 20 mL/h of 0.2% ropivacaine. (See chapter 28, "Local Anesthetics and Additives.")

4. Daily Management

All patients with CPNB catheters must be evaluated at least once daily. A tracking system should be used to ensure that all such patients are clinically monitored by providers experienced with CPNB. The hospital or unit acute pain service is usually responsible for this activity. Routine management of CPNB catheters includes the following measures:

- Evaluate vital signs (including fever) for the last 27 hours.
- Assess any changes in the patient's medications that could affect the CPNB infusion, such as antithrombotics and adjunct pain medications.
- Evaluate sleep, ability to do activities of daily living, pain score, and satisfaction with pain control.
- Inspect and palpate the catheter site for evidence of dislodgement or infection.
- Confirm that the correct local anesthetic medication is infusing in the correct patient.
- Confirm the desired infusion rate, bolus amount, lockout time, and local anesthetic bag volume.
- Evaluate the patient for signs or symptoms of local anesthetic toxicity (see chapter 52, "Regional Anesthesia Complications").
- Initiate heel precautions for patients with sciatic catheters, who may be at increased risk for pressure ulcers of the heel. Ideally the heel should be elevated and off the bed at all times.
- Determine if the patient needs additional pain medications.
- Determine if the patient should be weaned from the catheter, or if the catheter should be removed.
- Generate a daily clinical note on each patient, documenting management of the CPNB catheter.

5. Antithrombotic or Thrombolytic Therapy

For patients who have neuraxial or lumbar plexus catheters, follow the American Society of Regional Anesthesia (ASRA) guidelines for patients receiving antithrombotic or thrombolytic therapy.

The ASRA guidelines or smartphone app can be extremely helpful when considering whether or not to place other CPNBs. CPNB catheters may be placed or continued in patients receiving antithrombotic therapy at the discretion of the provider, after thorough discussion with the patient and primary care team regarding the risks and benefits of CPNB placement or continued CPNB use.

If a CPNB catheter appears infected, use clinical judgment to determine whether to wait the recommended amount of time after the antithrombotic medication before removing the catheter or to remove it immediately.

54

Interventional Chronic Pain Treatment

1. Introduction

Acute nonbattle injuries (NBIs) and chronic pain conditions that recur during war have been referred to as the "hidden epidemic" by the former surgeon general of the US Army, James Peake. Since statistics have been kept, the impact of NBIs on unit readiness has increased. In World War I, NBI was the fourth leading cause of soldier attrition. In World War II and the Korean conflict, NBIs were the third leading cause of morbidity. By the Vietnam War, NBIs had become the leading cause of hospital admissions, which they have remained ever since. However, increasing evidence demonstrates that in-theater management of NBIs and recurrent chronic pain syndromes can improve return-to-duty rates.

The current system of military treatment levels, designed to facilitate the rapid evacuation of wounded soldiers based on their medical condition and needs, was developed in World War II—predating the establishment of pain management as a medical specialty. No personnel are currently deployed specifically for pain management (acute or chronic) at level III combat support hospital (CSH) facilities in either Iraq or Afghanistan. Instead, anesthesiologists and other pain specialists are deployed in their primary specialties and are expected to provide pain management services as needed in addition to their regular full-time duties. This situation has resulted in a varying standard of pain management care in theaters of operation. The modern CSH has key infrastructure such as radiology services (e.g., fluoroscopy, radiography, computed tomography) and full surgical, laboratory, and pharmacy support, which can facilitate chronic pain clinical services if properly staffed.

The most common presenting complaints of NBI during Operation Iraqi Freedom have been radicular leg pain, axial low back pain (LBP), nonradicular leg pain, nonradicular arm pain, groin pain, noncardiac chest pain, and neck pain. The most common diagnoses conferred on these patients were lumbosacral radiculopathy, recurrence of postsurgical pain, lumbar facetogenic pain, myofascial pain, neuropathic pain, and lumbar degenerative disc disease.

The most common noninterventional treatments have been nonsteroidal anti-inflammatory drugs (NSAIDs; >90%); physical therapy referral (for back pain, neck pain, and leg pain); muscle relaxants (for spinal and myofascial pain); and anticonvulsants and tricyclic antidepressants (usually prescribed for radicular and other forms of neuropathic pain). The large majority of patients received at least one interventional procedure. The most frequently employed nerve blocks were lumbar transforaminal epidural

Table 54.1:
Procedures for Common Nerve Blocks Conducted in Theater

Injection	Injectate Volume* (mL)	Need for Fluoroscopy?	Comments
Cervical ESI	2–4	Yes	Use of local anesthetic controversial. Cervical TFESI may result in death or paraplegia and should not be done in austere environment.
Interlaminar lumbar ESI	3–5	Strongly advised	Performing blind ESI associated with a high likelihood of injectate failing to reach targeted area.
Transforaminal lumbar ESI	2–3	Yes	Superior outcomes compared to interlaminar ESI.
Intraarticular facet blocks	Cervical: 1 Lumbar: 1–2	Yes	Likelihood of relief higher in patients with acute inflammatory process.
Trochanteric bursa injection	3–5	No	Similar outcomes for fluoroscopically and landmark-guided injections.
Sacroiliac joint block	2–4	Yes	< 25% chance of intraarticular spread in landmark-guided injections.
Lateral epicondylar injection	0.5–1.5	No	Mixed results for treatment.
Subacromial bursa injection	4–10	Advised	May use posterior or anterolateral approach; 50%–80% accuracy rate for blinded injections.
Piriformis muscle injection	3–8	Yes	May use nerve stimulator to locate sciatic nerve (adjacent to muscle) if fluoroscopy is not available. Injection of local anesthetic may cause sciatic nerve weakness.
Carpal tunnel injection	1–2	No	Not superior to NSAID treatment after 2 months.
Greater occipital nerve injection	2–4	No	Difficult to clinically distinguish from referred cervical pain.

ESI: epidural steroid injection. NSAID: nonsteroidal antiinflammatory drug. TFESI: transforaminal epidural steroid injection.
*Volume of injectate consists of 1 to 2 mL of depot (long-acting) corticosteroid plus local anesthetic.

steroid injections (ESIs), trigger point injections, cervical ESIs, lumbar facet blocks, various groin blocks, and plantar fascia injections. Table 54.1 lists procedures for common nerve blocks conducted in theater. Significantly, when treated in theater, 94.7% of soldiers returned to their units. Differences in return-to-duty rates support aggressive pain management in forward-deployed areas.

2. Triaging Patients for Treatment

As a result of limited pain management resources, coupled with the risk involved with soldier transport, healthcare providers must triage NBI pain patients based on the anticipated risk-benefit ratio. Soldiers with acute or recurrent overuse injuries (e.g., tendonitis or bursitis) can usually be handled at a role I facility such as a battalion aid station. For soldiers who require more sophisticated interventions, the battalion or brigade surgeon must decide whether a medical evacuation to a CSH is warranted. This decision is based on several factors: the likelihood of quick resolution of the pain issue, the soldier's motivation to remain in theater, the soldier's military occupational specialty, the probability of recurrence, the commander's desire to keep the soldier in theater, the treatment capabilities at the CSH, and the risk of medical evacuation.

3. Chronic Pain Conditions Encountered in the Field

3.1. Low Back Pain

Low back pain is the most common complaint likely to be encountered by the pain practitioner deployed to the CSH. Its high incidence is probably caused by a combination of factors encountered in theater: the heavy loads service members must carry, frequent transportation over rough terrain in military vehicles with stiff suspensions, heavy individual body armor, sleep deprivation, and the high degree of psychosocial stressors faced by soldiers deployed to combat zones. Among the various causes of LBP, radiculopathy from nerve root irritation may be the most commonly encountered condition.

A mainstay interventional treatment for LBP is ESI. ESIs exert their beneficial effects through their anti-inflammatory properties, inhibition of the enzyme phospholipase A2, and suppression of ectopic discharges from injured neurons. Although ESIs have been successfully used to treat axial back pain, ideal candidates for the procedure are those with pain of less than 6 months' duration, leg pain greater than back pain, young age, intermittent pain, and absence of concomitant spinal stenosis. The use of fluoroscopic guidance is highly recommended for interlaminar ESIs and is required for transforaminal ESIs. ESIs performed without the fluoroscope have a high technical failure rate, even when performed by experienced practitioners. Transforaminal ESIs, although technically more challenging than interlaminar ESIs, are generally associated with superior outcomes because medication is deposited directly over the affected nerve root (Figure 54.1).

Patients suspected of radicular pain should receive computed tomography (CT) scans of the appropriate spine level. Whereas magnetic resonance imagery (MRI) is the gold standard for imaging soft tissue and disc anatomy, CT scans are sensitive at determining the presence of disc pathology. Although ESIs are considered by many practitioners to be the best interventional therapy for radicular pain, controversy exists regarding their long-term efficacy.

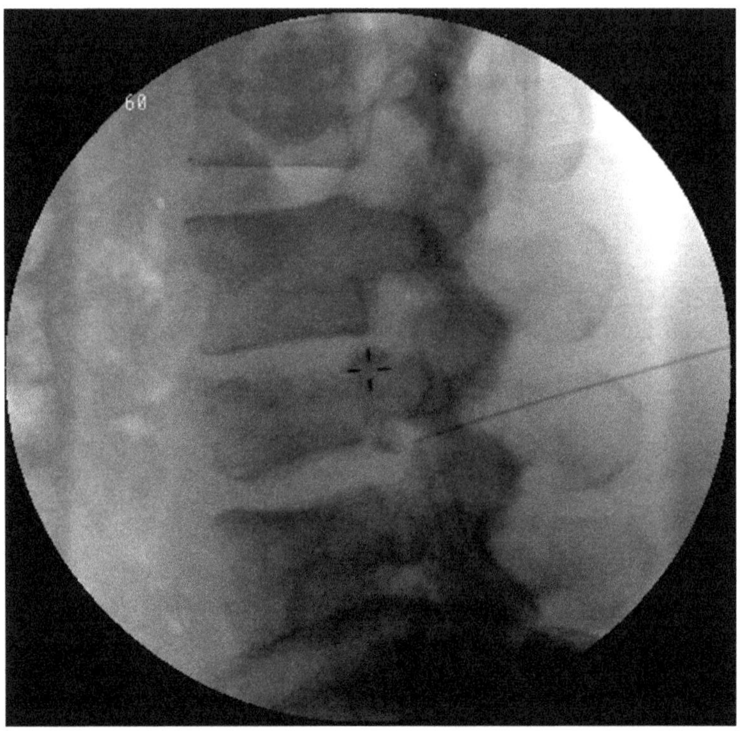

Figure 54.1 Lateral fluoroscopic view demonstrating needle position for L4–L5 transforaminal epidural steroid injection.

3.2. Zygapophyseal Joint Pain

Lumbar zygapophyseal (facet) joint pain accounts for approximately 15% of patients with chronic axial LBP. Typical presentation is a dull aching pain, usually bilateral, that radiates from the low back into the buttocks and thigh. Although the history and physical examination can be suggestive of facet joint pain, an analgesic response to fluoroscopically guided low-volume diagnostic blocks, of either the zygapophyseal joints themselves or the medial branches that innervate them, is the gold standard for diagnosis. The interventional treatment of facetogenic pain consists of either intra-articular injections with corticosteroid, which may benefit a small percentage of patients with an acute inflammatory component, or more frequently radiofrequency denervation of the nerves that innervate the painful joints. Because of the lack of radiofrequency capability, combination diagnostic/therapeutic intra-articular facet injections are recommended in theater. In patients with radiologic evidence of an acute inflammatory process, intra-articular corticosteroids may afford up to 3 months of excellent pain relief (Figure 54.2).

3.3. Sacroiliac Joint Pain

Sacroiliac (SI) joint pain is a frequent source of axial LBP, accounting for roughly 15% to 20% of cases. Compared with other causes of back pain, SI joint pain is more likely to result from a specific inciting event such as a fall, motor vehicle accident, or airplane jump. The primary pain generator in younger patients with documented SI joint pain tends to be extraarticular (i.e., surrounding ligaments or muscles). The typical presentation of SI joint pain is a unilateral aching pain in the low back or buttock. SI joint pain, typically associated with tenderness overlying the affected joint, is often reproducible. In patients with SI joint pain, multiple studies have demonstrated good intermediate- to long-term pain relief with intra-articular or periarticular injections of corticosteroid with local anesthetic. Previous studies have demonstrated that radiographic guidance is necessary to achieve accurate placement in or around the joint (Figure 54.3).

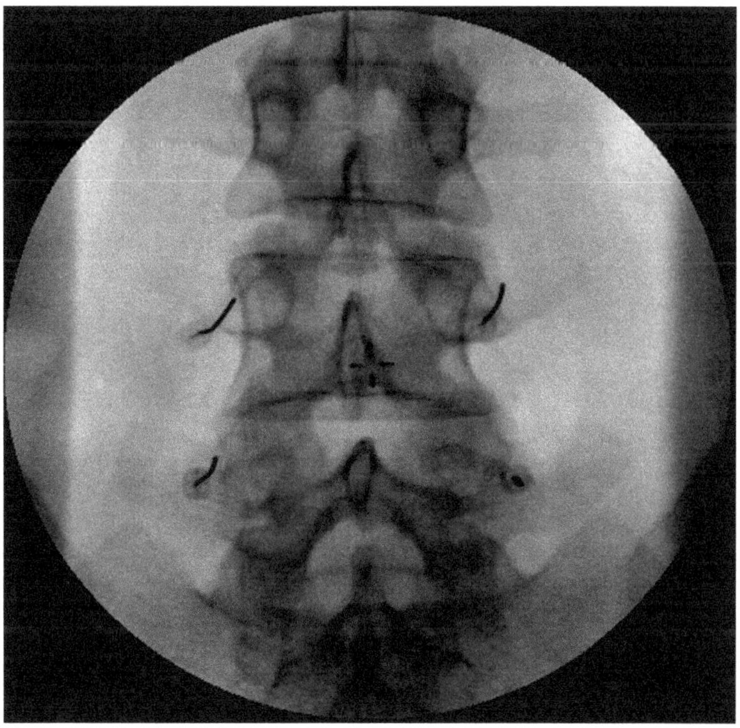

Figure 54.2 Anteroposterior fluoroscopic view demonstrating needle position for bilateral L3 and L4 facet joint (medial branch) nerve blocks.

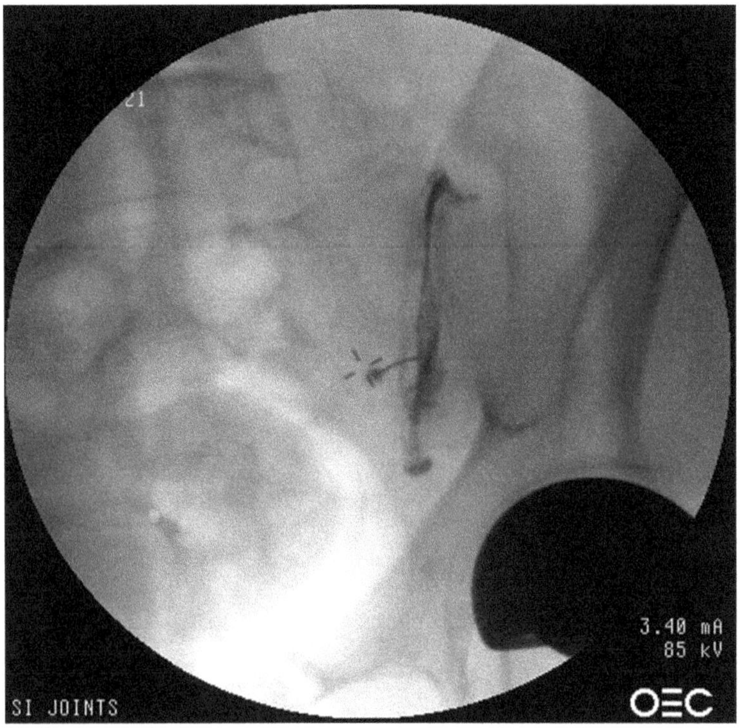

Figure 54.3 Anteroposterior fluoroscopic view demonstrating a right side sacroiliac joint injection.

3.4. Myofascial Pain

Myofascial pain accounts for a significant percentage of axial LBP cases, with an estimated prevalence of around 20%. Frequently, muscle spasm is superimposed on a more acute, underlying condition. The hallmark of treatment of myofascial pain is physical therapy to identify and treat the underlying cause, and pharmacotherapy with muscle relaxants and NSAIDs. When discrete bands of contracted muscle are palpable, trigger point injections can provide excellent relief.

3.5. Spinal Stenosis and Degenerative Disc Disease

Spinal stenosis and degenerative disc disease are other common causes of LBP, with a higher incidence among the elderly. Whereas ESIs can sometimes provide pain relief for these conditions, the benefit is often incomplete and transient. Less frequent sources of back and leg pain that need to be ruled out include osteomyelitis, vertebral fractures, and acute or worsening spondylolisthesis.

3.6. Cervical Spine Pain

An estimated 16% to 22% of adults suffer from chronic neck pain, with a higher prevalence seen in women. Among patients with chronic neck pain, approximately 30% report a history of neck injury, most commonly the result of a motor vehicle accident. In military pain clinics, neck pain and cervicogenic headaches account for about 10% to 15% of NBIs.

Numerous predisposing factors for neck pain are prevalent in soldiers, including prolonged static loads (from body armor), abnormal postures (secondary to body armor or in snipers), work-related stress, and full-force exertion. In patients with acute neck or upper thoracic pain, the etiology is likely to be myofascial in origin. In chronic axial neck pain or whiplash injury, the facet joints are the most common source of pain. Myofascial pain can be treated with muscle relaxants, NSAIDs, tricyclic antidepressants, short-term duty modification, and trigger point injections. For cervical facetogenic pain, intra-articular steroids can provide intermediate-term relief in patients with an acute inflammatory process (Figures 54.4 and 54.5).

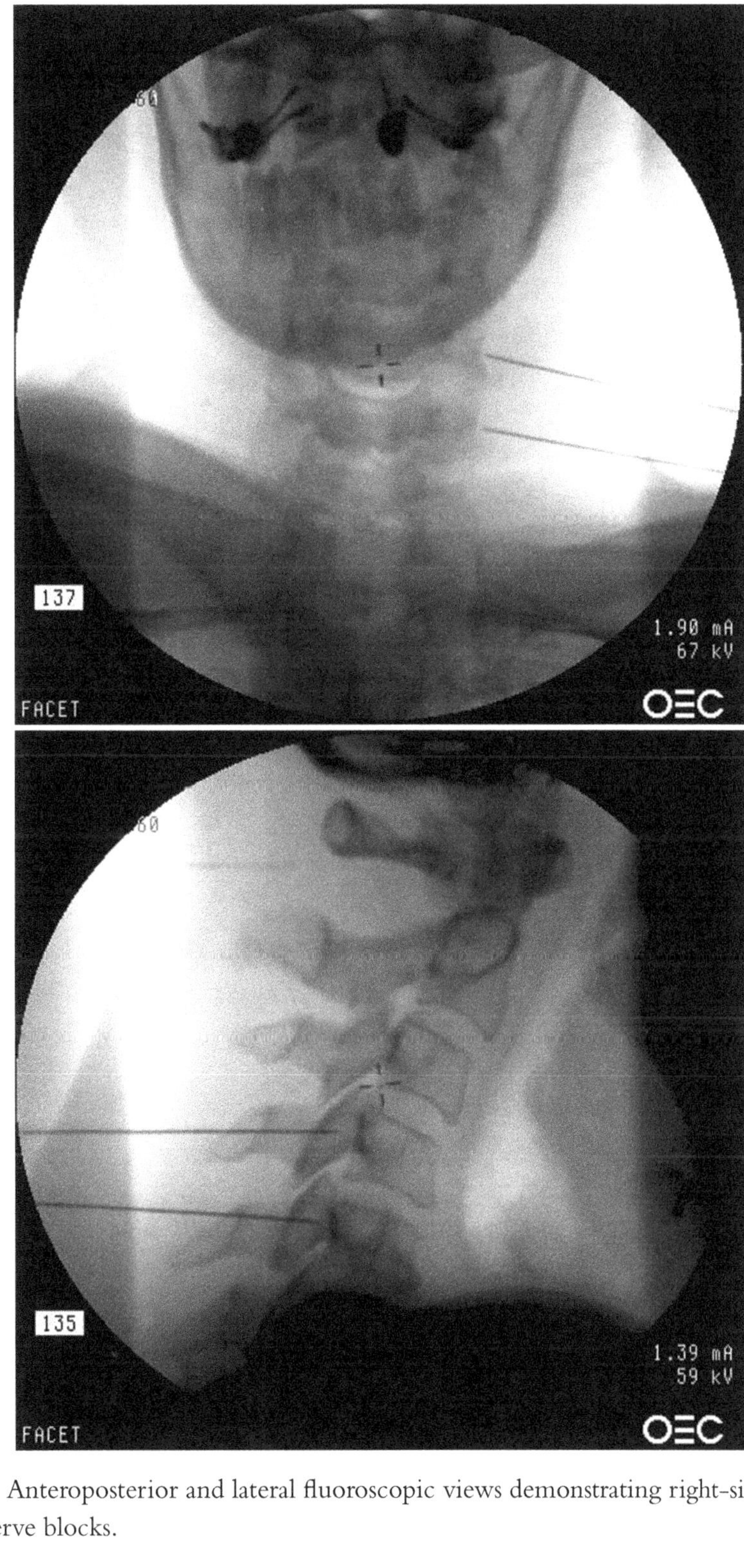

Figures 54.4 and 54.5 Anteroposterior and lateral fluoroscopic views demonstrating right-sided C4 and C5 facet joint (medial branch) nerve blocks.

Cervical radiculopathy typically manifests as neck pain radiating down one or both arms in a dermatomal distribution, sometimes accompanied by weakness and sensory changes. Similar to lumbar radicular pain, cervical radiculopathy can be treated with cervical ESIs (Figures 54.6 and 54.7). Because of reports of death and paralysis, cervical transforaminal ESIs are not recommended in an austere environment. Possible causes of cervicogenic headaches

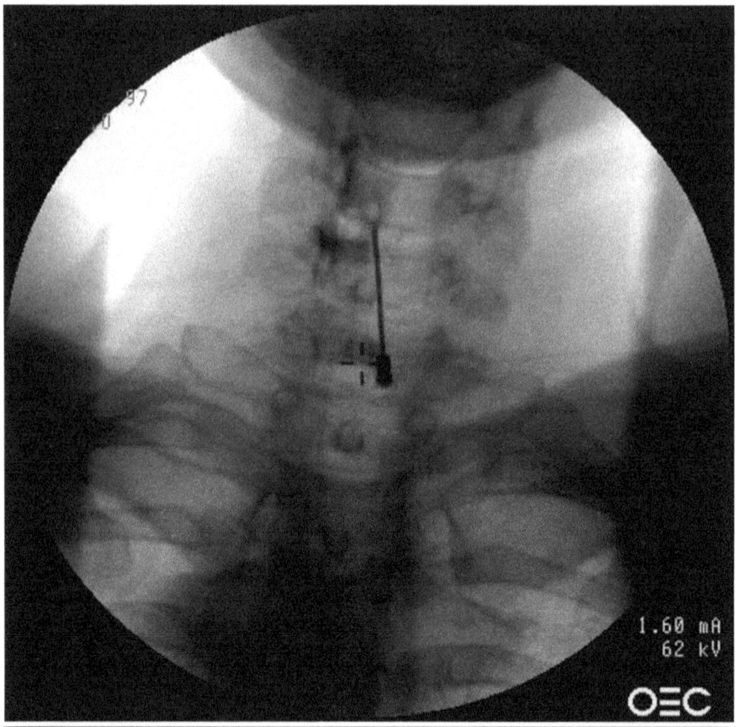

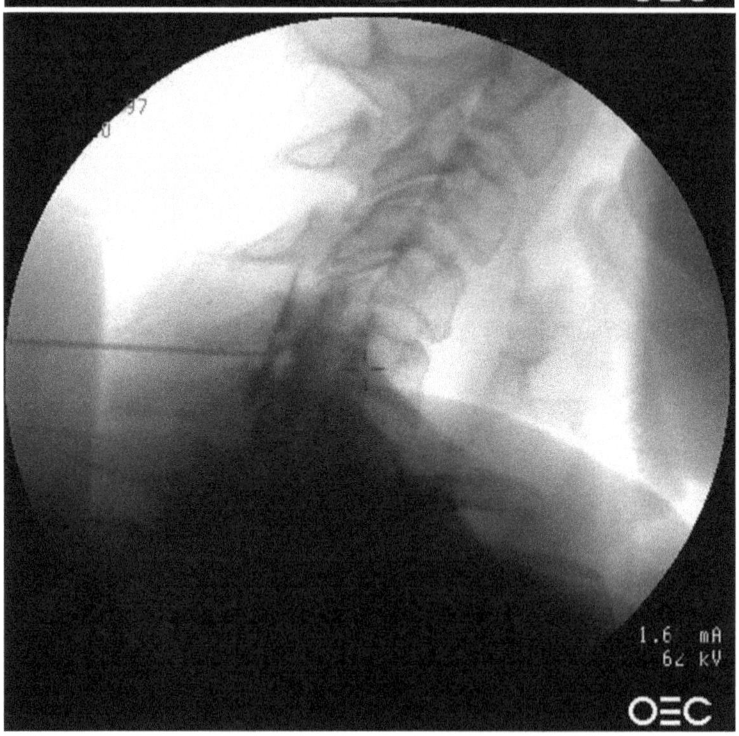

Figures 54.6 and 54.7 Anteroposterior and lateral fluoroscopic views demonstrating a C5–C6 epidural steroid injection.

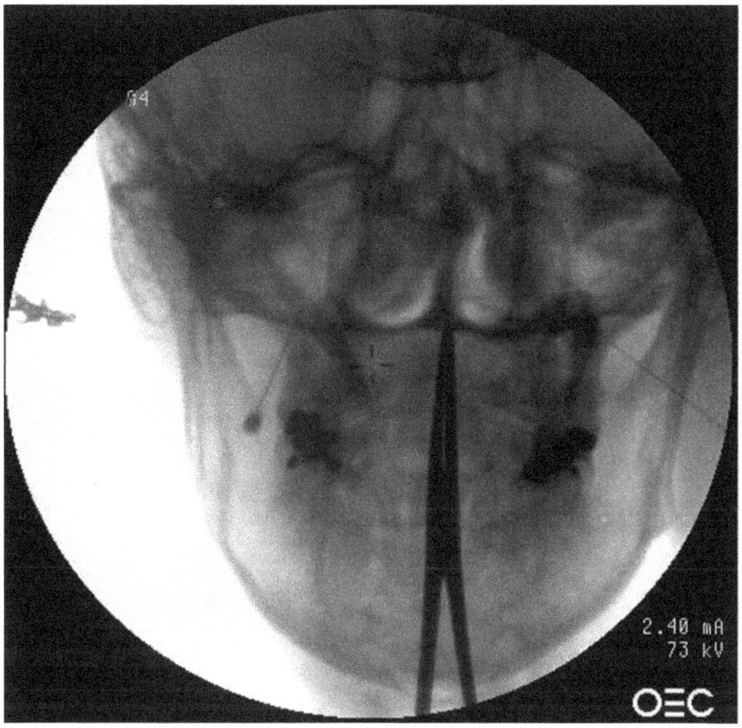

Figure 54.8 Needle position demonstrating bilateral greater occipital nerve blocks.

that may be amenable to injection therapy include atlanto-occipital and atlantoaxial joint pain. Occipital neuralgia, a frequent cause of occipital headaches, is best diagnosed and treated with injections containing local anesthetic and corticosteroid (Figure 54.8).

3.7. Nonradicular Leg Pain

Nonradicular leg pain (e.g., piriformis syndrome, plantar fasciitis, and greater trochanteric bursitis [TB]) accounts for approximately 10% of pain clinic visits from NBIs. Many of these conditions tend to be associated with overuse of the affected body part. Piriformis syndrome tends to present as unilateral buttock pain and, depending on the extent of sciatic nerve involvement, pain extending into the lower leg. The diagnosis of piriformis syndrome is predicated on a positive response to fluoroscopically guided intramuscular injection. In addition to their diagnostic utility, these injections can also be therapeutic.

TB is a clinical diagnosis characterized by the association of lateral hip pain, tenderness to palpation, and pain provocation by various movements. Sometimes called *pseudosciatica*, TB can radiate into the distal thigh but rarely extends below the knee. Risk factors for TB include coexisting lumbar spine pathology, gait and postural abnormalities, leg length discrepancy, female sex, and advanced age. It is important to note that a majority of patients clinically diagnosed with TB have no MRI evidence of bursa inflammation. In these patients, the true pain generator is often tendonitis, muscle tears, or trigger points (Figure 54.9).

Plantar fasciitis has a lifetime prevalence of almost 10% in the general population but tends to be more common in soldiers. Risk factors include excessive walking or running, especially in the early morning, on uneven surfaces, or wearing heavy backpacks; having flat feet or high arches; being overweight; and being middle age or older. Conservative treatments include rest, night splints or orthotics, stretching exercises, and NSAIDs. Corticosteroid injections may also relieve plantar fasciitis symptoms.

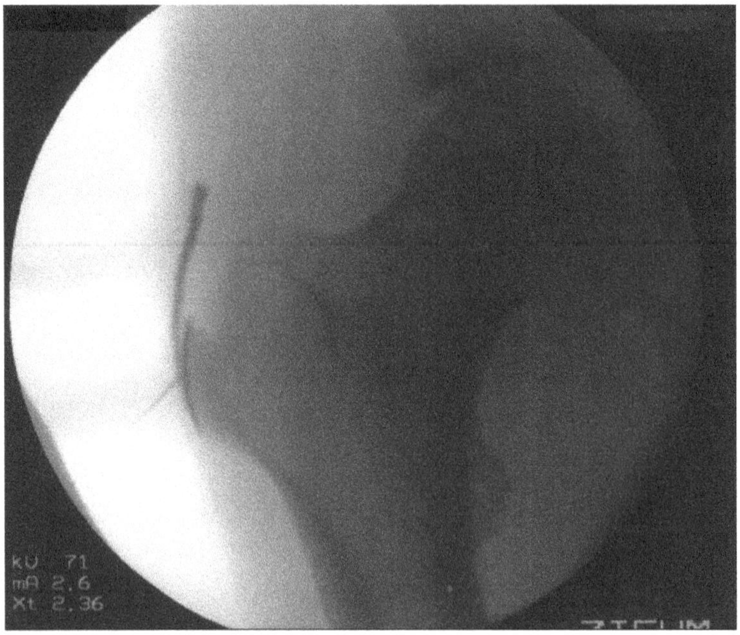

Figure 54.9 Anteroposterior fluoroscopic view demonstrating trochanteric bursa injection.

3.8. Less Common Pain Complaints

Nonradicular arm pain is less frequently encountered than nonradicular leg pain. Aside from complex regional pain syndrome, which is rarely encountered in soldiers at level III facilities, other causes of nonradicular arm pain include medial and lateral epicondylitis ("tennis elbow"), tendonitis, bursitis, and carpal tunnel syndrome. Injection of any of these overuse inflammatory conditions with corticosteroid and local anesthetic may result in significant pain relief and functional improvement. Since these injections are targeted by palpation and landmarks, they can usually be done in the field.

Finally, male groin pain, abdominal pain, and female pelvic pain are the least likely pain conditions to improve with the interventional therapy available in theater. Common to all these conditions are the diagnostic dilemma each poses, the lack of any reliable pharmacologic or interventional treatments, and the high prevalence of coexisting psychopathology. When a surgical scar is present, scar injections with corticosteroid and local anesthetic may afford pain relief by virtue of releasing entrapped nerves or suppressing ectopic discharges from injured neurons. Even in soldiers who will require medical evacuation, short-term relief can often be obtained with nerve blocks. Most of these blocks tend to be landmark-guided, so fluoroscopy is generally not necessary (see Table 54.1).

4. Summary

In modern combat, the most common cause of soldier attrition is not battle-related injuries, but rather acute and recurrent NBIs similar to those encountered in civilian pain clinics. Although recent evidence indicates that higher return-to-unit rates can be obtained with forward-deployed interventional pain management capabilities, these techniques are not always practical early in warfare.

Chronic pain management in the operational setting is fraught with a unique and often dynamic set of challenges, but the procedures can provide considerable benefit in a mature theater of war with deployment of personnel and equipment as described in this chapter.

Improving Surgical Pain Management with Multidisciplinary Care

55

1. Introduction

For the last two centuries, morphine has been the single most relied-upon drug for the management of acute surgical pain. Fortunately, modern advances in anesthesia and analgesia have revolutionized this pain management approach. Today, multidisciplinary treatment plans have been identified as a principal factor in both modern-day pain control and optimization of recovery after surgery. Despite numerous medical and technological advances, however, postsurgical pain is often undertreated. An understanding of the physiology and complex, multifaceted nature of pain is necessary to identify an optimal treatment plan, which often involves multiple therapeutic modalities. This balanced analgesic approach, known as multimodal analgesia, utilizes a combination of opioids, nonopioid analgesics, and nonpharmacologic approaches that target different pain processing sites of the peripheral and central nervous systems. The aim of multimodal analgesia is to optimize postoperative pain control while limiting the total amount of opioid and other medications administered to the patient, thereby minimizing adverse drug effects. This chapter will discuss recent advances in pain management and perioperative care that can improve the quality of postoperative recovery and reduce morbidity after major surgery.

2. Pathways and Types of Pain

The transduction of noxious stimuli involves both the peripheral and central nervous systems. It begins with peripheral nociceptors, which transmit signals along peripheral nerves through the dorsal root ganglia (Figure 55.1). Axons of myelinated A-fibers and unmyelinated C-fibers synapse in the dorsal horn of the spinal cord, and pain signals are transmitted to the thalamus and cerebral sensory cortex via the ascending spinothalamic tracts. Descending modulation of pain is mediated through the dorsal horn neurons. It has been recently discovered that spinal cord glial cell activation contributes to pain signal modification. Medications used to manage pain act at specific areas along this pathway to reduce the intensity of the pain experience.

The different types of pain include somatic, visceral, inflammatory-mediated, and neuropathic pain. Each type responds to different treatment modalities; understanding their distinctions will aid in developing specific therapeutic interventions to maximize patient benefit. Optimal pain management requires a careful appraisal of the source of pain, coupled with an appropriate selection of treatments for each patient. Complex pain cases require multimodal as well as interdisciplinary care. Coordination among

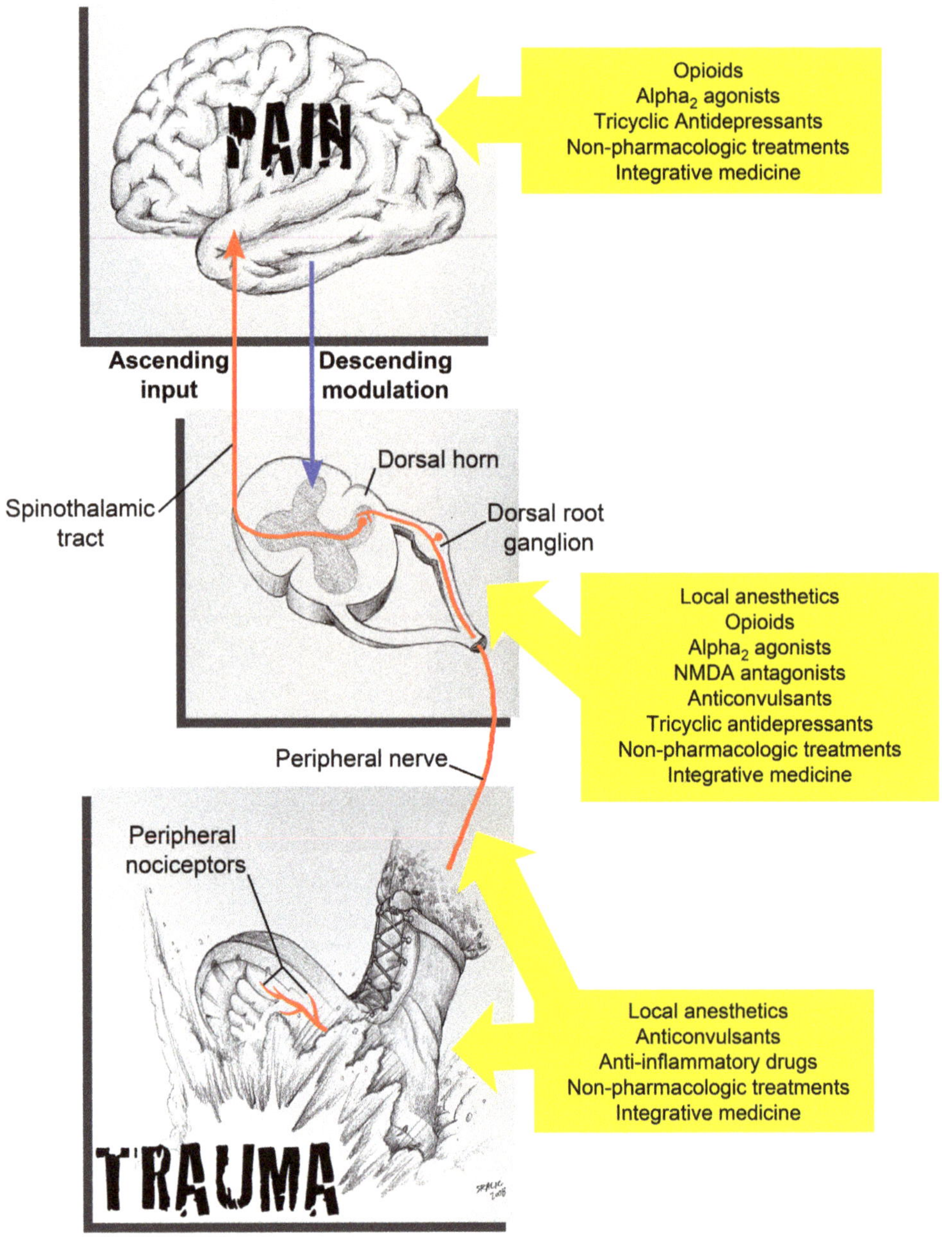

Figure 55.1 Transmission of pain signals.

healthcare providers before, during, and after a surgical procedure is a critical component of successful operative pain management.

Somatic pain and visceral pain result from stimulation of sensory receptors or nociceptors in response to noxious stimuli; they are distinguished by the location of their receptors and the nerve fibers that are stimulated. Somatic pain receptors are located within the skin and respond to environmental cues such as sharp, focused, and painful stimuli. Examples of this type of pain include incisional or cutaneous burn–related pain. Visceral receptors are located in visceral organs (bladder, ureter, small and large bowel, etc.) and respond to internal cues such as dilation of the bowel or inflammation from infection. Visceral fibers are slow-conducting unmyelinated C-fibers that join autonomic and somatic nerves entering the central nervous system. Visceral pain can either be localized to the site of tissue damage or be sensed at a distant anatomic region from the source of tissue injury, a phenomenon called *referred pain*. Neuropathic pain is related to the sensory perception of pain associated with peripheral or central nerves. Nerve injuries caused by stretching, compression, or cancer invasion are often the precursors to neuropathic pain, and may pose formidable treatment challenges.

Inflammatory mediators have been identified in pain pathways. Substance P, a neurotransmitter involved in the perception of pain, is also a mediator in the neuroinflammatory cascade. Interferons and cytokines (interleukin-1, interleukin-6, and tumor necrosis factor-α) are pro-inflammatory mediators thought to decrease the threshold for pain stimulation and increase the intensity of the response. Interruption of the inflammatory cascade is a potential adjunct for achieving optimal pain control.

3. Preoperative Patient Assessment

An adequate history and physical examination are critical to identifying the cause of a patient's pain as well as ensuring that appropriate treatment modalities are employed (Box 55.1). Assessment of pain should include several factors: location, severity, quality, radiation, duration of onset, aggravating and mollifying events, and associated symptoms. The healthcare provider must ascertain whether or not the patient experiences chronic pain or takes chronic medications such as narcotics, nonsteroidal anti-inflammatory drugs (NSAIDs), anxiolytics, or gabapentin. Patients with chronic pain or history of opioid use or drug abuse may have a tolerance of narcotic-based pain medications and may require substantially greater doses of narcotics than opioid-naive patients. Conversely, others may limit the amount of pain medication they take because of fear of drug dependency. Nonopioid analgesics are useful options in this context.

Acute, severe, and undertreated pain is associated with many adverse systemic effects, including increased myocardial oxygen demand, reduced functional residual capacity, hypoxemia, and gastrointestinal ileus. Some patients with severe, poorly controlled operative site pain may develop long-term central sensitization. This condition may serve as the basis for chronic pain syndromes wherein noxious stimuli are accompanied by an exaggerated pain response, or hyperalgesia, and painless stimuli are perceived as painful, a phenomenon known as *allodynia*.

Box 55.1 Preoperative Measures to Assess and Control Pain

- History and physical examination
  - specifics about pain: location, severity, quality of pain, radiation, onset and duration, aggravating and mollifying factors, and associated symptoms
  - history of chronic pain
  - medications: opioids, NSAIDs, anxiolytics, gabapentin, narcotics, antidepressants
  - history of drug use and abuse
- Patient education and reassurance that pain will be controlled
- Consider anxiolytics: midazolam (1–5 mg) 10 minutes prior to procedure
- Preemptive pain control
  - regional anesthesia with peripheral nerve blocks
  - neuraxial blockade (spinal, lumbar epidural, and thoracic epidural)
  - systemic medications (NSAIDs, opioids)

4. Pain Control at Each Operative Stage

4.1. Preoperative

The physiologic response to surgery involves a "sympathetic surge," a profound activation of the sympathetic nervous system that is thought to contribute to afferent pain signals. This stress response is a well-established sequence of physiologic and molecular events that include fever, tachycardia, tachypnea, hypertension, gastrointestinal ileus, hypercoagulability, protein catabolism, and immunosuppression. Circulating cytokines and neuroendocrine mediators are also involved. The response lasts approximately 3 to 4 days from the time of induction of general anesthesia.

The goal of preemptive pain control is to blunt the physiologic response to surgery as well as to decrease the level of overall pain. Specifically, effective preemptive analgesia reduces the surgical nociceptor input (pain) while simultaneously preventing an ensuing sensitization of the nervous system throughout the perioperative period. The efficacy of preemptive multimodal analgesia depends on the interruption of the transduction of noxious stimuli at multiple sites along the pain pathway. Sites targeted by preemptive analgesia include peripheral nociceptors, preganglionic peripheral nerves, the dorsal horn of the spinal cord, and the sensory cortex and limbic system (see Figure 55.1).

Adequate arterial perfusion and partial pressure of oxygen are critical to tissue healing; vasoconstriction is a threat to normal healing. Measures to control peripheral vasoconstriction should be initiated prior to the operation and include cessation of smoking; controlling fear, pain, and anxiety; correcting hypertension; maintaining normal circulating blood volume; and maintaining normothermia. Preoperative reassurance that pain will be treated aggressively to manage patient catastrophizing should be a goal of all members of the operative team. Administration of an anxiolytic at least 30 minutes before surgery has been shown to decrease both anxiety and postoperative pain throughout the first postoperative week in a randomized placebo-controlled trial of patients who had outpatient surgery under general anesthesia.

The use of perioperative NSAIDs in preemptive analgesia is preferred over narcotics to limit adverse side effects (nausea, vomiting, urinary retention, cognitive dysfunction, respiratory depression). The use of NSAIDs is often combined with infiltration of the wound with a long-acting local anesthetic (e.g., bupivacaine). Continuation of NSAID analgesia for at least 24 hours after surgery is considered essential in order to achieve effective postoperative control of peripheral nociceptive pain. In addition, NSAIDs may achieve a long-term effect by inhibiting sensitization of the central nervous system.

4.2. Intraoperative

Optimal preemptive pain control involves measures taken prior to the surgical incision and continues into the postoperative period (Box 55.2). Injection of medications into the subcutaneous tissue underlying the intended incision site reduces postoperative analgesic requirements. Long-acting local anesthetics such as bupivacaine are most commonly used, but ketorolac, tramadol, and morphine have also been used for preincisional analgesia.

Operative site infection is an established potent stimulus for pro-inflammatory cytokines and chemokines. Prophylactic antibiotics are administered within 60 minutes of incision, redosed during major operations, and continued for 24 hours postoperatively. Operations undertaken for infectious etiology, such as abscess, cholecystitis, appendicitis, and diverticulitis, should focus on control of the pathologic source. Infectious complications can be minimized by expeditious surgery; gentle tissue handling; maintenance of normothermia, partial pressure of oxygen, and perfusion pressures; judicious use of antibiotic irrigation; avoidance of fluid overload; and changing gloves and instruments before wound closure. Sympatholytic effects of epidural anesthesia reduce the physiologic stress response to surgery, improve perfusion, reduce hypoxemia, limit blood loss (thereby decreasing transfusion requirements), counteract the prothrombotic state of surgery, and optimize pain control and secondary sensitization.

Meticulous surgical technique and hemostasis are fundamental aspects of postoperative pain control. Blood within the intraperitoneal cavity irritates the peritoneum and causes visceral pain. Postsurgical hematomas that form in anatomically

Box 55.2 Intraoperative Measures By The Surgeon To Control Pain

- Preincision analgesia: subcutaneous injection prior to operation at incision site, use
  - bupivacaine (10–30 mL of 0.25%)
- Prevention of infection and systemic inflammatory cascade, includes
  - preoperative antibiotics 60 minutes prior to incision (appropriate to operation)
  - expeditious surgery
  - gentle tissue handling
  - maintenance of normothermia
  - adequate tissue perfusion (minimizing peripheral vasoconstriction)
  - adequate tissue oxygen partial pressure
  - judicious use of antibiotic irrigation
  - avoidance of fluid overload
  - different gloves, instruments, and possibly gowns prior to closure of incision
- Meticulous hemostasis (avoidance of operative site hematoma), prevents
  - visceral irritation
  - hematoma formation
- Intraoperative peritoneal or pleural administration of local anesthetics, use
  - bupivacaine (15 mL of 0.5% with 1:100,000 epinephrine; 2–5 mL per laparoscopic port site) or
  - ropivacaine (20 mL of 7.5 mg/mL; 4 mL per intercostal space)

confined areas, such as the groin, continually stimulate peripheral nociceptors, resulting in pain that is difficult to control. Unless it is resorbed over time, a pain hematoma may require reoperation for surgical evacuation.

Blockade of afferent pain signals not only blunts pain but also reduces the amount of postoperative narcotic required, ultimately improving the quality of recovery. Intraperitoneal and intrapleural administration of local anesthetic has been shown to control visceral pain better than systemic medication. Recent advances in minimally invasive surgery have translated into smaller surgical incisions, reduced stress response and narcotic requirement, and decreased wound complications, all of which lead to a more rapid postoperative recovery.

4.3. Postoperative

Parenteral analgesics are commonly administered postoperatively, because patients are often restricted from oral intake after major surgery. However, fast-track rehabilitation is challenging the surgical dogma that restricts oral intake for prolonged periods until passage of flatus or stool has been achieved. Opioid medications (e.g., morphine sulfate, fentanyl, Dilaudid [Abbott Laboratories, Abbott Park, Ill]) are among the most common perioperative analgesics administered because of their time-tested efficacy. However, adverse side effects, including sedation, nausea, pruritis, and impairment of gastrointestinal motility, make preemptive analgesia an attractive alternative. Multimodal perioperative analgesia that uses several different drug mechanisms of action facilitates dose reductions in all the pain medications used, early discontinuation of narcotic analgesics, and better analgesia while minimizing the unwanted side effects of any one drug class.

The method of narcotic delivery impacts the success of pain control. Nurse-administered, as needed, pain medication may result in unacceptable gaps in postoperative analgesia and may fail to establish a therapeutic baseline level of pain control. Intravenous patient-controlled anesthesia, which allows timely patient-directed narcotic administration, has a continuous baseline dosing function to limit the peaks of pain intensity in the postoperative period. Multiple studies have documented improved pain outcomes with patient-controlled anesthesia as compared with nurse-titrated medication, but no consensus has been reached about improvements in postoperative complications. Transdermal narcotic administration provides more consistent administration of medication but has a delayed onset of action.

The use of integrative health modalities (massage, acupuncture, virtual reality, etc.) is an underutilized and poorly studied nonpharmacologic adjunct to standard medication-based perioperative pain management techniques. The established efficacy and low risk profile of these approaches should cause providers to seek opportunities for use before medications whenever possible.

5. Summary

Comprehensive preoperative assessment by the surgeon and anesthesiologist is the key first step to optimizing operative outcomes. Many perioperative measures fundamental to optimizing patient outcomes are intuitive: gentle tissue handling, minimizing blood loss, preventing hypothermia, administering prophylactic antibiotics within 1 hour of incision, judicious antibiotic irrigation of contaminated sites, minimizing peripheral vasoconstriction, limiting use of drains, ensuring high arterial partial pressure of oxygen, minimizing fluid overload, limiting the physiologic stress response to surgery, and optimizing control of pain.

Emphasis on multidisciplinary approaches to pain management, including integrative health modalities, can significantly improve pain care plans beyond pharmacologic measures. Coordination among the primary team, anesthesia, acute pain nursing, pharmacy, mental health, physical and rehabilitative medicine, and the family is a vital component of any inpatient pain care activity. For example, although a dense block of a patient's upper extremity may provide excellent pain relief, if the patient has no motor function in the limb to participate in physical therapy, this modality may not be in the best interest of the patient's overall recovery and health. Effective acute pain management requires the existence of an acute pain service staffed with motivated professionals with a variety of skill sets dedicated to the effective treatment of pain using a multimodal approach.

Basic Pediatric Regional Anesthesia

56

1. Introduction

Military anesthesia providers often encounter pediatric patients in deployed medical settings. The application of regional anesthesia (RA) in children can be extremely useful in austere situations, particularly when limited resources are available (e.g., scarce oxygen supply, lack of postoperative analgesics, insufficient postoperative nursing expertise). Prior to providing any pediatric regional anesthetic, the provider should not only be experienced in the specific RA technique, but also be comfortable with pediatric anesthetic care. Most pediatric RA is done while the child is either heavily sedated or under general anesthesia. To provide safe anesthetic services to pediatric patients, medical staff must recognize the myriad physiologic and pharmacologic differences between pediatric and adult patients.

2. Differences Between Pediatric and Adult Patients

2.1. Safety

Multiple studies supported by the Pediatric Regional Anesthesia Network have demonstrated the safety of conducting RA in anesthetized children. The serious complication rate related to RA in children is very low; 2 large studies cite the rate as zero. However, complications are more likely to occur in children less than 6 months of age and in those having neuraxial RA.

2.2. Pharmacokinetics

Local anesthetics preferentially bind to α-1 acid glycoprotein (AAG) found in plasma. Neonates have very low levels of AAG, 20% to 40% of normal adult values. Normal levels are not reached until 1 year of age. Low levels of AAG lead to higher serum levels of unbound local anesthetic, and this "free" drug is responsible for toxicity. Infants also have decreased clearance and a longer elimination half-life of local anesthetic as compared with adults. All these factors contribute to the increased general risk of local anesthetic toxicity resulting from a preponderance of free drug circulating in the pediatric patient's plasma during RA.

2.3. Developmental and anatomic differences

Nerve myelination is not complete until 12 years of age. Incomplete myelination allows for better penetration of local anesthetic into the nerve fibers. Reduced milligram doses

Table 56.1:
Anatomic differences between pediatric and adult patients

Age	End of Spinal Cord	End of Dural Sac	Intercristal Line	CSF Volume	Intercranial vs.
					Spinal CSF (%)
Neonate	L2	S3	L5-S1	NA	NA
1 Year	L1	S2	L4-L5	4 mL/kg	50
Adult	L1	S2	L3-L4	2 mL/kg	25

from dilute local anesthetic solutions can provide a complete block in children. Also, loose fascial attachments around the nerves facilitate the spread of local anesthetic. Consequently, a regional block in children may spread farther than the provider intends. Additionally, because the local anesthetic spreads easily in children, the duration of the block may be shortened as compared with adults. In general, as the patient's age increases, local anesthetic latency of onset and duration of action increases as well. Table 56.1 lists anatomic differences between children and adults.

3. Pediatric Regional Anesthesia

All blocks should be conducted with intravenous access and with standard American Society of Anesthesiology (ASA) monitoring applied. Appropriate resuscitation equipment should also be available. In austere environments, adjustments to this standard may be necessary based on the availability of medical equipment.

3.1. Caudal block

Indications. Use for patients less than 8 years old to provide intraoperative and postoperative analgesia for pelvic, urologic, abdominal, and lower extremity surgery.
Positioning. Place the child in the lateral decubitus position with knees pulled up toward the chest.
Landmarks. Bilateral posterior superior iliac spine (PSIS) and sacral hiatus (SH). These 3 points should form an equilateral triangle. The SH is bounded by the sacral cornua. The sacral cornua are palpable on either side of the midline about 1 cm apart.
Technique. After sterile preparation and drape, insert a 20- or 22-gauge angiocatheter at a 45° angle to the skin over the SH. A "pop" will be felt as the needle passes through the sacrococcygeal membrane. Once the sacrococcygeal membrane is pierced, drop the needle angle to 20° to 40° from the skin and advance the needle and the catheter 2 to 4 mm. Then advance the catheter off the needle (the catheter should advance easily). A stimulating needle can also be used. If the stimulating needle is in the caudal space, anal sphincter activity will be visible with a stimulation of 1 to 10 mA. If using a stimulating needle, do not advance greater than 2 to 4 mm past the sacrococcygeal membrane to prevent risk of dural puncture. After aspiration test, local anesthetic should inject easily with no swelling of subcutaneous tissue.
Drug Dosing. See Table 56.2.

3.2. Thoracic epidural

Indications. Thoracic surgical procedures.
Positioning. Awake patients positioned in sitting position; anesthetized patients in lateral decubitus position with knees to chest.
Landmarks. Midline or paramedian. For midline technique, Tuohy needle insertion is between spinous processes. The Tuohy is inserted 1 to 2 cm lateral and inferior to the spinous processes for the paramedian approach. Ultrasound can be used to confirm anatomy.

Table 56.2:
Pediatric drug dosing for caudal or epidural blocks

Age	Bupivacaine	Ropivacaine	Clonidine	Fentanyl
Single Injection?				
< 1 Year	0.25%, 1 mL/kg	0.2%, 1.2 mL/kg	1.0–1.5 mcg/kg	2 mcg/mL
> 1 Year	0.25%, 1 mL/kg, max 20 mL⁺	0.2–0.5%, max 20 mL or 3.5 mg/kg	1.0–1.5 mcg/kg	2 mcg/mL
Continuous Injection				
< 3 Months	0.0625%–0.125%, 0.2 mg/kg/h	0.1%–0.2%, 0.2 mg/kg/h	0.12–0.2 mcg/kg/h	1–2 mcg/mL
< 1 Year	0.125%, 0.3 mg/kg/h	0.1–0.2%, 0.3 mg/kg/h	0.12–0.2 mcg/kg/h	1–2 mcg/mL
>1 Year	0.125%, 0.3–0.4 mg/kg/h	0.1%–0.2%, 0.4 mg/kg/h	0.12–0.2 mcg/kg/h	1–2 mcg/mL

⁺Thoracic epidural: reduce initial dose to 0.5 mg/kg.

Technique.

- Midline: The Tuohy needle is advanced cephalad incrementally using the loss of resistance with saline technique.
- Paramedian: The Tuohy needle is inserted until contact with the transverse process is made. The needle is then slightly withdrawn and advanced midline and cephalad until the ligamentum flavum is engaged and epidural space entered.

Drug Dosing. See Table 56.2. Initial bolus 0.3 to 0.5 mL/kg

3.3. Lumbar epidural

Indications. Use to provide anesthesia and/or continuous analgesia for abdominal or lower extremity surgery in children of any age.
Positioning. Place the child in the lateral decubitus position with knees pulled up toward the chest.
Landmarks. Intercristal line (posterior line between the superior aspect of the 2 iliac crests). Ultrasound can be used to confirm anatomy.
Technique. After sterile preparation and drape, insert a short, 18-gauge Tuohy or Crawford needle with a 20-gauge epidural catheter. Loss of resistance with saline is the preferred technique. Catheters can frequently be threaded from the lumbar to the thoracic level with the Tuohy bevel directed cephalad. If catheters will be threaded to the thoracic level, the distance must be measured prior to insertion. Depth to the epidural space can be determined as follows:

- Neonate ≈ 1 cm
- Children 10 kg–25 kg ≈ 1 mm/kg
- Children >25 kg: 0.8 + (0.05 × wt [kg]) = depth in cm

Drug Dosing. See Table 56.2. Initial bolus 0.3 to 0.5 mL/kg

3.4. Subarachnoid block

Indications. Lower abdominal and lower extremity procedures lasting less than 90 minutes. Subarachnoid block is an extremely effective and useful technique in resource-limited environments. Children have remarkable hemodynamic stability under spinal anesthesia.

Table 56.3:
Pediatric Spinal Dosing

Age	Bupivacaine (mg/kg)	Tetracaine* (mg/kg)	Ropivacaine (mg/kg)
Infants	0.5–1.0	0.5–1.0	0.5–1.0
1–7 yrs old†	0.3–0.5	0.3–0.5	0.5
>7 yrs old†	0.2–0.3	0.3	0.3–0.4

*With tetracaine, use epinephrine wash (epinephrine aspirated from vial and then fully expelled from the syringe prior to drawing up local anesthetic) to increase duration up to 120 minutes.

†Additives: clonidine 1–2 μg/kg for children > 1 year of age.

Positioning. Lateral decubitus or seated. Careful attention must be paid to avoid excessive neck flexion in young infants, which causes airway obstruction.

Technique. After sterile preparation, a short (1.5–2 in.) 25- or 22-gauge spinal needle should be used at the L4-L5 or L5-S1 interspace in infants. The L3-L4 interspace is acceptable in children greater than 1 year of age.

Drug Dosing. See Table 56.3. Hyperbaric or isobaric solutions should be used.

Possible Complications. Postdural puncture headaches are rare in children. Dose for blood patch: 0.3 mL/kg blood.

Teaching Points. Do not lift the child's legs in the air after the block or a high spinal will occur.

Although the local anesthetic dose may appear large, recall that children have a large cerebrospinal fluid volume relative to adults (see Table 56.1). The duration of the block increases with the patient's age.

3.5. Peripheral nerve block

Indications. Perioperative analgesia for upper extremity, lower extremity, abdominal, thoracic, or breast surgery.

Drug Dosing. Local anesthetics for these blocks are dosed by weight rather than by a set volume. Table 56.4 provides local anesthetic dosing for pediatric PNBs including recommendations of maximum allowable dosage. Children less than 8 years of age should receive 0.25% bupivacaine or 0.2% ropivacaine. If the peripheral nerve block (PNB) is placed after general anesthesia is induced, do not use neuromuscular blocking agents until after the block is placed. When performing a continuous peripheral nerve block, do not exceed the maximum doses listed in Table 56.4.

3.6. Upper Extremity Blocks

Before the more common use of ultrasound guidance, performing interscalene and supraclavicular nerve blocks in the pediatric population was less frequent due to the potential of adverse effects. These risks include pneumothorax, vertebral artery puncture with local anesthetic toxicity, epidural or intrathecal spread, phrenic nerve blockade, and recurrent laryngeal nerve blockade. Ultrasound technology has increased the frequency of these blocks, but due to the high risk of complications, these upper extremity blocks should only be performed by experts in pediatric RA.

3.7. Interscalene block

Positioning. Supine with the head turned away from the side of the block.

Landmarks. This block should only be performed using ultrasound in pediatric patients.

Table 56.4:
Pediatric drug dosing for individual single-injection nerve blocks

Body Area	Block	Dose (Do Not Exceed Maximum Allowable Dose)	Drug
Trunk			
	PVB	0.25–0.5 mL per side	0.2% ropivacaine or 0.25% bupivacaine with 1:400k epinephrine/mL⁺
	TAP	0.3–0.5 mL/kg	0.2% ropivacaine or 0.25% bupivacaine
	Rectus	0.2–0.4 mL/kg	0.2% ropivacaine or 0.25% bupivacaine
	Ilioinguinal iliohypogastric	0.2–0.4 mL/kg	0.2% ropivacaine or 0.25% bupivacaine⋆
Upper Extremity			
	Interscalene	0.1–0.3 mL/kg	0.2% ropivacaine or 0.25% bupivacaine⋆
	Supraclavicular	0.2–0.4 mL/kg	0.2% ropivacaine or 0.25% bupivacaine⋆
	Infraclavicular	0.2–0.4 mL/kg	0.2% ropivacaine or 0.25% bupivacaine⋆
	Axillary	0.2–0.4 mL/kg	0.2% ropivacaine or 0.25% bupivacaine⋆
Lower Extremity			
	Lumbar plexus	0.3–0.5 mL/kg	0.2% ropivacaine or 0.25% bupivacaine⋆
	Fascia iliaca	0.5–1 mL/kg	0.2% ropivacaine or 0.25% bupivacaine
	Femoral	0.2–0.3 mL/kg	0.2% ropivacaine or 0.25% bupivacaine⋆
	Lateral femoral cutaneous	0.1–0.2 mL/kg	0.2% ropivacaine or 0.25% bupivacaine⋆
	Adductor canal or saphenous	0.1–0.2 mL/kg	0.2% ropivacaine or 0.25% bupivacaine⋆
	Sciatic	0.3-0.6 mL/kg	0.2% ropivacaine or 0.25% bupivacaine⋆
	Ankle	1-3 mL/nerve	0.2% ropivacaine or 0.25% bupivacaine⋆

Maximum allowable dose of local anesthetic: do not use more than total dose of 3 mg/kg bupivacaine or 3.5 mg/kg ropivacaine.

⁺ Do not exceed 0.5 mcg/kg of epinephrine.

⋆In children >8 years of age **can** consider 0.5% ropivacaine. For children 12 years of age or greater **should** consider 0.5% ropivacaine. This does *not* apply for field blocks (TAP, rectus, fascia iliaca). Do not exceed the maximum allowable doses of local anesthetic.

PVB = paravertebral block; TAP = transverse abdominis plane block.

Technique. Same as adult, but use a 22-gauge, 5-cm needle. Use caution as risks for this block include vertebral artery puncture with local anesthetic toxicity, epidural or intrathecal spread, pneumothorax, phrenic nerve blockade, and recurrent laryngeal nerve blockade with unilateral vocal cord paralysis.

3.8. Parascalene block

The parascalene block was developed to provide a safer alternative in children to the interscalene or supraclavicular block, especially if ultrasound is unavailable.

Positioning. Place the patient supine with a rolled towel under the shoulder and arm at the side.

Landmarks. Midpoint of the clavicle, posterior border of the sternocleidomastoid, and the transverse process of C6. The level of C6 is at the same level as the cricoid cartilage. Draw a line between the transverse process of C6 and the midpoint of the clavicle (Figure 56.1).

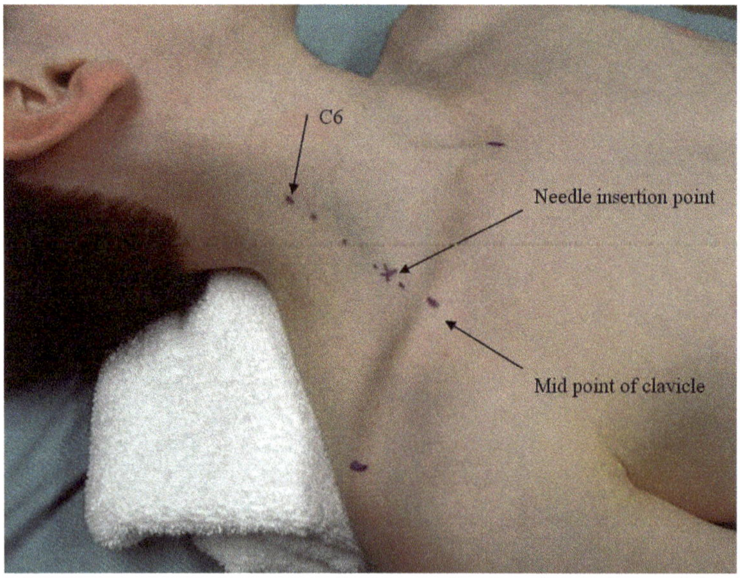

Figure 56.1 Parascalene block landmarks.

Technique. The needle puncture site is at the point between the lower one-third and upper two-thirds of this line. Insert the stimulating needle perpendicular to the skin and directed posteriorly until upper extremity twitches are noted. If no twitches are elicited, redirect the needle laterally. Then inject an appropriate dose (based on child's age and weight) of local anesthesia. Depth of plexus ≈ 1 to 2 cm.
Equipment. 22-gauge, 5-cm stimulating needle.

3.9. Supraclavicular block

Positioning. Supine with head turned away from block side.
Landmarks. This block should only be performed using ultrasound in pediatric patients.
Technique. Same as adult, but use a 22-gauge, 5-cm needle. Use caution as risks for this block include local anesthetic toxicity with inadvertent intravascular injection, pneumothorax, phrenic nerve blockade, and recurrent laryngeal nerve blockade with unilateral vocal cord paralysis.

3.10. Infraclavicular block

Positioning. Place the patient supine with the operative extremity at the side and head turned to the opposite side.
Landmarks and Techniques. Ultrasound is preferred. Two approaches are used in children for the infraclavicular block: (1) the deltopectoral groove approach, with the same the landmarks and technique as in an adult and (2) the midclavicular approach, in which the midpoint of the clavicle is the landmark. Insert the needle at a 45° angle to the skin, pointed toward the axilla. A 22-gauge, 5-cm needle is used for children under 40 kg.

3.11. Axillary block

Positioning. Same as adult.

Landmarks. Same as adult.

Technique. Ultrasound is preferred. Same as adult, but use a 22-gauge, 5-cm needle.

3.12. Lower extremity blocks

Lower extremity blocks include the femoral, lumbar plexus, and sciatic blocks.

3.13. Femoral block

The position, landmarks, and desired motor response with simulation are the same as in an adult. Use a 22-gauge, 5-cm or 1.5-in (3.8-cm) needle. Use of ultrasound is preferred.

3.14. Lumbar plexus block

Only practitioners with experience with this technique should use this block in children. Multiple techniques have been utilized for a lumbar plexus block. The technique described in the lumbar plexus block chapter (chapter 40, "Lumbar Plexus Block") of this book may also be utilized in the pediatric patient. An alternative is described in the following:
Positioning. Lateral decubitus position with the knees pulled up toward the chest.
Landmarks. Draw a line between the spinous process of L4 and the ipsilateral PSIS. The needle insertion point is at the point between the medial two-thirds and the lateral one-third of the line (Figure 56.2).
Technique. Advance a 5- or 10-cm stimulating needle parallel to the bed until quadriceps twitches are elicited. If the needle contacts the L5 process, withdraw and redirect it cephalad. Average depth to plexus: 2.5 cm (5-kg child) to 6.5 cm (50-kg child).

3.15. Sciatic block

Multiple approaches to the sciatic nerve block may be used in children. Which approach to use should be determined by provider experience with any particular technique. Ultrasound should be used if available.

- Posterior or classic sciatic block. The positioning, landmarks, and technique are the same as for an adult. Average distance to the nerve: 2 cm (5-kg child) to 4.5 cm (50-kg child).

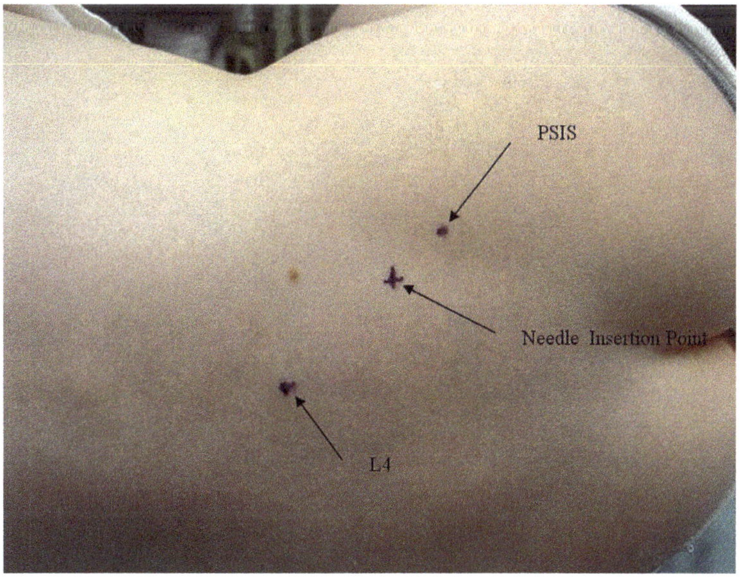

Figure 56.2 Lumbar plexus block landmarks. PSIS: posterior superior iliac spine.

- Raj or infragluteal sciatic block. The positioning, landmarks, and technique are the same as for an adult.
- Popliteal sciatic block. This is the most commonly reported as well as the safest approach to the sciatic nerve in children.

Positioning. The popliteal approach to the sciatic nerve can be done in the prone, lateral (operative leg up), or supine position, with an assistant elevating the leg. To appreciate the appropriate stimulation pattern of the tibial nerve, the patient's foot and ankle must be free to move.

Landmarks. The popliteal crease, the biceps femoris tendon, and the tendons of the semimembranosus and semitendinosus muscles define the sciatic nerve.

Technique. Bisect the triangle formed by the landmarks. The needle insertion point is 1 cm below the apex of the triangle and 0.5 cm lateral to the bisecting line. Needle length is 5 cm for a small child or 10 cm for a larger child. Direct the needle cephalad at a 70° angle to the skin until plantar flexion is elicited. Distance from the popliteal crease to the bifurcation of the sciatic nerve: 27+ (4 × age in years) = distance in mm.

3.16. Thoracic paravertebral block

Indications. Anesthesia and analgesia for breast and chest wall procedures.

Positioning. Sitting or lateral decubitus.

Landmarks. Spinous process. Needle insertion point is 1 to 2 cm lateral to the superior aspect of the spinous process.

Technique. Same as for an adult, but use a 22-gauge Tuohy needle. The insertion point should be 0.5 to 1 cm past the transverse process. Estimated depth to the paravertebral space: 20 + (0.5 × wt [kg]) = depth in mm.

3.17. Rectus sheath and transversus abdominus plane block

Positioning. Same as adult.

Landmarks. Same as adult.

Technique. Same as adult, but use a 22-gauge, 5-cm needle with ultrasound.

4. Injection Technique for Pediatric Regional Anesthesia

Use the following for all pediatric RA except the subarachnoid block:

- Aspirate prior to injection.
- For caudal and epidural RA: Inject test dose (0.1 mL/kg; max dose: 3 ml) of local anesthetic solution containing 1:200,000 or 1:400,000 of epinephrine.
- Look for signs of positive test dose.
- Inject the remaining volume of local anesthetic slowly (120–180 seconds).
- Aspirate every 3 to 5 mL.
- Continue to closely monitor electrocardiograph and blood pressure during injection.
- Carefully test dose any catheter prior to bolusing or starting a continuous infusion.

Air Transport of the Critically Injured Pain Patient

57

1. Introduction

Contemporary warfare has brought both advancements and new challenges for acute pain management in the combat setting. Although survivability has increased secondary to improvements in body armor, the necessarily exposed limbs of soldiers have become even more vulnerable to progressively more destructive explosive devices. The lethality of improvised explosive devices, explosively formed penetrators, and other weapons has clearly increased during the course of the current conflict. Rapid patient evacuation out of the battlefield, far-forward advanced surgical capabilities, and rapid air evacuation of combat wounded to critical care facilities outside of the war theater are the key factors resulting in a less than 10% died-of-wound rate. Historically, the relatively austere medical environment of the US Air Force (USAF) evacuation aircraft (Figure 57.1) made the management of acute pain in multitrauma patients particularly difficult. The lessons learned from military evacuation during recent conflicts can be used as a reference for civilian medical missions in response to natural disasters.

Today, the ability to evacuate patients from the battlefield has evolved into the most efficient transport and medically capable system in history. At the core of this system lies the USAF aeromedical evacuation system (AES). With the inclusion of the critical care air transport team (CCATT), the AES has been described as a 6000-mile-long intensive care unit in the sky, stretching from staging areas in the Middle East to the continental United States.

Although CCATTs focus on the critical care patient, the majority of injured soldiers require aeromedical evacuation (AE) transport without mechanical ventilation, inotropic medications, or other measures typically associated with critical care. However, these patients often have sustained massive injury, such as multiple amputations of limbs and complicated orthopedic injuries. Although "hemodynamically stable," these patients still have acute needs for in-flight monitoring and aggressive pain management.

The US military experience with evacuating casualties by air dates to World War I. Until recently, advances in pain management during evacuation have not kept pace with advances in casualty resuscitation and transport. This chapter will address the historical casualty transport capabilities of the military, advances in patient care en route, and the addition of advanced pain management during evacuation. Specific challenges encountered in patient care while traveling for hours for thousands of miles on military aircraft will also be addressed.

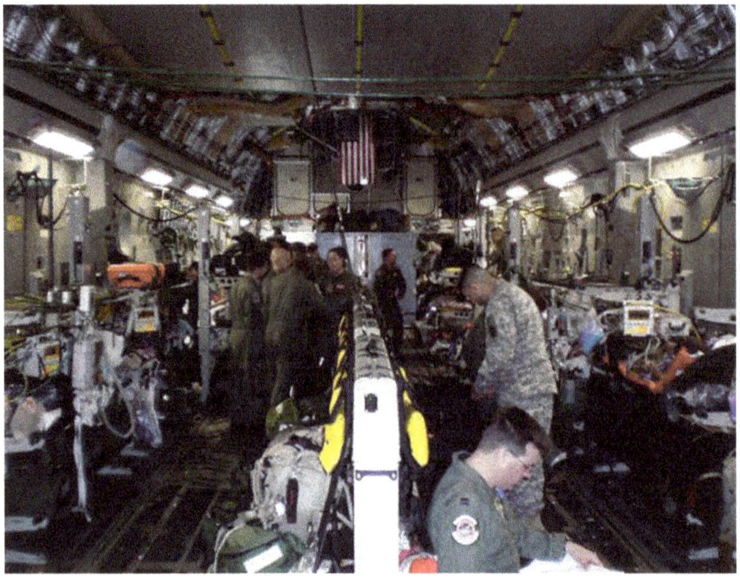

Figure 57.1 Interior of air evacuation aircraft.

2. Historical Transformation of the Air Force En Route Care Platform

The World War I air evacuation efforts led to the organization of an integrated AES by the US Army Air Corps during World War II. This system included nurses with specific AE training serving on cargo aircraft returning from the theater of battle.

By the 1990s, the AES included command and control functions, trained crews, mobile facilities for staging patients preflight, and extensive logistical support. The system could rapidly deploy, set up, and evacuate large numbers of stable casualties, but it lacked the intrinsic capability to manage critically ill casualties, instead relying on medical attendants, supplies, and equipment provided by the sending medical facility. The requirement to provide these resources was a particular challenge for small field hospitals with limited personnel, which cannot lose personnel without seriously degrading their capability. This problem became evident in Somalia when the surge of combat casualties on October 3–4, 1993 overwhelmed the medical response capabilities. As a result, casualties accumulated, and the most critical patients could not be immediately evacuated. Following Operation Desert Storm in 1990, calls were made for the addition of AE physicians and equipment capable of managing unstable patients in flight.

3. Joint En Route Care System

The current joint en route care system includes contributions from each of the US military services and, in many cases, from coalition military medical services as well. Casualties are evacuated through 5 roles of care with increasing capability, from self-care and buddy care with initial management at aid stations close to the point of injury, through advanced rehabilitative care at military and Veterans Administration medical centers in the United States.

Casualty evacuation (CASEVAC), a term used by all services, refers to the movement of unregulated casualties by nonmedical units aboard nonmedical ground vehicles, without en route care by medical professionals. The casualty is taken from the point of injury to the most appropriate medical facility, typically role I or role II facilities. The CASEVAC mission may involve care under fire, and speed and security are more important than advanced en route care. In the US military, CASEVAC is overwhelmingly an Army, Marine Corps, or Navy mission.

Medical evacuation (MEDEVAC) refers to a US Army capability involving designated rotary-wing aircraft and specially trained enlisted medical crew members. In MEDEVAC, casualties are transported aboard medical helicopters under the care of combat medics with advanced flight training. Constituting a paramedic level of care, this capability can be used from the point of injury to a medical facility, or between facilities.

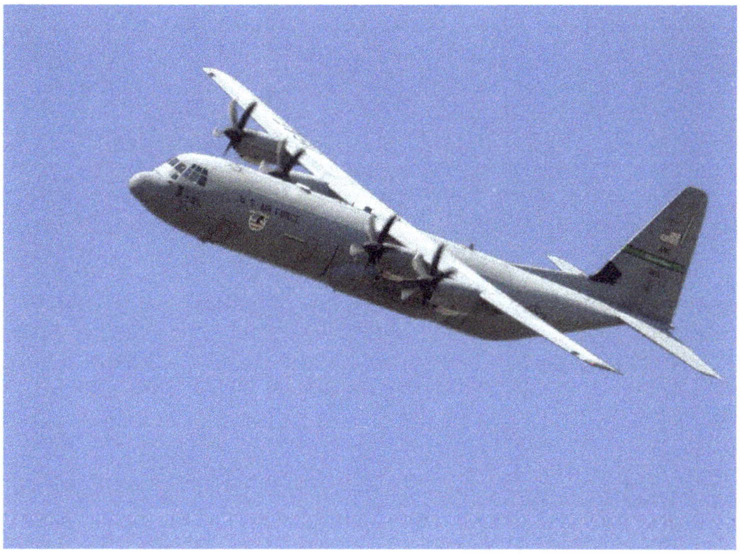

Figure 57.2 C-130 Hercules.

Strategic evacuation (STRATEVAC) is primarily the domain of the USAF. *Aeromedical evacuation system* refers to the regulated movement of casualties from role II or III through role V facilities by fixed-wing USAF aircraft. Staging facilities at hubs of the AES serve as buffers, allowing casualties to be housed, fed, and prepared for flight at a location from which they can be rapidly loaded as aircraft become available. Basic medical care and wound care, as well as basic (oral and intravenous [IV] bolus) pain control, are provided at these locations. Patients waiting at the hubs typically have minor injuries preventing them from immediately returning to duty. Aboard the aircraft, an AE crew, consisting of flight nurses and AE medical technicians who have undergone specialized training, manages the patients. The care given by an AE crew is limited by the large number of patients they are tasked to manage and their level of medical training. If a patient requires more than this basic level of care, the sending facility has historically been responsible for providing a medical attendant during evacuation. Today, for casualties who are critically ill or injured, the AES provides the medical attendants in the form of the CCATT.

The AE function can be categorized as tactical evacuation (TACEVAC) within a military theater of operations or STRATEVAC between theaters of operation. The most commonly used aircraft for TACEVAC is the C-130 Hercules (Figure 57.2), which is capable of operating from unimproved airfields and in hostile locations. The C-130 flies at 318 knots at 20,000 feet, with a maximum ceiling of 23,000 feet. It has the capacity for up to 74 litter patients but does not have onboard oxygen systems, mandating that oxygen be carried onboard as a portable liquid oxygen system or a compressed gas. The electrical system provides 400 Hz AC power through specially configured outlets, limiting its direct utility for medical devices. Therefore, AE/CCATT must rely on battery power, or power provided through an electrical converter, which limits the total amperage output for medical equipment use. Lighting and environmental control systems are minimal, requiring additional measures for patient warming and visualization of patient care. Lastly, access to patients is limited to 180°.

The C-17 Globemaster III (Figure 57.3) has the unique quality of being an excellent aircraft for both TACEVAC and STRATEVAC. It has a speed of 450 knots at an altitude of 28,000 feet, with an unrefueled range of 2400 nautical miles and unlimited range with aerial refueling. This range makes it useful for transoceanic missions. The C-17 can also utilize small, unimproved airfields with runways as short as 3500 feet and with a width of 90 feet. The aircraft's interior is well lit, and the system of litter stanchions provides 360° access to critical patients. The C-17 contains built-in systems that provide medical oxygen at 50 psi and 60 Hz AC electric power through standard US outlets. Currently the workhorse in patient transport, the C-17 can be rapidly configured from use as a cargo aircraft to accommodate 36 litter patients.

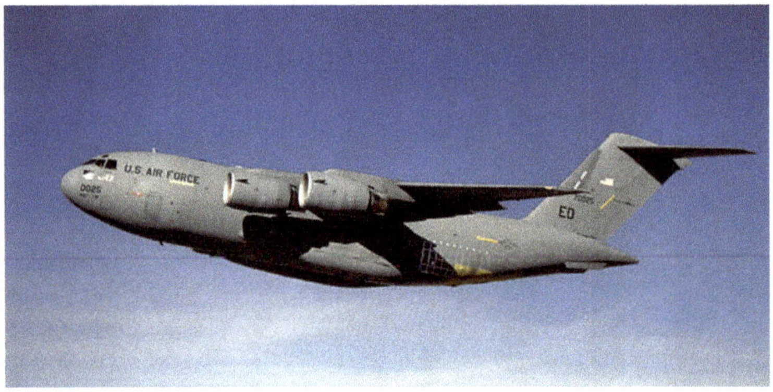

Figure 57.3 C-17 Globemaster III.

4. Pieces of the En Route Care Puzzle

The USAF is solely responsible for the transport of injured US military personnel from the theater of operation to their home station. This requires the ability to transport and provide ongoing care during long-distance flights lasting from 2 to 5 days. The system relies on available USAF aircraft that are temporarily converted into AE-capable platforms as the need arises. USAF teams involved in patient transport include the aircraft crew, AE medics, and the CCATT.

Until the mid-1990s, most if not all injured patients requiring AE transport had to be relatively stable for transport. Very little care was performed in the aircraft due to limited capabilities of the medical AE teams. For example, if a patient in Germany had an uncomplicated exploratory laparotomy, he or she would have to stay at the hospital where the surgery was performed until considered stable for transport, which would have been anywhere from 3 to 5 days postoperation. If patients required any special care or pain medicine other than oral or intermittent IV bolus, a medical attendant would have to travel with them to manage their care during transport. Early AE teams typically consisted of a mix of registered nurses and medical technicians, specifically trained for air transport of the medical patient. A typical AE team included 2 nurses and 3 technicians; an expanded team consisted of 3 nurses and 4 technicians. The personnel assigned to AE varied from outpatient clinic personnel to critical care personnel, and the patient care abilities and comfort levels of AE team members varied widely. Anything other than basic care was limited by the makeup of the AE team. The typical AE transport had a patient load of anywhere from 1 to more than 50 patients, depending on the types of patients, whether or not they were ambulatory, and the aircraft available. To support this method of AE, the holding capabilities of medical facilities in and out of theater had to be robust, which was logistically difficult to support and often not in the best interest of the patient.

During the 1980s and early 1990s, Dr Paul K. Carlton Jr, a surgeon and later the USAF surgeon general, developed capability for the rapid effective stabilization and transport of significantly injured or traumatized casualties. Carlton based his method on his experience at Wiesbaden, Germany, receiving casualties from the embassy bombing in Beirut, Lebanon. In 1994, Carlton and Dr Joseph C. Farmer, a medical intensivist, launched the CCATT program, consisting of teams with a critical care physician, critical care nurse, and respiratory therapist, accompanied by the supplies and equipment necessary to create a critical care environment that would move with the patient during evacuation. Team members were specifically trained to provide specialized care in the high-altitude, extreme aircraft environment, with emphasis on the "AE environment." The concept of CCATT is to manage stabilizing casualties—those who have undergone initial resuscitation but remain critically ill. A physician was included on the team to provide continuous medical decision-making so that therapies could be titrated to the patient's condition, new therapies started if required, and patients could continue progressing toward stability without interruption or setback for transport. Having a CCATT physician available during an AE mission also allowed better medical care for the non-CCATT patients, including pain management.

The timing of CCATT development allowed the US military healthcare system to adjust its doctrine in response to changing military strategy. During the Cold War, US forces prepared for large battles in predictable locations supported by established hospitals with the capacity to hold large numbers of casualties until they had completed convalescence and were returned to duty. After the Cold War ended, the US military became engaged in a large number of activities ranging from humanitarian and peacekeeping operations to combat. These operations often arose quickly, took place in unpredictable locations, and in some cases changed locations rapidly; establishing large-capacity hospitals whenever and wherever needed became impossible. Instead, the military needed to deploy small, high-capability, limited-holding-capacity facilities that could stabilize and evacuate casualties with far less logistic support. To accomplish this objective, medical personnel needed to be able to evacuate even unstable casualties safely, and CCATT offered that capability.

4.1. En route pain management

Despite advances made in the en route care system, one aspect in need of improvement involved patients who were not critical enough for CCATT, but had significant pain secondary to their injuries, which was worsened by the vibration, bouncing, and noise of the continuously moving aircraft transport environment. Due to the aircraft environment and external forces, patients frequently experienced inadequate pain control during bus transport and the aeroevacuation flight.

The aerospace environment presents numerous physiologic and psychological challenges, especially with trauma patients, to medical personnel. Altitude changes, extremes of temperature, noise, vibration, lighting, power, space, and flight equipment restrictions are just a few of the stresses placed on aeromedical personnel. Constant vibration and the cramped conditions aboard the aircraft can make a painful injury excruciating. Appropriate padding and securing of wounded extremities help to reduce pain and protect the patient from compression injuries. Some injured military members have even gone as far as posting signs saying, "Don't bump the stump!" Attention to such simple details goes far in the management of pain in this complex environment.

Until recently, oral medication and intermittent morphine (bolus IV) were essentially the only pain management therapies available for injured soldiers during transport. Medications for pain carried on a routine AE mission included acetaminophen; ibuprofen; Tylenol 3 (McNEIL-PPC Inc, Fort Washington, Pa); Percocet (Endo Pharmaceuticals, Chadds Ford, Pa); Demerol (Sanofi-Aventis, Bridgewater, NJ); and morphine. Patients were provided written orders for either oral pain medication or IV morphine. This was the AE standard of care until mid-2002. Despite having served the military well in the past, this type of pain management fails in today's complex evacuation systems.

In a typical AE mission, patients are held in a centralized location before transport via ambulance bus (AMBUS [Figure 57.4]) to the aircraft, where they are loaded as either ambulatory or litter patients. After taxi and takeoff, a safe altitude must be reached before patient care can be given, a process lasting about 60 minutes. At the end of the mission, all personnel must remain seated during approach, landing, and taxi, which also takes about 60 minutes. Unloading patients from the aircraft onto an AMBUS and transport lasting 60 to 90 minutes to the receiving facility is the next evacuation step. At the receiving facility, unloading patients from the AMBUS into the facility for admission and room assignment adds further time before patient care resumes. During the time of landing, taxi, loading, transport, unloading, and in-processing at the receiving facility, pain control received by the patient is minimal (Figure 57.5).

The problem of patients enduring extended time between administrations of pain medication was identified early in Operation Enduring Freedom and Operation Iraqi Freedom, secondary to the large numbers of patients arriving at the various receiving facilities (Landstuhl Regional Medical Center, Germany; Walter Reed Army Medical Center, Bethesda Naval Medical Center, and Malcolm Grow Medical Center, Andrews Air Force Base, in the Washington, DC, area; and Brook Army Medical Center, San Antonio, Tex) in extreme amounts of pain. An early attempt to combat this pain problem involved anesthesia pain teams meeting casualties as they arrived at receiving facilities. However, although the teams treated the immediate pain on arrival, the pain endured from aircraft approach to facility arrival was not treated. Anesthesia teams then began greeting the aircraft on arrival to provide pain medication (oral or IV) prior to AMBUS

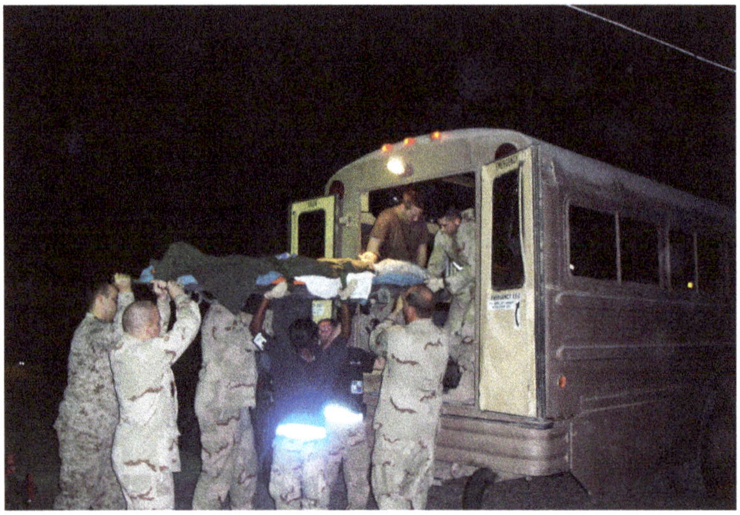

Figure 57.4 Loading patient into AMBUS.

loading and transport. Both measures helped significantly, but did not adequately address the issue of pain during transport as a whole, and the extended periods of time between dosing were not adequately resolved.

The casualty pain issues on AE flights prompted the triservice (Army, Navy, and USAF) anesthesia community to band together to identify and provide solutions to this problem of pain during transport. The result was the formation of the first triservice military organization specifically concentrating on management of pain in combat casualties—the Military Advanced Regional Anesthesia and Analgesia (MARAA) committee—organized in early 2002 to develop, recommend, and implement advanced pain initiatives to be placed in the AE environment.

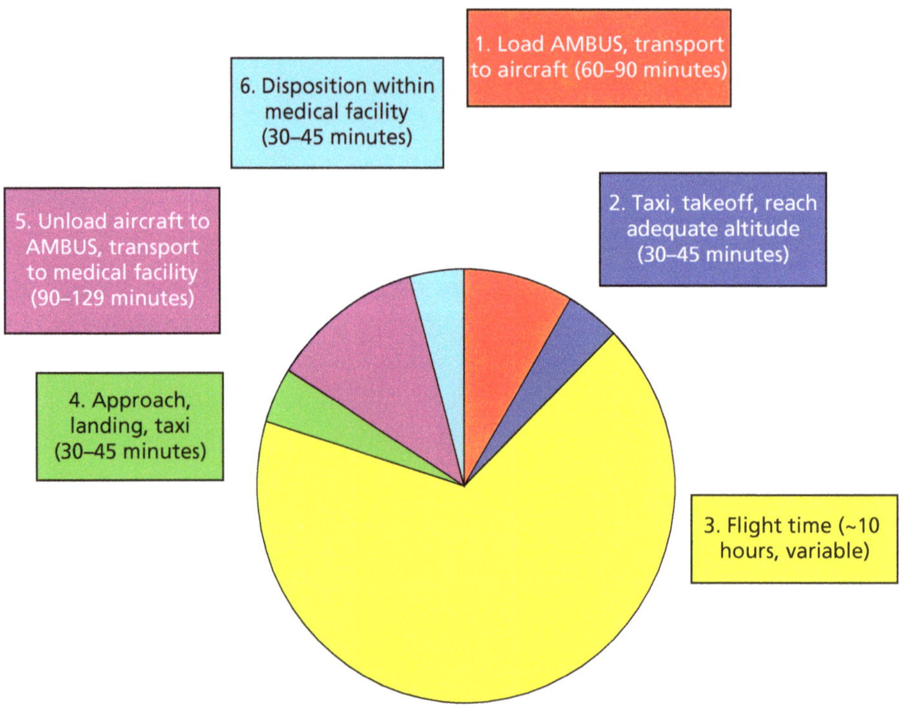

Figure 57.5 Proportionate stages of transport during air evacuation.

4.2. Military advanced regional anesthesia and analgesia initiatives

The first therapy advocated by MARAA was the continuous peripheral nerve block (CPNB), which had already proven successful for pain control, but was not allowed in the AES due to lack of a medical attendant to monitor the infusion. MARAA developed a training platform for CPNBs during AE and obtained airworthiness testing and approval for the Stryker PainPump (Stryker; Kalamazoo, Mich) for the infusions. The addition of CPNBs into the AES in 2003 significantly improved the pain management of many evacuating casualties. CPNB on military aircraft has enjoyed an excellent safety record in wounded soldiers since it was first introduced on October 7, 2003. To date, thousands of injured airmen, soldiers, sailors, and marines have benefited from this technique. However, CPNBs are appropriate only for a patient population with isolated extremity injuries, and MARAA continued developing further pain management techniques for the AES. Although none of the techniques would be considered new in a US medical facility, the application of these proven pain technologies in AE has greatly enhanced pain management in this difficult medical environment.

The second initiative was the institution of patient-controlled analgesia (PCA) for transport in 2004. PCA is common in civilian hospitals, where it is well monitored by trained nursing staff on a routine basis, whereas clinical capabilities in AE teams are unpredictable. MARAA realized that the pump selected for this mission had to be small, user-friendly, and safe and had to pass airworthy certification for acceptance onto military aircraft. In addition, the pump had to be relatively inexpensive and require no medical maintenance. MARAA members found the ambIT PCA pump (Summit Medical Products, South Sandy, Utah) to be the best interim choice for rapid implementation of this technology.

The third initiative by MARAA was epidural analgesia for AE patient care in late 2004. Implementation of epidural analgesia en route also required a user-friendly, fail-safe pump with simple instructions for monitoring and care. Today the pump utilized for all 3 pain management techniques is the ambIT infusion pump. Labels are provided in the packaging to identify the type of infusion, as well as instructions for troubleshooting and reprogramming the infusions if required. All pain techniques are followed and managed by the various military anesthesia departments while en route. More recently, nonpharmacologic adjuncts such as auricular acupuncture are routinely employed on evacuation flights to manage pain along with the other modalities mentioned.

4.3. En route patient packaging

AE mission variables include flight durations that range from 1 to more than 18 hours, significant physiologic flux demanding provider treatment flexibility, and a constantly changing mission pace that necessitates rapid assessment and prioritization of care in a medically austere environment. This practice is very different from the static hospital ward experience in the United States. Experience has shown that the independent, hands-on practitioner mind-set and skill sets of anesthesiologists and emergency physicians adapt well to the care of patients in the CCATT environment, specifically for ongoing resuscitation, required procedure, and pain management. The patient care approach these physicians bring into the development and maintenance of the CCATT program has also been a major benefit.

To package a patient for multihour transport, attention must be paid to multiple issues including prevention of pressure sores, prevention of further injury, spinal immobilization, prevention of injury from attached equipment, stabilizing extremity fractures, prevention of "blocked" extremity injury, external fixator padding and stabilization, and prevention of dislodgment of catheters or kinking of tubing, in addition to pain management. These duties are usually associated with nursing but are the responsibility of the caregiver team in the air transport arena. Patients typically require increases in pain medication during air transport because of the aircraft's constant motion, compared with the stable hospital environment. An easy technique to evaluate the effectiveness of the pain control (PCA, epidural, CPNB) is to shake the patient's hospital bed to see if it causes increased pain; if so, pain dosing during AE may need to be increased 10% to 20%.

4.4. Airworthy certification

Medical equipment on military aircraft must meet stringent criteria of airworthiness and interoperability. The major testing hurdles before approval for in-flight use include interface with the aircraft oxygen and electrical systems; assessment of how the device functions across the cabin altitude range of a typical mission (sea level to 8000 feet) and with rapid decompression to flying altitude; whether the device produces electromagnetic emissions that interfere with aircraft systems; whether electromagnetic emissions from the aircraft interfere with device function; and effect of vibration on the device. Another important consideration is how the equipment interfaces with that used by military ground facilities prior to AE transport. The goal is to eliminate the necessity of changing out patient-applied support devices such as IV drip sets, pressure transducers, disposable oximeter probes, monitoring equipment, and pain infusion pumps. Device swap-outs slow down urgent care, waste supplies, and introduce opportunities for error. Patient-applied support devices are designed to be left with the transported patient until no longer needed and then returned to the system. A robust logistics system tracks the devices while in use and then ensures their return into the en route care system.

5. Conclusion

Arguably the most significant advances in AE pain management in decades have been expansions in regional anesthesia strategies, both neuraxial and peripheral, in the military air transport arena. Patients are now routinely transported with epidural catheters, CPNB catheters, and PCA pumps. Indeed, the synergism of systemic opioid via PCA, combined with the targeted (but non-respiratory-depressant) effects of CPNB therapy, seems to offer the most powerful degree of pain relief available to multitrauma patients.

The evolution in AE pain management represents a revolutionary change in thinking about battlefield management of pain. Aggressive treatment of pain is now part of every wounded soldier's care plan. Certification of an airworthy portable infusion pump paved the way for implementation of PCA, epidural, and CPNB regional anesthesia during AE on military aircraft.

Ensuring that all acute pain management options are exercised as early as possible in the AE chain is critical. Building on the lessons of combat trauma, both military and civilian anesthesiologists can increase use of new pain management techniques for the acutely injured. The experience in pain management during combat AE has brought innovative and effective pain management solutions into common military use.

58

Novel Medical Acupuncture Treatments for Active Combat Units on the Battlefield

1. Introduction

Acupuncture has been employed in China since the second century BC to treat acute and chronic medical problems. The technique was introduced to Europe in the 16th century. In these regions, the benefits of acupuncture in treating musculoskeletal injuries are well documented, and acupuncture is widely practiced alongside mainstream Western medicine. Moreover, because of the convenience and cost-effectiveness in treating various training injuries among the military population, countries such as China, Japan, Korea, and France have incorporated acupuncture into their military medical armamentarium.

Although its introduction to American medicine has been very recent, acupuncture has steadily gained popularity. The alternative medical paradigm underlying acupuncture energetics (the use of acupuncture to move *qi*—pronounced "chi"—or life force within the human system) provides for a novel approach to treating difficult problems faced by physicians in such specialties as pain management, sports medicine, rheumatology, and internal medicine. Research has provided various possible explanations for acupuncture's effectiveness, including the release of enkephalins and endorphins during needle stimulation with activation or suppression of various areas of the brain found on functional magnetic resonance imaging (MRI).

Acupuncture offers unique advantages as an adjunct to traditional medicine in treating conditions such as post-traumatic stress disorder, phantom limb pain, and neuropathy. It is portable, cost-effective, and adaptable to harsh environments, and it requires minimal training. These qualities are particularly useful to battalion surgeons (physicians embedded with active infantry units). Typically, battalion surgeons work in a tactically isolated battle zone with limited medical resources and capability. In addition, as a sole provider for the battalion, the battalion surgeon has the daunting task of triaging all forms of trauma, as well as managing the day-to-day physical and mental health of the troops with the goal of maintaining critical mission readiness. An additional advantage acupuncture offers over traditional pain medications is the lack of side effects such as dizziness, somnolence, cardiac depression, gastrointestinal disturbance, and allergies that can potentially interfere with a soldier's ability to execute mission-critical tasks.

Many people who are unfamiliar with acupuncture have raised legitimate concerns over issues such as potential infection from needles, pain with needle insertion, and lack of evidence supporting acupuncture in the Western medical literature. Although acupuncture has been used in many Asian countries as a standard of medicine for more than 2000 years, it is only in the last several decades that the United States has been introduced to its conventions. Studies suggest that acupuncture needles, which are both sterile and disposable, involve minimal risk of infection. Also, because the needles are blunt tip and small bore (smaller than a 27-gauge needle), they typically cause minimal pain with insertion.

Acupuncture should not be thought of as a replacement for traditional medical treatment, but rather as an adjunct to enhance traditional medicine as part of a multimodal pain plan. It can potentially provide military pain management physicians with another medical tool to further improve the care of the troops on the battlefield. The remainder of this chapter does not provide a treatise on acupuncture energetics, but rather describes examples of several "tried and true" acupuncture treatments that have been effective during early 21st-century conflicts.

2. Acupuncture Needles

Acupuncture needles consist of a blunt-tip stainless steel shaft and coiled handle. Each needle is sterilely packaged inside a hollow guide tube and held in place with a small plastic chad (Figure 58.1).

The handles of acupuncture needles are often heated with a heat lamp or moxibustion to further amplify the treatment. Moxibustion is a technique that employs smoldering mugwort herb (moxa), rolled inside a long paper stick, to heat needles after they have been inserted. It requires well-ventilated space, and the herb has a pungent odor, so it is typically more suitable in field settings. Acupuncture treatment can also be done through ear access points with auricular pins (Figure 58.2).

3. Needle Insertion Technique

Although acupuncture needles do not cut the skin, practitioners may still prefer to wipe the skin with alcohol or iodine before insertion. Also, medical prudence must be exercised so that needles are not inserted into an area of dermatopathology (e.g., cellulitis, tinea pedis, eczema).

Various methods are used to insert acupuncture needles. One technique begins with holding the guide tube between the thumb and the index finger of the nondominant hand and placing it at the insertion site (Figure 58.3a). The chad is removed with the dominant hand, and with one gentle but firm tap on the end, the needle is inserted into the skin (Figure 58.3b). Once the epidermis is traversed, the practitioner uses brisk rotation of the coil of the needle while gently pushing the needle deep into the dermis, often into the muscular layer. The insertion of the needle is complete when the patient feels a deep aching sensation with rotation of the needle. At the same time, the provider will feel more resistance with each rotation of the needle, known as "needle grabbing," or *de qi* sensation, signifying, according to traditional Chinese theory, the engagement of the patient's acupuncture energetics.

The second method begins with removing the needle from the guide tube, holding it between the dominant thumb and the index finger like a pencil (Figure 58.4a), and aligning it along the length of the extended third finger (Figure 58.4b). While keeping the tip of the needle close to the tip of the third finger and using the finger as a guide, the needle is inserted in one motion. It is often useful to use the nondominant hand to stretch out the skin at the insertion site, so that insertion can be achieved perpendicularly to the skin. This technique can be more difficult than the first and often requires more practice to master; however, patients often find it more comfortable.

4. Battlefield Acupuncture

Auricular acupuncture was revolutionized in the United States by the battlefield acupuncture technique of Richard Niemtzow, a colonel in the US Air Force. In this technique, points on the ears are accessed with Aiguille Semi-Permanent (ASP) needles to activate corresponding areas in the brain that have been shown by functional MRI to modulate both acute and chronic pain, mainly the thalamus and cingulate gyrus, respectively (Figure 58.5). Preloaded in an injector, the ASP pins can be placed at the site of insertion by a gentle push of the guide tube. Because the pins can be left in the skin for 2 to 3 days, an alcohol pad should be used to clean the area before insertion.

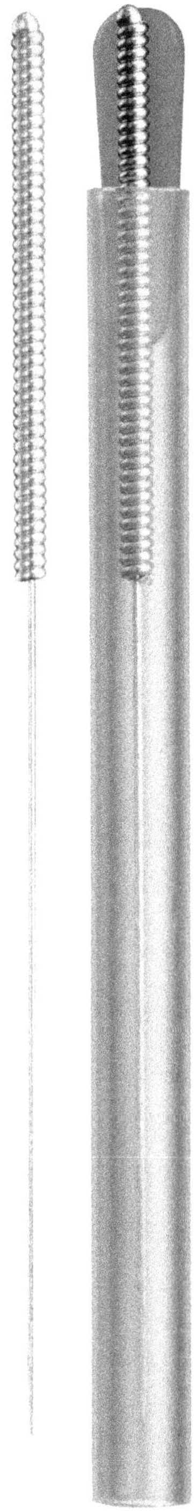

Figure 58.1 SEIRIN L-type acupuncture needle with insertion tube (SEIRIN-America, Weymouth, Mass). Each L-type needle has a 20-mm stainless steel handle with either a 30-mm, 40-mm, or 60-mm needle length (also made of stainless steel), and the gauge is available in 0.20 mm, 0.25 mm, or 0.30 mm, so the practitioner may choose the best size for each patient and each acupuncture point. Photograph: Courtesy of SEIRIN-America, Weymouth, Mass.

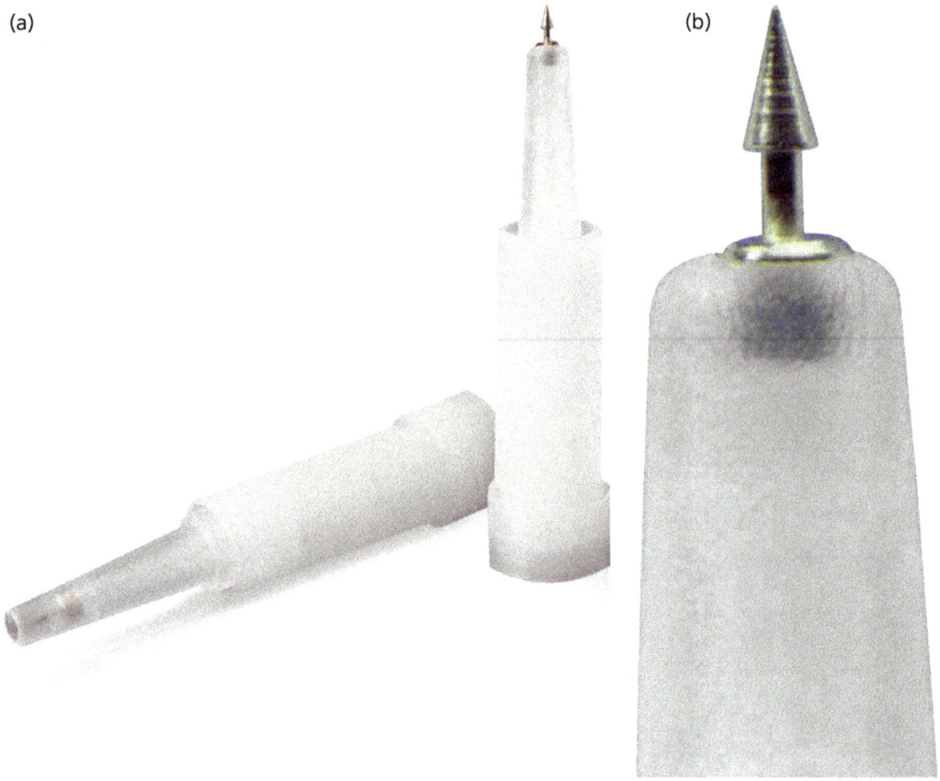

Figure 58.2 ASP brand auricular pins (Lhasa OMS Inc, Weymouth, Mass); inset: detail of tip. Photograph: Courtesy of SEIRIN-America, Weymouth, Mass.

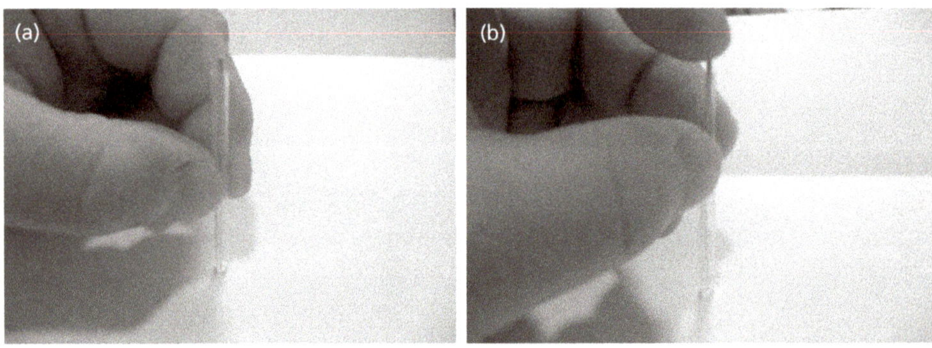

Figure 58.3 Acupuncture needle placement with guide tube.

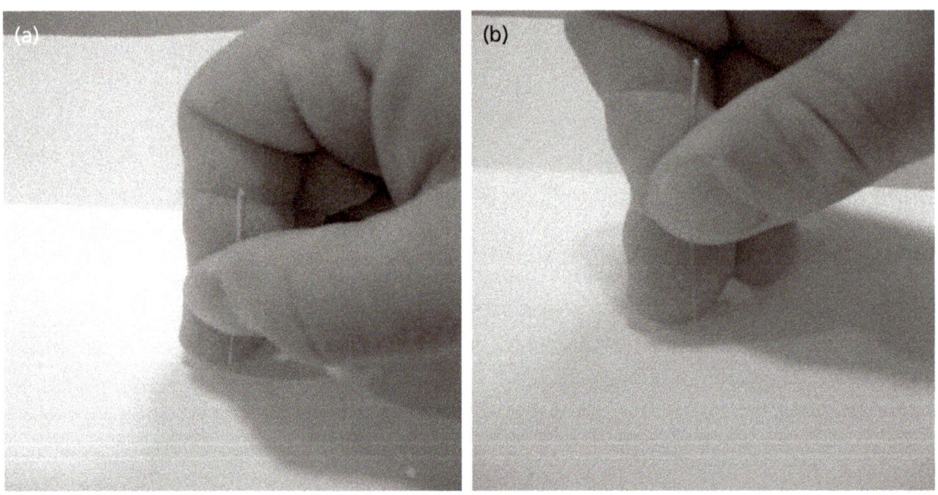

Figure 58.4 Acupuncture needle placement by hand.

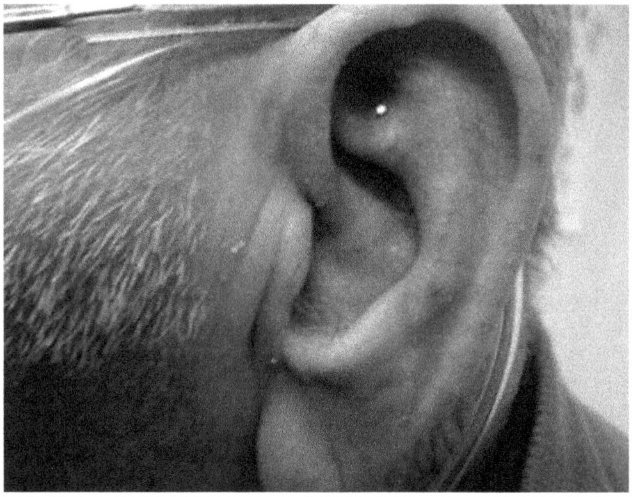

Figure 58.5 Battlefield acupuncture. Photograph: Courtesy of Colonel Richard Niemtzow.

5. Treatments

5.1. Severe heat exhaustion, heat stroke, shock, unconsciousness, acute muscular and lower back spasm

Acupuncture point: Governor vessel 26 (GV26), located on the face at the midline, at the junction of the upper third and lower two thirds of the distance from the nose to the lip (Figure 58.6).

GV26, a potent reviving point for patients with extreme heat exhaustion and shock, can be used in a mass casualty setting. Place the acupuncture needle into the GV26 point directed toward the center of the head and vigorously rotate it clockwise while achieving *de qi* sensation, which is usually felt at an approximate depth of 2 cm. Continue rotating the needle clockwise until the patient is revived, after which the needle should be removed. This procedure should only be instituted following standard trauma protocols initiated by the medical unit.

In addition to use in shock, the GV26 point can be used to revive patients following a vasovagal episode. GV26 is also an excellent point for relieving pain from acute muscle spasm. Physicians embedded in a mobile unit often have limited or difficult-to-access medical supplies. When a patient develops acute lower back or other muscular spasm and is unable to ambulate, placing a needle in GV26 and having the patient rotate it while slowly standing up and walking restores function within minutes, without parenteral or sedating medications.

5.2. Tension headaches, neck pain, shoulder pain

Acupuncture points (Figure 58.7):

- Small intestine 11 (SI11), located at the middle of the infraspinous fossa in the infraspinatus muscle.
- Small intestine 12 (SI12), located in the middle of the supraspinous fossa.
- Gallbladder 21 (GB21), located in the middle belly of the trapezius.
- Tripe heater 15 (TH15), located at the levator scapula insertion at the superior angle of the scapula.

These are outstanding points for relieving severe shoulder and neck strain and tension headaches. SI11 is inserted perpendicularly into the depression in the infraspinous fossa. SI12 is inserted at the middle of the supraspinous fossa, into the supraspinatus trigger point. GB21 is inserted into the middle belly of the trapezius. To reduce risk for pneumothorax, grasp the anterior and posterior belly of the trapezius muscle and lift it off the rib cage, so that the needle can be inserted parallel to the plane of the rib cage. TH15 is inserted into the levator scapula insertion at the superior scapular angle. The

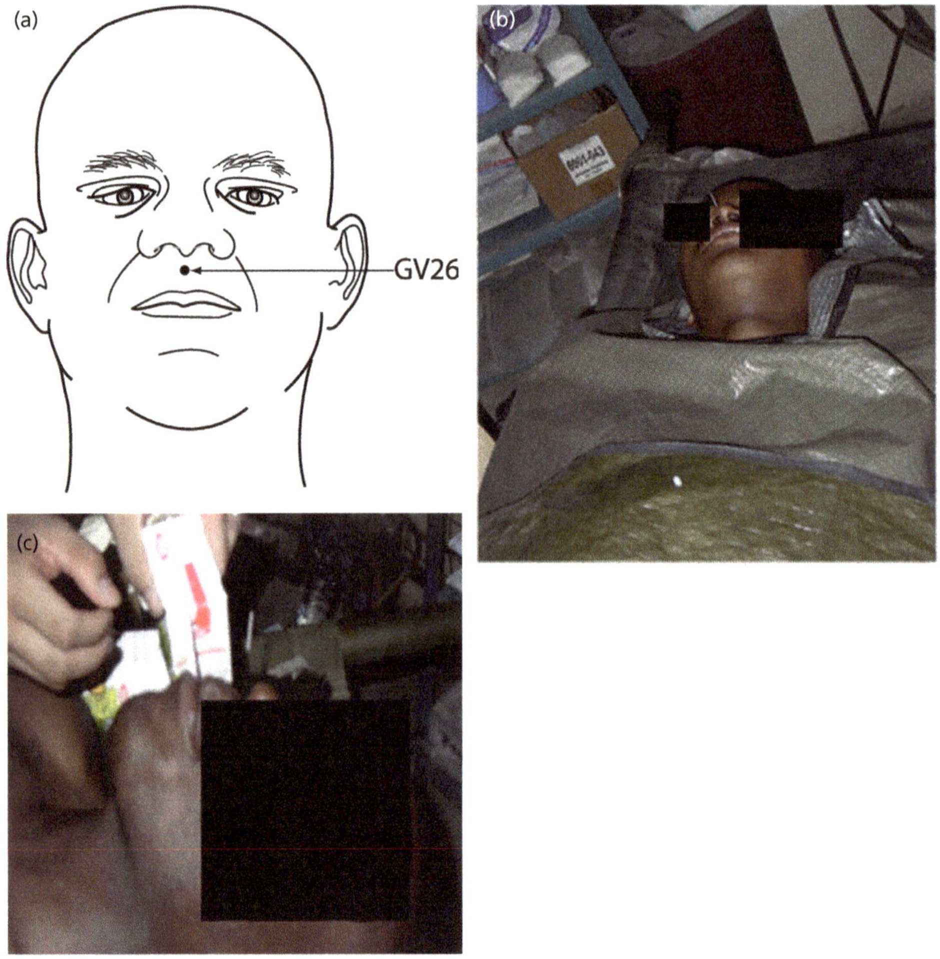

Figure 58.6 (b) Casualty being treated with governor vessel (GV26) point, needle placed. (c) Casualty being treated with governor vessel (GV26) point, needle placed.

depth of levator scapula can vary depending on the musculature of individuals, but the *de qi* sensation is typically felt before the needle is deeply inserted.

Often an area of erythema appears around the site after insertion of acupuncture needles into an activated trigger point. This is neither a side effect nor a histamine release; rather, the erythema correlates to the severity of the trigger tension. Once the trigger activation has been eased, normal skin color will return.

5.3. Hyperadrenergic states, combat stress, insomnia, anxiety, agitation

Acupuncture points:

- Liver 3 (LR3), located in the dorsum of the foot, on the first interosseous space of the metatarsus, in a depression distal to the intermetatarsal joint between the first and second metatarsal bones (Figures 58.8a and 58.8b).
- Heart 3 (HT3), located in the anterior antecubital region, at the ulnar end of the cubital crease (Figures 58.8c and 58.8d).
- Governor vessel 20 (GV20), located at the midsagittal point, a depression on the head at the intersection of lines drawn from the inferior earlobes through the superior apices of the bilateral earlobes (Figure 58.8e).

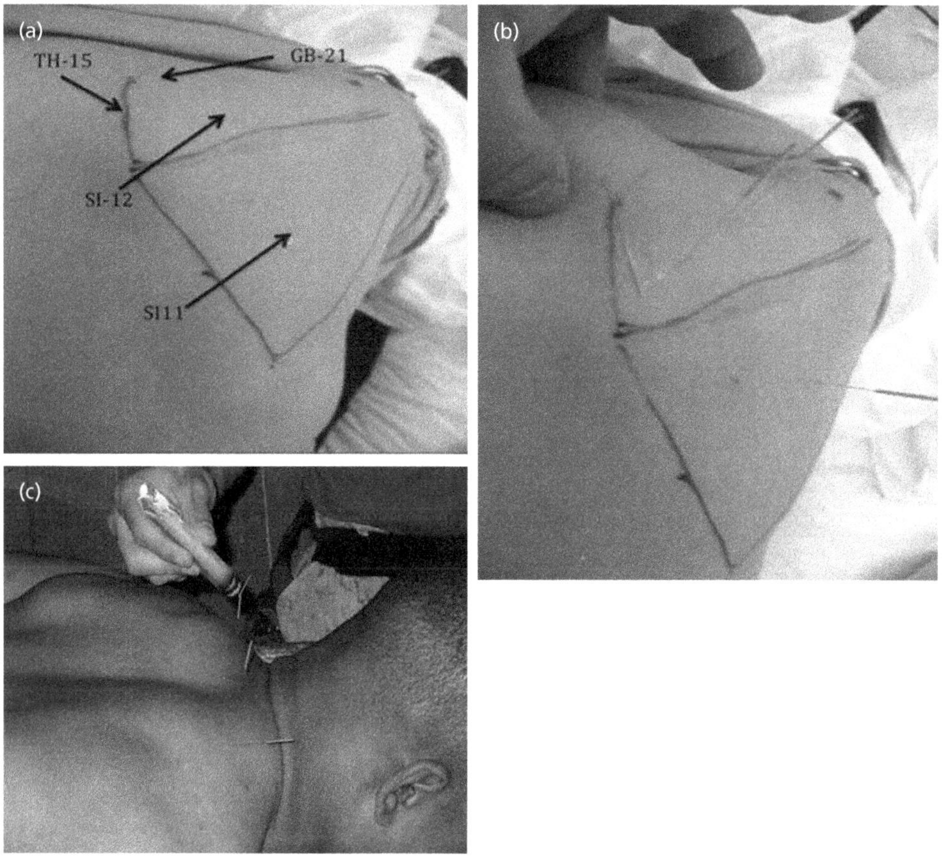

Figure 58.7 (a) Shoulder points gallbladder 21 (GB21), triple heater 15 (TH15), small intestine 12 (SI12), and small intestine 11 (SI 11) demonstrated. (b)Needles placed in points noted in figure 58.7a. Note the provider grasping the belly of the trapezius muscle to reduce the risk of pneumothorax. (c) Described acupuncture points being used in a casualty.

With the constant threat of enemy attacks and frequent combat missions, many troops develop early signs of combat stress such as insomnia, agitation, and panic attacks. Combinations of bilateral LR3, HT3, and GV20 provide a calming effect on panic symptoms, often allowing the patient to fall asleep. In fact, more patients preferred acupuncture to the traditional beta blockers, selective serotonin reuptake inhibitors, and zolpidem. LR3 can be found by sliding the thumb between the first and second interosseous space until it falls into a depression. HT3 is best accessed when the elbow is flexed. GV20 can be identified by placing the middle finger on the inferior end of the earlobe and the tips of the thumbs together over the midsagittal line while the hands traverse through the superior apices of each ear. Needles used at these points should not be heated, which could overstimulate an already hyperadrenergic state. If necessary, keep the patient warm with a warming blanket. Leave the needles in place for 15 to 20 minutes and then remove them. A successful protocol in the deployed setting involved repeating the treatment twice a week until the patients' symptoms abated.

5.4. Soft tissue injuries and ankle sprains

At many functional points and trigger points, typically found in muscles and depressions in the skin, the strain and stress of underlying tissues can be reduced with the insertion of acupuncture needles into the surrounding tissue (Figure 58.9). Enough acupuncture energetic points traverse the body that a needle placed subcutaneously or into the trigger points

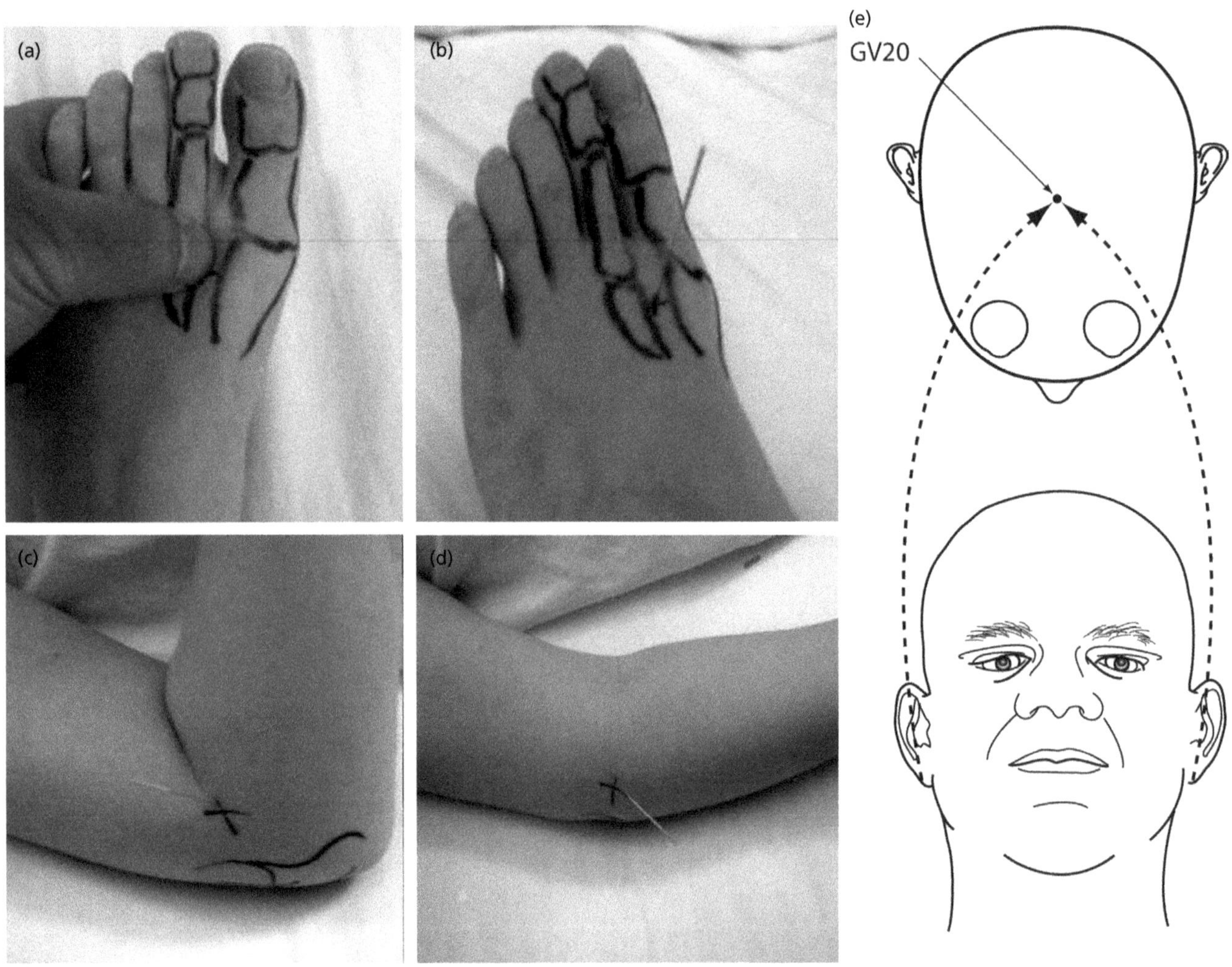

Figure 58.8 (a)Liver 3 (LR3) point location with the metatarsal bones outlined in the foot. (b) Liver 3 (LR3) point placed. (c)Heart 3 (HT3) point with needle placed at the ulnar end of the cubital crease.(d) Heart 3 (HT3) needle placed with the arm extended. Location of the governor vessel 20 (GV20) point.

of a muscle will reduce pain and swelling. The needles can be heated with moxibustion to improve efficacy and left in place for 15 to 20 minutes.

Traditional treatment of ankle sprains is not feasible in an active combat zone, due to the need for immobilization, lack of ice, and prolonged recovery period. An acupuncture protocol employing 3 or 4 needles inserted immediately into the soft tissue surrounding the area of edema and pain can reduce swelling within 24 hours and restore the patient's functional status. Most muscles strains were reduced with 1 to 2 needles placed into the most tender part of the muscles for 15 to 20 minutes, often with moxibustion.

5.5. Physical fatigue and emotional exhaustion

Acupuncture point: "Ming men" governor vessel 4 (GV4), located at the interspinal space of the L2 and L3 spinal processes (2 lateral depressions can be found by sliding thumbs bilaterally from the GV4 point Figure 58.10). Because this point is in the large paraspinal muscles, needles can be inserted deeper than usual. Insert the needles until the *de qi*

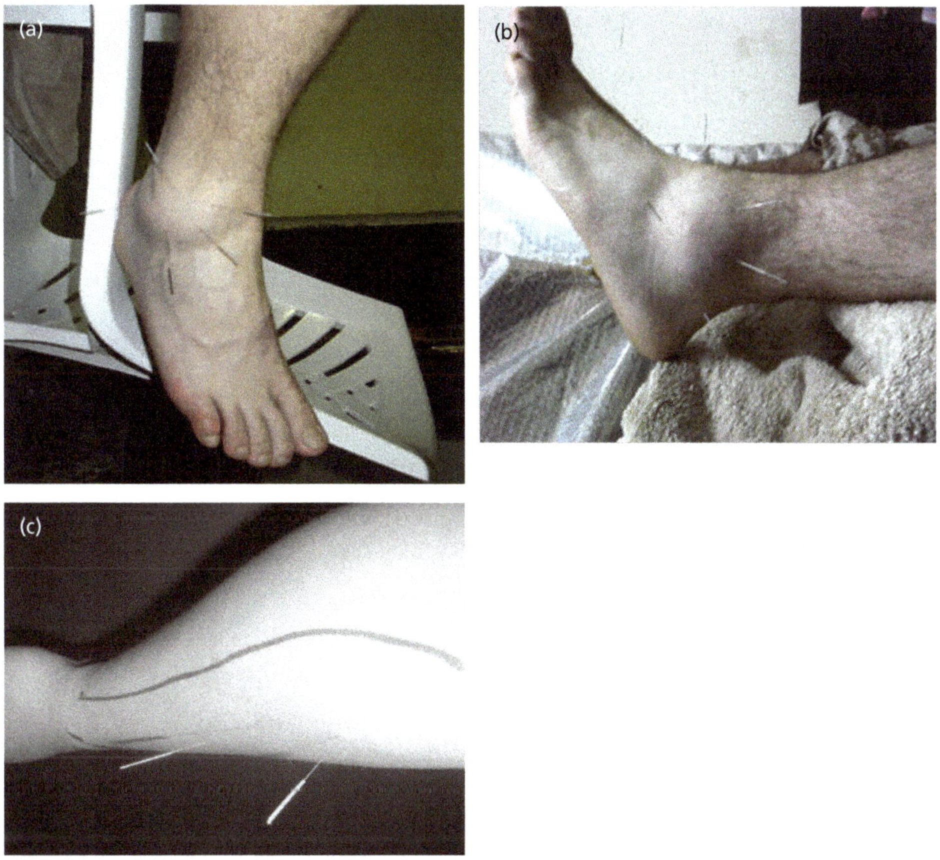

Figure 58.9 (a)Ankle sprain being treated with acupuncture needles. (b) Ankle sprain being treated with acupuncture needles. (c) Lower extremity muscle strain being treated with acupuncture needles.

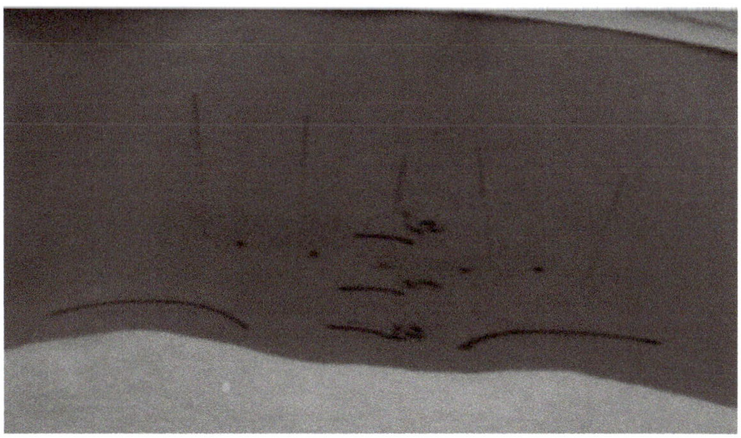

Figure 58.10 Needles placed in lower back between L2 and L3 spinous processes—governor vessel 4 (GV4) with additional needles laterally for back pain relief.

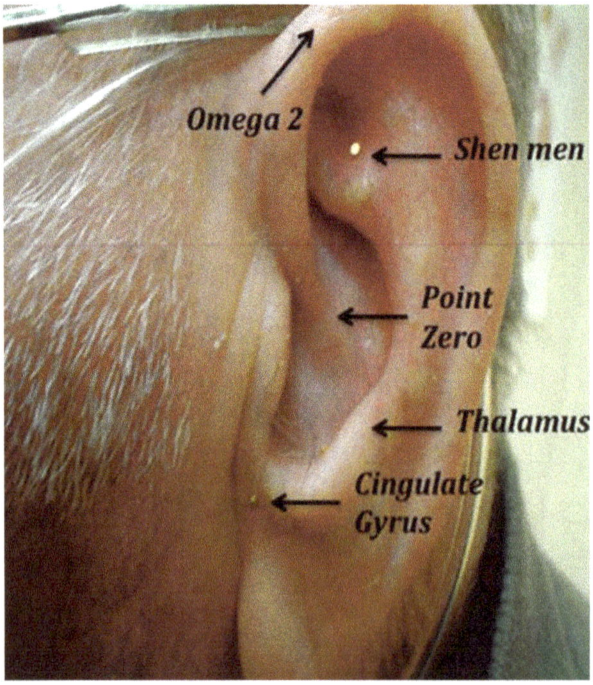

Figure 58.11 Auricular acupuncture points for the "battlefield acupuncture" protocol.

sensation is felt, heat them with moxa for 10 to 20 minutes, and remove them. With a steady swinging motion of the moxa from needle to needle, patients should feel energized, with their lower backaches relieved.

5.6. Chronic pain and recurring acute pain

Niemtzow's battlefield acupuncture can help individuals who require frequent referrals to specialists, are often placed on light-duty status, or have chronic pain syndromes but are otherwise capable of performing their duties. After cleaning the ear with an alcohol pad, the practitioner should place ASP pins starting with the cingulate gyrus, thalamus, and omega-2 points on one ear (Figure 58.11) and then the next ear. The "Shen men" point and point zero point typically provide a calming and balancing effect on the patient. While the pins are in place, the surrounding skin must be observed for any possible sign of infection. Patients should be reassured that the pins will come out by themselves.

Acute Pain Nursing

59

1. Introduction

Acute pain nursing is emerging as a specialty focus within the practice of pain management. As a subspecialty, acute pain (pain lasting up to 3 months) nursing encompasses care of patients following surgery, experiencing trauma, and with condition-or disease-specific pain. Pain management is a critical aspect of patient care, and to relieve pain and suffering is a primary responsibility shared among all healthcare professionals. Patient satisfaction with pain management is an important performance measure for healthcare organizations in the United States. The Joint Commission (TJC) promulgates regulatory standards for pain assessment and treatment across all transitions of care to ensure that all patients have the right to acceptable pain control. The American Society for Pain Management Nursing and the International Association for the Study of Pain (IASP) define core curriculum and competencies in pain management nursing, and interprofessional pain education competencies exist to prepare healthcare professionals in all areas of pain care. Nursing pain competencies span pain physiology and pathophysiology; pain measurement, pharmacology, nondrug, and integrated pain therapies, and patient education. Board certification is available for nurses through the American Nurse Credentialing Center of the American Nurses Association, Pain Management Nursing Certification. Nurses practicing as inpatient clinical nurses, on pain service teams, and in ambulatory pain centers and advance practice registered nurses (APRNs) are eligible for this certification.

Both military and civilian healthcare systems support specialized pain practice in acute pain medicine, regional anesthesia, and acute pain nursing. Some experts, however, have concerns that standards of care for acute pain (e.g., postoperative pain) are not as fully developed as those imposed for chronic pain (pain lasting >3 months). Nonetheless, healthcare organizations continue to expand acute pain services (APS) into clinical operations. This allows opportunities for acute pain nurses to practice as members of an APS collaborating with other pain management specialists to deliver quality pain care.

2. Mission

Acute pain nursing encompasses the mission set by the American Society for Pain Management Nursing to "advance and promote optimal nursing care for people affected by pain by promoting best nursing practices" (http://www.aspmn.org). Acute pain management nurses act as advocates for patients; apply evidence-based guidelines and best practices; ensure-high quality and safe care; and educate colleagues, patients, and families about effective pain modalities. Acute pain nurses are experts in the routine assessment of pain and delivery of acute pain interventions such as medication therapies, technology-supported pain care, and nondrug measures to relieve pain. They possess technical competencies in troubleshooting drug delivery devices, educate patient and families on pain and its consequences, and provide consultation to the patient's healthcare team. Acute pain nurses strive to effectively reduce the severity of acute pain and prevent its worsening over time that can ultimately lead to the development of chronic pain. Acute tissue injury causes inflammation and nerve damage, potentially evoking a cascade of electrophysiologic, structural, and neuropsychological responses. Increased neuronal firing of peripheral pain fibers can activate N-methyl-D-aspartate (NMDA) receptors in the dorsal horn of the spinal cord, increasing the likelihood of central sensitization, a complex pathological process contributing to chronic pain. Central sensitization, defined by the IASP, is an increased responsiveness of nociceptive neurons in the central nervous system. Unrelieved acute pain can transition to chronic pain through central sensitization; therefore, effectively controlling acute pain can prevent or reduce risks for acute pain contributing to chronic pain states.

3. Acute Pain Nurses: Roles and Responsibilities

Position descriptions for acute pain nurses practicing as members of an APS, as well as the composition and coverage responsibilities of their APS teams, can vary widely across institutions. The APS nurse model typically has a nurse or nurses directly supervised by a physician or APRN. APRNs who are members of APS, depending on institutional guidelines, often function independently and interdependently with collaborating physician colleagues. It is recommended that acute pain nurses be prepared with a minimum of a bachelor's degree in nursing (BSN). The demands of APS nurses require that they possess clinical experience, critical thinking and problem-solving skills, and effective interprofessional collaboration and communication skills. Acute pain nurses must be knowledgeable in the mechanisms of pain, pain assessment, pain therapies (e.g., pharmacologic, intervention-based treatments, and nondrug measures), and patient education, as well as promoting engagement of patients and families in pain management plans of care. Above all, acute pain nurses need to understand the underlying principles and nursing care required for multimodal analgesia. Multimodal analgesia combines classes of analgesics and pain interventions to target different pain mechanisms and pathways in the periphery and central nervous system (spinal cord and brain). Classes of analgesics include opioids, nonopioids (e.g., acetaminophen and NSAIDs), gabapentinoids (gabapentin and pregabalin), serotonin norepinephrine reuptake inhibitors, tricyclic antidepressants, NMDA receptor antagonists (e.g., ketamine), and alpha-2 agonists (e.g., clonidine). Multimodal analgesia also involves neuraxial (epidural and intrathecal) therapy, peripheral nerve blocks (PNBs), and intra-articular and wound infiltration with local analgesics. Integrative therapies such as physical (e.g., cold, massage, yoga, acupuncture) and behavioral and cognitive (e.g., cognitive-behavioral therapy, distraction, relaxation, visual imagery) modalities are also a part of multimodal interventions.

All nurses assume an integral role in the assessment of patients in pain, and they are uniquely positioned in hospital, ambulatory care, long-term care, and home settings to understand a patient's pain and its impact on biopsychosocial aspects of health and well-being. In acute care settings, nurses interact with patients 24 hours a day, 7 days a week, and they have ongoing responsibilities to assess pain; implement pain interventions; and monitor, evaluate, and document responses to these interventions. However, other patient care demands can often compete with nurses' time and ability to conduct comprehensive pain assessments and address the complex nature of pain. When nurse-to-patient ratios are strained and patient acuity is high, it can be extremely challenging to prioritize the delivery of optimal pain care. Nurses on general care units confront complex pain by managing or balancing the use of intravenous (IV) patient-controlled analgesia (PCA) and epidural analgesia with and without patient-controlled analgesia (PCEA), and the use of monitoring technology. PCA involves patient-activated analgesia through administration of an on-demand dose when needed. PCA devices can be programmed to deliver a basal rate (continuous infusion) and a demand dose within a programmable lockout interval. Safe patient monitoring with opioids, for example, use of pulse oximetry and end tidal carbon dioxide (CO_2), is essential to detect serious adverse events (e.g., unintended advancing sedation and respiratory depression from opioids). Monitoring practices are also important to ensure patient safety with multimodal analgesia regimens that include regional anesthesia or interventional techniques. Acute pain nurses on an APS provide support to nurses in all aspects of pain management to deliver optimal and safe pain care.

3.1. Pain assessment

TJC regulatory pain standards, guidelines and position statements from professional societies, and healthcare organization policies emphasize the need to regularly assess and reassess pain. Pain assessment not only should include a measure of pain intensity or severity but also should focus on pain locations(s), quality and character of pain, temporal factors affecting pain, and the biopsychosocial impact of pain. Because pain and its effects on an individual are highly subjective, it is critical to measure aspects of the pain experience with reliable and valid patient-reported scales and instruments. In practice, however, clinicians often make assumptions about a patient's pain without evaluating pain from the patient experiencing it. Common myths associated with pain assessment and barriers to pain management are outlined in Table 59.1, which highlights the importance of patient-reported pain outcomes. Moreover, healthcare professionals should recognize that for military populations and some cultures, stoicism is encouraged and may lead to underestimating the severity of pain and its impact.

In 2009, the Department of Defense (DoD) commissioned a Pain Management Task Force (PMTF) to examine pain assessment practices across multiple military, Veterans Health Administration (VHA), and civilian healthcare facilities. Interviews conducted with many clinicians revealed significant challenges associated with the lack of standard pain measures and variations in the use of scales and measures and their interpretations. The work of the PMTF culminated in 109 recommendations for improving pain care, several of which were focused on pain assessment practices. Some of the PMTF key recommendations were (1) focus on the warrior and family (sustain the force); (2) synchronize a culture of pain awareness, education, and proactive intervention (medical staff, patients, and leaders); (3) provide tools and infrastructure that support and encourage research advancements in pain management; and (4) build a full spectrum of best practices for the continuum of acute and chronic pain care. Subsequently, the PMTF designed a new pain scale, the Defense and Veterans Pain Rating Scale (DVPRS) (Figure 59.1). This scale integrated multiple features (word anchors, color coding, and facial expressions) imposed on a numeric rating scale of 0 to 10 to enhance and standardize pain measurement. The pain intensity scale is augmented with 4 supplemental questions to capture the biopsychosocial impact of how pain interferes with activity and sleep, affects mood, and contributes to stress. Psychometric testing performed on the DVPRS with military and veteran populations established reliability and validity for the scale. The DVPRS can be used to assess both acute and chronic pain, and it offers a uniform approach to collecting pain data across populations and healthcare settings. Acute pain management nurses in the military and VHA healthcare facilities are encouraged to use the DVPRS as a pain screening and assessment tool.

To achieve standardization in pain and pain-related patient-reported outcomes, one of the PMTF recommendations was to also create the Pain Assessment Screening Tool and Outcomes Registry (PASTOR) in collaboration with

Table 59.1:
Common myths and barriers to pain management

Myth	Truth
Nurses and physicians are the best judges of how much pain a patient is experiencing.	The patient's self-report of pain is the most valid indicator.
The same type of pain affects different people in the same way.	The same type of pain may affect people differently.
Patients who report pain get pain relief.	Stoicism is highly valued in many societies and the military.
All nurses and physicians know how to treat pain.	Although education of nurses and physicians is improving, pain is still undertreated.

(a)

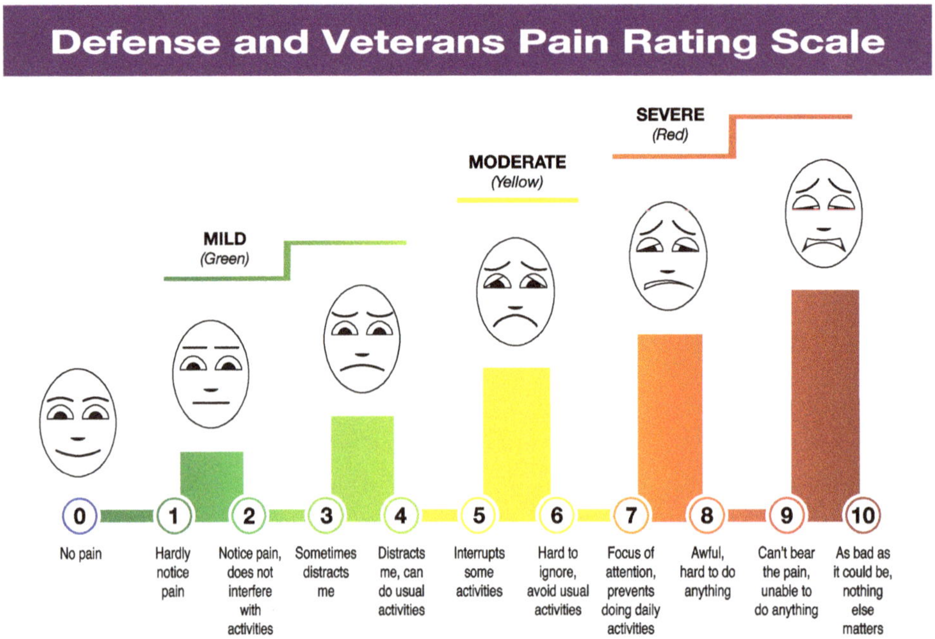

(b)

DoD/VA Pain Supplemental Questions

For clinicians to evaluate the biopsychosocial impact of pain

1. Circle the one number that describes how, during the past 24 hours, pain has interfered with your usual ACTIVITY:

0 — 1 — 2 — 3 — 4 — 5 — 6 — 7 — 8 — 9 — 10

Does not interfere — Completely interferes

2. Circle the one number that describes how, during the past 24 hours, pain has interfered with your SLEEP:

0 — 1 — 2 — 3 — 4 — 5 — 6 — 7 — 8 — 9 — 10

Does not interfere — Completely interferes

3. Circle the one number that describes how, during the past 24 hours, pain has affected your MOOD:

0 — 1 — 2 — 3 — 4 — 5 — 6 — 7 — 8 — 9 — 10

Does not affect — Completely affects

4. Circle the one number that describes how, during the past 24 hours, pain has contributed to your STRESS:

0 — 1 — 2 — 3 — 4 — 5 — 6 — 7 — 8 — 9 — 10

Does not contribute — Contributes a great deal

**Reference for pain interference: Cleeland CS, Ryan KM. Pain assessment: global use of the Brief Pain Inventory. Ann Acad Med Singapore 23(2): 129-138, 1994.*

Figure 59.1 Defense and Veterans Pain Rating Scale

the DoD and the VHA. PASTOR utilizes National Institutes of Health Patient-Reported Outcomes Measurement Information System (PROMIS®) measures and includes a comprehensive set of patient-reported pain outcomes representing domains such as pain interference, physical functioning, anxiety, depression, and fatigue. PASTOR is currently used both in research and in clinical care at military integrative pain management centers and other ambulatory practices.

3.2. Team-based care

Acute pain nurses are part of the interdisciplinary patient care team, and as such should participate in daily rounds with the APS and the primary patient care team. Pain plans of care should be developed in collaboration with both members of the APS and the patient's team of nurses, physicians, and a pharmacist, physical therapist, and social worker. This interprofessional collaboration allows each healthcare professional to contribute discipline-specific perspectives to the pain management plan and assures continuity of care and seamless transitions across levels of care throughout a patient's hospitalization and after discharge. In some hospitals, acute pain nurses may continue to follow patients after discharge from the APS. The primary goal of having an acute pain nurse remain involved is to maintain patient- and family-centered coordinated care and facilitate continuity of care. Moreover, sustained patient involvement from an acute pain nurse supports the primary patient team's ability to address ongoing pain issues, provide emotional support, meet the educational needs of patients and families, and promote self-care management of pain with integrative therapies.

3.3. Analgesic therapies

Acute pain nurses who are part of the APS must be knowledgeable about multimodal analgesia, technology-supported pain interventions (e.g., IV PCA, PCEA, regional anesthesia/analgesia), and safe patient monitoring. Given the current opioid crisis, it is imperative that all nurses caring for patients with acute pain understand the risks for opioid misuse and substance use disorder (SUD) with inpatient opioid administration and discharge prescriptions. SUD is defined by criteria in the fifth edition of the *Diagnostic and Statistical Manual of Mental Disorders* (*DSM-5*). The surgical team, the APS, and unit nurses must evaluate and discuss risks for opioid misuse and abuse on a case-by-case basis, clearly limiting opioid use for patients at high risk. Risks for opioid misuse and SUD appear in Figure 59.2. Opioid tolerance, occurring

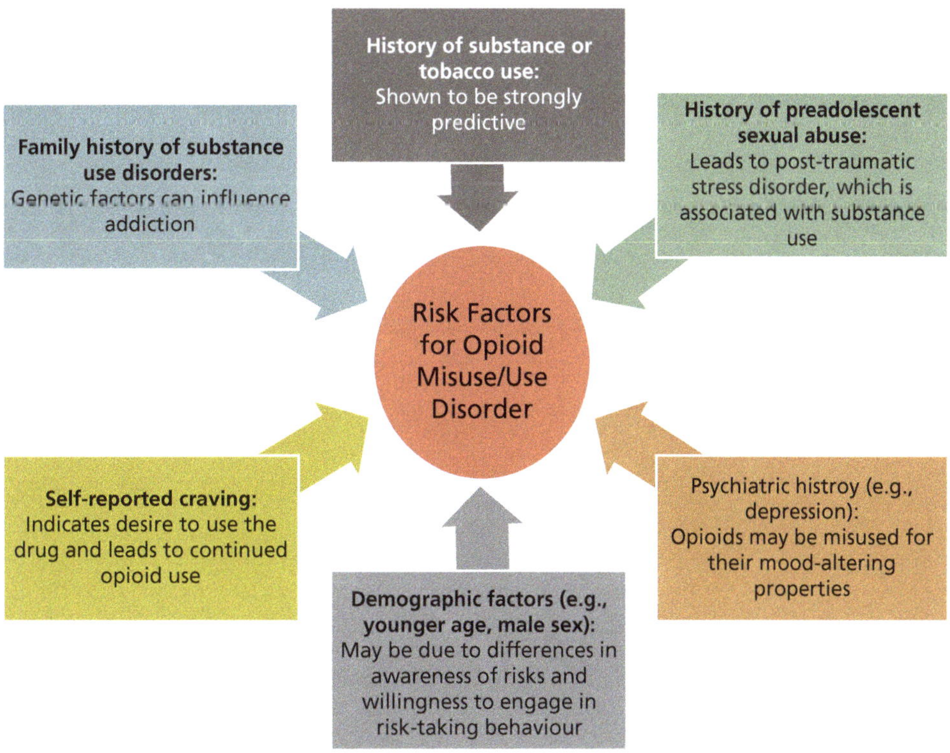

Figure 59.2 Risk factors for opioid misuse and SUD.

Reprinted with permission from Argoff CE, et al. Rational urine drug monitoring in patients receiving opioids for chronic pain: consensus recommendations. *Pain Med*. 2018;19(1):97–117.

when greater amounts are required to obtain an original degree of desired therapeutic effect, may be evident in patients with preexisting chronic pain treated with opioids. Tolerance to opioids is always considered when determining doses of opioids for management of acute pain. Acute pain nurses participate in decision-making to design individualized, appropriate, effective, and safe analgesic regimens.

Maximizing pain control with multimodal analgesia is evidence-based and best practice. Nurses need to understand the pharmacology of these agents, adverse effects, and synergistic effects to deliver safe medication administration. IV PCA and PCEA are also evidence-based practices for postoperative pain, and nurses must implement monitoring plans of care to prevent unintended advancing sedation and respiratory depression. This includes frequent assessments of respiratory rate, level of sedation using a reliable and valid sedation scale, and ventilation (e.g., pulse oximetry and end tidal carbon dioxide).

A major responsibility of acute pain nurses who are part of an APS is to oversee care of patients receiving regional anesthesia/analgesia involving the delivery of a local anesthetic to a defined part of the body. This is accomplished through an intermittent injection of a local anesthetic (peripheral nerve block) or continuous peripheral nerve block (CPNB) via a continuous infusion of a local anesthetic. Regional anesthesia/analgesia is the cornerstone of acute pain medicine/management practice, and similar to epidural analgesia reduces systemic analgesia requirements. Among the many benefits of regional anesthesia/analgesia, local neuromotor blockade mitigates the potential need for intraoperative and postoperative opioids (Figure 59.3). The APS nurse's involvement in the preoperative placement of the catheter offers the opportunity to meet the patient and become familiar with the health history and surgical plan. This is also an opportunity to strategically provide patient education, set realistic expectations for pain control, and alleviate concerns regarding pain management.

When appropriate, the acute pain nurse may suggest changes in pain treatment based on the patient's response. Further, the APS nurse provides a central coordinating role to oversee the efficiency of the overall APS team. In addition to participating in the administration and evaluation of pain management therapies, APS nurses also review all pain medications for possible interactions and contraindications (e.g., anticoagulation regimens in patients targeted for and with epidural and peripheral nerve catheters). Acute pain nurses typically participate in APS rounds, but they may also

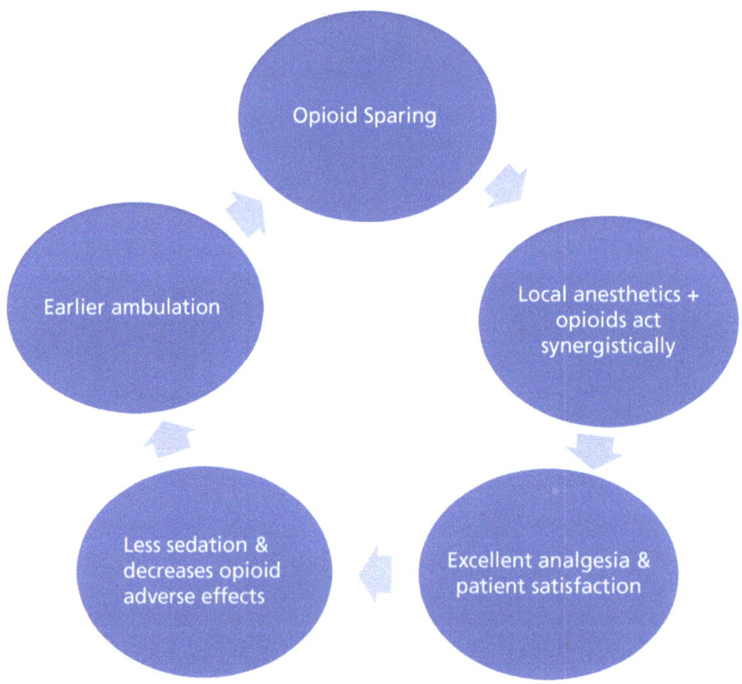

Figure 59.3 Benefits of regional anesthesia/analgesia.

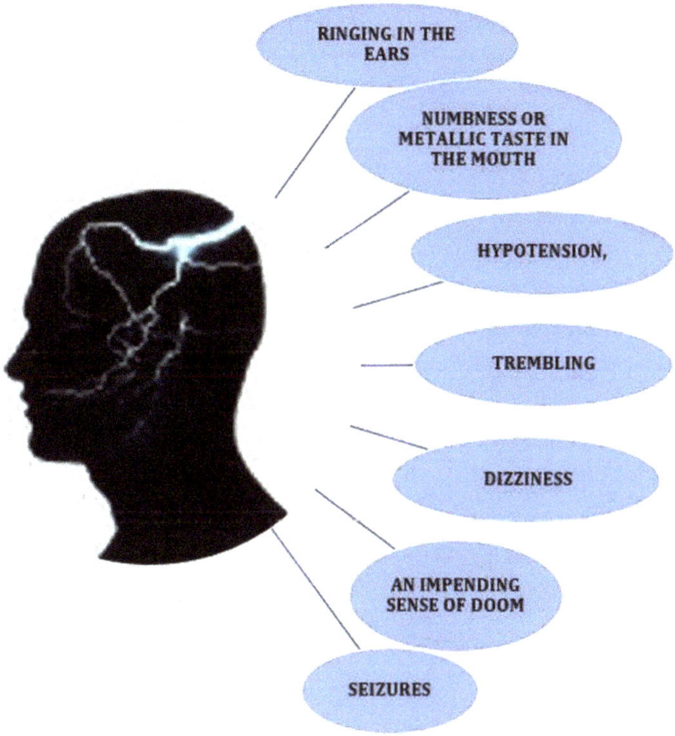

Figure 59.4 Signs of local anesthetic toxicity.

do rounds with the unit nursing staff to assess patients' response to therapy, troubleshoot technical problems with epidural or regional catheters or delivery devices, and identify any adverse events from regional anesthetic procedures. While complications from regional anesthesia are relatively uncommon, catheter dislodgement and malfunction can occur, which is often evident with leaking and/or swelling at the catheter insertion site and an increase in pain. Frequently assessing the treated extremity for color, capillary refill of distal digits, swelling, and allodynia (pain to a stimulus not typically painful such as touch) and hyperalgesia (an exaggerated pain response to a stimulus that is typically painful) minimizes risk for regional anesthesia complications. Acute pain nurses should also educate nurses caring for patients receiving regional anesthesia/analgesia about proper positioning of the treated extremity, measures for protecting the extremity and skin pressure reduction, and assistance with ambulation. Nurses should be familiar with the early signs and symptoms of local anesthetic toxicity before progressing to serious toxicity that can cause seizures (Figure 59.4). They should instruct patients and family members on all precautions to take while receiving regional anesthesia/analgesia.

4. Integration of Acute Pain Nursing and Clinical Environments

An important component of acute pain nursing is development of individualized patient plans of care and the integration of pain therapies that lead to the best possible outcomes. A model for patient-focused care with integrative approaches to pain management does exist for chronic pain. The Stepped Care Model for Pain Management (SCM-PM), developed by VHA investigators and tested in a VHA facility, emphasizes an individualized, stepwise approach to pain management that starts with conservative interventions and progressively escalates until pain becomes manageable by the patients. This model includes multimodal analgesia, physical therapy referral, pain management referral, chiropractic referral, and mental health referrals. Referrals for follow-up specialty pain care should be considered for patients with acute pain, especially those experiencing uncontrolled pain during hospitalization that does not resolve at discharge or progresses to persistent acute pain beyond the expected course of pain. Significant challenges for integrative pain programs include the lack of pain experts to provide integrative therapies and limited payer reimbursement for pain therapies during hospitalization and after discharge. These barriers affect the availability of comprehensive pain services delivered by APS and acute pain nurses.

5. Conclusion

Acute pain nurses play a vital and pivotal role in acute pain management. With fewer nurses entering the profession and a projected shortage of up to 1 million RNs by 2020, it will be important to expand the acute pain nurse workforce to support pain management practice. For the military, the integration of an APS in theater combat support hospitals (CSHs) poses a new challenge for future conflicts. A recent study of APS impact in a CSH at Camp Bastion, Afghanistan, showed that among 71 soldiers sustaining major combat extremity injuries there was a statistically significant reduction in pain intensity and increase in perceptions of pain relief with APS interventions. The DoD and VHA have invested in healthcare provider pain education resources with the launch of the Joint Pain Education Program (JPEP) (http://www.dvcipm.org/clinical-resources/joint-pain-education-project-jpep/). Model APS and integrative pain centers exist throughout the DoD, VHA, and civilian health systems that rely on the expertise and vast contributions of pain management nurses to specialized pain care. In moving forward, it will be essential to demonstrate the value of acute pain nurses in terms of improvements in patient-reported pain outcomes, increases in patient satisfaction scores, and reductions in length of hospitalization. These value-driven outcomes will influence decisions of healthcare leaders to allocate financial investments to support acute pain nurse positions.

5.1. Professional resources

American Pain Society
http://americanpainsociety.org
American Society for Pain Management Nursing Certification Preparation Materials
http://www.aspmn.org/certification/Pages/certificationpreparationmaterials.aspx
American Society for Pain Management Nursing Positions Statements
http://www.aspmn.org/Pages/positionstatements.aspx
Defense and Veterans Center for Integrative Pain Management
http://www.dvcipm.org
International Association for the Study of Pain (IASP) Curriculum Outline on Pain for Nursing
https://www.iasp-pain.org/Education/CurriculumDetail.aspx?ItemNumber=2052

Acute Pain in the Field

60

1. Introduction

Pain management in an austere environment depends on trained personnel who are motivated to aggressively treat acute pain. Lessons learned from military trauma pain care should be incorporated into civilian trauma systems. Efforts to improve perioperative pain management have centered on the development of acute pain service (APS) teams of healthcare professionals, usually directed by an anesthesiologist, who are organized and committed to the management of acute pain. The adoption of the APS model for effective pain management in austere environments by the US military is a logical approach. Without medical personnel organized specifically for the APS mission, pain treatment would revert to the low priority it has traditionally been given by surgeons and anesthesiologists. This is particularly true in the chaotic, high-stress, mass casualty medical environment of the battlefield or disaster scene.

Safe, effective, and efficient perioperative pain management depends on a multimodal approach to analgesia. Multimodal analgesia refers to the concept of using multiple analgesics and pain control technologies/techniques with different mechanisms of action. Not only will these components act synergistically to improve overall pain control, but this approach may also minimize the unwanted and possibly dangerous side effects of large doses of one medication. A significant advantage of multimodal analgesia in austere environments is the lower total dose needed for each drug component. Additionally, the multimodal analgesic approach offers a departure from the traditional opioid-only option in field medicine.

The following discussion and recommendations on commonly available pain medications are predicated on the existence of an APS. These guidelines are not intended to supersede medication package insert information or the physician's training in prescribing pain medication. The guidelines presented in this chapter are intended to serve as a starting point, but the physician must individualize acute pain care to each patient's needs and according to the environmental conditions.

2. Opioids

Morphine remains the gold standard analgesic to which all other medications are compared. The ease of morphine administration following the invention of hollow hypodermic needles and syringes in the 1850s enhanced use and acceptance of the drug as an effective treatment for traumatic pain. The use of morphine for pain was widespread during the American Civil War (1861–1865) and the Franco-Prussian War (1870–1871), but a lack of understanding of opioid use and side effects led to morphine addiction in many soldiers (known as "soldier's disease"). Despite the potential for life-threatening side effects, the success of opioids in treating pain in field medicine is beyond dispute. The challenge is to develop acute pain protocols and technologies that emphasize the beneficial pain relief properties of opioids while minimizing their side effects.

Casualty care advances in patients emerging from the conflicts in Iraq and Afghanistan have changed pain management attitudes and practices in the field environment. Although the lethality of weapons and severity of wounds continue to increase, casualty survival has never been higher. US military casualties from Iraq and Afghanistan currently have a 92% survival rate, compared with 76% during the Vietnam War, 67% during the Civil War, and 58% during the Revolutionary War. The increased survival rate results from many factors, including emphasis on early, advanced, far-forward surgical care; improved surgical and critical care techniques; availability of blood products; advances in body and vehicle armor; improved communication within the treatment/evacuation chain; and rapid ground and air evacuation to major medical facilities within and outside of the war zone. A severely injured soldier in Afghanistan could be moved from the point of injury to Walter Reed National Military Medical Center within 24 hours. The rapid movement of casualties in particular has rendered opioid-based pain management protocols less appealing: the crowded, low-light, deafening, jolting environment of evacuation aircraft makes monitoring difficult and magnifies the difficulties of opioid-only pain control therapy. Healthcare providers in this situation are less likely to use adequate doses of morphine because of valid patient safety concerns. The high numbers of healthcare providers in the evacuation chain and long evacuation distances further complicate opioid use. Many of these issues can be addressed by a multimodal pain therapy protocol, tailored to the austere medicine scenario, in which opioids are only part of the overall pain medication plan (Tables 60.1 and 60.2).

3. N-Methyl-D-Aspartate Receptor Antagonists

Of the N-methyl-d-aspartate (NMDA) antagonists, ketamine is the most commonly used and well-known example for use in austere conditions. It has been used extensively and exclusively for anesthesia in war casualties in a variety of conflicts and conditions. Ketamine's cardiovascular stimulating and bronchodilator activity, multiple routes of administration, coupled with its profound amnestic and analgesic properties make it particularly useful in austere environments. For perioperative pain management, ketamine has been shown to provide an additive analgesic effect when used with other medications preemptively, in epidural catheters, and as an intravenous (IV) infusion following major surgery. Small-dose ketamine has been found to be a safe adjuvant to opioids or primary analgesic when reduced narcotic use is desirable. Ketamine, rather than opioids, is the preferred analgesic in patients with current or impending circulatory or pulmonary instability in the latest US military Tactical Combat Casualty Care (TCCC) guidelines. Despite historical findings, recent evidence shows that ketamine is safe to use in head injury/traumatic brain injury patients who can complain of pain. A common concern among providers is ketamine's association with bad dreams, hallucinations, dizziness, dysphoria, disorientation, and confusion. However, evidence indicates no significant increase in central nervous system symptoms in patients receiving ketamine (via patient-controlled analgesia, IV infusion, continuous IV infusion, or epidural) compared with patients receiving opioids alone. Dissociation does not begin until doses higher than 0.5 mg/kg IV are given. Subanesthetic concentrations of ketamine can provide postoperative antihyperalgesia, analgesia, and an opioid-sparing effect when used in combination with opioid medications by reducing the development of opioid tolerance and recovering opioid antinociception from a tolerant state (Table 60.3).

4. α_2-Agonists

Clonidine and dexmedetomidine are α_2-adrenergic agonists that can produce a significant analgesic effect when used alone or in combination with other analgesics, without the respiratory depression associated with opioids. Both clonidine's and dexmedetomidine's analgesic properties have been demonstrated whether the drug is administered intravenously, intrathecally, epidurally, intraarticularly, or as an adjunct to local anesthetics in a peripheral nerve block. The versatility of these agents in providing anesthesia in a variety of clinical scenarios suggests they would be useful additions to the field

Table 60.1:
Suggested Dosages of Opioids for Acute Pain Control in the 70-Kg Opioid-Naive Military Casualty

Opioid	Intravenons/ Intramuscular*	PCA†	Oral	Epidural‡	Intrathecar‡	Plasma Half-life	Comments§
Morphine	5-15 mg every 3-4 h	1-2 mg every 6-12 min	10-30 mg every 2-3h	1-4 mg	100-300 µg	3 h (1-5 h)	Principal medical alkaloid of opium; causes active metabolites, respiratory depression, and increased intracranial pressure
Hydromorphone	2-3 mg every 3-4 h	0.2-0.8 mg every 8-12 min	2-3 mg every 4-6 h	0.5-1 mg	100-200 µg	2-3 h	Semisynthetic opioid, approximately 5 times more potent than morphine and a useful alternative
Fentanyl	25-100 µg every 5 min titrated to effect at bedside	25-50 µg every 8-12 min, rare applications	Sublingual preparation available	50-100 µg	12.5-25 µg	7 h (3-12 h)	Synthetic; novel delivery technologies are in development
Meperidine	75-150 mg every 2-3 h	10 mg every 6-12 min, rare applications	100-300 mg every 3 h	NA	NA	3-5 h	Toxic metabolite normeperidine can lead to seizures; increased risk of abuse due to rapid onset and associated "rush"
Methadone	5-10 mg every 8-12 h short term use	NA	5-15 mg every 8-12 h short-term use	NA	NA	24-36 h	Synthetic; exhibits NMDA receptor antagonist activity; long half-life provides more stable analgesia compared to more frequently dosed opioids; usually reserved for level 4 use
Codeine	15-60 mg every 4 h IM only	NA	30-60 mg every 4 h	NA	NA	2-4 h	Antitussive; combined with acetaminophen as Tylenol-3[Y]; ineffective in 10% of Caucasians

(continued)

Table 60.1: Continued

Opioid	Intravenons/ Intramuscular*	PCA†	Oral	Epidural‡	Intrathecar‡	Plasma Half-life	Comments§
Oxycodone	NA	NA	10–20 mg every 4–6 h	NA	NA	3–4.5 h	Combined with aspirin as Percodan¶ and acetaminophen as Percocet**; high abuse potential
Tramadol	50–100 mg every 4–6 h	NA	50–150 mg every 4–6 h	NA	NA	5–7 h	Respiratory depression is not a common side effect; can decrease the seizure threshold

*Generally, the intramuscular administration of opioids should be avoided in favor of intravenous administration.
†PCA is a preferred method for opioid pain control when equipment is available and the patient is able to operate the PCA device.
‡Epidural/intrathecal infusions of narcotics should be avoided in patients who may be transported to the next level of care within 24 hours.
§Naloxone is an opioid antagonist that reverses systemic opioid effects (analgesia, sedation, respiratory depression, etc) and should be available when opioids are used. Naloxone doses (0.2-0.04 mg) are titrated to desired effect every 2 to 3 minutes. The effect is dose dependent, lasting 20 to 60 minutes.
ᵞJohnson & Johnson, New Brunswick, NJ.
¶DuPont Pharmaceuticals, Wilmington, Del.
**Endo Pharmaceuticals, Chadds Ford, Pa.
IM: intramuscular
NA: not applicable
NMDA: *N*-methyl d-aspartate
PCA: patient-controlled analgesia

medicine medication list (Table 60.4). Dose-related side effects of clonidine include bradycardia, hypotension, and sedation. Dexmedetomidine, which is 7 times more selective for α_2-adrenergic receptors though of shorter duration than clonidine, has also been used for cooperative sedation in intubated patients, making it useful for long-transports. Sedation mimics a non–rapid eye movement (NREM) sleep secondary to effects in the brain that lead to decreased histamine release. An important consideration when using these medications in austere conditions is their propensity to suppress antidiuretic hormone release from the pituitary gland, causing diuresis and promoting hypovolemia, and thermoregulatory responses promoting the development of hypothermia.

Table 60.2: Equianalgesic opioid conversion

Opioid	Intra venous (mg)	Oral (mg)	Epidural (mg)	Intrathecal (mg)
Morphine	1	3	0.1	0.01
Hydromorphone	0.2	0.6	0.02	0.002
Meperidine	10	3	NA	NA
Fentanyl	0.01	0.03	0.001	0.0001

NA: not applicable.

Table 60.3:
Suggested dosages of ketamine for acute pain control in the military casualty*

Route	Dosage
Intravenous/intramuscular dose	150–300 mcg/kg loading
Continuous infusion	1–14 mcg/kg/min
Oral	0.5 mg/kg
Epidural	30–60 mg
Intrathecal	NA
Tactical Combat Casualty Care Guideline recommendations for ketamine[b]	
IV[c] or IO	Give initial 20 mg and repeat q20min as required
IM	Give initial 50 mg and repeat q30min as required
IN (if nasal atomizer available)	Give initial 50 mg and repeat q30min as required

Notes:
NA: Not applicable. Remove weapons from any casualty given ketamine. Onset is in 1 min if IV, 5 min if IM or IN.
[a]The more active S-ketamine enantiomer is available. Ketamine is underutilized for acute pain control. Plasma half-life is 2.5 to 3 hours.
[b]From Wedmore IS, Butler FK Jr. Battlefield Analgesia in Tactical Combat Casualty Care. Wilderness Environ Med. 2017 Jun;28(2S):S109-S116.
[c] Give IV over 30 to 60 seconds to avoid rare apnea.

Table 60.4:
Suggested dosages of α2-adrenergic receptor agonists for acute pain management in the military casualty

α2-Adrenergic Receptor Agonist	Intravenous/ Intramuscular	Continuous Infusion	Oral	Epidural	Intrathecal	Plasma Half-life	Comments
Clonidine*	2–5 mcg/kg	0.3 mcg/kg/h following loading bolus	2–5 mcg/kg	3 mcg/kg added to local anesthetic	15–30 mcg added to local anesthetic	12–16 h	Hypotension, sedation, and bradycardia are important side effects; additive effect when used with opioids
Dexmedetomidine**	1 mcg/kg	0.4 mcg/kg/h following loading bolus	NA	NA	NA	2 h	Pure α2-adrenergic agonist; increases incidence of sedation and bradycardia

NA: Not applicable.
*Clonidine, 1 mcg/kg, added to local anesthetic injected for peripheral nerve blocks prolongs block analgesia with minimal (sedation) to no side effects.
**Dexmedetomidine increases incidence of bradycardia, sedation, and diuresis.

5. Nonsteroidal Anti-Inflammatory Drugs

Non-steroidal anti-inflammatory drugs (NSAIDs) are an important class of medications for austere environment analgesia when used as part of a multimodal pain management plan (Table 60.5). Acetaminophen (paracetamol) lacks some of the side effects associated with other NSAIDs, such as impaired platelet function, renal function, and bone growth. Acetaminophen enhances the analgesic effects of other NSAIDs and opioids when used concurrently. Oral NSAIDs block prostaglandin synthesis by inhibiting cyclooxygenase enzyme (COX-1, COX-2), thus reducing the inflammatory as well as the nociceptive response following injury. COX-2 selective NSAIDs (COX-2s) lack the antiplatelet effects of nonselective NSAIDs but have similar analgesic effects, making them the preferred moiety in a field setting. Prolonged use of any NSAIDs is associated with increased cardiovascular events, while COX-2s have a lower rate of gastric irritation. The opioid-sparing effects of COX-2s decrease the probability of respiratory depression and oversedation, and for short-term use in a field setting, their advantages as adjunct analgesics far outweigh their disadvantages. Long shelf life, ease of transport, and low abuse potential are additional benefits of NSAIDs in an austere environment. Meloxicam, a 90% COX-2 selective NSAID, along with acetaminophen make up the Combat Wound Medication Pack (CWMP)

Table 60.5:
Suggested doses of nonsteroidal anti-inflammatory drugs for acute pain management in the military casualty

NSAID	Intravenous/ Intramuscular	Oral	Plasma Half-life	Comments
Acetaminophen	NA	325–1300 mg every 4–8 h up to 4,000 mg/day	1–4 h	Does not produce gastric irritation or alter platelet aggregation; weak anti-inflammatory; hepatotoxic in large doses
Ketorolac	30 mg, then 15–30 mg every 6 h	10 mg every 4–6 h	5 h	30 mg intravenous is equivalent to 10 mg of morphine; moderate anti-inflammatory activity; may cause life-threatening bronchospasm in asthma patients
Acetylsalicylic acid (aspirin)	NA	325–650 mg every 4–6 h	2–3 h	Antipyretic; low-intensity pain; effective platelet activation inhibitor; useful for acute angina or myocardial infarction; can induce asthma in up to 20% of asthma patients
Ibuprofen	NA	400–800 mg every 8 h	2 h	Higher incidence of serious gastrointestinal events than selective COX-2 inhibitor celecoxib
Naproxen	NA	250–500 mg every 12 h	12–15 h	Longer half-life allows twice-daily dosing
Indomethacin	NA	25–50 mg every 8 h	4.5 h	Potent anti-inflammatory
Celecoxib	NA	400 mg loading dose followed by 100–200 mg daily	11 h	Highly selective COX-2 inhibitor; lower incidence of serious gastrointestinal events than nonselective COX inhibitors ibuprofen and naproxen; lower incidence of renal events than ibuprofen
Meloxicam	NA	7.5–15 mg every day	15–20 h	90% selective for COX-2 inhibition; longer half-life allows for daily dosing

Notes: COX: cyclooxygenase; NA: not applicable; NSAID: nonsteroidal anti-inflammatory drugs.

and are a first-line therapy for patients with mild to moderate pain per TCCC guidelines. Celecoxib, another COX-2, is also available but is contraindicated in patients with sulfa allergy, although the data to support this are lacking. Parenteral preparations of ibuprofen and ketorolac are also available for patients unable to take oral medication, with the preceding limitations in mind.

6. Anticonvulsants

Anticonvulsant medications such as gabapentin and pregabalin (gabapentinoids) are used in acute pain management as antihyperalgesic drugs to prevent the induction and maintenance of pain sensitization of the spinal cord, dorsal horn, and peripheral nerves following trauma (Table 60.6). In theory, preemptive analgesia, using a multimodal approach, can prevent or at least attenuate the unwanted neurophysiologic and biochemical consequences of untreated pain. Gabapentinoids have been shown to significantly reduce perioperative opioid requirements across almost all surgery types with minimal side effects. When combined with opioids, gabapentinoids have a synergistic analgesic effect, possibly due to combined inhibition of nociceptor neurotransmitter release. Research has shown gabapentinoids may also reduce or prevent opioid tolerance and recover opioid antinociception in tolerant states, possibly through trafficking effects of NMDA receptors. Gabapentin and pregabalin are currently used routinely in the pain management of US military casualties returning from Iraq and Afghanistan. Side effects include sedation and dizziness, although these usually resolve with repeated administration. Conclusive evidence supports the inclusion of these medications in a field pain medicine plan and perhaps warrants a future role alongside acetaminophen and COX-2 selective NSAIDs in the CWMP.

7. Tricyclic Antidepressants

Tricyclic antidepressants have been used to manage neuropathic pain for more than 30 years. Medications of this class act through the inhibition of norepinephrine and serotonin reuptake into postganglionic sympathetic nervous system nerve endings, enhancing the antinociceptive effects of these neurotransmitters. These medications can be used following traumatic injury in combination with other pain medications as part of a multimodal approach. Dosages that contribute to analgesia are significantly lower than those used to treat depression. Early application of tricyclic antidepressants may have some benefit in preventing acute pain progression into chronic pain states, and these medications are first-line agents in the treatment of neuropathic pain (Table 60.7).

Table 60.6:
Suggested dosages of anticonvulsants for acute pain management in the military casualty

Anticonvulsant	Oral Dosage	Plasma Half-life	Comments
Gabapentin (Neurontin*)	100–300 mg every 8 h gradually increased as needed up to 3600 mg daily in 3 divided doses	5–7 h	Therapeutic effect on neuropathic pain believed to be due to action on voltage-gated N-type calcium ion channels; somnolence and fatigue are side effects; does not appear to interact with other medications
Pregabalin (Lyrica*)	75 mg every 12 h increased as needed up to 600 mg daily in 2 or 3 divided doses	5–6 h	Similar to gabapentin but more potent; fewer dose-related side effects

*Pfizer Inc, New York, NY.

Table 60.7: Suggested Dosages of Tricyclic Antidepressants for Acute Pain Management in the Military Casualty

Tricyclic Antidepressant	Oral	Plasma Half-life	Comments
Amitriptyline (Elavil*)	10-150 mg daily	12-24 h	Anticholinergic and sedative side effects; will enhance the response to other central nervous system depressants
Nortriptyline	25 mg every night up to a maximum of 150 mg every day	18-60 h	Fewer side effects; overactive or agitated patients may exhibit greater agitation

*Zeneca Pharmaceuticals, Wilmington Del.

8. Other Pain Medications

Other nonopioid medications, such as adenosine, droperidol, magnesium, neostigmine, opioid antagonists, and mixed opioid agonist/antagonists, have been used successfully in the management of postsurgical pain. However, the clinical advantages and disadvantages of these unconventional therapies still require further clarification before recommendations for use in an austere medical environment can be made. In addition to peripheral nerve blocks, local anesthetics can be very effective in the management of pain through subcutaneous injections around a wounded area or direct infusion into a wound using a catheter.

9. Future Pain Control Methods and Equipment

Research and development of methods other than IV opioids for pain management in battlefield scenarios continue. Oral sufentanil developed by AcelRx Pharmaceuticals (USA) is another non-IV opioid being developed that has several features that make it more advantageous than oral transmucosal fentanyl citrate (OTFC). Nearly all of its analgesic effect comes from buccal absorption, due to increased potency facilitating smaller (3-mm diameter) tablets that dissolve within 5 minutes, minimizing salivation and risk of swallowing. Any swallowed portion has <10% bioavailability. Onset of pain relief after a single 30-mcg dose is typically between 15 and 30 minutes, with a steady context-sensitive half-time of 2 to 2.5 hours even after multiple repeated doses, allowing for as needed dosing every 3 hours. The 15-mcg dose has a context-sensitive half-life of 81 to 100 minutes and is available from a patient-controlled analgesia (PCA) dispenser every 20 minutes. Sufentanil also has no active metabolites. Both doses, 15 mcg as part of a PCA dispenser and single 30-mcg doses, are currently approved for use in Europe to treat acute pain in non-opioid-tolerant patients, and initial approvals have been obtained in the US. Oral sufentanil is poised to become the oral opioid of choice for acute moderate to severe pain on the battlefield due to its more favorable pharmacokinetic profile and reduced effects on respiration compared with OTFC.

Ketamine can be delivered intranasally, when a nasal atomizer is available; Johnson & Johnson (USA) is currently conducting phase 3 trials on intranasal S-ketamine with anticipated FDA approval filing in 2019 for treatment of depression. However, regarding cognitive effects in high-stress environments, more information is needed before wider adoption on the battlefield.

Finally, nonpharmacologic management of pain through proper splinting of fractures and protection of wounds from further injury continues to be a vital consideration in any acute pain management plan. This is especially true during patient transport, when inadvertent impact or vibration can lead to extreme discomfort. Furthermore, there is a role for other integrative health modalities (e.g., acupuncture and massage) as adjuncts for managing pain. Auricular acupuncture is presently being used for pain in US Air Force evacuation flights. The psychological benefits derived from healthcare provider attention to patient comfort during evacuation can greatly enhance the effectiveness of the multimodal pain care plan.

Further Reading

Foreword by Kent and Tighe

Keyes KM, Galea S. *Population Health Science*. New York: Oxford University Press; 2016.

Frazier HS, Mosteller F. *Medicine Worth Paying For: Assessing Medical Innovations*. Cambridge, MA. Harvard University Press; 1995.

Chapter 1

Kellermann A, Elster E, Babington C, Harris R, eds. *Out of the Crucible: How the US Military Transformed Combat Casualty Care in Iraq and Afghanistan*. Washington, DC: Government Printing Office; 2017.

Chapter 3

Bailard NS, Ortiz J, Flores RA. Additives to local anesthetics for peripheral nerve blocks: evidence, limitations, and recommendations. *Am J Health-Syst Pharm*. 2014 Mar 1;71(5): 373–85.

Gitman M, Barrington MJ. Local anesthetic systemic toxicity: a review of recent case reports and registries. *Reg Anesth Pain Med*. 2018;43:124 130.

Neal JM, Barrington MJ, Fettiplace MR, Gitman M, Memtsoudis SG, Mörwald EE, Rubin DS, Weinberg G The third American Society of Regional Anesthesia and Pain Medicine practice advisory on local anesthetic systemic toxicity: executive summary 2017. *Reg Anesth Pain Med*. 2018 Feb;43(2):113–123.

Chapter 4

Klein SM, Melton MS, MG Warren, Nielsen KC. Peripheral nerve stimulation in regional anesthesia. *Reg Anesth Pain Med*. 2012;37:383–392.

Neal JM. Ultrasound-guided regional anesthesia and patient safety update of an evidence-based analysis. *Reg Anesth Pain Med*. 2016;41:195–204.

Chapter 5

Mian A, Chaudhry I, Huang R, Rizk E, Tubbs RS, Loukas R. Brachial plexus anesthesia: a review of the relevant anatomy, complications, and anatomical variations. *Clinl Anat*. 2014;27:210–221.

Tran DQ, Elgueta MF, Aliste J, Finlayson RJ. Diaphragm-sparing nerve blocks for shoulder surgery. *Reg Anesth Pain Med*. 2017 Jan–Feb;42(1):32–38.

Van Geffen GJ, Moayeri N, Bruhn J, Scheffer GJ, Chan VW, Groen GJ. Correlation between ultrasound imaging, cross-sectional anatomy, and histology of the brachial plexus. *Reg Anesth Pain Med*. 2009;34:490–497.

Chapter 6

Leblanc I, Chterev V, Rekik M, Boura B, Costanzo A, Bourel P, Combes M, Philip I. Safety and efficiency of ultrasound-guided intermediate cervical plexus block for carotid surgery. *Anaesth Crit Care Pain Med.* 2016 Apr;35(2):109–114.

Sait Kavaklı A, Kavrut Öztürk N, Umut Ayoğlu R, Sağdıç K, Çakmak G, İnanoğlu K, Emmiler M. Comparison of combined (deep and superficial) and intermediate cervical plexus block by use of ultrasound guidance for carotid endarterectomy. *J Cardiothorac Vasc Anesth.* 2016 Apr;30(2):317–322.

Chapter 7

Fredrickson MJ, Leightley P, Wong A, Chaddock M, Abeysekera A, Frampton C. An analysis of 1505 consecutive patients receiving continuous interscalene analgesia at home: a multicentre prospective safety study. *Anaesthesia.* 2016 Apr;71(4):373–379.

Rajpal G, Winger DG, Cortazzo M, Kentor ML, Orebaugh SL. Neurologic outcomes after low-volume, ultrasound-guided interscalene block and ambulatory shoulder surgery. *Reg Anesth Pain Med.* 2016 Jul–Aug;41(4):477–481.

Salviz EA, Xu D, Frulla A, Kwofie K, Shastri U, Chen J, Shariat AN, Littwin S, Lin E, Choi J, Hobeika P, Hadzic A. Continuous interscalene block in patients having outpatient rotator cuff repair surgery: a prospective randomized trial. *Anesth Analg.* 2013 Dec;117(6):1485–1492.

Chapter 8

Park SK, Lee SY, Kim WH, Park HS, Lim YJ, Bahk JH. Comparison of supraclavicular and infraclavicular brachial plexus block: a systemic review of randomized controlled trials. *Anesth Analg.* 2017 Feb;124(2):636–644.

Chapter 9

Chin KJ, Singh M, Velayutham V, Chee V. Infraclavicular brachial plexus block for regional anaesthesia of the lower arm. *Anesth Analg.* 2010 Oct;111(4):1072.

Petrar SD, Seltenrich ME, Head SJ, Schwarz SK. Hemidiaphragmatic paralysis following ultrasound-guided supraclavicular versus infraclavicular brachial plexus blockade: a randomized clinical trial. *Reg Anesth Pain Med.* 2015 Mar–Apr;40(2):133–138.

Chapter 10

Barrington MJ, Gledhill SR, Kluger R, Clarke AL, Wong DM, Davidson H, Thomas R. A randomized controlled trial of ultrasound versus nerve stimulator guidance for axillary brachial plexus block. *Reg Anesth Pain Med.* 2016 Nov–Dec;41(6):671–677.

Chapter 11

Eichenberger U, Stöckli S, Marhofer P, Huber G, Willimann P, Kettner SC, Pleiner J, Curatolo M, Kapral S. Minimal local anesthetic volume for peripheral nerve block: a new ultrasound-guided, nerve dimension-based method. *Reg Anesth Pain Med.* 2009 May–Jun;34(3):242–246.

Macaire P, Singelyn F, Narchi P, Paqueron X. Ultrasound- or nerve stimulation-guided wrist blocks for carpal tunnel release: a randomized prospective comparative study. *Reg Anesth Pain Med.* 2008 Jul–Aug;33(4):363–368.

Chapter 12

Bashandy GM, Abbas DN. Pectoral nerves I and II blocks in multimodal analgesia for breast cancer surgery: a randomized clinical trial. *Reg Anesth Pain Med.* 2015 Jan–Feb;40(1):68–74.

Blanco R. The "pecs block": a novel technique for providing analgesia after breast surgery. *Anaesthesia.* 2011 Sep;66(9):847–848.

Kunigo T, Murouchi T, Yamamoto S, Yamakage M. Injection volume and anesthetic effect in serratus plane block. *Reg Anesth Pain Med.* 2017 Nov–Dec;42(6):737–740.

Kunigo T, Murouchi T, Yamamoto S, Yamakage M. Spread of injectate in ultrasound-guided serratus plane block: a cadaveric study. *JA Clin Rep*. 2018;4(1):10.

Mayes J, Davison E, Panahi P, Patten D, Eljelani F, Womack J, Varma M. An anatomical evaluation of the serratus anterior plane block. *Anaesthesia*. 2016 Sep;71(9):1064–1069.

Perez MF, Duany O, de la Torre PA. Redefining PECS blocks for postmastectomy analgesia. *Reg Anesth Pain Med*. 2015 Nov–Dec;40(6):729–730.

Woodworth GE, Ivie RMJ, Nelson SM, Walker CM, Maniker RB. Perioperative breast analgesia: a qualitative review of anatomy and regional techniques. *Reg Anesth Pain Med*. 2017 Sep–Oct;42(5):609–631.

Chapter 13

Chin KJ, Adhikary S, Sarwani N, Forero M. The analgesic efficacy of pre-operative bilateral erector spinae plane (ESP) blocks in patients having ventral hernia repair. *Anaesthesia*. 2017 Apr;72(4):452–460.

Chin KJ, Malhas L, Perlas A. The erector spinae plane block provides visceral abdominal analgesia in bariatric surgery: a report of 3 cases. *Reg Anesth Pain Med*. 2017 May–Jun;42(3):372–376.

Forero M, Adhikary SD, Lopez H, Tsui C, Chin KJ. The erector spinae plane block: a novel analgesic technique in thoracic neuropathic pain. *Reg Anesth Pain Med*. 2016 Sep–Oct;41(5):621–627.

Hernandez MA, Palazzi L, Lapalma J, Forero M, Chin KJ. Erector spinae plane block for surgery of the posterior thoracic wall in a pediatric patient. *Reg Anesth Pain Med*. 2018 Feb;43(2):217–219.

Chapter 14

Fanelli A, Ghisi D, Melotti RM. An update around the evidence base for the lower extremity ultrasound regional block technique. *F1000Research*. 2016;5:F1000 Faculty Rev-104.

Salinas FV. Evidence basis for ultrasound guidance for lower-extremity peripheral nerve block: update 2016. *Reg Anesth Pain Med*. 2016 Mar–Apr;41(2):261–274.

Chapter 15

Amiri HR, Zamani MM, Safari S. Lumbar plexus block for management of hip surgeries. *Anesth Pain Med*. 2014 Jul 8;4(3):e19407.

Karmakar MK, Li JW, Kwok WH, Hadzic A. Ultrasound-guided lumbar plexus block using a transverse scan through the lumbar intertransverse space: a prospective case series. *Reg Anesth Pain Med*. 2015 Jan–Feb;40(1):75–81.

Karmakar MK, Li JW, Kwok WH, Soh E, Hadzic A. Sonoanatomy relevant for lumbar plexus block in volunteers correlated with cross-sectional anatomic and magnetic resonance images. *Reg Anesth Pain Med*. 2013 Sep–Oct;38(5):391–397.

Chapter 16

Chan EY, Fransen M, Parker DA, Assam PN, Chua N. Femoral nerve blocks for acute postoperative pain after knee replacement surgery. *Cochrane Database Syst Rev*. 2014 May 13; 5(5): CD009941.

Hussain N, Ferreri TG, Prusick PJ, Banfield L, Long B, Prusick VR, Bhandari M. Adductor canal block versus femoral canal block for total knee arthroplasty: a meta-analysis: what does the evidence suggest? *Reg Anesth Pain Med*. 2016 May–Jun;41(3):314–320.

Terkawi AS, Mavridis D, Sessler DI, Nunemaker MS, Doais KS, Terkawi RS, Terkawi YS, Petropoulou M, Nemergut EC. Pain management modalities after total knee arthroplasty: a network meta-analysis of 170 randomized controlled trials. *Anesthesiology*. 2017 May;126(5):923–937.

Chapter 17

Burckett-St Laurant D, Peng P, Girón Arango L, Niazi AU, Chan VW, Agur A, Perlas A. The nerves of the adductor canal and the innervation of the knee: an anatomic study. *Reg Anesth Pain Med*. 2016 May–Jun;41(3):321–327.

Gautier PE, Hadzic A, Lecoq JP, Brichant JF, Kuroda MM, Vandepitte C. Distribution of injectate and sensory-motor blockade after adductor canal block. *Anesth Analg*. 2016 Jan;122(1):279–282.

Grevstad U, Mathiesen O, Valentiner LS, Jaeger P, Hilsted KL, Dahl JB. Effect of adductor canal block versus femoral nerve block on quadriceps strength, mobilization, and pain after total knee arthroplasty: a randomized, blinded study. *Reg Anesth Pain Med*. 2015 Jan–Feb;40(1):3–10.

Nader A, Kendall MC, Manning DW, Beal M, Rahangdale R, Dekker R, De Oliveira GS Jr, Kamenetsky E, McCarthy RJ. Single-dose adductor canal block with local infiltrative analgesia compared with local infiltrate analgesia after total knee arthroplasty: a randomized, double-blind, placebo-controlled trial. *Reg Anesth Pain Med*. 2016 Nov–Dec;41(6):678–684.

Runge C, Børglum J, Jensen JM, Kobborg T, Pedersen A, Sandberg J, Mikkelsen LR, Vase M, Bendtsen TF. The analgesic effect of obturator nerve block added to a femoral triangle block after total knee arthroplasty: a randomized controlled trial. *Reg Anesth Pain Med*. 2016 Jul–Aug;41(4):445–451.

Yoshida T, Nakamoto T, Kamibayashi T. Ultrasound-guided obturator nerve block: a focused review on anatomy and updated techniques. *Biomed Res Int*. 2017;2017:7023750.

Chapter 18

Abdallah FW, Chan VW, Koshkin A, Abbas S, Brull R. Ultrasound-guided sciatic nerve block in overweight and obese patients: a randomized comparison of performance time between the infragluteal and subgluteal space techniques. *Reg Anesth Pain Med*. 2013 Nov–Dec;38(6):547–552.

Hara K, Sakura S, Yokokawa N, Tadenuma S. Incidence and effects of unintentional intraneural injection during ultrasound-guided subgluteal sciatic nerve block. *Reg Anesth Pain Med*. 2012 May–Jun;37(3):289–293.

Yamamoto H, Sakura S, Wada M, Shido A. A prospective, randomized comparison between single- and multiple-injection techniques for ultrasound-guided subgluteal sciatic nerve block. *Anesth Analg*. 2014 Dec;119(6):1442–1448.

Chapter 19

Uz A, Apaydin N, Cinar SO, Apan A, Comert B, Tubbs RS, Loukas M. A novel approach for anterior sciatic nerve block: cadaveric feasibility study. *Surg Radiol Anat*. 2010 Nov;32(9):873–878.

Chapter 20

Domingo-Triado V, Selfa S, Martinez F, et al. Ultrasound guidance for lateral midfemoral sciatic nerve block: a prospective, comparative, randomized study. *Anesth Analg*. 2007;104:1270–1274.

Chapter 21

Barbosa FT, Barbosa TR, da Cunha RM, Rodrigues AK, Ramos FW, de Sousa-Rodrigues CF. Anatomical basis for sciatic nerve block at the knee level. *Braz J Anesthesiol*. 2015 May–Jun;65(3):177–179. doi:10.1016/j.bjane.2014.03.010. Epub 2015 Mar 18.

Monahan AM, Madison SJ, Loland VJ, Sztain JF, Bishop ML, Sandhu NS, Bellars RH, Khatibi B, Schwartz AK, Ahmed SS, Donohue MC, Nomura ST, Wen CH, Ilfeld BM. Continuous popliteal sciatic blocks: does varying perineural catheter location relative to the sciatic bifurcation influence block effects? A dual-center, randomized, subject-masked, controlled clinical trial. *Anesth Analg*. 2016 May;122(5):1689–1695.

Silverman ER, Vydyanathan A, Gritsenko K, Shaparin N, Singh N, Downie SA, Kosharskyy B. The anatomic relationship of the tibial nerve to the common peroneal nerve in the popliteal fossa: implications for selective tibial nerve block in total knee arthroplasty. *Pain Res Manag*. 2017;2017:7250181.

Soberón JR, McInnis C, Bland KS, Egger AL, Patterson ME, Elliott CE, Treuting RJ, Osteen K. Ultrasound-guided popliteal sciatic nerve blockade in the severely and morbidly obese: a prospective and randomized study. *J Anesth.* 2016 Jun;30(3):397–404.

Tiyaprasertkul W, Bernucci F, González AP, Leurcharusmee P, Yazer MS, Techasuk W, Arnuntasupakul V, de la Garza DC, Finlayson RJ, Tran DQ. A randomized comparison between single- and triple-injection subparaneural popliteal sciatic nerve block. *Reg Anesth Pain Med.* 2015 Jul–Aug;40(4):315–320.

Chapter 22

Chin KJ, Wong NW, Macfarlane AJ, Chan VW. Ultrasound-guided versus anatomic landmark-guided ankle blocks: a 6-year retrospective review. *Reg Anesth Pain Med.* 2011 Nov–Dec;36(6):611–618.

López AM, Sala-Blanch X, Magaldi M, Poggio D, Asuncion J, Franco CD. Ultrasound-guided ankle block for forefoot surgery: the contribution of the saphenous nerve. *Reg Anesth Pain Med.* 2012 Sep–Oct;37(5):554–557.

Chapter 23

Krediet AC, Moayeri N, van Geffen GJ, Bruhn J, Renes S, Bigeleisen PE, Groen GJ. Different approaches to ultrasound-guided thoracic paravertebral block: an illustrated review. *Anesthesiology.* 2015 Aug;123(2):459–474.

Malekpour M, Hashmi A, Dove J, Torres D, Wild J. Analgesic choice in management of rib fractures: paravertebral block or epidural analgesia? *Anesth Analg.* 2017 Jun;124(6):1906–1911.

Pace MM, Sharma B, Anderson-Dam J, Fleischmann K, Warren L, Stefanovich P. Ultrasound-guided thoracic paravertebral blockade: a retrospective study of the incidence of complications. *Anesth Analg.* 2016 Apr;122(4):1186–1191.

Chapter 24

Abrahams M, Derby R, Horn JL. Update on ultrasound for truncal blocks: a review of the evidence. *Reg Anesth Pain Med.* 2016 Mar–Apr;41(2):275–288.

Allcock E, et al. Continuous transversus abdominis plane (TAP) block catheters in a combat surgical environment. *Pain Medicine* 2010;11(9):1426–1429.

Baeriswyl M, Kirkham KR, Kern C, Albrecht E. The analgesic efficacy of ultrasound-guided transversus abdominis plane block in adult patients: a meta-analysis. *Anesth Analg.* 2015;121(6):1640–1654.

Ma N, Duncan JK, Scarfe AJ, Schuhmann S, Cameron AL. Clinical safety and effectiveness of transversus abdominis plane (TAP) block in post-operative analgesia: a systematic review and meta-analysis. *J Anesth.* 2017 Jun;31(3):432–452.

Chapter 25

Blanco R, Ansari T, Girgis E. Quadratus lumborum block for postoperative pain after caesarean section. *Eur J Anaesthesiol.* 2015;32:812–818.

Blanco R, Ansari T, Riad W, Shetty N. Quadratus lumborum block versus transversus abdominis plane block for postoperative pain after cesarean delivery: a randomized controlled trial. *Reg Anesth Pain* Med. 2016 Nov–Dec;41(6):757–762.

Carline L, McLeod GA, Lamb C. A cadaver study comparing spread of dye and nerve involvement after three different quadratus lumborum blocks. *Br J Anaesth.* 2016 Sep;117(3):387–394.

Dam M, Moriggl B, Hansen CK, Hoermann R, Bendtsen TF, Børglum J. The pathway of injectate spread with the transmuscular quadratus lumborum block: a cadaver study. *Anesth Analg.* 2017 Jul;125(1):303–312.

El-Boghdadly K, Elsharkawy H, Short A, Chin KJ. Quadratus lumborum block nomenclature and anatomical considerations. *Reg Anesth Pain Med.* 2016 Jul–Aug;41(4):548–549.

Ueshima H, Otake H, Lin JA. Ultrasound-guided quadratus lumborum block: an updated review of anatomy and techniques. *Biomed Res Int.* 2017;2017:2752876.

Chapter 26

Kellermann A, Elster E, Babington C, Harris R, ed. *Out of the Crucible: How the US Military Transformed Combat Casualty Care in Iraq and Afghanistan.* Washington, DC: Government Printing Office; 2017.

Chapter 28

Bailard NS, Ortiz J, Flores RA. Additives to local anesthetics for peripheral nerve blocks: evidence, limitations, and recommendations. *Am J Health-Syst Pharm.* 2014 Mar 1;71: 373–385.

Gitman M, Barrington MJ. Local anesthetic systemic toxicity: a review of recent case reports and registries. *Reg Anesth Pain Med.* 2018;43:124–130.

Neal JM, Barrington MJ, Fettiplace MR, Gitman M, Memtsoudis SG, Mörwald EE, Rubin DS, Weinberg G, The third American Society of Regional Anesthesia and Pain Medicine practice advisory on local anesthetic systemic toxicity: executive summary 2017. *Reg Anesth Pain Med.* 2018 Feb;43(2):113–123.

Chapter 29

Klein SM, Melton MS, MG Warren, Nielsen KC. Peripheral nerve stimulation in regional anesthesia. *Reg Anesth Pain Med.* 2012;37:383–392.

Neal JM. Ultrasound-guided regional anesthesia and patient safety update of an evidence-based analysis. *Reg Anesth Pain Med* 2016;41:195–204.

Chapter 30

Mian A, Chaudhry I, Huang R, Rizk E, Tubbs RS, Loukas R: Brachial plexus anesthesia: a review of the relevant anatomy, complications, and anatomical variations. *Clin Anat.* 2014;27:210–221.

Tran DQ, Elgueta MF, Aliste J, Finlayson RJ. Diaphragm-sparing nerve blocks for shoulder surgery. *Reg Anesth Pain Med.* 2017 Jan–Feb;42(1):32–38.

Van Geffen GJ, Moayeri N, Bruhn J, Scheffer GJ, Chan VW, Groen GJ. Correlation between ultrasound imaging, cross-sectional anatomy, and histology of the brachial plexus. *Reg Anesth Pain Med.* 2009;34:490–497.

Chapter 31

Leblanc I, Chterev V, Rekik M, Boura B, Costanzo A, Bourel P, Combes M, Philip I. Safety and efficiency of ultrasound-guided intermediate cervical plexus block for carotid surgery. *Anaesth Crit Care Pain Med.* 2016 Apr;35(2):109–114.

Sait Kavaklı A, Kavrut Öztürk N, Umut Ayoğlu R, Sağdıç K, Çakmak G, İnanoğlu K, Emmiler M. Comparison of combined (deep and superficial) and intermediate cervical plexus block by use of ultrasound guidance for carotid endarterectomy. *J Cardiothorac Vasc Anesth.* 2016 Apr;30(2):317–322.

Chapter 32

Fredrickson MJ, Leightley P, Wong A, Chaddock M, Abeysekera A, Frampton C. An analysis of 1505 consecutive patients receiving continuous interscalene analgesia at home: a multicentre prospective safety study. *Anaesthesia.* 2016 Apr;71(4):373–379.

Rajpal G, Winger DG, Cortazzo M, Kentor ML, Orebaugh SL. Neurologic outcomes after low-volume, ultrasound-guided interscalene block and ambulatory shoulder surgery. *Reg Anesth Pain Med.* 2016 Jul–Aug;41(4):477–481.

Salviz EA, Xu D, Frulla A, Kwofie K, Shastri U, Chen J, Shariat AN, Littwin S, Lin E, Choi J, Hobeika P, Hadzic A. Continuous interscalene block in patients having outpatient rotator cuff repair surgery: a prospective randomized trial. *Anesth Analg.* 2013 Dec;117(6):1485–1492.

Chapter 33

Park SK, Lee SY, Kim WH, Park HS, Lim YJ, Bahk JH. Comparison of supraclavicular and infraclavicular brachial plexus block: a systemic review of randomized controlled trials. *Anesth Analg*. 2017 Feb;124(2):636–644.

Chapter 34

Chin KJ, Singh M, Velayutham V, Chee V. Infraclavicular brachial plexus block for regional anaesthesia of the lower arm. *Anesth Analg*. 2010 Oct;111(4):1072.

Petrar SD, Seltenrich ME, Head SJ, Schwarz SK. Hemidiaphragmatic paralysis following ultrasound-guided supraclavicular versus infraclavicular brachial plexus blockade: a randomized clinical trial. *Reg Anesth Pain Med*. 2015 Mar–Apr;40(2):133–138.

Chapter 35

Barrington MJ, Gledhill SR, Kluger R, Clarke AL, Wong DM, Davidson H, Thomas R. A randomized controlled trial of ultrasound versus nerve stimulator guidance for axillary brachial plexus block. *Reg Anesth Pain Med*. 2016 Nov–Dec;41(6):671–677.

Chapter 36

Eichenberger U, Stöckli S, Marhofer P, Huber G, Willimann P, Kettner SC, Pleiner J, Curatolo M, Kapral S. Minimal local anesthetic volume for peripheral nerve block: a new ultrasound-guided, nerve dimension-based method. *Reg Anesth Pain Med*. 2009 May–Jun;34(3):242–246.

Macaire P, Singelyn F, Narchi P, Paqueron X. Ultrasound- or nerve stimulation-guided wrist blocks for carpal tunnel release: a randomized prospective comparative study. *Reg Anesth Pain Med*. 2008 Jul–Aug;33(4):363–368.

Chapter 37

Bashandy GM, Abbas DN. Pectoral nerves I and II blocks in multimodal analgesia for breast cancer surgery: a randomized clinical trial. *Reg Anesth Pain Med*. 2015 Jan–Feb;40(1):68–74.

Blanco R. The "pecs block": a novel technique for providing analgesia after breast surgery. *Anaesthesia*. 2011 Sep;66(9):847–848.

Kunigo T, Murouchi T, Yamamoto S, Yamakage M. Injection volume and anesthetic effect in serratus plane block. *Reg Anesth Pain Med*. 2017 Nov–Dec;42(6):737–740.

Kunigo T, Murouchi T, Yamamoto S, Yamakage M. Spread of injectate in ultrasound-guided serratus plane block: a cadaveric study. *JA Clin Rep*. 2018;4(1):10.

Mayes J, Davison E, Panahi P, Patten D, Eljelani F, Womack J, Varma M. An anatomical evaluation of the serratus anterior plane block. *Anaesthesia*. 2016 Sep;71(9):1064–1069.

Perez MF, Duany O, de la Torre PA. Redefining PECS blocks for postmastectomy analgesia. *Reg Anesth Pain Med*. 2015 Nov–Dec;40(6):729–730.

Woodworth GE, Ivie RMJ, Nelson SM, Walker CM, Maniker RB. Perioperative breast analgesia: a qualitative review of anatomy and regional techniques. *Reg Anesth Pain Med*. 2017 Sep–Oct;42(5):609–631.

Chapter 38

Chin KJ, Adhikary S, Sarwani N, Forero M. The analgesic efficacy of pre-operative bilateral erector spinae plane (ESP) blocks in patients having ventral hernia repair. *Anaesthesia*. 2017 Apr;72(4):452–460.

Chin KJ, Malhas L, Perlas A. The erector spinae plane block provides visceral abdominal analgesia in bariatric surgery: a report of 3 cases. *Reg Anesth PainMed*. 2017 May–Jun;42(3):372–376.

Forero M, Adhikary SD, Lopez H, Tsui C, Chin KJ. The erector spinae plane block: a novel analgesic technique in thoracic neuropathic pain. *Reg Anesth Pain Med*. 2016 Sep–Oct;41(5):621–627.

Hernandez MA, Palazzi L, Lapalma J, Forero M, Chin KJ. Erector spinae plane block for surgery of the posterior thoracic wall in a pediatric patient. *Reg Anesth Pain Med.* 2018 Feb;43(2):217–219.

Chapter 39

Fanelli A, Ghisi D, Melotti RM. An update around the evidence base for the lower extremity ultrasound regional block technique. *F1000Research.* 2016;5:F1000 Faculty Rev-104.

Salinas FV. Evidence basis for ultrasound guidance for lower-extremity peripheral nerve block: update 2016. *Reg Anesth Pain Med.* 2016 Mar–Apr;41(2):261–274.

Chapter 40

Amiri HR, Zamani MM, Safari S. Lumbar plexus block for management of hip surgeries. *Anesth Pain Med.* 2014 Jul 8;4(3):e19407.

Karmakar MK, Li JW, Kwok WH, Hadzic A. Ultrasound-guided lumbar plexus block using a transverse scan through the lumbar intertransverse space: a prospective case series. *Reg Anesth Pain Med.* 2015 Jan–Feb;40(1):75–81.

Karmakar MK, Li JW, Kwok WH, Soh E, Hadzic A. Sonoanatomy relevant for lumbar plexus block in volunteers correlated with cross-sectional anatomic and magnetic resonance images. *Reg Anesth Pain Med.* 2013 Sep–Oct;38(5):391–397.

Chapter 41

Chan EY, Fransen M, Parker DA, Assam PN, Chua N. Femoral nerve blocks for acute postoperative pain after knee replacement surgery. *Cochrane Database Syst Rev.* 2014 May 13;5(5):CD009941.

Hussain N, Ferreri TG, Prusick PJ, Banfield L, Long B, Prusick VR, Bhandari M. Adductor canal block versus femoral canal block for total knee arthroplasty: a meta-analysis: what does the evidence suggest? *Reg Anesth Pain Med.* 2016 May–Jun;41(3):314–320.

Terkawi AS, Mavridis D, Sessler DI, Nunemaker MS, Doais KS, Terkawi RS, Terkawi YS, Petropoulou M, Nemergut EC. Pain management modalities after total knee arthroplasty: a network meta-analysis of 170 randomized controlled trials. *Anesthesiology.* 2017 May;126(5):923–937.

Chapter 42

Burckett-St Laurant D, Peng P, Girón Arango L, Niazi AU, Chan VW, Agur A, Perlas A. The nerves of the adductor canal and the innervation of the knee: an anatomic study. *Reg Anesth Pain Med.* 2016 May–Jun;41(3):321–327.

Gautier PE, Hadzic A, Lecoq JP, Brichant JF, Kuroda MM, Vandepitte C. Distribution of injectate and sensory-motor blockade after adductor canal block. *Anesth Analg.* 2016 Jan;122(1):279–282.

Grevstad U, Mathiesen O, Valentiner LS, Jaeger P, Hilsted KL, Dahl JB. Effect of adductor canal block versus femoral nerve block on quadriceps strength, mobilization, and pain after total knee arthroplasty: a randomized, blinded study. *Reg Anesth Pain Med.* 2015 Jan–Feb;40(1):3–10.

Nader A, Kendall MC, Manning DW, Beal M, Rahangdale R, Dekker R, De Oliveira GS Jr, Kamenetsky E, McCarthy RJ. Single-dose adductor canal block with local infiltrative analgesia compared with local infiltrate analgesia after total knee arthroplasty: a randomized, double-blind, placebo-controlled trial. *Reg Anesth Pain Med.* 2016 Nov–Dec;41(6):678–684.

Runge C, Børglum J, Jensen JM, Kobborg T, Pedersen A, Sandberg J, Mikkelsen LR, Vase M, Bendtsen TF. The analgesic effect of obturator nerve block added to a femoral triangle block after total knee arthroplasty: a randomized controlled trial. *Reg Anesth Pain Med.* 2016 Jul–Aug;41(4):445–451.

Yoshida T, Nakamoto T, Kamibayashi T. Ultrasound-guided obturator nerve block: a focused review on anatomy and updated techniques. *Biomed Res Int.* 2017;2017:7023750.

Chapter 43

Abdallah FW, Chan VW, Koshkin A, Abbas S, Brull R. Ultrasound-guided sciatic nerve block in overweight and obese patients: a randomized comparison of performance time between the infragluteal and subgluteal space techniques. *Reg Anesth Pain Med.* 2013 Nov–Dec;38(6):547–552.

Hara K, Sakura S, Yokokawa N, Tadenuma S. Incidence and effects of unintentional intraneural injection during ultrasound-guided subgluteal sciatic nerve block. *Reg Anesth Pain Med.* 2012 May–Jun;37(3):289–293.

Franco CD. Posterior approach to the sciatic nerve in adults: is Euclidean geometry still necessary?. *Anesthesiology*. 2003 Mar 1;98(3):723–728.

Yamamoto H, Sakura S, Wada M, Shido A. A prospective, randomized comparison between single- and multiple-injection techniques for ultrasound-guided subgluteal sciatic nerve block. *Anesth Analg.* 2014 Dec;119(6):1442–1448.

Chapter 44

Uz A, Apaydin N, Cinar SO, Apan A, Comert B, Tubbs RS, Loukas M. A novel approach for anterior sciatic nerve block: cadaveric feasibility study. *Surg Radiol Anat.* 2010 Nov;32(9):873–878.

Chapter 45

Domingo-Triado V, Selfa S, Martinez F, et al. Ultrasound guidance for lateral midfemoral sciatic nerve block: a prospective, comparative, randomized study. *Anesth Analg.* 2007;104:1270–1274.

Chapter 46

Barbosa FT, Barbosa TR, da Cunha RM, Rodrigues AK, Ramos FW, de Sousa-Rodrigues CF. Anatomical basis for sciatic nerve block at the knee level. *Braz J Anesthesiol.* 2015 May–Jun;65(3):177–179. doi:10.1016/j.bjane.2014.03.010. Epub 2015 Mar 18.

Monahan AM, Madison SJ, Loland VJ, Sztain JF, Bishop ML, Sandhu NS, Bellars RH, Khatibi B, Schwartz AK, Ahmed SS, Donohue MC, Nomura ST, Wen CH, Ilfeld BM. Continuous popliteal sciatic blocks: does varying perineural catheter location relative to the sciatic bifurcation influence block effects? A dual-center, randomized, subject-masked, controlled clinical trial. *Anesth Analg.* 2016 May; 122(5):1689 1695.

Silverman ER, Vydyanathan A, Gritsenko K, Shaparin N, Singh N, Downie SA, Kosharskyy B. The anatomic relationship of the tibial nerve to the common peroneal nerve in the popliteal fossa: implications for selective tibial nerve block in total knee arthroplasty. *Pain Res Manag.* 2017;2017:7250181.

Soberón JR, McInnis C, Bland KS, Egger AL, Patterson ME, Elliott CE, Treuting RJ, Osteen K. Ultrasound-guided popliteal sciatic nerve blockade in the severely and morbidly obese: a prospective and randomized study. *J Anesth.* 2016 Jun;30(3):397–404.

Tiyaprasertkul W, Bernucci F, González AP, Leurcharusmee P, Yazer MS, Techasuk W, Arnuntasupakul V, de la Garza DC, Finlayson RJ, Tran DQ. A randomized comparison between single- and triple-injection subparaneural popliteal sciatic nerve block. *Reg Anesth Pain Med.* 2015 Jul–Aug; 40(4):315–320.

Chapter 47

Chin KJ, Wong NW, Macfarlane AJ, Chan VW. Ultrasound-guided versus anatomic landmark-guided ankle blocks: a 6-year retrospective review. *Reg Anesth Pain Med.* 2011 Nov–Dec;36(6):611–618.

López AM, Sala-Blanch X, Magaldi M, Poggio D, Asuncion J, Franco CD. Ultrasound-guided ankle block for forefoot surgery: the contribution of the saphenous nerve. *Reg Anesth Pain Med.* 2012 Sep–Oct;37(5):554–557.

Chapter 48

Krediet AC, Moayeri N, van Geffen GJ, Bruhn J, Renes S, Bigeleisen PE, Groen GJ. Different approaches to ultrasound-guided thoracic paravertebral block: an illustrated review. *Anesthesiology*. 2015 Aug;123(2):459–474.

Malekpour M, Hashmi A, Dove J, Torres D, Wild J. Analgesic choice in management of rib fractures: paravertebral block or epidural analgesia? *Anesth Analg*. 2017 Jun;124(6):1906–1911.

Pace MM, Sharma B, Anderson-Dam J, Fleischmann K, Warren L, Stefanovich P. Ultrasound-guided thoracic paravertebral blockade: a retrospective study of the incidence of complications. *Anesth Analg*. 2016 Apr;122(4):1186–1191.

Chapter 49

Abrahams M, Derby R, Horn JL. Update on ultrasound for truncal blocks: a review of the evidence. *Reg Anesth Pain Med*. 2016 Mar–Apr;41(2):275–288.

Allcock, Edward, et al. Continuous transversus abdominis plane (TAP) block catheters in a combat surgical environment. *Pain Medicine* 2010;11(9):1426–1429.

Baeriswyl M, Kirkham KR, Kern C, Albrecht E. The analgesic efficacy of ultrasound-guided transversus abdominis plane block in adult patients: a meta-analysis. *Anesth Analg*. 2015;121(6):1640–1654.

Ma N, Duncan JK, Scarfe AJ, Schuhmann S, Cameron AL. Clinical safety and effectiveness of transversus abdominis plane (TAP) block in post-operative analgesia: a systematic review and meta-analysis. *J Anesth*. 2017 Jun;31(3):432–452.

Chapter 50

Blanco R, Ansari T, Girgis E. Quadratus lumborum block for postoperative pain after caesarean section. *Eur J Anaesthesiol*. 2015;32:812–818.

Blanco R, Ansari T, Riad W, Shetty N. Quadratus lumborum block versus transversus abdominis plane block for postoperative pain after cesarean delivery: a randomized controlled trial. *Reg Anesth Pain Med*. 2016 Nov–Dec;41(6):757–762.

Carline L, McLeod GA, Lamb C. A cadaver study comparing spread of dye and nerve involvement after three different quadratus lumborum blocks. *Br J Anaesth*. 2016 Sep;117(3):387–394.

Dam M, Moriggl B, Hansen CK, Hoermann R, Bendtsen TF, Børglum J. The pathway of injectate spread with the transmuscular quadratus lumborum block: a cadaver study. *Anesth Analg*. 2017 Jul;125(1):303–312.

El-Boghdadly K, Elsharkawy H, Short A, Chin KJ. Quadratus lumborum block nomenclature and anatomical considerations. *Reg Anesth Pain Med*. 2016 Jul-Aug;41(4):548–549.

Ueshima H, Otake H, Lin JA. Ultrasound-guided quadratus lumborum block: an updated review of anatomy and techniques. *Biomed Res Int*. 2017;2017:2752876.

Chapter 51

Cameron CM, Scott DA, McDonald WM, Davies MJ. A review of neuraxial epidural morbidity: experience of more than 8,000 cases at a single teaching hospital. *Anesthesiology*. 2007 May;106(5):997–1002.

Perlas A, Chaparro LE, Chin KJ. Lumbar neuraxial ultrasound for spinal and epidural anesthesia: a systematic review and meta-analysis. *Reg Anesth Pain Med*. 2016 Mar–Apr;41(2):251–260.

Chapter 52

Barrington MJ, Snyder GL. Neurologic complications of regional anesthesia. *Curr Opin Anaesthesiol*. 2011 Oct;24(5):554–560.

Barrington MJ, Watts SA, Gledhill SR, Thomas RD, Said SA, Snyder GL, Tay VS, Jamrozik K. Preliminary results of the Australasian Regional Anaesthesia Collaboration: a prospective audit of more than 7000 peripheral nerve and plexus blocks for neurologic and other complications. *Reg Anesth Pain Med*. 2009 Nov–Dec;34(6):534–541.

Ben-David B. Complications of regional anesthesia: an overview. *Anesthesiol Clin North America*. 2002 Sep;20(3):665–667, ix. Review.

Borgeat A, Ekatodramis G, Kalberer F, Benz C. Acute and nonacute complications associated with interscalene block and shoulder surgery: a prospective study. *Anesthesiology*. 2001 Oct;95(4):875–880.

Brull R, Hadzic A, Reina MA, Barrington MJ. Pathophysiology and etiology of nerve injury following peripheral nerve blockade. *Reg Anesth Pain Med*. 2015 Sep–Oct;40(5):479–490.

Brull R, McCartney CJ, Chan VW, El-Beheiry H. Neurological complications after regional anesthesia: contemporary estimates of risk. *Anesth Analg*. 2007 Apr;104(4):965–974.

Candido KD, Sukhani R, Doty R Jr, Nader A, Kendall MC, Yaghmour E, Kataria TC, McCarthy R. Neurologic sequelae after interscalene brachial plexus block for shoulder/upper arm surgery: the association of patient, anesthetic, and surgical factors to the incidence and clinical course. *Anesth Analg*. 2005 May;100(5):1489–1495

Gauss A, Tugtekin I, Georgieff M, Dinse-Lambracht A, Keipke D, Gorsewski G. Incidence of clinically symptomatic pneumothorax in ultrasound-guided infraclavicular and supraclavicular brachial plexus block. *Anaesthesia*. 2014 Apr;69(4):327–336

Horlocker TT, Vandermeuelen E, Kopp SL, Gogarten W, Leffert LR, Benzon HT. Regional anesthesia in the patient receiving antithrombotic or thrombolytic therapy: American Society of Regional Anesthesia and Pain Medicine Evidence-Based Guidelines (Fourth Edition). *Reg Anesth Pain Med*. 2018 Apr;43(3):263–309.

Jacob AK, Mantilla CB, Sviggum HP, Schroeder DR, Pagnano MW, Hebl JR. Perioperative nerve injury after total knee arthroplasty: regional anesthesia risk during a 20-year cohort study. *Anesthesiology*. 2011 Feb;114(2):311–317

Kim DH, Murovic JA, Tiel RL, Kline DG. Intrapelvic and thigh-level femoral nerve lesions: management and outcomes in 119 surgically treated cases. *J Neurosurg*. 2004 Jun;100(6):989–996.

Neal JM, Barrington MJ, Brull R, Hadzic A, Hebl JR, Horlocker TT, Huntoon MA, Kopp SL, Rathmell JP, Watson JC. The second ASRA practice advisory on neurologic complications associated with regional anesthesia and pain medicine: executive summary 2015. *Reg Anesth Pain Med*. 2015 Sep–Oct;40(5):401–430.

Welch MB, Brummett CM, Welch TD, Tremper KK, Shanks AM, Guglani P, Mashour GA. Perioperative peripheral nerve injuries: a retrospective study of 380,680 cases during a 10-year period at a single institution. *Anesthesiology*. 2009 Sep;111(3):490–497.

Chapter 53

Ilfeld BM. Continuous peripheral nerve blocks: an update of the published evidence and comparison with novel, alternative analgesic modalities. *Anesth Analg*. 2017 Jan;124(1):308–335.

Wood P, Gill M, Edwards D, Clifton P, Bullock C, Aldington D. Clinical and microbiological evaluation of epidural and regional anaesthesia catheters in injured UK military personnel. *J R Army Med Corps*. 2016 Aug;162(4):261–265.

Chapter 54

Hauret KG, Pacha L, Taylor BJ, Jones BH. Surveillance of disease and nonbattle injuries during US Army operations in Afghanistan and Iraq. *US Army Med Dep J*. 2016 Apr–Sep;(2-16):15–23.

Hauret KG, Taylor BJ, Clemmons NS, Block SR, Jones BH. Frequency and causes of nonbattle injuries air evacuated from Operations Iraqi Freedom and Enduring Freedom, U.S. Army, 2001–2006. *Am J Prev Med*. 2010 Jan;38(1 suppl):S94–107.

Sharma AK, Vorobeychik Y, Wasserman R, Jameson J, Moradian M, Duszynski B, Kennedy DJ; Standards Division of the Spine Intervention Society. The effectiveness and risks of fluoroscopically guided lumbar interlaminar epidural steroid injections: a systematic review with comprehensive analysis of the published data. *Pain Med*. 2017 Feb 1;18(2):239–251.

Chapter 55

Buckenmaier CC III, Rupprecht C, McKnight G, McMillan B, White RL, Gallagher RM, Polomano R. Pain following battlefield injury and evacuation: a survey of 110 casualties from the wars in Iraq and Afghanistan. *Pain Med*. 2009 Nov;10(8):1487–1496.

Carli F, Kehlet H, Baldini G, Steel A, McRae K, Slinger P, Hemmerling T, Salinas F, Neal JM. Evidence basis for regional anesthesia in multidisciplinary fast-track surgical care pathways. *Reg Anesth Pain Med*. 2011 Jan–Feb;36(1):63–72.

Danninger T, Opperer M, Memtsoudis SG. Perioperative pain control after total knee arthroplasty: an evidence based review of the role of peripheral nerve blocks. *World J Orthop.* 2014;5(3):225–232.

Kopp SL, Børglum J, Buvanendran A, Horlocker TT, Ilfeld BM, Memtsoudis SG, Neal JM, Rawal N, Wegener JT. Anesthesia and analgesia practice pathway options for total knee arthroplasty: an evidence-based review by the American and European Societies of Regional Anesthesia and Pain Medicine. *Reg Anesth Pain Med.* 2017 Nov–Dec;42(6):683–697.

Miller TE, Thacker JK, White WD, Mantyh C, Migaly J, Jin J, Roche AM, Eisenstein EL, Edwards R, Anstrom KJ, Moon RE, Gan TJ; Enhanced Recovery Study Group. Reduced length of hospital stay in colorectal surgery after implementation of an enhanced recovery protocol. *Anesth Analg.* 2014 May;118(5):1052–1061.

Chapter 56

Guay J, Suresh S, Kopp S. The use of ultrasound guidance for perioperative neuraxial and peripheral nerve blocks in children: a Cochrane Review. *Anesth Analg.* 2017 Mar;124(3):948–958.

Lam DK, Corry GN, Tsui BC. Evidence for the use of ultrasound imaging in pediatric regional anesthesia: a systematic review. *Reg Anesth Pain Med.* 2016 Mar–Apr;41(2):229–241.

Muhly WT, Gurnaney HG, Ganesh A. Regional anesthesia for pediatric knee surgery: a review of the indications, procedures, outcomes, safety, and challenges. *Local Reg Anesth.* 2015;8:85–91.

Stein AL, Baumgard D, Del Rio I, Tutiven JL. Updates in pediatric regional anesthesia and its role in the treatment of acute pain in the ambulatory setting. *Curr Pain Headache Rep.* 2017 Feb;21(2):11.

Taenzer AH, Walker BJ, Bosenberg AT, Martin L, Suresh S, Polaner DM, Wolf C, Krane EJ. Asleep versus awake: does it matter? Pediatric regional block complications by patient state: a report from the Pediatric Regional Anesthesia Network. *Reg Anesth Pain Med.* 2014 Jul–Aug;39(4):279–283.

Chapter 57

Mora AG, Ganem VJ, Ervin AT, Maddry JK, Bebarta VS. En route use of analgesics in nonintubated, critically ill patients transported by U.S. Air Force critical care air transport teams. *Mil Med.* 2016 May;181(5 suppl):145–151.

Chapter 58

Chen CC, Yang CC, Hu CC, Shih HN, Chang YH, Hsieh PH. Acupuncture for pain relief after total knee arthroplasty: a randomized controlled trial. *Reg Anesth Pain Med.* 2015 Jan–Feb;40(1):31–36.

Fox LM, Murakami M, Danesh H, Manini AF. Battlefield acupuncture to treat low back pain in the emergency department. *Am J Emerg Med.* 2018 Feb 27. pii:S0735-6757(18)30175-X

King HC, Hickey AH, Connelly C. Auricular acupuncture: a brief introduction for military providers. *Mil Med.* 2013 Aug;178(8):867–874.

Jan AL, Aldridge ES, Rogers IR, Visser EJ, Bulsara MK, Niemtzow RC. Does ear acupuncture have a role for pain relief in the emergency setting? A systematic review and meta-analysis. *Med Acupunct.* 2017 Oct 1;29(5):276–289.

Chapter 59

Naqib D, Purvin M, Prasad R, Hanna IM, Dimitri S, Llufrio A, Hanna MN. Quality improvement initiative to improve postoperative pain with a clinical pathway and nursing education program. *Pain Manag Nurs.* 2018 Jul 26.

Chapter 60

Allcock E, Spencer E, Frazer R, Applegate G, Buckenmaier C III. Continuous transversus abdominis plane (TAP) block catheters in a combat surgical environment. *Pain Med.* 2010 Sep;11(9):1426–1429.

Clifford JL, Fowler M, Hansen JJ, Cheppudira B, Nyland JE, Salas MM, McGhee LL, Petz LN, Loyd DR. State of the science review: advances in pain management in wounded service members over a decade at war. *J Trauma Acute Care Surg*. 2014 Sep;77(3 suppl 2):S228–S236.

Croll SM, Griffith SR. Acute and chronic pain on the battlefield: lessons learned from point of injury to the United States. *US Army Med Dep J*. 2016 Apr–Sep;(2-16):102–105.

Gadsden J, Warlick A. Regional anesthesia for the trauma patient: improving patient outcomes. *Local Reg Anesth*. 2015;8:45–55.

Plunkett A, Turabi A, Wilkinson I. Battlefield analgesia: a brief review of current trends and concepts in the treatment of pain in US military casualties from the conflicts in Iraq and Afghanistan. *Pain Manag*. 2012 May;2(3):231–238.

Index

CPSIA information can be obtained
at www.ICGtesting.com
Printed in the USA
BVHW020524111121
621259BV00006B/16

9 780190 856649